1.

NEUROREGENERATION

NEUROREGENERATION

Editor

Alfredo Gorio, Ph.D.
*Department of Medical Pharmacology
University of Milan
Milan, Italy*

Raven Press ● New York

Raven Press, Ltd., 1185 Avenue of the Americas, New York, New York 10036

© 1993 by Raven Press, Ltd. All rights reserved. This book is protected by copyright. No part of it may be reproduced, stored in a retrieval system, or transmitted, in any form or by any means, electronic, mechanical, photocopying, recording, or otherwise, without prior written permission of the publisher.

Made in the United States of America

Library of Congress Cataloging-in-Publication Data

Neuroregeneration / editor, Alfredo Gorio.
     p. cm.
     Includes bibliographical references and index.
     ISBN 0-88167-952-6
     1. Nervous system—Regeneration.   I. Gorio, Alfredo.
     [DNLM: 1: Nerve Regeneration.   WL 102 N5058]
RC347.N483   1992
612.8—dc20
DNLM/DLC
for Library of Congress   92-49715
                                                                                         CIP

   The material contained in this volume was submitted as previously unpublished material, except in the instances in which some of the illustrative material was derived.

   Great care has been taken to maintain the accuracy of the information contained in the volume. However, neither Raven Press nor the editor can be held responsible for errors or for any consequences arising from the use of the information contained herein.

9 8 7 6 5 4 3 2 1

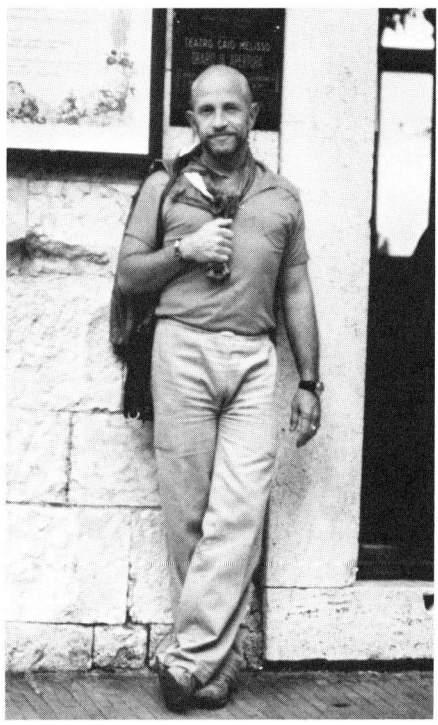

This book is dedicated to the memory of Michael Goldberger, who died in Philadelphia on January 15, 1992. He helped to establish the study of neural plasticity after injury.

Michael's contributions to the field were many and his scientific interests were focused on some of the major themes of this volume. Most important was the parallel application of careful anatomical and behavioral methods to the study of the reorganization of the spinal cord and the recovery of locomotion that normally takes place after spinal injury. He had just begun studies using transplants of fetal tissue into injured spinal cord and was able to see the first results showing enhanced axonal growth and dramatically improved locomotor function. This work was the culmination of a career dedicated to neural plasticity.

Michael is greatly missed by his many friends, colleagues, and students. In particular, he is missed by those whose work has been influenced by his always imaginative and often provocative approaches to the most important scientific questions.

The photograph was taken in Spoleto, Italy, in 1985, during a conference on Development and Plasticity of the Mammalian Spinal Cord organized by Michael Goldberger, Alfredo Gorio, and Marion Murray.

Contents

Contributors ... ix
Preface ... xi

1. Historical Bases for an Introduction to Neuroregeneration ... 1
   Alfredo Gorio, Anna Maria Di Giulio, and Paolo Mantegazza

2. Axonal Dynamics and Regeneration ... 7
   Scott T. Brady

3. The Fate of Denervated Neurons: Transneuronal Degeneration, Dendritic Atrophy, and Dentritic Remodeling ... 37
   Oswald Steward and Edwin W Rubel

4. Supporting Cells: Central and Peripheral ... 61
   Jean De Vellis

5. Adhesive Molecules of the Cell Surface and Extracellular Matrix in Neural Regeneration ... 77
   Salvatore Carbonetto and Samuel David

Peripheral Nervous System

6. Neurotrophic Function in Normal Nerve and in Peripheral Neuropathies ... 101
   Bruce G. Gold and Peter S. Spencer

7. Human Schwann Cells in Culture: Recent Advances and Relevance to Nerve Pathology ... 123
   Elio Scarpini, Pierluigi Baron, and Guglielmo Scarlato

8. Nerve-Muscle Trophic Interaction ... 145
   Alberto Cangiano, Mario Buffelli, and Efrem Pasino

Central Nervous System

9. Nonregenerative Approaches to Spinal Cord Injury ... 169
   Wise Young

10. Traumatic Brain Injury: The Pathobiology of Injury and Repair ... 185
    John T. Povlishock

11. Molecular Cascades in Adaptive versus Pathological Plasticity ... 217
    Carl W. Cotman, Brian J. Cummings, and Christian J. Pike

12. Sprouting and Regeneration in the Spinal Cord: Their Roles in Recovery of Function After Spinal Injury ... 241
    Michael M. Goldberger, Marion Murray, and Alan Tessler

13. Neurotrophic Factors and CNS Regeneration 265
    Theo Hagg, Jean-Claude Louis, and Silvio Varon

14. Pharmacology of Neuronal Regeneration 289
    Alfredo Gorio, Anna Maria Di Giulio, and Paolo Mantegazza

15. Future Directions on Neuroregeneration Research:
    Concluding Remarks 321
    Alfredo Gorio, Anna Maria Di Giulio, and Paolo Mantegazza

Subject Index 325

Contributors

Pierluigi Baron, M.D. *Institute of Neurology, Dino Ferrari Center for Neuromuscular Diseases, University of Milan, Via Sfarza 35, 20122 Milan, Italy*

Scott T. Brady, Ph.D. *Department of Cell Biology and Neuroscience, University of Texas Southwestern Medical Center, 5323 Harry Hines Boulevard, Dallas, Texas 75235*

Mario Buffelli, Ph.D. *Institute of Human Physiology, Medical School, University of Verona, Strada le Grazie, 37134 Verona, Italy*

Alberto Cangiano, Ph.D. *Institute of Human Physiology, Medical School, University of Verona, Strada le Grazie, 37134 Verona, Italy*

Salvatore Carbonetto, Ph.D. *Neuroscience Research Center, McGill University, Montreal General Hospital, Research Institute, 1650 Cedar Avenue, Montreal, Quebec H3G 1A4, Canada*

Carl W. Cotman, Ph.D. *Department of Psychobiology, University of California, Steinhaus Hall, Room 249, Irvine, California 92717*

Brian J. Cummings, Ph.D. *Department of Psychobiology, University of California, Steinhaus Hall, Irvine, California 92717*

Samuel David, Ph.D. *Neuroscience Research Center, McGill University, Montreal General Hospital, Research Institute, 1650 Cedar Avenue, Montreal, Quebec H3G 1A4, Canada*

Jean De Vellis, Ph.D. *UCLA, Neurochemistry Group 68-225 MRRC, 760 Westwood Plaza, Los Angeles, California 90024*

Anna Maria Di Giulio, Ph.D. *Department of Medical Pharmacology, Faculty of Medicine, University of Milan, Via Vanvitelli, 20129 Milan, Italy*

Bruce G. Gold, Ph.D. *Center for Research in Occupational and Environmental Toxicology, Oregon Health Sciences University, 3181 S. W. Sam Jackson Road, Portland, Oregon 97201*

Michael M. Goldberger, Ph.D. (Deceased) *Department of Anatomy, Medical College of Pennsylvania, 3200 Henry Avenue, Philadelphia, Pennsylvania 19129*

Alfredo Gorio, Ph.D. *Department of Medical Pharmacology, Faculty of Medicine, University of Milan, Via Vanvitelli 32, 20129 Milan, Italy*

CONTRIBUTORS

Theo Hagg, Ph.D., M.D.   Department of Biology, M-001, University of California, San Diego, School of Medicine, La Jolla, California, 92093

Jean-Claude Louis, Ph.D., M.D.   Department of Biology, M-001, University of California, San Diego, La Jolla, California 92093

Paolo Mantegazza, Ph.D.   Department of Medical Pharmacology, Faculty of Medicine, University of Milan, Via Vanvitelli 32, 20129 Milan, Italy

Marion Murray, Ph.D.   Department of Anatomy and Neurobiology, The Medical College of Pennsylvania, Philadelphia, Pennsylvania 19129

Efrem Pasino, Ph.D.   Institute of Human Physiology, Medical School, University of Verona, Strada le Grazie, 37134 Verona, Italy

Christian J. Pike, Ph.D.   Department of Psychobiology, University of California, Steinhaus Hall, Irvine, California 92717

John T. Povlishock, Ph.D.   Department of Anatomy, Medical College of Virginia, 12th Street and Marshall, Richmond, Virginia 23298

Edwin W Rubel, Ph.D.   Virginia Merrill Bloedel Hearing Research Center; and Department of Otolaryngology–Head and Neck Surgery, The University of Washington, School of Medicine, Seattle, Washington 98195

Guglielmo Scarlato, M.D.   Institute of Neurology, Dino Ferrari Center for Neuromuscular Diseases, University of Milan, Via Sfarza 35, 20122 Milan, Italy

Elio Scarpini, M.D.   Institute of Neurology, Dino Ferrari Center for Neuromuscular Diseases, University of Milan, Via Sfarza 35, 20112 Milan, Italy

Peter S. Spencer, Ph.D., MRCPath   Center for Research in Occupational and Environmental Toxicology, Oregon Health Sciences University, 3181 S. W. Sam Jackson Road, Portland, Oregon 97201

Oswald Steward, Ph.D.   Departments of Neuroscience and Neurosurgery, University of Virginia Health Sciences Center, Box 230 Medical Center, Charlottesville, Virginia 23298

Alan Tessler, M.D.   Department of Anatomy and Neurobiology, The Medical College of Pennsylvania, Philadelphia, Pennsylvania 19129

Silvio Varon, M.D., Eng.D.   Department of Biology M-001, University of California, San Diego, La Jolla, California 92093

Wise Young, Ph.D., M.D.   Department of Neurosurgery, New York University Medical Center, 550 First Avenue, New York, New York 10016

Preface

This book discusses various aspects of neuroregeneration, a key problem related to nervous system repair. We have solicited the efforts of outstanding basic scientists actively involved in the study of the aspects of neuroregeneration in which regeneration and restoration of synaptic contacts in the nervous system are the goal. We have focused our attention on the developments of neurobiology of regeneration in the 1980s and early 1990s. The wealth of literature and data on brain transplants and trophic factors as related to neuroregeneration are synthesized, as are the intriguing and exciting developments from studies of glial cells, axonal growth, and adhesion molecules. This concise book, focused on the mammalian nervous system under pathophysiological stress and in trauma, will be of interest to neuroscientists, developmental biologists, cell biologists, neurologists, and pathologists.

Alfredo Gorio

Acknowledgment

The Editor and the Publisher acknowledge the Kent Waldrep National Paralysis Foundation for supporting the publication of the color photographs in Chapter 8, *Nerve-Muscle Trophic Interaction,* by Alberto Cangiano, Mario Buffelli, and Efrem Pasino, and Chapter 14, *Pharmacology of Neuronal Regeneration,* by Alfredo Gorio, Anna Maria Di Giulio, and Paolo Mantegazza.

1
Historical Bases for an Introduction to Neuroregeneration

Alfredo Gorio, Anna Maria Di Giulio, and Paolo Mantegazza

Department of Medical Pharmacology, Faculty of Medicine, University of Milan, 20129 Milan, Italy

As long as 250 years ago, the abbot Felice Fontana, the personal medical doctor of the Grand Duke of Tuscany, made several original observations on the structure and regeneration of nerves, which are probably among the earliest known in the field. Most of his efforts were dedicated to wax works of anatomical reconstructions of the human body and to the effects of various poisons such as curare. His observations on the nervous system were rather reduced in number but not in importance; he showed that inside the small cylinders constituting the nerve there was a dense fluid containing small bodies capable of movements. This might have been the first description of mitochondria (1). In the same part of the book, he reported that the continuity of a rabbit hypoglossal nerve was reconstituted some time after sectioning as revealed by the microdissection of the nerve fibers (Fig. 1). He interpreted the repair process as a consequence of the reproduction of the injured tissue (1).

Neuroregeneration studies jumped forth in a very significant way with the studies of Ramón y Cajal (2) and J. F. Tello (3) and with the consolidation of the neuron theory. The improved morphological techniques allowed a correct analysis of regenerating nerves so that the theory of nerve autoregeneration was set aside, while putting forth the true mechanisms of nerve regeneration (3). The autoregeneration theory of lesioned nerves claimed that, in the distal stump, the generation of the newly forming axon occurs in a discontinuous manner depending on Schwann cells without the involvement of the neuron cell body (4). This hypothesis was supported by the observations of several investigators that produced evidence of anastomosis between different axons in culture as if an axon might be capable of interacting and then sealing in continuity with another (5,6). As Ramón y Cajal and colleagues strongly argued, such a conclusion was likely reached because fixatives and impregnation methods employed were not sufficiently appropriate for preserving the integrity of the entire regenerating axons, so that no axonal continuity between proximal and distal stump could have been observed by the authors supporting this hypothesis. Tello proved that lesioned nerves regenerate by forming sprouts that elongate, crossing the site of injury and penetrating the distal stump up to the denervated organ (3). By describing this process Tello suggested that the regenerating axons might have been attracted throughout the distal stump to the denervated target by some substances liberated by denervation (3). The in vitro suggestions of interaxonal anastomosis were likely due to juxtaposition of axons with no cytoplasmic fusion. In spite of this very minor confusing

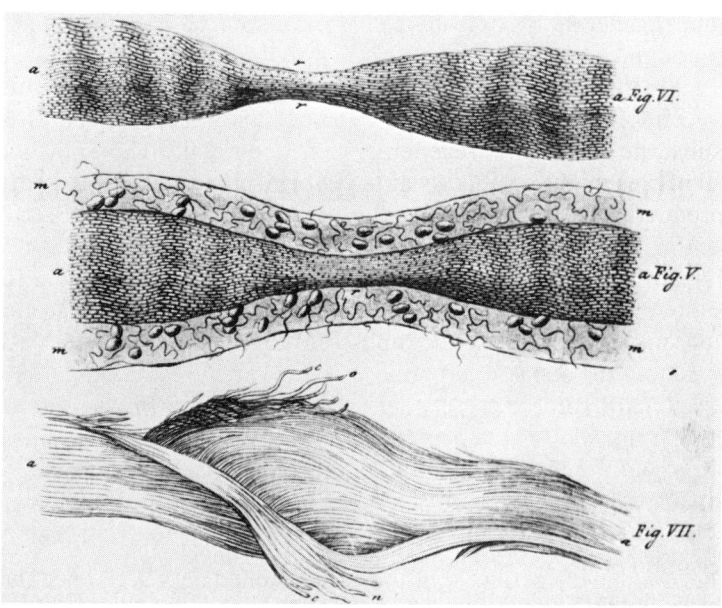

FIG. 1. The original picture shows a lesioned rabbit hypoglossal nerve 30 days after section. The microdissection of the nerve fibers shows the reconstituted integrity at the site of lesion. (From Fontana, ref. 1).

observation, the introduction of in vitro techniques for studying the nervous system was extremely brilliant and timely. Harrison invented the tissue culture technique by placing some small pieces of embryonic frog neural tube in a drop of lymph. This method allowed the direct visualization of neurite outgrowth confirming Cajal's observation that the leading portion of the growing neurites was a flat tip that grew by extending and retracting some fine extensions (7). While making these studies in vitro, Harrison also noted a relationship between cell movements and their interaction with the substrate (8), which was defined later by Weiss as "contact guidance" (9). It is now well accepted that gradients of adhesiveness are important for cell movement and neurite elongation. The filopodia of the growth cone explore the culture dish surface, which is capable of influencing the direction of growth. It is likely that neurites grow following selective adhesive pathways in vitro and in vivo as well (see Chapter 5, this volume). It is well established that adhesion to a proper substrate might be fundamental during development of the nervous system; however, if a proper environment is supplied also CNS neurons may regenerate after injury. Ramón y Cajal described how, after a wound lesion to the brain, axons form a retraction club, and if the lesion is close to the cell body the retrograde change is followed by death of the injured neuron (2). Cajal also noted that even in the most favorable cases no regeneration across the lesion site could take place, unless a piece of peripheral nerve were placed into the wound. The latter experiment was carried out by Tello who demonstrated that this procedure stimulated axonal regeneration in such a way that the peripheral nerve was invaded by regenerating neurites originating from CNS neurons (10). The author drew the conclusion that Schwann cells promoted rejuvenation of CNS axons. More recent experiments showed that peripheral nerves implanted into the brain or spinal cord could supply such an appropriate environment for neurite growth that regeneration could be extended for several millimeters bridging two parts of CNS quite distant (11). It has also been shown recently that in addition to an appropriate substrate for axonal regeneration peripheral nerves might be able to supply a local production of trophic factors, thereby preventing retrograde degeneration and neuronal death and enhancing regeneration (see Chapters 6 and 13, this volume). The suggestion made by Tello and supported by Cajal about the distal target organ production of agents favorable to regeneration received a tremendous advancement with the work of Viktor Hamburgher and Rita Levi Montalcini. Their powerful contribution to neuronal regeneration was dual: the description of neuronal death during embryonic development and the discovery of the protein nerve growth factor. Already early in the century it was known that the ablation of a limb bud from embryos caused the loss of sensory and motor neurons (12) and that the implantation of an extra limb bud caused an increase of innervating neurons (13). Rita Levi Montalcini and Viktor Hamburgher showed that cell death occurs normally during embryonic development and not only after limb removal (14). Subsequently Hamburgher defined how the size of the peripheral field of innervation quantitatively settles the number of surviving motor neurons, while the others degenerate after failing to find an appropriate peripheral territory (15). It is now well known that at least for certain neuronal populations the process of cell death is regulated by the availability of a target-derived trophic factor. Nerve growth factor was the first of such trophic agents to be characterized. A graduate student in Hamburgher laboratory transplanted a mouse sarcoma tumor into a chick embryo seeking an easier way of augmenting the periphery to be innervated. He discovered that the tumor was invaded by axon bundles and that the ipsilateral dorsal root ganglia were enlarged (16). Pursuing this observation further, Levi Montalcini and Hamburgher discovered that also the sympathetic ganglia were affected by the tumor, and that the effect was likely due to a diffusible substance since the tumor was also effective when applied onto the chorioallantoic membrane. The trophic substance was named nerve growth factor (17–19). In the attempt to purify the active agent, Levi Montalcini and Cohen used snake venom for its phosphodiesterase activity in digesting nucleic acid, but the in vitro assay showed that the blank preparation containing the snake venom was even more effective than the tumor extracts (20,21). Both venom and tumor extracts contained a protein, which now we know to be nerve growth factor (22). Later it was found that the mammalian salivary gland, which corresponds to the snake venom gland, contained large amounts of nerve growth factor, and it became the most important source for the purification of the trophic factor (23). With sufficient quantities of the factor available, this field of research increased greatly, particularly in the last 20 years; recently other agents with putative trophic activity have also been purified and may represent future treatments of degenerative disorders of the nervous system (see Chapters 6, 13, and 14, this volume). In addition to the trophic effects exerted by the targets on innervation, there are several suggestions indicating a trophic regulation of the target by the innervation. The nerve-muscle interactions in normal conditions and during nerve regeneration are a good example of such a phenomenon (see Chapter 8, this volume). In addition, as T.J. Todd had recognized in 1823, the limb regeneration in some amphibians is dependent upon the presence of the nerve, otherwise the blastema would remain stationary or degenerate (24). Marcus Singer showed also that the nerve trophic effect upon limb regeneration depends on the number of axons present rather than on their nature; below a certain threshold number of axons no trophic effects can be observed (25). Even from the very early works the reciprocal trophic regulation of both pre- and postsynaptic connecting systems was evident. Langley interpreted his reinnervation experiments by suggesting that there might exist a chemical relation between regenerating axons and denervated target, so that a chemical affinity would determine the synaptic reformation (26). The hypothesis of chemoaffinity was rejuvenated several years later by Sperry (27); however, it is apparent now that chemical interactions are among the several factors involved in synapse formation during development and reinnervation. The process of synaptogenesis can take place along the entire life span as evidenced by the constant dendrite and synaptic remodeling (see Chapter 3, this volume). In a paper published in 1884 Exner showed an example of such a phenomenon. By resecting a portion of the nerve innervating the circothyroid muscle he caused a partial denervation; some time later he observed that denervation was not permanent and likely the surviving nerve fibers had formed new end organs innervating the denervated muscle fibers (28). These data on functional recovery after partial denervation were reconfirmed a few years later (29,30), and the morphological examination showed that new axons were formed by outgrowth from the node of Ranvier or from nerve terminals of the surviving axons (31,32). The persistent ability of axons to modify or enlarge the territory of innervation by means of new branches and synapses, and their capacity to regrow and regenerate following axotomy, stimulated many scientists to pursue this field of research as briefly indicated above. Among them a special mention goes to Paul Alfred Weiss who gave a great contribution to this field of research by discovering the axoplasmic transport. The concept of materials flowing down the axons was already disputed at Cajal's time; in search for a mechanism responsible for nerve growth, Weiss showed accumulation of materials at a point of mechanical constriction on the nerve (33). The interpretation of the experiment was correct and provided the basis for further studies that established axonal transport as the intrinsic machinery responsible for axonal regeneration (see Chapter 2, this volume).

REFERENCES

1. Fontana F. *Treatise on the venom of the viper; . . . To which are annexed observations on the primitive structure of the animal body. Different experiments on the reproduction of the nerves.* Florence, 1787. Transl. from the French by J. Skinner. London: Murray.
2. Ramón y Cajal S. *Degeneration and regeneration of the nervous system.* 2 vol. Translated by R M May. London: Oxford Press; 1928.
3. Tello JF. Dégéneration et régénération des plaques motrices, etc. *Trav Lab Rech Biol Univ Madrid* 1907; V: 117–149.
4. Bethe A. *Zur theorie und praxis der verheilung durchtrennten nerven.* Volume in honor of Doctor Cajal, 1992.
5. Levi G. Ricerche sperimentali sopra elementi nervosi sviluppati in vitro. *Arch Exp Zellforsch Besonders Gewebezuecht* 1926;2: 244–272.
6. Levi G. *Trattato di Istologia.* 1927.
7. Harrison RG. The outgrowth of the nerve fiber as a mode of protoplasmic movement. *J Exp Zool* 1910; 9: 787–846.
8. Harrison RG. The reaction of embryonic cells to solid structures. *J Exp Zool* 1914; 17: 521–544.
9. Weiss P. Guiding principles in cell locomotion and cell aggregation. *Exp Cell Res* 1961; Suppl 8: 260–281.
10. Tello JF. La influencia del neurotropismo en la regeneracion de los centros nerviosos. *Trab Lab Invest Biol Univ Madrid* 1911: vol IX.
11. Aguayo A, David S, Richardson P, Bray G. Axonal elongation in peripheral and central nervous system transplants. *Adv Cell Neurobiol* 1982; 3: 215–234.
12. Shorey M L. The effect of the destruction of peripheral areas on the differentiation of the neuroblasts. *J Exp Zool* 1909; 7: 25–63.
13. Detwiler SR. On the hyperplasia of nerve centers resulting from excessive peripheral loading. *Proc Natl Acad Sci USA* 1920; 6: 96–101.
14. Hamburger V, Levi Montalcini R. Proliferation, differentiation and degeneration in the spinal ganglia of chick embryo under normal and experimental conditions. *J Exp Zool* 1949; 111: 457–501.
15. Hamburger V. Regression versus peripheral control of differentiation in motor hypoplasia. *Am J Anat* 1958; 102: 365–409.
16. Bueker ED. Implantation of tumors in the hind limb field of the embryonic chick and the developmental response of the lumbosacral nervous system. *Anat Rec* 1948; 102: 369–390.
17. Levi Montalcini R, Hamburger V. Selective

growth-stimulating effects of mouse sarcoma on the sensory and sympathetic nervous system of the chick embryo. *J Exp Zool* 1951; 116: 321–361.
18. Levi Montalcini R, Hamburgher V. A diffusible agent of mouse sarcoma, producing hyperplasia of sympathetic ganglia and hyperneurotization of viscera in the chick embryo. *J Exp Zool* 1953; 123: 233–287.
19. Levi Montalcini R. Effects of mouse tumor transplantation on the nervous system. *Ann NY Acad Sci* 1953; 55: 330–343.
20. Levi Montalcini R, Meyer H, Hamburgher V. In vitro experiments on the effects of mouse sarcoma 180 and 37 on the spinal and sympathetic ganglia of the chick embryo. *Cancer Res* 1954; 14: 49–57.
21. Levi Montalcini R, Cohen S. In vitro and in vivo effects on a nerve growth-stimulating agent isolated from snake venom. *Proc Natl Acad Sci USA* 1956; 42: 695–699.
22. Cohen S, Levi Montalcini R. A nerve growth stimulating factor isolated from snake venom. *Proc Natl Acad Sci USA* 1956; 42: 571–574.
23. Cohen S. Purification and metabolic effects of a nerve growth-promoting protein from the mouse salivary gland and its neurocytotoxic antiserum. *Proc Natl Acad Sci USA* 1960; 46: 302–311.
24. Todd TJ. On the process of reproduction of the members of the aquatic salamander. *Q J Sci Lit Arts* 1823; 16: 84–96.
25. Singer M. Induction of regeneration of the forelimb of the postmetamorphic frog by augmentation of the nerve supply. *J Exp Zool* 1952; 126: 419–471.
26. Langley JN. Note on regeneration of pre-ganglionic fibres of the sympathetic. *J Physiol (Lond)* 1895; 18: 280–284.
27. Sperry RW. Chemoaffinity in the orderly growth of nerve fiber patterns and connections. *Proc Natl Acad Sci USA* 1963; 50: 703–710.
28. Exner S. Die Innervation des Kehlkopfes. Sitzungsber. Akad Wiss Wien, Math-Naturwiss, Abt 1, 1885; 89: 63–118.
29. Van Harreveld A. Reinnervation of denervated muscle fibers by adjacent functioning motor units. *Am J Physiol* 1945; 144: 447–493.
30. Weiss P, Edds MV. Spontaneous recovery of muscle following partial denervation. *Am J Physiol* 1946; 145: 587–607.
31. Edds MV. Experiments on partially deneurotized nerves. *J Exp Zool* 1949; 111: 211–226
32. Edds MV. Collateral regeneration of residual motor axons in partially denervated muscles. *J Exp Zool* 1950; 113: 517–552
33. Weiss P, Hiscoe HB. Experiments on the mechanisms of nerve growth. *J Exp Zool* 1948; 107: 315–396

2

Axonal Dynamics and Regeneration

Scott T. Brady

Department of Cell Biology and Neuroscience, University of Texas Southwestern Medical Center, Dallas, Texas 75235

A single neuron may achieve remarkable dimensions: in an adult human, some axons extend for a meter or more. Greater than 99.9% of cell volume in these large neurons is associated with axonal and dendritic arbors, but effectively all protein synthesis occurs in the remaining volume: the perikaryon, which may represent less than 0.1% of the total neuronal volume. The scale on which neurons must operate is orders of magnitude greater than that of other cell types. As a result, neuronal growth and maintenance depend critically on the timely, efficient delivery of material to specific cellular domains. The dynamics underlying neuronal growth encompass the synthesis, packaging, sorting, targeting, and translocation of those components required for neuronal function. Obviously, an understanding of the molecular mechanisms associated with neuronal dynamics is critical to any description of neuronal growth and regeneration.

Axonal dynamics can in large part be considered in the context of axonal transport, which subsumes packaging, sorting, targeting, and translocation of materials in the axon. While a substantial literature exists regarding axonal transport in intact and regenerating neurons, a comprehensive review of that literature is beyond the scope of this chapter. However, insights into the mechanisms of axonal transport have led to a new perspective on axonal dynamics, particularly in the context of regeneration. This new information includes determination of the molecular identity for motors involved in transport, identification of potential mechanisms for regulating transport, and characterization of the influence of different axonal environments on transport. Some of these recent developments may eventually lead to new approaches for stimulation of CNS regeneration, but they already represent a substantive contribution to our understanding of the mechanisms of regeneration.

Identifying the molecular basis for the striking differences in regenerative potential of CNS and PNS axons remains a central question in axonal dynamics. These differences are apparent even when comparing different branches of single neurons that extend into both CNS and PNS millieus. Since the microenvironments associated with CNS and PNS glia differ in many respects, most attempts to explain the lack of effective CNS regeneration have focused on variations in the glial environment. Consistent with this, CNS axons will regenerate given a suitable PNS environment. Observations such as these provide compelling evidence that functional CNS regeneration is possible given the correct environment (1–4).

The molecular mechanisms which underly regeneration must be understood if we are to devise a means for stimulating functional regeneration in CNS tracts. While many aspects of CNS and PNS responsible for observed differences in regeneration remain to be defined, some important elements in the glial environment are beginning to be characterized (5–7). Rather less progress has been made in determining the molecular mechanisms through which glial environments affect neuronal responses. The molecular differences between an axon in a PNS environment and a comparable axon (or even the same axon) in a CNS environment remain poorly understood. Those neuronal and axonal parameters which are modulated during regeneration must be identified, and the mechanisms by which the microenvironment affects axonal dynamics need to be characterized.

The goal of this chapter is to provide a contemporary perspective on those aspects of axonal dynamics related to regeneration. Several key questions need to be answered to accomplish this. Some of these questions now have answers, while others will require further study. Four broad areas of interest will be considered. First, structural elements of the axon that underly axonal dynamics will be summarized, i.e., those that form the molecular basis of neuronal architecture. Second, the essential characteristics of axonal transport will be described, with an emphasis on our current understanding of the molecular mechanisms of transport. Third, our current understanding of regulatory mechanisms for axonal transport and for the targeting of transported materials to specific neuronal domains will be characterized. Finally, a description of the cellular and molecular consequences of disrupting the glial environment on axonal dynamics will provide a basis for understanding the pathways by which glia modulate axonal architecture and axonal dynamics. Through consideration of these four areas an integrated view may emerge of how axonal dynamics serve to create a functioning neuron and contribute to regeneration of damaged nerve fibers.

STRUCTURAL AND MOLECULAR BASES OF NEURONAL MORPHOLOGY

Neuronal morphologies require that cytoskeletal, cytoplasmic, and membranous elements be assembled in a characteristic manner. The biochemical specialization for each of these elements in the neuron can be quite striking. Composition of proteins in axonal compartments differ qualitatively and quantitatively from dendritic and perikaryal compartments. Most of these protein constituents are synthesized in a specialized region of the perikarya which we have referred to as translational cytoplasm (8). Translational cytoplasm typically includes the protein synthetic machinery and associated structures for processing of those proteins, such as the Golgi complex. Most translational cytoplasm is in the perikaryon near the nucleus, but some of components of translational cytoplasm can be found in dendritic compartments.

Axons, dendrites, and more peripheral regions of the perikaryon contain those expressed products unique to that neuron. Such regions include functional domains, which can be grouped into the general category of expressional cytoplasm (8). Different types of expressional cytoplasm, along with specialized regions of neuronal membrane, are arranged to form distinct functional compartments. The components of a specialized dendritic or axonal compartment are generally delivered via intracellular transport. Even in dendrites, where there is some local protein synthesis, only selected mRNAs are transported into dendrites (9).

Dendritic and Axonal Protein Synthesis

While intracellular transport is highly developed in neurons, a wide variety of polypeptides must be delivered to the axonal and dendritic compartments. This has led to continued interest in local synthesis of proteins in domains relatively distant from the perikaryon. Although the axon has the capacity for some synthesis and processing of lipids and carbohydrates, protein synthesis is generally thought to be restricted to cell bodies and some dendrites. This conclusion is based on the absence of identifiable components for protein synthesis in axons.

Several laboratories (10–12) have devoted considerable time and resources to the detection of protein synthesis in certain large axons (i.e., the squid giant axon and Mauthner cell axons), but the evidence for even a small amount of protein synthesis remains equivocal. Some axons do contain various RNA species, including tRNA (13,14), but ribosomal RNA is undetectable in mature axons. Ultrastructural studies have consistently failed to detect polysomes in axons (15), although they can be readily identified in some dendritic regions (16). The tRNA may play an important role in regeneration as a mechanism for posttranslational modification of axonal proteins (14) and the small amounts of incorporation that have occasionally been reported probably result from this mechanism. Even if a small amount of protein synthesis does exist in some axons, there are no axonal proteins that need to be synthesized in the axon. All necessary axonal proteins can be transported from the cell body. Until a specific function and defined set of polypeptides can be associated with a functionally significant amount of axonal protein synthesis, contributions to axonal dynamics from axonal protein synthesis can be ignored.

A more substantial contribution to the axon following injury may be transfer of glial proteins into the axon (17–19). Although the process has primarily been studied in the giant axon of the squid, there is reason to think that the phenomenon is more general (17). The primary proteins transferred appear to be members of the stress protein family (20). Stress proteins are highly conserved polypeptides whose synthesis is induced in a wide variety of tissues as a response to many types of stress, including heat shock, and are thought to interact with partially denatured proteins (21,22). Synthesis of these proteins is poorly induced in neurons, but glia exhibit a significant stress response (20,23). One attractive model is that the glia supply stress proteins to axonal regions lacking protein synthesis.

In dendritic regions where polysomes can be readily demonstrated, the amount of protein synthesized is modest when compared to that occurring in the cell body. Most dendritic proteins originate in the perikaryon and must be transported to the sites of utilization (16,24,25). When considering protein synthesis in dendrites, a useful comparison can be made with mitochondria, which also have a limited capacity for protein synthesis. Genes for most mitochondrial proteins are nuclear genes and the polypeptides must be synthesized in the translational cytoplasm of the cell body. Polypeptides destined for mitochondria are then transported into a mitochondrion. While there are no mRNAs that have been localized exclusively to the dendrites, dendritic mRNAs do represent a subset of neuronal mRNAs (9,249). The physiological roles played by translation of selected proteins in the dendritic compartment remains uncertain. The hypothesis that these mRNAs code for polypeptides whose levels must change in response to synaptic input is attractive (25).

Membrane Components

Much of contemporary neurobiology has focused on specializations in neuronal membranes. The number of distinct membrane compartments identifiable in neurons is quite large, consistent with the number of discrete activities of a neuron. Receptors and ion channels are a key to the excitability of neurons. As a result, the locations in which receptors or channels are placed play a critical role in neuronal function. Numerous examples may be cited. Saltatory conduction of the action potential occurs efficiently because sodium channels have been concentrated at nodes of Ranvier while potassium channels are largely confined to internodal regions of the axolemma. Similarly, synaptic vesicles must be concentrated in the presynaptic terminal, available for mobilization and release. Receptors to specific neurotransmitters must be localized to appropriate postsynaptic domains, whether they serve as excitatory, inhibitory, or modulatory synapses.

In particular, the plasmalemma is divided into many domains, each exhibiting a specialized function and a characteristic composition. Presynaptic and postsynaptic membrane specializations are an obvious example of functionally distinct domains, but many others can be distinguished. Postsynaptic specializations on dendritic spines may be quite different from postsynaptic regions in the vicinity of a presynaptic terminal involved in modulation of synaptic function. Along the axon itself, morphological, biochemical, and electrophysiological differences in the plasmalemma can be seen at the axon hillock, nodes of Ranvier, and internodes. Each has a characteristic composition of ion channels and structural proteins that must be maintained for generation and conduction of the action potential.

Despite the importance of proper placement for membrane proteins, surprisingly little is known about the mechanisms for directing or targeting membrane components to a particular function domain of the neuron. Similarly, our understanding of how these specialized domains are maintained is limited. In part, the explanation may reflect disposition of different transport vesicle populations within the neuron, each of which may carry the specific protein and lipid components needed for a given functional domain. Certainly, populations of vesicles can be defined in the axon that are precursors to synaptic vesicles or peptidergic vesicles, carrying neurotransmitters or peptides along with associated enzymes and regulatory proteins (26,27). Other populations of membrane bounded organelles can be seen to contain sodium channel (28), presynaptic receptors (29), or other membrane components. Precedents exist for sorting of proteins to specific membrane compartments at the level of the Golgi complex within the cell body (30). In neurons, however, after assembly intracellular membranous organelles must be moved considerable distances into an axonal or dendritic compartment before being delivered to specialized domains. Movement to the distal regions of a neuron is accomplished via mechanisms of axonal transport, to be discussed in the next section. Mechanisms for delivery of membrane components to the correct location are not well defined, but plausible mechanisms for targeting membrane proteins to specific domains in axons or growing neurites have begun to emerge that may lead to models of general utility.

Cytoskeletal Structures

Three categories of cytoskeletal elements play distinct roles in neuronal growth: microtubules, neurofilaments, and microfilaments. Each consists of a diverse set of polypeptides that are combined in various permutations to fill specific niches within the biochemical ecology of the nervous system. Sometimes plasticity is critical, while at other times morphological stability is needed. The importance of cytoskeletal structures for neurite outgrowth and neuronal morphologies have been well documented, but specific roles played by the different classes of cytoskeletal elements are not as well delineated. There are overlapping functions between classes, and isoforms exist within each class of cytoskeletal protein that may subtly change local properties of the cytoskeleton. The role of specializations in the cytoskeleton and cytomatrix for neuronal growth and regeneration has been recently reviewed (31). While considerable progress has been made toward characterizing the components, the molecular mechanisms for modulation of the neuronal cytoskeleton in vivo are poorly characterized, whether during neurite outgrowth in development and regeneration or in maintainance of a mature fiber.

Microtubules serve at least two main roles in the mature nervous system. First, they provide a structural framework for the axon (32,33), playing an important role in determining the size and morphology of neuronal processes. In small unmyelinated fibers and in many dendrites, both of which have few neurofilaments, microtubules act as the primary structural element. This role is particularly important in insect and crustacean axons, which lack intermediate filaments entirely. As a result, in the arthopod nervous system microtubules are the primary structural components. A second critical role for microtubules is connected with intracellular transport. Two of the three classes of molecular motors identified in the nervous system mediate microtubule-based motility: Both kinesins and dyneins move materials along microtubule tracks (34). The properties of these motors and their role in axonal transport will be considered later.

Neuronal microtubules found in different intracellular compartments (axons, dendrites, etc.) are biochemically and physiologically diverse, but there are no obvious ultrastructural differences in their appearance. The primary subunits of the microtubule are alpha and beta tubulins. There are multiple genes for both alpha and beta tubulins, including brain specific isoforms (35). Expression of brain isoforms is developmentally regulated and may vary in different neuronal populations (184). The expression of various isoforms is differentially affected during regeneration (36,37). The primary sequences of different isoforms is highly conserved, with limited variability in specific domains such as the carboxyl terminal (35). In addition to primary sequence variants, the tubulins are subject to a variety of posttranslational modifications. The most common modifications in neurons are acetylation (38) and detyrosination (39), but some isoforms may be phosphorylated as well (40). The physiological significance of tubulin posttranslational modifications is not well understood, because the in vitro properties of resulting tubulin and microtubules are largely unaffected. These posttranslational modifications largely correlate in vivo with the increased stability of microtubules, but this is because the modifying enzymes work preferentially on tubulin assembled into microtubules (40-43). As a result, the longer a microtubule has been polymerized (i.e., the more stable it is), the greater the extent of modification. The posttranslational modifications are rapidly removed for the tubulin following depolymerization (43). The microtubules in axonal and dendritic compartments differ in their composition and dynamics, so the extent of posttranslational modification also differs (42).

Although stable microtubules are typically acetylated and detyrosinated, these two modifications to tubulin do not directly confer stability on the microtubules (43-45). While modification may affect stability indirectly (see below), the assembly/disassembly kinetics of microtubules made with modified tubulins are essentially indistinguishable from those made with unmodified tubulins. In addition to the better-characterized modifications, there is evidence for additional types of posttranslational modification to tubulins (46). Even within a single microtubule, there may be distinct domains with different composition and degrees of stability (41). Domains of increased stability are preserved as short microtubule segments when other microtubule segments have been depolymerized (47). Such stable microtubule segments may serve to nucleate and organize microtubules in the axon, particularly during regeneration (41,47). The various modifications may play a direct or an indirect role in the stabilization of axonal microtubules (41,46,48).

The stability of assembled microtubules plays a critical role in effective regeneration. Axonal microtubules apparently must be disassembled as part of the reorganization of the cytoskeleton for neurite outgrowth, then must be reassembled for neurite extension. As a result, microtubules play critical roles in regeneration (31,48). They serve both for transporting required materials to the growth cone and as the primary structural element in growing neurites. The importance of the tubulins in regeneration can be inferred from changes in tubulin associated with regeneration. Specific tubulin genes are upregulated during axonal growth or regeneration (36,49,50) and there are characteristic changes in the axonal transport of tubulin (51–53).

In addition to the tubulins, a heterogeneous group of microtubule-associated proteins (MAPs) have been described (54,55). MAPs do not include every protein which can interact with microtubules. The rigorous definition states that a MAP binds to microtubules rather than free tubulin and cycles with microtubules through multiple assembly/disassembly reactions at a constant stoichiometry. MAPs must also be associated with microtubules in situ. Some MAPs are specific to particular cellular populations, and many MAPs are neuron specific. Some MAPs have differential distributions even within a neuron. For example, the high molecular weight MAP known as MAP2 is restricted to dendritic compartments (56–59,177). MAP2 mRNA is specifically transported into dendrites where MAP2 may be locally synthesized (9,24,249), but may also be transported. Another class of neuronal MAPs, tau proteins, exhibit a characteristic pattern of phosphorylation with a different site of phosphorylation for axonal tau than for tau in cell bodies and dendrites (60). There are also MAPs which are widely distributed, being found in both neuronal and nonneuronal tissues (54,55).

One function of MAPs in all cells is thought to be stimulation microtubule formation and stabilization of existing microtubules. Some MAPs may contribute to the formation of stable microtubules (61) or may preferentially associate with stable microtubules. Although MAPs are often described as forming microtubule crossbridges, there is no evidence that MAPs crosslink microtubules to other microtubules or to nonmicrotubule structures. While transient interactions with microtubules certainly occur, microtubules are not bound together into a crosslinked network. As a result, microtubules can slide relative to one another (62,63), a property which is likely to be important for their axonal transport.

The roles played by MAPs during regeneration and growth have not been characterized as extensively as those for tubulin. Enhanced expression of tau proteins in tissue culture cells has been reported to stimulate formation of neurite-like processes (64,65). However, these effects may reflect increased stabilization and bundling of microtubules in nonneuronal cells, owing to overexpression of tau proteins (65,66). The microtubule bundles seen in these situations are not characteristic of normal neurons and may not reflect a normal function of tau (66). Expression of antisense oligonucleotides to tau in primary cultures of cerebellar neurons appears to interfere with neurite formation (58) and tau is thought to aid in the stabilization of neurites (64–66). MAPs are differentially expressed during development (67–70), but less is known about changes in the expression of specific MAPs during regeneration (71). Since microtubules in vivo invariably include MAPs, a more detailed consideration of changes in MAPs during regeneration is merited.

Intermediate filaments of the nervous system are the cytoskeletal elements with the greatest metabolic stability (72). As a result, they are especially well suited for a cytoarchitectonic role. In recent years, our understanding of intermediate filament biology has increased substantially. The biochemistry and molecular genetics of intermediate filaments have provided considerable insight into both the structure and function of these cytoskeletal elements.

The predominant intermediate filaments of neurons are those formed from the neurofilament triplet proteins (73,74). Each of the triplet polypeptides are synthesized from a different mRNA coded by a separate gene (75). The apparent molecular weights for neurofilament subunits vary widely, but the mammalian forms range from 180 to 200 kD for the high molecular weight subunit (NFH), from 130 to 170 kD for the medium subunit (NFM), and from 60 to 70 kD for the low molecular weight subunit (NFL) (76). Intermediate filaments formed by these three subunits are 100 nm in diameter and many micrometers in length. The individual subunits are typically highly phosphorylated, with NFM and NFH having unusually high phosphorylation levels (77,78). In some species, the NFH tails may have 50 or more repeats of a consensus phosphorylation site and levels of NFH phosphorylation indicate that most or all may be phosphorylated in vivo.

The amount of neurofilaments in an axon play an important role in determining the caliber of that axon (32,33,79–81). Different populations of neurons may vary in the amount of neurofilaments and/or level of neurofilament phosphorylation (82). Neurofilaments have characteristic sidearms, unique among intermediate filaments. The NF sidearms are formed primarily by NFM and NFH carboxyl terminal regions, which contain the repeated consensus phosphorylation sites (83,84). Although all three subunits contribute to the central core of the filament, the sidearms are often labeled by antibodies that recognize only NFM- and NFH-subunits (85). NFM and NFH are required to form filaments with sidearms during in vitro assembly studies (86,87). Phosphorylation of the sidearms appears to alter the surface charge on the neurofilament and increase the spacing between adjacent neurofilaments (88). Although many reports refer to the sidearms as crossbridges between neurofilaments, the only evidence for such crossbridges comes from electron micrographs. However, direct studies of neurofilament interactions provide no evidence of crosslinks between neurofilaments or between neurofilaments and other cytoskeletal structures in the axon (89,90). Indeed, the amount of charged phosphate groups on the surface of a typical phosphorylated neurofilament makes it difficult to imagine a stable interaction of neurofilaments with other structures of like charge.

Neurofilament protein expression and phosphorylation are both regulated during development and regulation (36,91,92). One hallmark of the cell body response to an axonal lesion in classes of neurons that regenerate well is downregulation of neurofilament triplet expression, frequently coupled with the upregulation of specific tubulin isotypes (36,50,53,93,94). Although a variety of other synthetic changes occur, these are among the most dramatic. Moreover, in CNS neurons which fail to mount an effective regenerative response, the changes in expression for neurofilament proteins and tubulins are reduced in magnitude or are absent (95). Since changes in cytoskeletal protein expression will not produce alterations in the cytoskeletal composition of the axon until after the growth cone has formed and extended for some distance (96, and see below in discussion of axonal transport), such changes do not immediately affect neurite growth. The changes in cytoskeletal protein expression may reflect the activation of a cellular program for neurite growth. One research area of particular importance for the near future is the identification of mechanisms for regulating expression of neurofilament proteins and tubulins during development and regeneration. These may provide a key to more general mechanisms for regulating neurite growth.

In addition to the neurofilament triplet polypeptides, several additional intermediate filament subunit proteins can be identified in neurons. Intermediate filament proteins form a superfamily with five classes of proteins, including the nuclear lamins

(72). The neurofilament triplet polypeptides are class IV intermediate filament proteins. Class IV intermediate filaments are expressed only in neurons and have a characteristic domain structure that can be recognized in both primary sequence and intron structure in the genes. Class III intermediate filaments are a diverse family that includes, among others, vimentin (characteristic of fibroblasts and many embryonic tissues, including embryonic neurons) and glial filament acidic protein. Recently, class III intermediate filament proteins that are unique to neurons have also been described, including peripherin (97–99), and a 66 kD protein (100). Each of these are expressed in distinct neuronal populations with a characteristic pattern of expression during development (101–105). Peripherin can coassemble with the neurofilament triplet polypeptides both in vitro and in vivo (106), but it is not known whether this is the general case for neuronal class III intermediate filaments. The physiological roles played by neuron-specific class III intermediate filament polypeptides remains uncertain. Since class III intermediate filaments are more readily disassembled than class IV intermediate filaments (72), addition of class III neuronal intermediate filament proteins may contribute to the plasticity of neuronal morphologies. Consistent with this possibility is the observation that peripherin is not downregulated along with the neurofilament triplet during regeneration (107).

Actin microfilaments are particularly concentrated in presynaptic terminals, dendritic spines, growth cones, and the subplasmalemmal cortex. Although concentrated in these regions, microfilaments are also present throughout the cytoplasm of the neuron in the form of short filaments 4–6 nm diameter (108). In the axonal cytoplasm, microfilaments are most apparent in the vicinity of axonal microtubules and near the plasma membrane. While many microfilament-associated proteins in the nervous system (actin, actin-binding proteins) are well documented, less is known about their distribution and normal function. The prominent actin bundles seen in fibroblasts or other nonneuronal cells in culture and not characteristic of neurons, and most neuronal actin microfilaments are less than 1 μm in length (108,109).

One location containing longer microfilaments and more elaborate organization is the growth cone, which contains bundles of microfilaments in the filopodia as well as a more dispersed actin network (for review, see 110). Neurofilaments are largely excluded from the growth cone, typically extending no further than the neck of the growth cone (111). In contrast, microtubules and microfilaments play complementary roles in the growth cone itself (110,112). Microfilaments are critical in sprouting, but appear less critical for elongation, at least over short distances. Disruption of microtubules in the distal neurite does not affect sprouting, but does inhibit neurite elongation.

An elegant series of experiments using fluorescent tubulin in cultured embryonic *Xenopus* neurons (62,113,114) has examined the behavior of individual microtubules in the growth cone. The microtubules exhibit a large repertoire of different behaviors, which are consistent with roles in both elongation and consolidation of growth. Microtubules also play a role in the steering of growth cones (114), a critical element in choosing the correct path during development or regeneration. Microfilament function in the growth cone has been studied with fluorescent probes and video microscopy (110), but details remain sketchy. However, it is likely that interactions between the microfilaments and microtubules are responsible for most growth cone motility.

MOLECULAR MECHANISMS OF AXONAL TRANSPORT

Thousands of different polypeptides, lipids, neuropeptides, and carbohydrates are required in axonal and dendritic arbors. Since protein synthesis in these domains is limited or absent, axonal transport processes represent the primary mechanism for delivering proteins to their sites of utilization. Although the phenomenon of axonal transport has been described in considerable detail since the original demonstration by Weiss and Hiscoe (115), the underlying molecular mechanisms are still the subject of investigation and often of debate.

Four major components of axonal transport can be typically defined along with some minor components. Two forms of fast axonal transport exist, one in the anterograde and one in the retrograde direction. Both directions of fast transport represent the movement of membrane bounded organelles along microtubules at rates ranging from 100 to 400 mm/day or 1 to 5 μm/second (for reviews, see 116–118). Slow axonal transport has two major components, both representing movement of cytoplasmic constituents (119–121). The cytoplasmic and cytoskeletal elements of the axon in axonal transport move at rates at least two orders of magnitude slower than fast transport. Slow Component a (SCa) comprises largely cytoskeletal proteins, neurofilaments, and microtubule protein. Slow Component b (SCb) represents a complex and heterogeneous rate component, including hundreds of distinct polypeptides ranging from cytoskeletal proteins such as actin (and tubulin in some nerves, see 119,123–126) to soluble enzymes of intermediary metabolism (such as the glycolytic enzymes, see 241–243). Many characteristics of axonal transport have been described and these provide the foundation for our understanding of mechanisms.

Structural Hypothesis of Axonal Transport

The diversity of polypeptides in each axonal transport rate component and the coherent movement of proteins having many different molecular weights produces a conundrum (119,121,126). How can so many different polypeptides move down the axon as a group? In theory, one could propose that each protein has a motor of its own. In that case, each rate component might represent movements due to a specific class of motors or to variable affinities for a smaller number of motors. However, the relatively small numbers of motor molecules and the logistical difficulties associated with such a model effectively preclude this possibility.

The Structural Hypothesis (127) was formulated in response to the observation that rate components of axonal transport move as discrete waves, each with a characteristic rate and a distinctive composition. The hypothesis is deceptively simple: "Proteins in axonal transport do not move as individual polypeptides. Instead, polypeptides move as part of cytological structures or in association with a cytological structure. Therefore, axonal transport represents the movement of cytological structures." The only assumption made is that the number of elements which can interact with transport motor complexes are limited, so transported material must be packaged appropriately to be moved. The different rate components result from packaging of transported material into different cytologically identifiable structures. In other words, membrane-associated proteins move as membrane bounded organelles (vesicles, mitochondria, etc.), while tubulin and MAPs move as microtubules, and neurofilaments move as neurofilaments.

There has been some confusion in the literature about specific predictions of the Structural Hypothesis. Some critics have argued that this model requires movement of a crosslinked microtubule/neurofilament complex in the form of a solid axoplasmic column. However, the evidence for a crosslinked complex of microtubules and neurofilaments is not compelling, being both indirect and inconsistent with available direct analyses. The Structural Hypothesis specifically predicts that individual microtubules and neurofilaments move rather than tubulin dimers or neurofilament monomers, but makes no assumptions about higher order interactions between cytoskeletal structures (127). A variant on the Structural Hypothesis even proposes that cytoskeletal proteins move in the form of small oligomers rather than polymers (128), although there is no evidence for the presence of such oligomers in vivo. To the limits of detection under in vivo conditions, neurofilaments exist only as the polymer and tubulin exchanges between dimer and polymer (129). Since a number of observations indicate that microtubules and neurofilaments can move in vivo as intact polymers, there is no compelling reason to postulate additional oligomeric forms.

Movement of Cytoskeletal Structures

The coherent movement of neurofilaments and microtubule proteins (73,119,126) was strong evidence for the Structural Hypothesis. Particularly striking evidence was provided by pulse-labeling experiments in which neurofilament proteins moved as a bell-shaped wave with little or no trailing of neurofilament protein (119). Similarly, the coherent transport of tubulin and MAPs (130) makes sense only if microtubules are moved, since MAPs do not interact with unpolymerized tubulin.

Nixon and Logvinenko (131) reported that small amounts of neurofilament protein are deposited in the axons of mouse optic nerve, although they also found that most neurofilament protein moves to the end of the axons. This study remains the only report of significant deposition of neurofilament protein in the axon and is at odds with a substantial literature which finds that neurofilament proteins move to the terminals where they are degraded (51,73,119, 124,125,132–135). A number of factors help to explain the single anomalous report (131): 1) the small size of the mouse optic system reduces both temporal and spatial resolution; 2) conclusions were based on a quantitation of NFL from a band of the appropriate molecular weight, even though a number of other axonal proteins have similar molecular weights (125,133); and 3) the normalization procedure used seriously overestimated amounts left behind the main peak of transported neurofilament protein. Studies on the turnover of neurofilament protein during transport indicate that little loss of material occurs until reaching the vicinity of the nerve terminals, where it is rapidly degraded (132,133).

A striking demonstration of microtubule movement has recently been provided by Kirschner and his colleagues. Reinsch et al. (113) injected tubulin labeled with caged fluorescein into a *Xenopus* oocyte, then allowed the embryo to develop. Early embryonic neurons were cultured and the caged fluorescent tubulin could be locally photoactivated. With this method, patches of fluorescent tubulin could be seen to move down the axon. As predicted by the Structural Hypothesis, the fluorescent patches remained discrete during movements in the anterograde direction at slow transport rates. Observations of fluorescent tubulin and microtubules could also be made using rhodamine tubulin (62,114). Under favorable conditions, individual fluorescent microtubules could be detected in the neurites or growth cones (62,113,114), and these microtubules were pulled and even bent in conjunction with growth cone movements. When combined with studies of axonal transport using radiolabels (see 116,119, 127, for reviews) and direct observations of individual microtubules with video microscopy (63), there is little doubt that microtubules and neurofilaments can and do move in the axon in a manner consistent with the Structural Hypothesis.

Movement of Membrane Bounded Organelles

Biochemical and morphological studies established that the material moving in fast axonal transport was associated with membrane bounded organelles (for review of the early literature, see 136,137). A variety of materials could be shown in fast transport. In anterograde transport, materials being moved include membrane-associated enzyme activities, neurotransmitters, and neuropeptides. Many of the materials moving down the axon in anterograde transport are returned in retrograde transport (138), in some cases following modification in the terminal (13). In addition, a number of exogenous materials taken up in the distal regions of the axon are moved back to the cell body by retrograde transport. Exogenous materials in retrograde transport include neurotrophic factors, such as nerve growth factor (140), and viral particles invading the nervous system (141). The uptake of neurotrophic factors may play a critical role in the process of regeneration (142).

Electron microscopic analysis of materials accumulated at a ligation or crush demonstrated that the organelles moving in the anterograde direction were morphologically distinct from those moving in the retrograde direction (143–145). Consistent with the ultrastructural differences, radiolabel (139) and immunocytochemical (27) studies indicate that there are both quantitative and qualitative differences between anterogradely and retrogradely moving material. The differences between anterograde and retrograde transport indicate that some processing or repackaging events must occur as part of turnaround in axonal transport. Turnaround processing appears to involve a proteolytic event, because certain protease inhibitors inhibit turnaround without affecting anterograde and retrograde transport (146).

Biochemical and morphological approaches made considerable progress toward a description of the materials being transported in fast axonal transport, but were ill suited for identifying the molecular motors involved in translocation. A different technology was required that permitted direct observation of organelle movements and precise control of experimental conditions. Such experiments became possible with the advent of video microscopic techniques (147).

An early use of video-enhanced contrast (VEC) microscopy was to characterize the bidirectional movement of membrane bounded organelles in giant axons from the squid *Loligo pealeii* (148). Years before, Bear et al. (149) had demonstrated that axoplasm could be extruded from the giant axon as an intact cylinder. Properties of the isolated axoplasm had been characterized in some detail (150), making VEC-DIC microscopic analysis of axoplasm a natural choice. Remarkably, fast axonal transport continued unabated in isolated axoplasm for hours (151). Isolated axoplasm from the giant axon has no plasma membrane or other permeability barriers, but can be readily maintained in an active state. Combining VEC-DIC microscopy with isolated axoplasm permitted rigorous dissection of the mechanisms for fast axonal transport using biochemical and pharmacological approaches (151,152). A number of insights into axonal transport mechanisms have resulted from these studies. Most importantly, studies in isolated axoplasm have led to the identification of several families of molecular motors that may be involved in axonal transport.

Motors in the Nervous System

Until 1985, our knowledge of molecular motors in vertebrate cells of any type was restricted to myosins and flagellar dyneins. Myosins had been identified in nervous tissue, but myosin functions were uncertain. Since the preponderance of evidence indicated that fast axonal transport was microtubule-based, there was considerable interest in dyneins in cell cytoplasm. Despite a number of studies, no evidence emerged for a functional cytoplasmic dynein. Worse yet, the characteristic properties of fast organelle movements appeared inconsistent with both myosins and dyneins (152,153).

Myosins and dyneins can be distinguished pharmacologically by differential susceptibility to inhibitors ATPase activity, but the spectrum of inhibitors active against fast axonal transport failed to match the properties of either myosin or dynein (152,153). The most striking difference between inhibitor effects on axonal transport and on myosin/dynein motors was seen in the effect of a nonhydrolyzable analogue of ATP. Adenylyl-imidodiphosphate (AMP-PNP) is a weak competitive inhibitor of both myosin and dynein, requiring a 10–100-fold excess of analogue. In contrast, within minutes of AMP-PNP perfusion into isolated axoplasm, both anterograde and retrograde axonal transport stop (152–154). Inhibition by AMP-PNP occurs even in the presence of stoichiometric concentrations of ATP (153, 154). Organelles moving in both directions freeze in place and remain attached to microtubules. AMP-PNP weakens the interaction of myosin with microfilaments and of dynein with microtubules, but stabilizes the binding of membrane bounded organelles to microtubules (see review in 34). Thus, the effects of AMP-PNP indicated that movement of membrane bounded organelles in fast axonal transport must involve a new type of motor, unrelated to the myosins or dyneins (154).

A New Class of Motor Molecules

The effects of AMP-PNP demonstrated the existence of a new type of mechanochemical ATPase and provided a basis for identifying its constituent polypeptides. Binding of the ATPase to microtubules should be increased by AMP-PNP and decreased by ATP (153,154). Polypeptides meeting this criterion were soon identified (155,156). The new ATPase was named kinesin, based initially on an ability to move microtubules across glass coverslips as first described in axoplasmic extracts by Allen et al. (157). Studies soon established that kinesin was a microtubule-activated ATPase with minimal basal activity (156,157). This combination of ATPase activity and motility in vitro confirmed that kinesin was a new class of microtubule-based motor.

Kinesin has now been identified in a variety of organisms and tissues, leading to an extensive characterization of many biochemical, pharmacological, immunochemical, and molecular properties (for review, see 34,159). Electron microscopic and biophysical analyses reveal kinesin as a long, rod-shaped protein, approximately 80 nm in length (160–164). Neuronal kinesin is a heterotetramer with two heavy chains (molecular weight 115–130 kD) and two light chains (62–70 kD) (161,162). Localization of antibodies specific for kinesin subunits by high resolution electron microscopy that bovine brain kinesin indicates that the two heavy chains are arranged in parallel, forming the heads and much of the shaft, while light chains are localized to the fan-shaped tail region (164).

A variety of approaches have demonstrated that the ATP-binding and microtubule-binding domains of kinesin are in the head regions of the heavy chains. While the light chains in the tail region of kinesin appear involved in binding to membranes (see review in 34). When in vitro motility assays are employed for analysis of brain kinesins, movements are directed toward the plus ends of microtubules. Since axonal microtubules are oriented with their plus ends distal from the cell body, this movement would be appropriate for a motor which moves organelles in the anterograde direction.

Neuronal kinesin appears associated with a variety of membrane bounded organelles, including synaptic vesicles, mitochondria, coated vesicles, and lysosomes (165–168). The interaction of kinesin and other molecular motors with membrane surfaces is not well understood. In the case of kinesin, the interaction is thought to involve the light chains of kinesin along with the carboxyl terminals of the heavy chains (164,169).

The kinesins have now been shown to be a family of related proteins with a highly conserved domain that includes the ATP- and microtubule-binding domains (170). Many of these kinesin-related polypeptides appear associated with cell division, and kinesin-related proteins in vertebrate tissues are not well characterized. However, the discovery that claret[nd], a kinesin-related protein from *Drosophila,* can move structures toward the minus end of microtubules (171) increases the number of potential functions that kinesin might serve in nervous tissue, perhaps including a role in retrograde transport.

Dyneins

As an indirect result of the discovery of kinesin, one of the high molecular weight microtubule-associated proteins of brain, MAP1C (172), was the long sought cytoplasmic form of dynein (173,174). MAP1C dynein and kinesin can both be isolated from bovine brain by incubation of microtubules with nucelotide-free soluble extracts. Both are bound to microtubules under these conditions and released by ATP (174–177). MAP1C dynein moved microtubules in vitro with a polarity opposite of that seen with kinesin (175) and was identified as a two-headed cytoplasmic dynein using both structural and biochemical criteria (174,178). Concurrently, a similar protein was identified in nematodes (179).

MAP1C dyneins form a 40 nm long complex of molecular weight 1.6×10^6 daltons, which includes two heavy chains and a number of light chains (178,180,181). Less information is available about the distribution and properties of MAP1C dyneins than for kinesin. Immunocytochemical studies in nonneuronal cells showed immunoreactivity on mitotic spindles (182,183). In addition, Pfarr et al. (182) reported that a punctate pattern of immunoreactivity was also present in interphase cells, which was thought to reflect dynein bound to membranous organelles. Dyneins are widely thought to be the motor for fast retrograde axonal transport (175,181) but are also a candidate for a motor in slow axonal transport (34).

Myosins

Myosins were the first molecular motors identified, and in recent years interest in nonmuscle myosins has increased. Nonmuscle myosins may be categorized as belonging to one of three classes (185–187). Myosin II proteins include the thick filaments of smooth and skeletal muscle, but is also present at significant levels in nonmuscle cells. Two heavy chains of myosin II form a dimer which can interact with other myosin II dimers to form bipolar filaments. Under tissue culture conditions, many cells contain bundles of actin microfilaments known as stress fibers, which exhibit a characteristic distribution of myosin II into distinct patterns that may be sarcomeric equivalents (187). Many of traditional roles for myosins in contractile events are thought to involve myosin II in nonneuronal cells, such as the contractile ring in mitosis. Although brain myosin II was one of the first nonmuscle myosins to be described (188–190), relatively little is known about the function of myosin II in neurons.

Myosin I proteins have a single, smaller heavy chain that does not form filaments, but possesses a homologous actin-activated ATPase domain (191,192). The most exciting aspect of myosin I is an ability to interact directly with membrane surfaces (193,194) that may generate movements of plasma membrane components or intracellular organelles. Myosin I has now been purified from mammalian neural tissues (195). Both myosin I and myosin II molecules have been proposed to have a role in the motility of lamelipodia at the leading edge of growth cones.

Recently, Mercer et al. (186) showed that the murine coat color mutant *dilute* was a novel myosin heavy chain distinct from both myosins I and II. There are complex neurological deficits in *dilute* mutants (186), which suggests that the various myosins may have narrowly defined functions. Despite intensive study of myosins I and II (185,187,191), relatively little is known about neuronal functions for the myosins. Axonal transport of myosin-like proteins has been described (196), but little further progress has been made on the functions of myosin II in the mature nervous system. Even less is known about myosin I in the nervous system. However, myosins are likely to play roles in growth cone motility, synaptic plasticity, and even neurotransmitter release (for review see 110).

Matching Motors to Physiological Functions

The most distinctive characteristic of kinesins is nucleotide-sensitive binding to microtubules which is stabilized by AMP-PNP (154–156). By comparison, the affinities of myosin for microfilaments and dynein for microtubules are reduced following treatment with either ATP or AMP-PNP. Whereas nucleotide binding favors release of myosin or dynein, it enhances binding of kinesin. In most other respects, the three classes of mechanochemical ATPases are similar in biochemical and pharmacological sensitivity (34). For example, myosin, dynein, and kinesin all remain in a bound rigor state without nucleotides. There are few instances in our understanding of neuronal function for which we understand fully the role played by molecular motors. The proliferation of different motor molecules and their isoforms even raises the possibility that some physiological activities may involve multiple classes of motor molecules.

REGULATION AND TARGETING OF AXONALLY TRANSPORTED MATERIALS

Since synthesis of proteins occurs at some distance from many functional domains of a neuron, transport to distal regions of the neuron is necessary but not sufficient for proper function. Specific materials must also be delivered to their proper site of utilization and should not be left in inappropriate locations. For example, a synaptic vesicle has no known function in axons or the cell body, so they must be delivered to the presynaptic terminals along with other components necessary for regulated neurotransmitter release. The traditional picture places the presynaptic terminal at the end of an axonal process. This image implies that a synaptic vesicle need only move along the axonal microtubules until it reaches microtubule ends in the presynaptic terminal. However, many CNS synapses are not at the end of an axon. Numerous terminals may occur sequentially along a single axon, making *en passant* contacts with multiple target cells along the way. Targeting of synaptic vesicles then becomes a more complex problem.

In dorsal ganglion cells, the problem is compounded, because a single process leaves the cell body which then branches. The central branch leads to presynaptic terminals in the spinal cord, while the peripheral branches ends in a specialized sensory structure that does not release neurotransmitters. As a result, precursors to synaptic vesicles must be assembled in the cell body and exported into the axon. Synaptic vesicles should move preferentially into the central branch for eventual delivery to the presynaptic terminals. An equivalent problem exists in neuronal cell bodies with both dendritic and axonal processes. Some aspect of the membrane proteins themselves may be important for sorting. Transfection of hippocampal neurons with various viral proteins that are differentially sorted in epithelial cells displays a comparable degree of polarized sorting in neurons between axonal and dendritic compartments (197). As a result, efficient mechanisms must exist for both sorting and targeting to specific domains of the neuron. Virtually nothing can be stated about sorting mechanisms except that they must exist because axons and dendrites have distinct morphologies and biochemical composition.

Progress has been made toward identification of targeting mechanisms, and some general principles have begun to emerge. Since cytoplasmic constituents move only in the anterograde direction, differential metabolism appears to be the key to targeting of cytoplasmic and cytoskeletal proteins. Concentration of actin and other proteins in the presynaptic terminal can be explained by the slower turnover of such proteins in the presynaptic terminal relative to neurofilament proteins and tubulin (132,133,198). Proteins with slow degradative rates in the terminal accumulate and reach a higher steady-state concentration. Alteration of the rate of degradation for a protein will cause a change in the rate of accumulation for that protein. For example, inhibition of calpains will cause the appearance of neurofilament rings in the presynaptic terminal (199). Differential turnover may be accomplished by the activity of proteases with appropriate specificities or by posttranslational modifications that affect susceptibility to degradation. The latter mechanism has been proposed as a mechanism for differential distribution of MAPs in the axon and dendrites (200). Tau is phosphorylated on different sites in axons and in dendrites (60), but at present there is no evidence that this difference affects tau stability in vivo. MAP2 is absent from axons (56,57,59) and exogenous MAP2 appears to be preferentially degraded in axonal compartments (200). However, MAP2 may also be synthesized locally in dendrites (9,249), so the relative contribution of various mechanisms remains uncertain.

A different mechanism for targeting has been proposed for membrane components in the axon. The phosphoprotein synapsin, which is concentrated in the presynaptic terminal (201,202) may provide one mechanism for targeting of synaptic vesicles to the terminal. Synapsin is subjected to repeated cycles of phosphorylation and dephosphorylation. Dephosphorylated synapsin binds tightly to synaptic vesicles and actin microfilaments, while phosphorylation releases synapsin from both of them (203–206). McGuiness et al. (207) showed that concentrations of dephosphorylated synapsin comparable to those found in the synaptic terminal inhibit fast axonal transport in isolated axoplasm, while phosphorylated synapsin at similar concentrations has no effect on transport. The inhibition appears to require the presence of actin microfilaments.

Phosphorylation/dephosphorylation cycles may serve to target synaptic vesicles to presynaptic terminals by changing the affinity of synapsin for microfilaments and the synaptic vesicle. Synapsin is concentrated in the microfilament-rich presynaptic terminal (201,208,209). When a synaptic vesicle precursor in fast axonal transport passes through a region rich in dephosphorylated synapsin, the vesicle will be crosslinked to the available microfilament matrix by synapsin. Such crosslinked vesicles would be removed from fast axonal transport and are effectively targeted to a synapsin-rich domain, the presynaptic terminal. Crosslinked synaptic vesicles are part of the reserve pool of vesicles typically present near the center of a terminal. Calcium-activated kinases may subsequently mobilize the crosslinked vesicles for transfer to the active zones and neurotransmitter release (210,211). As will be discussed in the next section, variations on this motif mechanism may be a general mechanism for targeting membrane bounded organelles to specific domains.

Turnaround processes or conversion from anterograde to retrograde transport may also play a role in defining the composition of distal portions of the axon. Morphological (143–145) and biochemical (139) studies have demonstrated that the organelles returning in retrograde transport differ from those in anterograde transport. Repackaging of membrane components is apparently required for turnaround, consistent with observations that initiation of the return process takes several hours (138,139). Sahenk and Lasek (146) demonstrated that some protease inhibitors would inhibit turnaround without affecting either anterograde or retrograde movements, leading to an accumulation of organelles in the terminal. The protease(s) involved have not been identified, but the specificities of the effective protease inhibitors implicate a thiol protease. This eliminates the calcium-activated protease calpain, which appears to be involved in neurofilament degradation. Calpains are serine proteases and would not be inhibited by a specific inhibitor of thiol proteases.

Consistent with reports that proteases are involved in turnaround of membrane bounded organelles, protease treatment of purified synaptic vesicles can affect the directionality of their movements in axoplasm. Synaptic vesicles which have been purified and fluorescently tagged can be introduced into isolated axoplasm (212) or the squid giant synapse (213). These fluorescent synaptic vesicles will move predominantly in the anterograde direction. Treatment of these synaptic vesicles with proteases prior to labeling can block movement altogether or produce vesicles that move predominantly in the retrograde direction (212; unpublished observations by Leopold, Llinas, Sugimori, Lin, and Brady).

GLIAL MODULATION OF NEURONAL FUNCTION

The recognition that axonal structures are intrinsically dynamic provides a basis for understanding the plasticity of the nervous system during development and regeneration. As specific molecular mechanisms are identified for transport or reorganization of a neuronal structure, they are usually considered independent of other concurrent mechanisms for axonal dynamics. Considering each form of axonal dynamics separately tends to conceal relationships between various aspects of neuronal growth or maintenance. When movement of membrane bounded organelles along microtubules is considered, the concurrent movement of microtubules can easily be forgotten. Altering the cytoskeletal elements of an axon invariably changes the membranous organelle traffic associated with that cytoskeleton as well as neuronal morphologies. Many details of these interrelationships remain to be discovered, but a rough picture has evolved. A consideration of how the glial microenvironment affects the axon can usefully illustrate the complex interdependence of the various forms of axonal dynamics.

Traditionally, the relationship between myelinating glial cells and the axon has been couched in terms of the response by glial cells to changes in the axon during development. The thickness of the myelin sheath and the length of the internode were considered to be dependent on axonal caliber (214), while axonal caliber was a function of a variety of physiological factors. Changes in synthesis of cytoskeletal proteins in the perikaryon in response to developmental programs, connection with suitable targets, and availability of neurotrophic substances, among others, have been reported to affect axonal caliber. The number of microtubules and neurofilaments (32) supplied to the axon via slow axonal transport (80,96,215–217) were considered to be the effective determinants of axonal diameter, and caliber was altered by effects on the axonal cytoskeleton. During maturation of the axon, the role of the myelinating glia was thought to be primarily reactive. Myelination was initiated by contact with the axon and then myelin thickness increased as axonal caliber changed.

Some effects of glia on neuronal growth have been demonstrated. For example, oligodendrocytes have been shown to express surface molecules which inhibit neurite growth (5,6,218,219), but oligodendrocytes have not differentiated at the time of initial neurite outgrowth during development (220–222). Any inhibition by oligodendrocytes and CNS myelin would be significant during regeneration, but not during development. Treatment of CNS tissue with antibodies to these myelin-associated growth inhibitors will neutralize the inhibition of growth by white matter (7,218), indicating an intrinsic ability of CNS neurons to regenerate that is also apparent when a PNS environment is provided for CNS axons (1–4). This suggests that blocking the action of restrictive elements in the glial environment using either direct or indirect means may provide a therapeutically useful treatment.

Recently, several observations have indicated that myelinating glia can directly alter neuronal architecture as well. Myelination may locally induce increased axonal caliber in regions underlying the myelin. In mixed primary cultures of Schwann cells and neurons, focal myelination of axons results in a local increase in axonal caliber (223,224). Similarly, focal demyelination of axons in vivo results in a local reduction of axonal diameter (88,225–228) and changes in the organization of axonal cytoskeletal elements (88,225,229,230). These observations suggest that the interaction between Schwann cells and axons is more complex than prevailing views would indicate. A more detailed consideration of this phenomenon has begun to reveal the underlying molecular mechanisms.

In the demyelinating mutant Trembler mouse, the thickness of the peripheral myelin sheath is reduced and the axonal diameters are smaller. Aguayo et al. (225) grafted a segment of Trembler nerve into a normal mouse and allowed normal axons to regenerate through the Trembler segment. Axonal regions within the Trembler segment exhibited the characteristic reduction in myelin and in axonal caliber associated with the Trembler phenotype (88,225,226). The spatially restricted effects on both myelination and axonal caliber indicated that the genetic lesion was associated with the Trembler Schwann cells and suggested that an interaction between axons and Schwann cells might alter the shape and function of the underlying axons. Since axonal diameter depends largely on the cytoskeleton and slow axonal transport, we compared the properties of slow transport in the sciatic nerve of control and Trembler mice (231).

Slow transport in sciatic nerve of normal mice exhibited rates for SCa and SCb that were similar to those previously measured in rat. However, overall slow transport in Trembler mouse sciatic nerve was significantly slower than that in normal mice. In Trembler, the rate of neurofilament proteins was significantly slower (1.15 mm/d as compared to 1.38 mm/d in the control). Most proteins in SCb were also transported more slowly in Trembler than control: including actin and calmodulin (2.29 mm/d as compared to 2.73 mm/d in control) as well as spectrin (2.01 mm/d as compared to 2.54 mm/d in control). In contrast, the average rate of transport for tubulin was increased with a rate of 1.73 mm/d for Trembler as compared to 1.56 mm/d in the control mice.

The importance of slow axonal transport in regeneration is indicated by the correlation between rates for regeneration and for SCb (232,233). Regeneration of motor axons in Trembler mice was evaluated to determine whether regeneration was changed by the disruption of Schwann cell/axon interactions (231). The rate of regeneration was significantly slower in Trembler (1.7 mm/d) than control motor axons (2.29 mm/d). Decreases in SCb rates in Trembler nerves correlated well with observed decreases in the rate of regeneration in Trembler. Motor axons in Trembler sciatic nerve regenerated 15–25% more slowly than in controls, comparable to the decreases (16–21%) seen in Trembler SCb rates.

Despite the decrease in overall rate, the elongation of fibers during regeneration began sooner in Trembler (1.6 d) than in control nerves (2.5 d). By contrast, the initial delay in elongation of fibers in Trembler is 35–43% shorter than in a normal mouse. The shorter delay before elongation of neurites begins in Trembler implies that these demyelinated axons are already primed and ready for growth to begin. Changes in both the time of initial delay and rates of regeneration have been previously described, but not in this combination. When a conditioning lesion is administered before the test lesion, normal regeneration starts after a shorter delay, but then proceeds at a faster rate (234–237). Reductions in the delay before initiation of the elongation phase of regeneration following a conditioning lesion have been attributed to a priming of the neuron. The conditioning procedure induces a reorganization in the neuron with respect to expression of neuronal proteins and to cytoskeletal organization in the axon (52). The effect is presumed to result from alterations in the trophic signals moving retrogradely back to the cell body. This has the net result of putting the nerve into a "regeneration" mode. Nerve function and synthetic activity are redirected toward elongation and formation of new axons. The reorganization of neuronal protein synthesis due to a conditioning lesion persists for several weeks. Associated increases in the rate of SCb and increases in the amount of tubulin moving with SCb persist until synaptogenesis and remyelination of the new fibers. As a result, when the nerve is subjected to a second lesion during that period, there is no need to go through the reorganization process and regeneration starts with minimal delay.

Shorter delays in regeneration and increases in the fraction of SCb tubulin imply that Trembler nerves never attain a state of full maturity. The machinery for neurite elongation is ready to be used without delay, so Trembler nerves are perpetually in a modified "regeneration" mode. Myelination apparently "matures" the underlying axon and reduces plasticity of the fiber. The situation is likely to be more complex, because of the slower rates of axonal elongation during regeneration and slow axonal transport in Trembler. Factors that control the rates of slow transport in the axon are not primed to increase transport and regeneration rates in Trembler as they are in the conditioning lesion paradigm. The separation of these two axonal parameters in Trembler suggests that distinct regulatory pathways exist that are subject to independent modulation by experimental manipulations.

The cytoskeletal organization in Trembler axons was also significantly altered (88,226,229,231). The most notable change was in the neurofilaments. While the average cross-sectional area of axons in the Trembler is less than in control nerves, the density of neurofilaments was increased by a factor of 2 (from 168 ± 28 NF/μm^2 to 398 ± 51 NF/μm^2 in Trembler). Since the amount of neurofilament protein does not change, the ultrastructural changes seen in Trembler suggest that biochemical properties of the axonal cytoskeleton might also be affected. Quantitative immunoblots with antibodies that distinguish between phosphorylated and nonphosphorylated neurofilaments demonstrated a biochemical change in Trembler axons. Neurofilaments are highly phosphorylated in normal axons (83). While the total amount of neurofilament protein was comparable in Trembler and normal mice, neurofilaments in Trembler were enriched in dephosphorylated epitopes and reduced in the highly phosphorylated forms (88). This reduced phosphorylation of NFH and NFM permits the neurofilaments in Trembler axons to be packed more densely (88,226).

When segments of Trembler nerve are grafted into normal nerve, rates of slow axonal transport remain normal in proximal portions of the nerve with normal myelination. When the transported materials enter the Trembler segment, axonal transport of neurofilaments is significantly slowed (88,226). In contrast, when a normal sciatic nerve segment is grafted into a normal mouse, there are no changes in slow axonal transport rates upon entering the grafted segment. As axons enter the Trembler graft segment, axonal neurofilaments also become more densely packed and dephosphorylated epitopes increase. Neurofilament packing densities in Trembler graft segments are indistinguishable from Trembler nerves while densities in proximal segments are the same as in intact normal nerves. Similarly, the phosphorylation patterns are normal in proximal segments and identical with Trembler in the Trembler graft segments (88).

Although the genetic lesion in Trembler appears associated with Schwann cells rather than neurons, a variety of axonal properties are altered. Many of these properties are related to neuronal growth. Rates for slow axonal transport and regeneration, organization of axonal cytoskeletal elements, and the phosphorylation of neurofilaments were all affected in axons surrounded by Trembler Schwann cells. Disruption of myelination by Schwann cells locally modifies fundamental properties of the neuron, producing quantitative and qualitative changes in both axonal dynamics and structure. The ability of Schwann cells to modulate axonal characteristics indicates that glia/axon interactions may play an important role in regulating axonal shape and function. While the specific pathway for transmission of information between Schwann cell and axon has yet to be identified, the implications for axonal regeneration are profound.

A simple model can be proposed that would explain the effects of Schwann cell-neuron interactions on axonal dynamics (see Fig. 1). Myelination would specifically inhibit an axonal phosphatase or activate an axonal kinase in those regions of an axon surrounded by myelin. The resulting changes in neurofilament phosphorylation produce changes in the packing density of neurofilaments and axonal caliber. At the same time, rates for both slow axonal transport and regeneration are affected, leading to a reduction in axonal plasticity and its potential for regeneration. Such a model predicts that the phosphorylation state of axonal proteins in myelinated axons is modulated by receptor-mediated second messenger systems activated during the cell-cell interactions between myelin and axolemma. One promising direction for future research is identification of the components for this putative receptor-mediated system. Once determined, pharmacological manipulations of this pathway in a nerve may be useful for facilitating axonal regeneration.

A second intriguing possibility is suggested by the structure of nodes of Ranvier in the PNS. Beginning in the paranodal regions where compact myelin is lost, the diameter of the axon is dramatically reduced and the packing density of neurofilaments is increased in the node (238). The characteristic architecture of a PNS node suggests that interruption of Schwann cell myelination even for the short distance corresponding to a node of Ranvier may change the phosphorylation state of axonal neurofilaments. Since phosphatases and kinases generally have multiple substrates (239, 240), the phosphatase/kinase system modulated by myelination may change the phosphorylation state of proteins other than neurofilaments at a node of Ranvier as well. Given the example of synapsin targeting synaptic vesicles to the presynaptic terminal, other phosphoproteins may function to target different classes of membrane bounded organelles to other functional domains in the neuron.

Sodium channels are enriched in the the node of Ranvier and potassium channels are preferentially in the internodal membrane. This must be accomplished by a targeting mechanism, because the lateral movement of membrane proteins in the axonal plasmalemma appears to be limited (244). If a dephosphorylated targeting protein for sodium channel carrier vesicles serves as a nodal equivalent to synapsin,

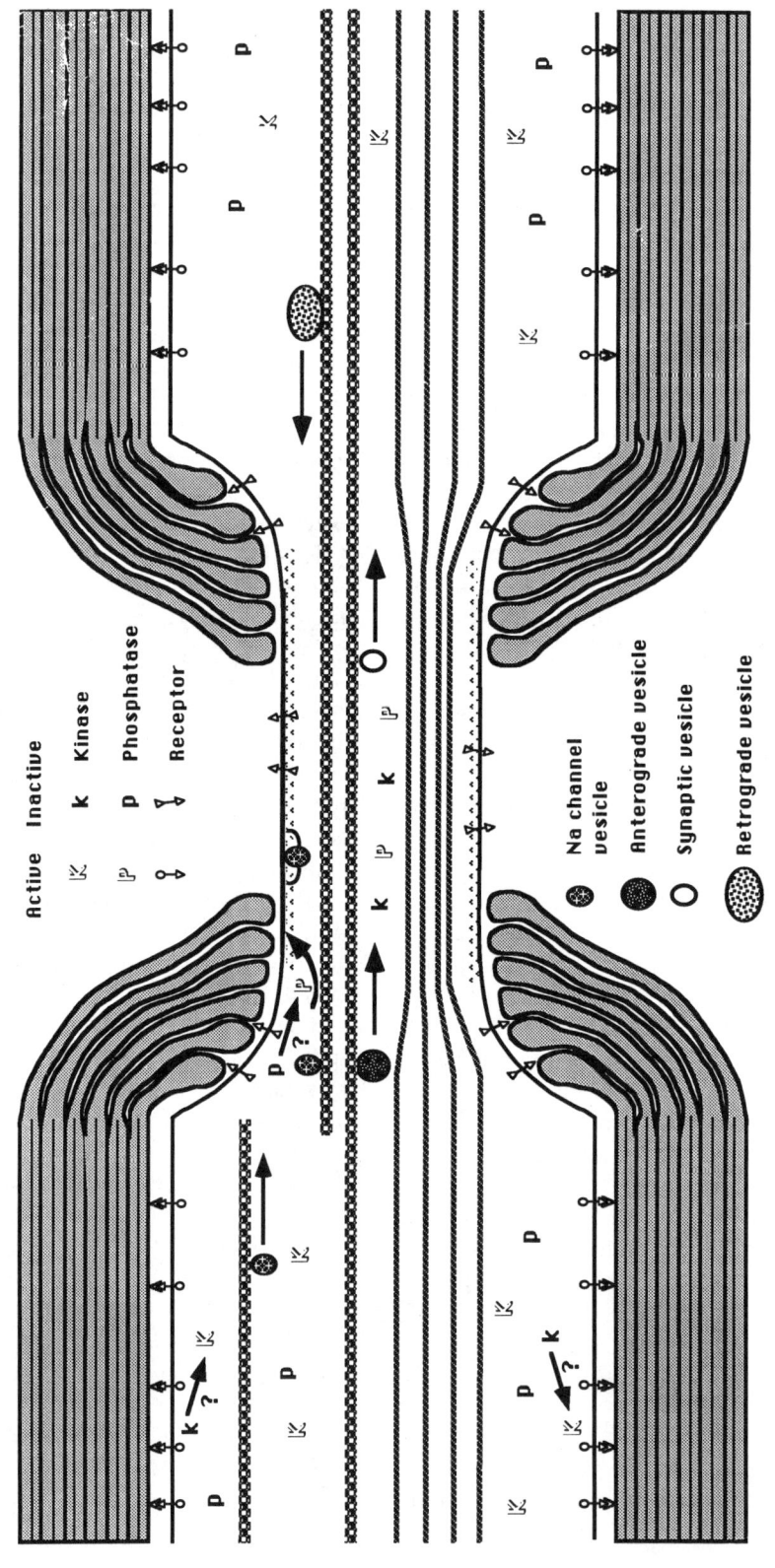

then a gap in myelination would lead to dephosphorylation and binding of vesicles containing sodium channels (see Fig. 1). This would lead to insertion of sodium channels only in regions of the axolemma free of myelin, at a node of Ranvier, or all along an unmyelinated axon. If this model proves to be correct, then myelinating Schwann cells can be said to shape the functional architecture of an axon and will play a critical role in regulating axonal dynamics. Experiments are currently underway to test the predictions of this model.

The effects of myelinating Schwann cells on axonal parameters related to regeneration raises questions about the effects of oligodendrocytes on CNS axons. Preliminary studies in the CNS using the Shiverer mutant and a Shiverer transgenic model (245, and unpublished observations of Brady,

---

FIG. 1. Axonal dynamics at the node of Ranvier in a myelinated axon from the PNS. Axons are in a constant flux with many different and concurrent dynamic processes. This diagram illustrates a few of the many dynamic events occurring in an intact myelinated axon from the PNS at steady state. For successful regeneration after a lesion, additional mechanisms must be triggered to induce formation of a growth cone and to reorganize the local axonal cytoskeleton for neurite elongation.

Axonal transport moves both cytoskeletal structures and membrane bounded organelles from cell body toward the periphery (from right to left in this diagram). At the same time, some membrane bounded organelles return to the cell body by retrograde transport (retrograde vesicle). Membrane bounded organelles are moved along microtubules to motor proteins such as the kinesins (34). Each class of organelles must be directed to the correct functional domain of the neuron. Synaptic vesicles must continue until reaching a presynaptic terminal where they can participate in synaptic transmission. In contrast, other membrane organelles must be targeted specifically to axonal domains. For example, sodium channels must be concentrated at nodes of Ranvier for saltatory conduction to occur.

Examples of cytoskeletal transport illustrated here include microtubules (rods in the upper half of the axon) and neurofilaments (bundle of rope-like rods in the lower half of the axon) representing the cytoskeleton. They move only in the anterograde direction as discrete elements and are degraded in the distal regions of an axon. Although they presumably interact with each other transiently during transport, the distribution of these structures in axonal cross-sections suggests that they move independent of one another (90). In axonal segments without compact myelin, such as the node of Ranvier or following focal demyelination, there appears to be a net dephosphorylation of the neurofilament sidearms which allows the neurofilaments to become more densely packed (88). Other changes may occur locally in the axon as a result of gaps in the compact myelin. The interaction of compact myelin with the axolemma is thought to activate a receptor mediated second messenger in the axon which alters the balance between a kinase (K indicates an active kinase; k is an inactive kinase) and a phosphatase (P indicates an active phosphatase; p is an inactive phosphatase) activity (88).

Since kinases and phosphatases typically have multiple substrates (239,240), this observation suggests a mechanism for targeting membrane bounded organelles to a specific axonal domain. Changes in the phosphorylation of cytoplasmic and/or membrane proteins may change the affinities of crosslinking proteins. Studies on the action of synapsin I in squid axoplasm (207) indicate that dephosphorylated synapsin can apparently crosslink synaptic vesicles to an actin microfilament matrix. When a synaptic vesicle encounters the dephosphorylated synapsin and actin-rich matrix of a presynaptic terminal, the vesicle is trapped at the terminal by inhibition of further axonal transport, effectively targeting the synaptic vesicle to a presynaptic terminal. A similar mechanism may act in other contexts. For example, if an analogous vesicle-binding protein is present at nodes of Ranvier in a high affinity state (i.e., dephosphorylated), transport vesicles for nodal sodium channels (Na channel vesicle) which contain appropriate binding sites could specifically interact. When the Na channel vesicle encounters such a dephosphorylated crosslinker protein at a node of Ranvier, the Na channel transport vesicle is effectively targeted to the nodal membrane. While no direct evidence exists for such a mechanism, such a model is consistent with known characteristics of axonal dynamics.

de Waegh, Readhead, and Hood) indicate that myelinating cells alter properties of the axon in the CNS as well, but the effects are not the same as those seen in the PNS. In slow axonal transport within the Shiverer mouse optic nerve, neurofilaments were found to move faster in Shiverer nerves (approximately 0.27 mm/day) than in control nerves (0.17 mm/day) (245). Interestingly, the rate of SCb transport is also increased by approximately 20–25%. The genetic lesion in Shiverer has been identified as a deletion in the myelin basic protein gene, which has been cloned and sequenced (246,247). This made feasible the generation of transgenic Shiverer mice in which the myelin basic protein gene was replaced (248). These transgenic Shiverer mice partially recover their ability to myelinate CNS axons, although the thickness of the myelin sheath is only 30–35% of that in the normal mouse. When slow axonal transport is analyzed in the optic nerve of transgenic Shiverer mice, the rates of both SCa and SCb have returned to normal. Studies are currently underway to complete the characterization of axonal parameters in CNS axons of Shiverer and transgenic Shiverer mice. However, these preliminary observations already document a specific physiological difference between axons in a CNS environment and those in the PNS.

A variety of neuronal parameters are specifically affected by the glial microenvironment in the PNS. There are clear differences in the molecular response of axonal elements to PNS and CNS glial environments. Characteristic changes in slow axonal transport, cytoskeletal organization, and neurofilament phosphorylation have been evaluated in Trembler and/or Shiverer mice. These same parameters are already known to be important determinants of plasticity and regeneration in nerve fibers. At present, we do not know the regulatory pathway by which demyelination of axons in the Trembler mutant affects cytoskeletal organization, neurofilament phosphorylation, or regeneration, but further studies should illuminate basic modes of regulating axonal growth and regeneration at the molecular level. The use of a genetic approach in the form of these two mutant mice strains is particularly powerful, because they present genetic disruptions of specific cell-cell interactions without the many confounding pathologies that result from experimental manipulation using surgical or pharmacological approaches.

CONCLUSIONS AND SUMMARY

Many of the neuronal constituents important in growth and regeneration have now been identified. Cytoskeletal structures and membrane bounded organelles establish the functional architecture of the axon, while regulatory pathways serve to modulate these elements in response to the local environment. Enough molecular motors have been identified to move materials from their site of synthesis to the locations needed, but many questions remain about the targeting and sorting of transported materials. The interaction between neurons and glial cells in general, and the myelinating glia in particular, represents a complex relationship that affects many physiologically important aspects of the nervous system. While the importance of axonal surroundings to regeneration is well documented, relatively little has been known about the cellular and molecular responses of neurons to different glial microenvironments of the CNS and PNS. The changes noted in the axonal cytoskeleton following demyelination constitute a specific molecular response of the axon to its environment. Continued exploration of the pathways for regulating axonal structures and the molecular bases of axonal transport will provide the basis for understanding the dynamics of the nervous system. Description of glial modulation of the functional architecture of axons is the first step to formulation of a synthesis which will bring together the various pieces of axonal dynamics as a physiological entity.

ACKNOWLEDGMENTS

This work was supported in part by grants from the National Institutes of Health (NS23320 and NS23868) and by a grant from the Welch Foundation.

REFERENCES

1. Aguayo A, David S, Gray G. Influence of the glial environment on the elongation of axons after injury: transplantation studies in adult rodents. *J Exp Biol* 1981; 95: 231–240.
2. Benley M, Aguayo A. Extensive elongation of axons from rat brain into peripheral nerve graft. *Nature* 1982; 296: 150–152.
3. Richardson PM, McGuinness UM, Aguayo AJ. Axons from CNS neurones regenerate into PNS grafts. *Nature* 1980; 284: 264–265.
4. Vidal-Sanz M, Bray G, Villegas-Perez M, Thanos S, Aguayo A. Axonal regeneration and synapse formation in the superior colliculus by retinal ganglion cells in the adult rat. *J Neurosci* 1987; 7: 2894–2909.
5. Caroni P, Schwab M. Two membrane protein fractions from rat central myelin with inhibitory properties for neurite growth and fibroblast spreading. *J Cell Biol* 1988a; 106: 1281–1288.
6. Savio T, Schwab M. Rat CNS white matter, but not gray matter, is nonpermissive for neuronal cell adhesion and fiber outgrowth. *J Neurosci* 1989; 9: 1126–1133.
7. Schnell L, Schwab M. Axonal regeneration in the rat spinal cord produced by an antibody against myelin associated neurite growth inhibitors. *Nature* 1990; 343: 269–272.
8. Lasek RJ, Brady ST. The axon: a prototype for studying expressional cytoplasm. *Cold Spring Harbor Symp Quant Biol* 1982; XLVI: 113–124.
9. Garner CC, Tucker R, Matus A. Selective localization of messenger RNA for cytoskeletal protein MAP2 in dendrites. *Nature* 1988; 336: 674–677.
10. Giuditta A, Dettbarn WD, Brzin M. Protein synthesis in the isolated giant axon of the squid. *Proc Natl Acad Sci USA* 1968; 59: 1286–1287.
11. Giuditta A, Metafora S, Felsami A, Del Rio A. Factors of protein synthesis in the axoplasm of squid giant axons. *J Neurochem* 1977; 28: 1393–1395.
12. Koenig E. Synthetic mechanisms in the axon: IV. *In vitro* incorporation of ^3H precursors into axonal protein and RNA. *J Neurochem* 1967; 14: 437–446.
13. Black MM, Lasek R. The presence of transfer RNA in the axoplasm of the squid giant axon. *J Neurobiol* 1977; 8: 229–237.
14. Ingoglia NA, Chakraborty G, Shyne-Athwal S. Posttranslational protein modifications by amino acids are critical reactions in nerve regeneration. In: Smith RS, Bisby M, eds. *Axonal transport.* New York: Alan R. Liss, Inc.; 1987: 435–457. (Chan-Palay V, Palay SL, eds; *Neurology and Neurobiology;* vol 25).
15. Peters A, Palay SL, Webster HD. *The fine structure of the nervous system: neurons and their supporting cells.* New York: Oxford University Press; 1991.
16. Steward O, Fass B. Polyribosomes associated with dendritic spines in the denervated dentate gyrus: evidence for local regulation of protein synthesis during reinnervation. *Prog Brain Res* 1983; 58: 131–136.
17. Lasek RJ, Tytell MA. Macromolecular transfer from glia to the axon. *J Exp Biol* 1981; 95: 153–165.
18. Lasek RJ, Gainer H, Przybylski R. Transfer of newly synthesized proteins from Schwann cells to the squid giant axon. *Proc Natl Acad Sci USA* 1974; 71: 1188–1192.
19. Lasek RJ, Gainer H, Barker J. Cell to cell transfer of glial proteins to the squid giant axon: the glial-neuron protein transfer hypothesis. *J Cell Biol* 1977; 74: 501–523.
20. Tytell M, Greenberg SG, Lasek RJ. Heat shock-like protein is transferred from glia to axon. *Brain Res* 1986; 363: 161–164.
21. Lindquist SA. The heatshock response. *Annu Rev Biochem* 1986; 55: 1151–1191.
22. Pelham H. Speculations on the functions of the major heat shock and glucose-regulated proteins. *Cell* 1986; 46: 5–9.
23. Greenberg SG, Lasek RJ. Comparison of labelled heat-shock proteins in neuronal and non-neuronal cells of *Aplysia californica*. *J Neurosci* 1985; 5: 1239–1245.
24. Davis L, Burger B, Banker GB, Steward O. Dendritic transport: quantitative analysis of the time course of somatodendritic transport of recently synthesized RNA. *J Neurosci* 1990; 10: 3056–3068.
25. Steward O, Davis L, Reeves TM, Banker G. Microcompartmentation of the protein synthetic machinery of neurons: polyribosome localization under postsynaptic sites. In: Smith RS, Bisby M, eds. *Axonal transport.* *Neurol Neurobiol* 1987; 25: 521–544.
26. Dahlström A, Heiwall P-O. Intraaxonal transport of transmitters in mammalian neurons. *J Neural Transm [Suppl]* 1975; 12: 97–114.
27. Dahlström A, Kling-Peterson T, Bööj S, Lundmark K, Larsson P-A. Quantification of axon ally transported material using cytofluorometric scanning. *J Microsc* 1989; 155: 61–80.
28. Lombet A, Laduron P, Mourrem C, Jacomet Y, Lazdunsky M. Axonal transport of the voltage dependent Na^+ channel protein identified by its tetrodotoxin binding site in rat sciatic nerves. *Brain Res* 1985; 345: 153–158.
29. Laduron PM. Axonal transport of presynaptic receptors. In: Smith RS, Bisby MA, eds. *Axonal transport.* New York: Alan R. Liss, Inc.; 1987: 347–363.
30. Stone GC, Hammerschlag R. Molecular mech-

anisms involved in sorting of fast-transported proteins. In: Smith RS, Bisby M., eds. *Axonal transport*. New York: Alan R. Liss, Inc.; 1987: 15–36.
31. Brady ST. Cytotypic specializations of the neuronal cytoskeleton and cytomatrix: implications for neuronal growth and regeneration. In: Haber B, Gorio A, de Vellis J, Perez-Polo JR, eds. *Cellular and molecular aspects of neural development and regeneration*. New York: Springer-Verlag: 1988: 311–322.
32. Friede RL, Samorajski T. Axon caliber related to neurofilaments and microtubules in sciatic nerve fibers of rats and mice. *Anat Rec* 1970; 167: 379–388.
33. Lasek RJ. Studying the intrinsic determinants of neuronal form and function. In: Lasek RJ, Black MM, eds. *Intrinsic determinants of neuronal form and function*. New York: Alan R. Liss, Inc.; 1988: 1–60.
34. Brady ST. Molecular motors in the nervous system. *Neuron* 1991; 7: 521–533.
35. Sullivan KF. Structure and utilization of tubulin isotypes. *Annu Rev Cell Biol* 1988; 4: 687–716.
36. Hoffman P, Cleveland D. Neurofilament and tubulin gene expression recapitulates the developmental program during axonal regeneration: induction of a specific β-tubulin isotype *Proc Natl Acad Sci USA* 1988; 85: 4530–4533.
37. Miller FD, Naus CCG, Durand M, Bloom FE, Milner RJ. Isotypes of α-tubulin are differentially regulated during neuronal maturation. *J Cell Biol* 1987; 105: 3065–3073.
38. Black MM, Keyser P. Acetylation of α-tubulin in cultured neurons and the induction of α-tubulin acetylation in PC12 cells by treatment with nerve growth factor. *J Neurosci* 1987; 7: 1833–1842.25.
39. Raybin D, Flavin M. Modification of tubulin by tyrosylation in cells and extracts and its effects on assembly *in vitro*. *J Cell Biol* 1977; 73: 492–504.
40. Gard DL, Kirschner M. A polymer dependent increase in phosphorylation of β-tubulin accompanies differentiation of a mouse neuroblastoma cell line. *J Cell Biol* 1985; 100: 764–774.
41. Baas PW, Black MM. Individual microtubules in the axon consist of domains that differ in both composition and stability. *J Cell Biol* 1990; 111: 495–509.
42. Baas PW, Slaughter T, Brown A, Black MM. Microtubule dynamics in axons and dendrites. *J Neurosci Res* 1991; 30: 134–153.
43. Black MM, Baas PW, Humphries S. Dynamics of α-tubulin deacetylation in intact neurons. *J Neurosci* 1989; 9: 358–368.
44. Khawaja S, Gunderson GG, Bulinski JC. Enhanced stability of microtubules enriched in detyrosinated tubulin is not a direct function of detyrosination level. *J Cell Biol* 1988; 106: 141–150.
45. Maruta H, Greer K, Rosenbaum JL. The acetylation of alpha-tubulin and its relationship to the assembly and disassembly of microtubules *J Cell Biol* 1986; 103: 571–579.
46. Brady ST, Tytell M, Lasek RJ. Axonal tubulin and axonal microtubules: biochemical evidence for cold stability. *J Cell Biol* 1984; 99: 1716–1724.
47. Sahenk Z, Brady ST. Axonal tubulin and axonal microtubules: morphologic evidence for stable regions on axonal microtubules. *Cell Motil Cytoskel* 1987; 8: 155–164.
48. Brady ST, Black MM. Axonal transport of microtubule proteins: cytotypic variation of tubulin and MAPs in neurons. *Ann NY Acad Sci* 1986; 466: 199–217.
49. Miller FD, Tetzlaff W, Bisby MA, Fawcett JW, Milner RJ. Rapid induction of the major embryonic α-tubulin mRNA Tα1, during nerve regeneration in adult rats. *J Neurosci* 1989; 9: 1452–1463.
50. Wong J, Oblinger M. A comparison of peripheral and central axotomy effects on neurofilament and tubulin gene expression in rat dorsal root ganglion neurons. *J Neurosci* 1990; 10: 2215–2223.
51. Hoffman P, Lasek RJ. Axonal transport of the cytoskeleton in regenerating motor neurons: consistency and changes. *Brain Res* 1980; 202: 317–333.
52. McQuarrie I, Lasek RJ. Transport of cytoskeletal elements from parent axons into regenerating daughter axons. *J Neurosci* 1989; 9: 436–446.
53. Oblinger M, Lasek RJ. Axotomy induced alterations in the synthesis and transport of neurofilaments and microtubules in dorsal root ganglion cells. *J Neurosci* 1988; 8: 1747–1758.
54. Matus A. Microtubule-associated proteins: their potential role in determining neuronal morphology. *Annu Rev Neurosci* 1988; 11: 29–44.
55. Olmsted J. Microtubule associated proteins. *Annu Rev Cell Biol* 1986; 2: 421–457.
56. Bernhardt R, Matus A. Light and electron microscopic studies of the distribution of microtubule associated protein 2 in rat brain: a difference between dendritic and axonal cytoskeletons. *J Comp Neurol* 1984; 226: 203–221.
57. Caceres A, Binder LI, Payne MR, Bender P, Rebhun L, Steward O. Differential subcellular localization of tubulin and microtubule associated protein MAP2 in brain tissue as revealed by immunocytochemistry with monoclonal hybridoma antibodies. *J Neurosci* 1983b; 4: 394–410.
58. Caceres A, Kosik KS. Inhibition of neurite polarity by tau antisense oligonucleotides in primary cerebellar neurons. *Nature* 1990; 343: 461–462.
59. de Camilli P, Miller PE, Navone F, Theurkauf NE, Vallee RB. Distribution of microtubule-associated protein-2 in the nervous system of the rat studied by immunofluorescence. *Neuroscience* 11: 1984; 11: 819–846.
60. Papasozomenos SC, Binder LI. Phosphoryla-

tion determined two distinct species of tau in the central nervous system. *Cell Motil Cytoskel* 1987; 8: 210–226.
61. Margolis R, Rauch C. Characterization of rat brain crude extract microtubule assembly: correction of cold stability with the phosphorylation of a microtubule associated 64K protein. *Biochemistry* 1981; 20: 4451–4458.
62. Tanaka EM, Kirschner M. Microtubule behavior in the growth cones of living neurons during axon elongation. *J Cell Biol* 1991; 115: 345–364.
63. Weiss DG, Langford GM, Seitz-Tutter D, Keiler F. Dynamic instability and motile events of native microtubules from squid axoplasm. *Cell Motil Cytoskel* 1988; 10: 285–295.
64. Drubin D, Kirschner M. Tau protein function in living cells. *J Cell Biol* 1986; 103: 2739–2746.
65. Kanai Y, Takemura R, Oshima T, Mori H, Ihara Y, Yanigasawa M, Masaki T, Hirokawa N. Expression of multiple tau isoforms and microtubule bundle formation in fibroblasts transfected with a single tau cDNA. *J Cell Biol* 1989; 109: 1173–1184.
66. Baas PW, Pienkowski TP, Kosik KS. Processes induced by tau expression in Sf9 cells have an axon-like microtubule organization. *J Cell Biol* 1991; 115: 1333–1344.
67. Francon J, Lennon A, Fellous A, Maveck A, Pierre M, Nunez J. Heterogeneity of microtubule associated proteins and brain development. *Eur J Biochem* 1982; 129: 465–471.
68. Kosik KS, Orecchio LD, Bekalis S, Neve RL. Developmentally regulated expression of specific tau sequences. *Neuron* 1989; 2: 1389–1397.
69. Nunez J. Differential expression of microtubule components during brain development. *Dev Neurosci* 1986; 8: 125–141.
70. Tucker RP. The roles of microtubule associated proteins in brain morphogenesis: a review. *Brain Res Rev* 1990; 15: 101–120.
71. Oblinger MM, Argasinski A, Wong J, Kosik KS. Tau gene expression in DRG neurons during development and regeneration. *J Neurosci* 1991; 11: 2453–2459.
72. Steinert PM, Roop DR. Molecular and cellular biology of intermediate filaments. *Annu Rev Biochem* 1988; 57: 593–625.
73. Hoffman P, Lasek RJ. The slow component of axonal transport identification of major structural polypeptides of the axon and their generality among mammalian neurons. *J Cell Biol* 1975; 66: 351–366.
74. Lasek RJ, Hoffman P. The neuronal cytoskeleton, axonal transport, and axonal growth. In Goldman R, Pollard T, Rosenbaum J, eds. *Cell motility*. Cold Spring Harbor Conference on Cell Proliferation, 1976; 3: 1021–1049.
75. Czosnek H, Soifer D, Wisniewski H. Studies on the biosynthesis of neurofilament protein. *J Cell Biol* 1980; 85: 726–734.
76. Lee VM-Y, Carden M, Schlaepfer W. Structural similarities and differences between neurofilament proteins from five different species as revealed using monoclonal antibodies. *J Neurosci* 1986; 6: 2179–2186.
77. Jones S, Williams R. Phosphate content of mammalian neurofilaments *J Biol Chem* 1982; 257: 9902–9905.
78. Julien JP, Mushynski WE. Multiple phosphorylation sites in mammalian neurofilament polypeptides. *J Biol Chem* 1982; 257: 10467–10470.
79. Hoffman P, Griffin J, Price D. Control of axonal caliber by neurofilament transport. *J Cell Biol* 1984; 99: 705–714.
80. Hoffman P, Griffin J, Gold B, Price D. Slowing of neurofilaments transport and the radial growth of developing nerve fibers. *J Neurosci* 1985a; 5: 2920–2929.
81. Hoffman PN, Cleveland D, Griffin J, Landes P, Cowan N, Price D. Neurofilament gene expression: a major determinant of axonal caliber. *Proc Natl Acad Sci USA* 1987; 84: 3472–3476.
82. Szaro BG, Whitnall MH, Gainer H. Phosphorylation dependent epitopes on neurofilament proteins and neurofilament densities differ in axons in the corticospinal and primary sensory dorsal tracts in the rat spinal cord. *J Comp Neurol* 1990; 302: 220–235.
83. Lee VM-Y, Otvos L, Carden M, Hollosi M, Dietzschold B, Lazzarini R. Identification of the major multiphosphorylation site in mammalian neurofilaments. *Proc Natl Acad Sci USA* 1988; 85: 1998–2002.
84. Lee VM-Y, Otvos L, Schmidt MS, Trojanowski J. Alzheimer's disease tangles share immunological similarities with multiphosphorylation repeats in the two large neurofilament proteins *Proc Natl Acad Sci USA* 1988; 85: 7384–7388.
85. Hirokawa N, Glicksman M, Willard M. Organization of mammalian neurofilament polypeptides within the neuronal cytoskeleton. *J Cell Biol* 1984; 98: 1523–1536.
86. Hisanaga S-H, Hirokawa N. Structure of the the peripheral domains of neurofilaments revealed by low angle rotary shadowing. *J Mol Biol* 1988; 202: 297–305.
87. Liem R, Hutchinson S. Purification of the neurofilament triplet: filament assembly from the 70,000 dalton subunit. *Biochemistry* 1982; 21: 3221–3226.
88. de Waegh SM, Lee VM-Y, Brady ST. Modulation of neurofilament phosphorylation, axonal caliber, and slow axonal transport by myelinating schwann cells. *Cell* 1982; (in press).
89. Brown A, Lasek RJ. The cytoskeleton of the squid giant axon. In: Gilbert DL, Adelman WJ, Jr., Arnold JM, eds. *Squid as experimental animals*. New York: Plenum Publishing Corp.; 1990: 235–302.
90. Price R, Paggi P, Lasek RJ, Katz M. Neurofilaments are spaced randomly in the radial dimension of axons. *J Neurocytol* 1988; 17: 55–62.
91. Carden MJ, Trojanowski JQ, Schlaepfer WW, Lee VM-Y. Two stage expression of neurofilament polypeptides during rat neurogenesis with

early establishment of adult phosphorylation patterns. *J Neurosci* 1987; 7: 3489–3504.
92. Willard M, Simon C. Modulations in neurofilament axonal transport during development of rabbit retinal ganglion cells. *Cell* 1983; 35: 551–559.
93. Oblinger MM, Szumlas RA, Wong J, Liuzzi FJ. Changes in cytoskeletal gene expression affect the composition of regenerating axonal sprouts elaborated by dorsal root ganglion neurons *in vivo*. *J Neurosci* 1989; 9: 2645–2653.
94. Wong J, Oblinger M. Changes in neurofilament gene expression occurs after axotomy of dorsal root ganglion neurons: an in situ hybridization study. *Metab Brain Dis* 1987; 2: 291–303.
95. Mickucki SA, Oblinger MM. Corticospinal neurons exhibit a novel pattern of cytoskeletal gene expression after injury. *J Neurosci Res* 1991; 30: 213–225.
96. Hoffman P, Thompson G, Griffin J, Price D. Changes in neurofilament transport coincide temporally with alternations in the caliber of axons in regenerating motor fibers. *J Cell Biol* 1985; 101: 1332–1340.
97. Leonard DGB, Gorham JD, Cole P, Greene LA, Ziff EB. A nerve growth factor-regulated messenger RNA encodes a new intermediate filament protein. *J Cell Biol* 1988; 106: 181–193.
98. Parysek LM, Chisolm RL, Ley CA, Goldman RD. A type III intermediate filament gene is expressed in mature neurons. *Neuron* 1988; 1: 395–401.
99. Portier MM, de Nechaud B, Gros F. Peripherin: a new member of the intermediate filament protein family. *Dev Neurosci* 1984; 6: 335–344.
100. Chiu F-C, Barnes EA, Das K, Haley J, Socolow P, Macaluso FP, Fant J. Characterization of a novel 66 kD subunit of mammalian neurofilaments. *Neuron* 1989; 2: 1435–1445.
101. Escurat M, Djabali K, Gumpel M, Gros F, Portier MM. Differential expression of two neuronal intermediate filament proteins, peripherin and low molecular mass neurofilament protein (NF-L) during the development of the rat. *J Neurosci* 1990; 10: 764–784.
102. Gorham JD, Baker H, Kegler D, Ziff EB. The expression of the neuronal intermediate protein peripherin in the rat embryo. *Dev Brain Res* 1990; 57: 235–248.
103. Parysek LM, Goldman RD. Distribution of a novel 57kDa intermediate filament (IF) protein in the nervous system. *J Neurosci* 1988; 8: 555–563.
104. Troy CM, Brown K, Greene LA, Shelanski ML. Ontogeny of the neuronal intermediate filament protein peripherin in the mouse embryo. *Neuroscience* 1990; 36: 217–237.
105. Galinovic-Schwartz V, Peng D, Chiu FC, Van de Water TR. Temporal pattern of innervation in the developing mouse inner ear: an immunocytochemical study of a 66 kD subunit of mammalian neurofilaments. *J Neurosci Res* 1991; 30: 124–133.
106. Parysek LM, McReynolds MA, Goldman RD, Ley CA. Some neural intermediate filaments contain both peripherin and neurofilament proteins. *J Neurosci Res* 1991; 30: 80–91.
107. Wong J, Oblinger M. Differential regulation of peripherin and neurofilament gene expression in regenerating rat DRG neurons. *J Neurosci Res* 1990; 27: 332–341.
108. Fath K, Lasek RJ. Two classes of actin microfilaments are associated with the inner cytoskeleton of axons. *J Cell Biol* 1987; 107: 613–621.
109. Letourneau PC, Ressler AH. Differences in the organization of actin in the growth cones compared with neurites of cultured neurons from chick embryos. *J Cell Biol* 1983; 97: 963–973.
110. Smith SJ. Neuronal cytomechanics: the actin-based motility of growth cones. *Science* 1988; 242: 708–715.
111. Shaw G, Osborne M, Weber K. Neurofilaments, microtubules, and microfilament-associated proteins in cultured dorsal root ganglion cells. *Eur J Cell Biol* 1981; 24: 20–27.
112. Yamada KM, Spooner BS, Wessells NK. Axon growth: roles of microfilaments and microtubules. *Proc Natl Acad Sci USA* 1970; 66: 1206–1212.
113. Reinsch SS, Mitchison TJ, Kirschner M. Microtubule polymer assembly and transport during axonal elongation. *J Cell Biol* 1991; 115: 365–380.
114. Sabry JH, O'Connor TP, Evans L, Toroian-Raymond A, Kirschner M, Bentley D. Microtubule behavior during guidance of pioneer growth cones *in situ*. *J Cell Biol* 1991; 115: 381–396.
115. Weiss P, Hiscoe H. Experiments in the mechanism of nerve growth. *J Exp Zool* 1948; 107: 315–395.
116. Brady S. Axonal transport methods and applications. In: Boulton A, Baker G, eds. *Neuromethods, general neurochemical techniques.* 1985: 419–476.
117. Hammerschlag R, Brady ST. Cytoskeleton and axonal transport. In: Siegel G, Agranoff BW, Albers RW, Molinoff P, eds. *Basic neurochemistry,* Fourth Edition. New York: Raven Press; 1989: 457–478.
118. Vallee RB, Bloom GS. Mechanisms of fast and slow axonal transport. *Annu Rev Neurosci* 1991; 14: 59–92.
119. Black MM, Lasek RJ. Slow component of axonal transport: two cytoskeletal networks. *J Cell Biol* 1980; 86: 616–623.
120. Brady ST, Lasek RJ. The slow components of axonal transport: movements compositions and organization. In: Weiss D, ed. *Axoplasmic transport.* New York: Springer-Verlag; 1982: 206–217.
121. Garner JA, Lasek RJ. Cohesive axonal transport of the slow component b complex of polypeptides. *J Neurosci* 1982; 2: 1824–1835.
122. Lasek RJ, Garner JA, Brady ST. Axonal transport of the cytoplasmic matrix. *J Cell Biol* 1984; 99: 212–221.
123. Black MM, Lasek RJ. Axonal transport of ac-

tin: slow component b is the principal source of actin for the axon. *Brain Res* 1979; 171: 402–413.
124. McQuarrie I, Brady ST, Lasek RJ. Diversity in the axonal transport of structural proteins: major differences between optic and spinal axons in the rat. *J Neurosci* 1986; 6: 1593–1605.
125. Oblinger MM, Brady ST, McQuarrie IG, Lasek RJ. Differences in the protein composition of the axonally transported cytoskeleton in peripheral and central mammalian neurons. *J Neurosci* 1987; 7: 453–462.
126. Tytell M, Black MM, Garner JA, Lasek RJ. Axonal transport: each of the major rate components consist of distinct macromolecular complexes. *Science* 1981; 214: 179–181.
127. Lasek RJ, Brady ST. The structural hypothesis of axonal transport: two classes of moving elements. In: Weiss D, ed. *Axoplasmic transport.* Berlin: Springer-Verlag; 1982: 397–405.
128. Weisenberg RC, Cianci C. ATP-induced gelation-contraction of microtubules assembled *in vitro. J Cell Biol* 1984; 99: 1527–1533.
129. Black MM, Keyser P, Sobel E. Interval between the synthesis and assembly of cytoskeletal proteins in cultured neurons. *J Neurosci* 1986; 6: 1004–1012.
130. Tytell M, Brady ST, Lasek RJ. Axonal transport of a subclass of tau proteins: evidence for the regional differentiation of microtubules in axons. *Proc Natl Acad Sci USA* 1983; 81: 1570–1574.
131. Nixon RA, Logvinenko KB. Multiple fates of newly synthesized neurofilaments: evidence for a stationary neurofilament network distributed nonuniformly along axons of retinal ganglion cells. *J Cell Biol* 1986; 102: 647–659.
132. Garner JA. Differential turnover of tubulin and neurofilaments in central nervous system neuron terminals. *Brain Res* 1988; 458: 309–318.
133. Paggi P, Lasek RJ. Axonal transport of cytoskeletal proteins in oculomotor axons and their residence times in the axon terminals. *J Neurosci* 1987; 7: 2397–2411.
134. Tashiro T, Kurokawa M, Komiya Y. Two populations of axonally transported tubulin differentiated by their interactions with neurofilaments. *J Neurochem* 1984; 43: 1220–1225.
135. Tashiro T, Komiya Y. Organization of cytoskeletal proteins transported in the axon. In: Smith RS, Bisby MA, eds. *Axonal transport.* New York: Alan R. Liss, Inc.; 1987: 201–221.
136. Grafstein B, Forman DS. Intracellular transport in neurons. *Physiol Rev* 1980; 60: 1167–1283.
137. Brady ST. Basic properties of fast axonal transport and the role of fast axonal transport in axonal growth. In: Elam J, Cancalon P, eds. *Axonal transport in neuronal growth and regeneration.* New York: Plenum Press; 1983: 13–29.
138. Bisby MA. Retrograde axonal transport of endogenous proteins. In: Weiss D, ed. *Axoplasmic transport.* New York: Springer-Verlag; 1982: 193–205.
139. Martz D, Garner JA, Lasek RJ. Protein changes during anterograde to retrograde conversion of axonally transported vesicles. *Brain Res* 1989; 476: 199–203.
140. Stoeckel K, Thoenen H. Retrograde axonal transport of nerve growth factor: specificity and biological importance. *Brain Res* 1975; 85: 337–341.
141. Lycke E, Kristensson K, Svennerholm B, Vahline A, Ziegler R. Uptake and transport of Herpes simplex virus in neurites of rat dorsal root ganglia cells in culture. *J Gen Virol* 1984; 65: 55–64.
142. Heumann R, Korsching S, Bandtlow C, Thoenen H. Changes in nerve growth factor synthesis in nonneuronal cells in response to sciatic nerve transsection. *J Cell Biol* 1987; 104: 1623–1631.
143. Fahim M, Lasek RJ, Brady ST, Hodge A. Identification of the membranous organelles moving in fast axonal transport in squid giant axon: a correlative electron microscopy and video microscopy study. *J Neurocytol* 1985; 14: 689–704.
144. Smith RS. The short term accumulation of axonally transported organelles in the region of localized lesions of single myelinated axons. *J Neurocytol* 1980; 9: 39–65.
145. Tsukita S, Ishikawa H. The movement of membranous organelles in axons: electron microscopic identification of anterogradely and retrogradely transported organelles. *J Cell Biol* 1980; 84: 513–530.
146. Sahenk Z, Lasek RJ. Inhibition of proteolysis blocks anterograde-retrograde conversion of axonally transported vesicles. *Brain Res* 1988; 460: 199–203.
147. Allen RD, Allen NS, Travis JL. Video-enhanced contrast, differential interference contrast (AVEC-DIC) microscopy: a new method capable of analyzing microtubule related movement in the reticulopodial netowork of *Allogromia laticollaris. Cell Motil* 1981; 1: 291–302.
148. Allen RD, Metuzals J, Tasaki I, Brady ST, Gilbert SP. Fast axonal transport in squid giant axon. *Science* 1982; 218: 1127–1129.
149. Bear R, Schmitt FO, Young JZ. Investigations on the protein constituents of nerve axoplasm. *Proc R Soc Lond [Biol]* 1937; 123: 520–529.
150. Lasek RJ. The structure of axoplasm. *Curr Top Membr Transp* 1984; 22: 39–53.
151. Brady ST, Lasek RJ, Allen RD. Fast axonal transport in extruded axoplasm from squid giant axon. *Science* 1982; 218: 1129–1131.
152. Brady ST, Lasek RJ, Allen RD. Video microscopy of fast axonal transport in isolated axoplasm: a new model for study of molecular mechanisms. *Cell Motil* 1985; 5: 81–101.
153. Brady ST. Fast axonal transport in isolated axoplasm from the squid giant axon. In: Smith RS, Bisby MA, eds. *Axonal transport.* New York: Alan R. Liss, Inc.; 1987: 113–137. (Chan-Paley V, Palay SL, eds; *Neurology and Neurobiology,* vol 25).
154. Lasek RJ, Brady ST. AMP-PNP facilitates at-

tachment of transported vesicles to microtubules in axoplasm. *Nature* 1985; 316: 645–647.
155. Brady ST. A novel brain ATPase with properties expected for the fast axonal transport motor. *Nature* 1985; 317: 73–75.
156. Vale RD, Reese TS, Sheetz MS. Identification of a novel force-generating protein, kinesin, involved in microtubule-based motility. *Cell* 1985; 42: 39–50.
157. Allen RD, Weiss DG, Hayden JH, Brown DT, Fujiwake H, Simpson M. Gliding movement of and bidirectional transport along single native microtubules from squid axoplasm: evidence for an active role of microtubules in cytoplasmic transport. *J Cell Biol* 1985; 100: 1736–1752.
158. Kuznetsov SA, Gelfand VI. Bovine brain kinesin is a microtubule-activated ATPase. *Proc Natl Acad Sci USA* 1986; 83: 8530–8534.
159. Bloom GS. Motor proteins for cytoplasmic microtubules. *Curr Opin Cell Biol* 1992; (in press).
160. Amos LA. Kinesin from pig brain studied by electron microscopy. *J Cell Sci* 1987; 87: 105–111.
161. Bloom GS, Wagner MC, Pfister KK, Brady ST. Native structure and physical properties of bovine brain kinesin and identification of the ATP-binding subunit polypeptide. *Biochemistry* 1988; 27: 3409–3416.
162. Kuznetsov SA, Vaisberg EA, Shanina NA, Magretova NA, Chernyak NM, Gelfand VI. The quartenary structure of bovine brain kinesin. *EMBO J* 1988; 7: 353–356.
163. Scholey JM, Heuser J, Yang JT, Goldstein LSB. Identification of globular mechanochemical heads of kinesin. *Nature* 1989; 338: 355–357.
164. Hirokawa N, Pfister KK, Yorifuji H, Wagner MC, Brady ST, Bloom GS. Submolecular domains of bovine brain kinesin identified electron microscopy and monoclonal antibody decoration. *Cell* 1989; 56: 867–878.
165. Hollenbeck PJ. The distribution, abundance, and subcellular localization of kinesin. *J Cell Biol* 1989; 108: 2335–2342.
166. Hollenbeck PJ, Swanson JA. Radial extension of macrophage tubular lysosomes supported by kinesin. *Nature* 1990; 346: 864–866.
167. Leopold PL, McDowall A, Pfister KK, Bloom GS, Brady ST. Association of kinesin with membrane bounded organelles of defined function. *Cell Motil Cytoskel* 1992; (in press).
168. Pfister KK, Wagner MC, Stenoien DS, Brady ST, Bloom GS. Monoclonal antibodies to kinesin heavy and light chains stain vesicle-like structures, but not microtubules, in cultured cells. *J Cell Biol* 1989; 108: 1453–1463.
169. Cyr JC, Pfister KK, Bloom GS, Slaughter C, Brady ST. Molecular genetics of kinesin light chains: generation of isoforms by alternative splicing. *Proc Natl Acad Sci USA* 1991; 88: 10114–10118.
170. Endow SA, Hatsumi M. A multimember kinesin gene family in *Drosophila*. *Proc Natl Acad Sci USA* 1991; 88: 4424–4427.

171. Walker RA, Salmon ED, Endow SA. The *Drosophila claret* segregation protein is a minus-end directed motor molecule. *Nature* 1990; 347: 780–782.
172. Bloom GS, Schoenfeld TA, Vallee RB. Widespread distribution of the major polypeptide component of MAP 1 (microtubule associated protein 1) in the nervous system. *J Cell Biol* 1984; 98: 320–330.
173. Paschal BM, Shpetner HS, Vallee RB. MAP1C is a microtubule-activated ATPase which translocates microtubules in vitro and has dynein-like properties. *J Cell Biol* 1987; 105: 1273–1282.
174. Shpetner HS, Paschal BP, Vallee RB. Characterization of the microtubule-activated ATPase of brain cytoplasmic dynein (MAP1C). *J Cell Biol* 1987; 107: 1001–1009.
175. Paschal BM, Vallee RB. Retrograde transport by the microtubule-associated protein MAP1C. *Nature* 1987; 330: 181–183.
176. Paschal BM, Obar RA, Vallee RB. Interaction of brain cytoplasmic dynein and MAP2 with a common sequence at the C terminus of tubulin. *Nature* 1989; 342: 569–572.
177. Caceres A, Payne MR, Binder LI, Steward O. Immunocytochemical localization of actin and microtubule-associated protein (MAP2) in dendritic spines. *Proc Natl Acad Sci USA* 1983; 80: 1738–1742.
178. Vallee RB, Wall JS, Paschal BM, Shpetner JS. Microtubule associated protein 1C from brain is a two headed cytosolic dynein. *Nature* 1988; 332: 561–563.
179. Lye J, Porter ME, Scholey JM, McIntosh JR. Identification of a microtubule-based cytoplasmic motor in the nematode, *Caenorhabditis elegans*. *Cell* 1987; 51: 309–318.
180. Vallee RB, Shpetner HS. Motor proteins of cytoplasmic microtubules. *Annu Rev Biochem* 1990; 59: 909–932.
181. Vallee RB, Shpetner JS, Paschal BM. The role of dynein in retrograde axonal transport. *Trends Neurosci* 1989; 12: 66–70.
182. Pfarr CM, Coue M, Grissom PM, Hays TS, Porter ME, McIntosh JR. Cytoplasmic dynein is localized to kinetochores during mitosis. *Nature* 1990; 345: 263–265.
183. Steuer ER, Wordeman L, Schroer TA, Sheetz MP. Localization of cytoplasmic dynein to mitotic spindles and kinetochores. *Nature* 1990; 345: 266–268.
184. Lewis SA, Lee MG, Cowan NJ. Five mouse tubulin isotypes and their regulated expression during development. *J Cell Biol* 1985; 101: 852–861.
185. Korn ED, Hammer JA. Myosins of nonmuscle cells. *Annu Rev Biophys Chem* 1988; 17: 23–45.
186. Mercer JA, Seperack PK, Strobel MC, Copeland NG, Jenkins NA. Novel myosin heavy chain encoded by murine *dilute* coat colour locus. *Nature* 1991; 349: 709–713.
187. Spudich JA. In pursuit of myosin function. *Cell Reg* 1989; 1: 1–11.

188. Berl S, Puszkin S, Nicklas WJK. Actomyosin-like protein in brain. *Science* 1973; 179: 441–446.
189. Kuczmarski ER, Rosenbaum JL. Chick brain actin and myosin: Isolation and characterization. *J Cell Biol* 1979; 80: 341–355.
190. Puszkin S, Berl S, Puszkin E, Clarke DD. Actomyosin-like protein isolated from mammalian brain. *Science* 1968; 161: 170–171.
191. Korn ED, Hammer JA. Myosin I. *Curr Opin Cell Biol* 1990; 2: 57–61.
192. Pollard TD, Doberstein SK, Zot HG. Myosin-I. *Annu Rev Physiol* 1991; 53: 653–681.
193. Adams RJ, Pollard T. Binding of myosin 1 to membrane lipids. *Nature* 1989; 340: 566–568.
194. Miyata H, Bowers B, Korn ED. Plasma membrane association of *Acanthamoeba* myosin 1. *J Cell Biol* 1989; 109: 1519–1528.
195. Barylko B, Wagner MC, Reiszes O, Albanesi JP. Mammalian myosin 1: purification and characterization of myosin I from bovine adrenal medulla. *Proc Natl Acad Sci USA* 1992; (in press).
196. Willard M. The identification of two intra-axonally transported polypeptides resembling myosin in some respects in the rabbit visual system. *J Cell Biol* 1977; 75: 1–11.
197. Dotti CG, Simons K. Polarized sorting of viral glycoproteins to the axon and dendrites of hippocampal neurons in culture. *Cell* 1990; 62: 63–72.
198. Garner JA, Mahler HR. Biogenesis of presynaptic terminal proteins. *J Neurochem* 1987; 49: 905–915.
199. Roots B. Neurofilament accumulation induced in synapses by leupeptin. *Science* 1983; 221: 971–972.
200. Okabe S, Hirokawa N. Rapid turnover of microtubule associated protein MAP2 in the axon revealed by microinjection of biotinylated MAP2 into cultured neurons. *Proc Natl Acad Sci USA* 1989; 86: 4127–4131.
201. de Camilli P, Benfenati F, Valtorta F, Greengard P. The synapsins. *Annu Rev Cell Biol* 1990; 6: 433–460.
202. Nestler EJ, Greengard P. Synapsin I: a review of its distribution and biological regulation. *Prog Brain Res* 1986; 69: 322–339.
203. Bahler M, Greengard P. Synapsin I bundles F-actin in a phosphorylation-dependent manner. *Nature* 1987; 326: 704–707.
204. Bahler M, Benfenati F, Valtorta F, Czernick AJ, Greengard P. Characterization of synapsin I fragments produced by cysteine-specific cleavage: a study of their interactions with F-actin. *J Cell Biol* 1989; 108: 1841–1849.
205. Benfenati F, Bahler M, Jahn R, Greengard P. Interactions of synapsin I with small synaptic vesicles: distinct sites in synapsin I bind to vesicle phospholipids and vesicle proteins. *J Cell Biol* 1989; 108: 1863–1872.
206. Huttner WB, Scheibler W, Greengard P, de Camilli P. Synapsin I (protein I), a nerve terminal-specific phosphoprotein. III. Its association with synaptic vesicles studied in a highly purified synaptic vesicle preparation. *J Cell Biol* 1983; 96: 1374–1388.
207. McGuinness TL, Brady ST, Gruner J, Sugimori M, Llinas R, Greengard P. Phosphorylation-dependent inhibition by synapsin I of organelle movement in squid axoplasm. *J Neurosci* 1989; 9: 4138–4149.
208. de Camilli P, Cameron R, Greengard P. Synapsin I (protein I), a nerve terminal-specific phophoprotein. I. Its general distribution in synapses of the central and peripheral nervous system demonstrated by immunofluorescence in frozen and plastic sections. *J Cell Biol* 1983; 96: 1337–1354.
209. de Camilli P, Harris M, Huttner WB, Greengard P. Synapsin I (protein I), a nerve terminal-specific phosphoprotein. II. Its specific association with synaptic vesicles demonstrated by immunocytochemistry in agarose-embedded synaptosomes. *J Cell Biol* 1983b; 96: 1355–1373.
210. Greengard P, Browning MD, McGuinness TL, Llinas R. Synapsin I, a phosphoprotein associated with synaptic vesicles: possible role in regulation of neurotransmitter release. In: Ehrlick YH, Lenox RH, Korneeki E, Berry WO, eds. *Molecular mechanisms of neuronal responsiveness*. New York: Plenum Press; 1987: 135–153.
211. Llinas R, McGuinness TL, Leonard CS, Sugimori M, Greengard P. Intraterminal injection of synapsin I or calcium/calmodulin-dependent protein kinase II alters neurotransmitter release at the squid giant synapse. *Proc Natl Acad Sci USA* 1985; 82: 3035–3039.
212. Schroer TA, Brady ST, Kelly R. Fast axonal transport of foreign vesicles in squid axoplasm. *J Cell Biol* 1985; 101: 568–572.
213. Llinas R, Sugimori M, Lin J-W, Leopold PL, Brady ST. ATP-dependent directional movement of rat synaptic vesicles injected into the presynaptic terminal of the squid giant synapse. *Proc Natl Acad Sci USA* 1989; 86: 5656–5660.
214. Fraher JP. Quantitative studies on the maturation of central and peripheral parts of individual ventral motoneuron axons: I. Myelin sheath and axon caliber. *J Anat* 1978; 126: 509–533.
215. Hoffman P, Koo E, Muma N, Griffin J, Price D. Role of neurofilaments in the control of axonal caliber in myelinated nerve fibers. In: Lasek RJ, Black MM, eds. *Intrinsic determinants of neuronal forms and functions*. New York: Alan R. Liss, Inc.; 1988; 389–402.
216. Lasek RJ, Oblinger M, Drake P. Molecular biology of neuronal geometry: expression of neurofilament genes influences axonal diameter. *Cold Spring Harbor Symp Quant Biol* 1983; 18: 731–744.
217. Wujek L, Lasek RJ, Gambetti P. The amount of slow axonal transport is proportional to the radial dimensions of the axon. *J Neurocytol* 1986; 15: 75–83.
218. Caroni P, Schwab M. Antibody against myelin associated inhibitor of neurite growth neutral-

izes nonpermissive substrate properties of CNS white matter. *Neuron* 1988; 1: 85–96.
219. Schwab M, Caroni P. Oligodendrocytes and CNS myelin are nonpermissive substrates for neurite growth and fibroblast spreading in vitro. *J Neurosci* 1988; 8: 2381–2393.
220. Caroni P, Schwab M. Codistribution of neurite growth inhibitors and oligodendrocytes in rat CNS: appearance follows nerve fiber growth and precedes myelination. *Dev Biol* 1989; 136: 287–295.
221. Miller RH, David S, Patel R, Abney ER, Raff MC. A quantitative immunohistochemical study of macroglial cell development in the rat optic nerve: in vivo evidence for two distinct astrocyte populations. *Dev Biol* 1985; 111: 35–41.
222. Miller RH, Ffrench-Constant C, Raff MC. The macroglial cells of the rat optic nerve. *Annu Rev Neurosci* 1989; 12: 517–534.
223. Pannese E, Ledda M, Matsuda S. Nerve fibers with myelinated and unmyelinated portions in dorsal root spinal roots. *J Neurocytol* 1988; 17: 693–700.
224. Windebank AJ, Wood P, Bunge R, Dyck P. Myelination determines the caliber of dorsal root ganglion neurons in culture. *J Neurosci* 1985; 5: 1563–1569.
225. Aguayo A, Attiwell M, Trecarten J, Perkins S, Bray G. Abnormal myelination in transplanted Trembler mouse Schwann cells. *Nature* 1977; 265: 73–75.
226. de Waegh SM, Brady ST. Local control of axonal properties: neurofilaments and axonal transport in homologous and heterologous nerve grafts. *J Neurosci Res* 1991; 30: 201–212.
227. Perkins S, Aguayo A, Bray G. Behaviour of Schwann cells from Trembler mouse unmyelinated fibers transplanted into myelinated nerves. *Exp Neurol* 1981; 71: 515–526.
228. Pollard J, McLeod J. Nerve grafts in the Trembler mouse: an electrophysiological and histological study. *J Neurol Sci* 1980; 46: 373–383.
229. Low PA. Hereditary hypertrophic neuropathy in the Trembler mouse part 1: histological studies electron microscopy. *J Neurol Sci* 1976; 30: 343–368.
230. Parhad I, Clark A, Griffin J. The effect of impairment of slow transport on axonal caliber. In: Smith RS, Bisby MA, eds. *Axonal transport*. New York: Alan R. Liss, Inc.; 1987; 473–492.
231. de Waegh SM, Brady ST. Slow axonal transport in Trembler mouse: altered cytoskeletal dynamics in a myelin deficient mouse model. *J Neurosci* 1990; 10: 1855–1865.
232. Lasek RJ, McQuarrie I, Wujek J. The central nervous system regeneration problem: neuron and environment. In: Gorio A, et al. eds. *Posttraumatic peripheral nerve regeneration: experimental basis and clinical implication*. New York: Raven Press; 1981: 59–70.
233. Wujek J, Lasek RJ. Correlation of axonal regeneration and slow component b in two branches of a single axon. *J Neurosci* 1983; 3: 243–251.
234. Forman D, McQuarrie IG, Labore F, Wood D, Stone L, Braddock C, and Fuchs D. Time course of the conditioning lesion effect on axonal regeneration. *Brain Res* 1980; 182: 180–185.
235. McQuarrie I. The effect of a conditioning lesion on the regeneration of motor axons. *Brain Res* 1978; 152: 597–602.
236. McQuarrie I, Grafstein B. Effect of a conditioning lesion on optic nerve regeneration in goldfish. *Brain Res* 1981; 216: 253–264.
237. McQuarrie I. Effect of a conditioning lesion on axonal transport during regeneration: the role of slow transport. *Adv Neurochem* 1984; 6: 185–209.
238. Berthold C. Some aspects of the ultrastructural organization of peripheral myelinated axons in the cat. In: Weiss D, ed. *Axoplasmic transport*. New York: Springer-Verlag; 1982: 40–54.
239. Cohen P. The structure and regulation of protein phosphatases. *Annu Rev Biochem* 1989; 58: 453–508.
240. Nairn AC, Hemmings HC, Greengard P. Protein kinases in the nervous system. *Annu Rev Biochem* 1985; 54: 931–976.
241. Brady ST, Tytell M, Heriot K, Lasek RJ. Axonal transport of calmodulin: a physiological approach to identification of long term association between proteins. *J Cell Biol* 1981; 89: 607–614.
242. Brady ST, Lasek RJ. Nerve specific enolase and creatine phosphokinase in axonal transport: soluble proteins and the axoplasmic matrix. *Cell* 1981; 23: 515–523.
243. Oblinger MM, Foe LG, Kwiatkowska D, Kemp RG. Phosphofructokinase in the rat nervous system: regional differences in activity and characteristics of axonal transport. *J Neurosci Res* 1988; 21: 25–34.
244. Griffin JW, Price DL, Drachman DB, Morris JR. Incorporation of transported glycoproteins into axolemma during regeneration. *J Cell Biol* 1981; 88: 205–214.
245. de Waegh SM, Brady ST. Altered slow axonal transport in optic nerve of Shiverer mutant mice. *Soc Neurosci Abstr* 1988; 14: 118.
246. Roach A, Boylan K, Horvath S, Prusiner SB, Hood L. Characterization of the cloned cDNA representing rat myelin basic protein: absence of expression in brain of Shiverer mutant mice. *Cell* 1983; 34: 799–806.
247. Roach A, Takahashi N, Pravtcheva D, Ruddle F, Hood L. Chromosomal mapping of mouse myelin basic protein gene and structure and transcription of the partially deleted gene in Shiverer mutant mice. *Cell* 1985; 42: 149–155.
248. Readhead C, Popko B, Takahashi N, Shine HD, Saavedra RA, Sidman RL, Hood L. Expression of a myelin basic protein gene in transgenic Shiverer mice: correction of the dysmyelinating phenotype. *Cell* 1987; 48: 703–712.
249. Tucker R, Garner CC, Matus A. In situ localization of microtubule-associated protein mRNA in the developing and adult rat brain. *Neuron* 1989; 2: 1245–1256.

3

The Fate of Denervated Neurons

Transneuronal Degeneration, Dendritic Atrophy, and Dendritic Remodeling

Oswald Steward[*] and Edwin W Rubel[†]

Departments of Neuroscience and Neurosurgery, University of Virginia Health Sciences Center, Charlottesville, Virginia 22908; †Virginia Merrill Bloedel Hearing Research Center and the Department of Otolaryngology–Head and Neck Surgery, University of Washington, Seattle, Washington 98195

Neurons that lose their normal synaptic inputs following injury or disease experience one of three fates: 1) they may die through a process of transneuronal degeneration; 2) they may survive with reduced total input; or 3) they may be reinnervated in whole or in part. In the case of neurons of the CNS, reinnervation usually occurs as a result of the elaboration of new contacts from afferent systems that terminate near the denervated sites.

From the point of view of developing strategies to promote CNS repair following injury, it is of considerable importance to understand the factors that determine which of these fates neurons experience. Obviously, in the case of neurons that die following denervation, it would be useless to develop strategies to foster the regeneration of axons that would normally innervate these cells—no targets would be present for the regenerated axons to reinnervate. Instead, the first concern is developing a means to preserve the denervated target cells. Thus, the first order of business is understanding the processes which lead to the degeneration of the denervated target cells.

In the case of neurons which survive, a key issue is whether the postsynaptic cells remain receptive to new innervation. In this regard, two important questions are the following: 1) What happens to the denervated portion of the postsynaptic cell's receptive surface (i.e., is it preserved? does it undergo atrophy?); and 2) If there is an atrophy of portions of the denervated postsynaptic cell, can these surfaces be regenerated in order to accommodate new inputs?

The present review will focus on three experimental models that have provided partial answers to these questions. In the first section, we will consider a situation in which denervation leads to transneuronal degeneration. Using the model system provided by the auditory system of the chick, we will summarize the evidence that defines the signals that initiate the response, and the cellular processes involved. In the second section, we will discuss a situation in which denervation of one portion of a dendritic arbor leads to the selective atrophy of that dendritic domain. We will also discuss the evidence that indicates that because this atrophy occurs rapidly, reinnervation is prevented. In the third section, we will review how neurons remodel their receptive surface during reinnervation, focusing on the well-characterized example of reinnervation that occurs in the dentate gyrus of adult rats. Although these different examples offer unique experimental advantages because of the special properties of the systems, the conclusions derived may be applicable to other systems with similar properties.

MECHANISMS OF TRANSNEURONAL DEGENERATION IN THE CNS

The best-characterized examples of transneuronal degeneration and atrophy in the CNS involve sensory systems. Well-known examples include the changes that occur in central visual pathways following manipulations that disrupt visual input, or changes in the organization of the somatosensory cortex in response to manipulations of the periphery. While these studies have provided considerable information about the changes in connectivity that occur in response to changes in afferent input, less is known about the cellular mechanisms that bring about the changes in connectivity. In particular, there is little information about the cellular processes within postsynaptic cells that are actually under afferent control. In part, this is because little is known about how the manipulations (i.e., the elimination of input from one eye, the deprivation of pattern vision, digit removal, whisker removal, etc.) actually affect the pattern and quantitative extent of neuronal activity over the involved pathways. Also, the requisite cellular and molecular studies have not yet been carried out, and may be difficult because of the nature of the systems involved.

A system that has been very useful for studies of cellular events that may be under afferent control is the auditory system of the chick. One advantage of the auditory system is that it is possible to precisely manipulate afferent activity and to quantitatively define the effects of these manipulations on postsynaptic activity (for a review, see 1). Moreover, the components of the system are well suited to at least some types of cellular and molecular studies.

The auditory portion of the eighth nerve terminates in several sites including the cochlear nuclei. These nuclei represent the first synaptic station in the transmission of auditory information to higher brain areas. Most of the work in the chick auditory system has involved nucleus magnocellularis (NM), which is the avian homolog of the anteroventral cochlear nucleus. Eighth nerve afferents form large calyx endings known as end bulbs of Held on neurons of NM. These inputs are excitatory. While NM neurons receive a small number of synaptic connections from other sources, the eighth nerve afferents provide by far the bulk of the innervation of these cells (Fig. 1).

Because of this synaptology, it is not surprising that the activity of NM neurons is tightly coupled with the activity of the eighth nerve axons. Thus, the "spontaneous" activity of NM cells that is present even in quiet settings is totally eliminated when the cochlea is removed, or when the activity of eighth nerve fibers is silenced by injecting small amounts of tetrodotoxin (TTX) into the perilymphatic fluid of the cochlea (2). In terms of the effects on the *activity* of NM neurons, the results of cochlea removal are comparable at all ages after innervation has first been established. However, the consequences of the change in activity on neurons depends critically upon the age at the time of the injury (see below).

A number of studies have demonstrated that some NM neurons die if deprived of input from the cochlea in young chicks. There are several features of this transneuronal degeneration that are noteworthy. First, the cells die very rapidly. Following cochlea removal, the neurons that will die begin to exhibit a number of characteristic changes within a few hours (see below), and disappear within 2–3 days (3). Second, only about 1/3 of the denervated cells ac-

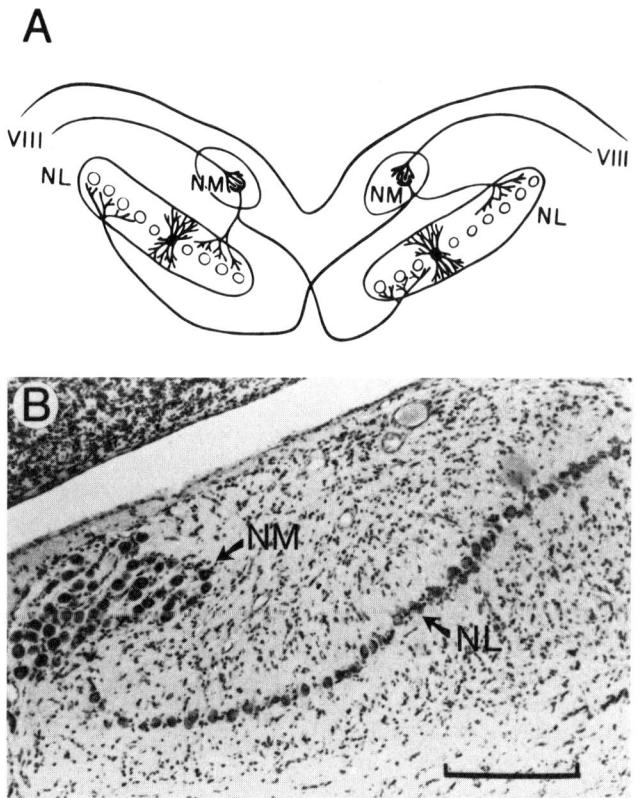

FIG. 1. *Organization of the brainstem auditory projections in the chick.* The cochlear ganglion cells give rise to eighth nerve axons, which project to two main sites in the brainstem—nucleus magnocellularis *(NM)* and nucleus angularis *(NA)*. Axons from NM neurons project to the dorsal dendritic lamina of nucleus laminaris *(NL)* ipsilaterally and to the ventral dendritic lamina on the contralateral side. From (18).

tually die, despite the fact that all neurons of the nucleus receive input from the cochlea. There is also some animal-to-animal variability in the proportion of cells that die, suggesting that some unknown variables determine the fate of individual cells. Third, there is an age-dependency in the response. Transneuronal degeneration after cochlea removal occurs until about 6 weeks of age in the chick; however, there is minimal cell death as a result of cochlea removal in adult chickens. When the cochlea is removed in embryonic chicks, NM cells develop normally until the time at which eighth nerve axons would normally form synapses; then the neurons undergo the same changes as denervated neurons. In other species, transneuronal cell death also occurs in adult animals.

Studies of the chick auditory system have suggested two generalizations about how afferents influence their targets. First, a distinction can be made between *informational* and *trophic* coupling between afferents and their target cells. Information coupling involves the transmission of information within a time frame of milliseconds to seconds, depends upon the action of well-characterized neurotransmitter systems, and is present from the time that the synapse is first established throughout the life of the organism. Trophic coupling on the other hand involves the transmission of information over a much longer interval; the actual time constant of the minimal "bit" of information must still be defined, but it is clearly on the order of minutes, hours, or perhaps days. Because of the differential sensitivity to deafferentation as a function of age, either the degree of trophic coupling or the signal for the coupling must vary at different life stages.

Cellular Events Leading to Transneuronal Degeneration

Studies of the chick auditory system have provided some interesting clues about the cellular events leading to transneuronal degeneration. NM neurons that degenerate following cochlea removal can be identified within hours after removing the cochlea because of the disappearance of Nissl substance within the cell bodies (3). Since Nissl stains are essentially RNA stains, this observation suggested that alterations in protein synthesis might play an important role in the process of cell death.

Studies of cellular protein synthesis early in the course of transneuronal degeneration confirmed this suspicion (4). Cellular protein synthesis was evaluated autoradiographically at various times after removing the cochlea, by injecting chicks intravenously with ^{3}H-leucine. The chicks were allowed to survive for 30 minutes, and were then perfused with aldehyde fixatives and prepared for autoradiography. Using this technique, the sites and extent of protein synthesis can be evaluated. These studies revealed that protein synthesis ceased entirely within some of the denervated neurons within 3–6 hours after the removal of the cochlea (Fig. 2). Not surprisingly, the cells with disrupted protein synthesis were the same ones in which Nissl staining was reduced.

Subsequent studies revealed that the transneuronal degeneration came about because of a cessation of afferent activity rather than as a result of some degenerative change in eighth nerve axons. It is possible to totally block eighth nerve activity without damaging the middle ear or cochlea by introducing TTX into the perilymph. A single injection of TTX totally blocks eighth nerve activity for 3–8 hours, and multiple injections can block activity for longer periods. Single injections of TTX that blocked eighth nerve activity produced the same sorts of decreases in protein synthesis as removal of the cochlea (2). Multiple injections over a 48 hour period (four at 12 hour intervals) led to essentially the same degree of cell death in NM as occurred following cochlea removal. Thus, all of the effects of cochlea removal can be duplicated by blocking the activity of eighth nerve axons.

Importantly, it is not simply the generation of action potentials in the postsynaptic neurons that is important. This conclusion is based on neurophysiological studies that compare the consequences of orthodromic and antidromic activation of NM neurons in brainstem preparations maintained in vitro. Orthodromic activation via stimulation of the eighth nerve increased protein synthesis in NM neurons; antidromic stimulation did not (5). These results suggest that transneuronal regulation occurs through the action of an agent that is released by the presynaptic terminal in an activity-dependent fashion. It remains to be determined whether it is the neurotransmitter itself or some other molecule that is co-released which actually is the transcellular signal.

Rapid Destruction of the Protein Synthetic Machinery of the Neuron During Transneuronal Cell Death

Because the cessation of protein synthesis in NM neurons was so rapid, it was of considerable interest to try to define the events occurring within the affected cells. The autoradiographic technique provided the means to address this question because it was possible to identify individual cells

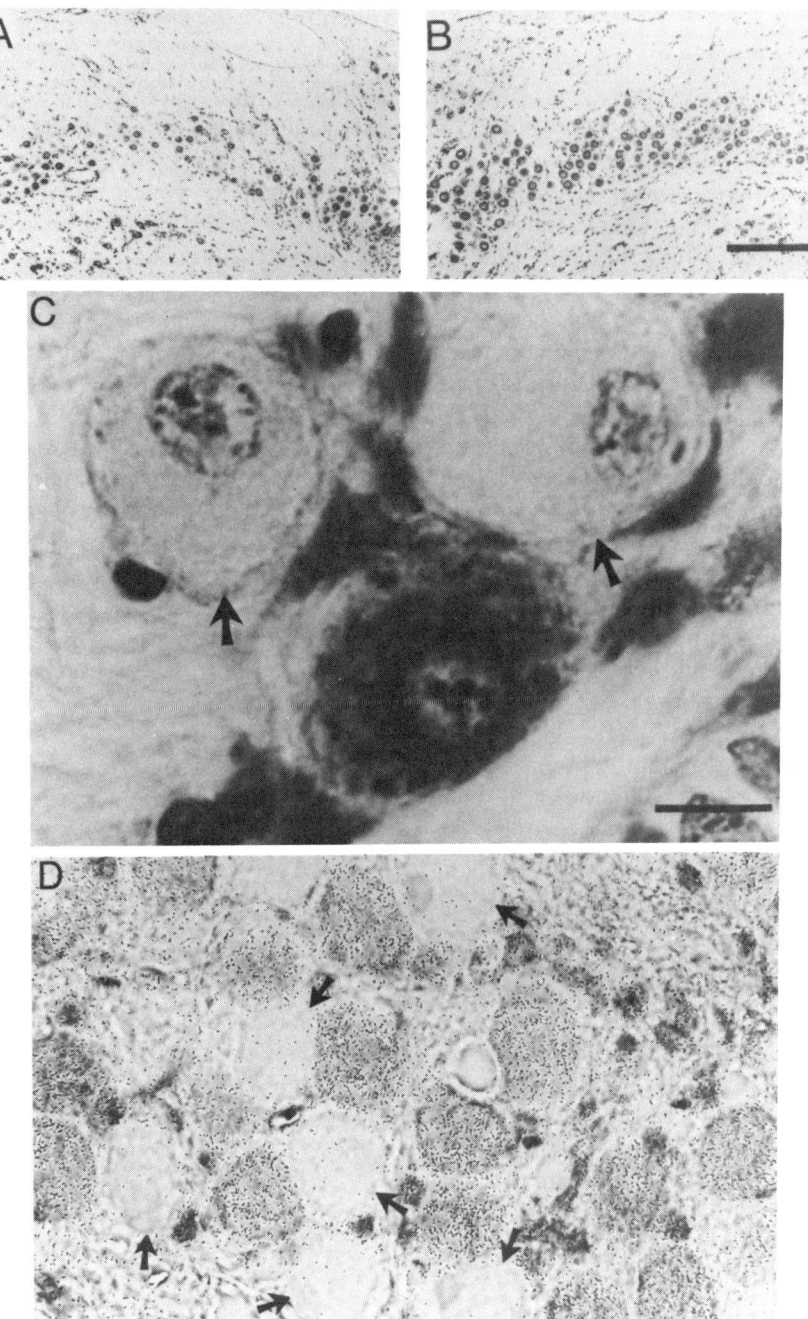

FIG. 2. Transneuronal degeneration of neurons in the auditory brainstem after cochlea removal. Following removal of the cochlea, about 30% of the neurons in the ipsilateral nucleus magnocellularis die (**A** and **B** illustrate Nissl stained sections through the nucleus ipsi, and contralateral to the cochlea removal, respectively). Early in the course of the degeneration, there is a dramatic decrease in Nissl staining of the cells destined to die (*arrows* indicate the "ghost" cells in **C**). Accompanying this decrease in Nissl staining is a dramatic decrease in protein synthetic activity, as documented autoradiographically in **D**. Animals were injected intraveneously with ^{3}H-leucine, and euthanized 30 minutes later. The extent of protein synthesis is revealed by the distribution of silver grains over neuronal somata. The neurons that exhibit decreases in Nissl staining were essentially unlabeled. A–C are from (3); D is from (4). The composite photograph has appeared in previous reviews (21,34,35).

that were affected very early after the cochlea removal, and evaluate these cells at the electron microscopic level.

For these studies, chicks were allowed to survive for 1.5, 3, or 6 hours after cochlea removal. In order to identify cells that had ceased protein synthesis, animals were injected intravenously with ^{3}H-leucine 30 minutes prior to being euthanized and perfused for combined autoradiographic and electron microscopic evaluation. Paired 1 μm and 60 nm sections were taken through the deafferented and control sides of the brain; the 1 μm sections were prepared for light microscopic autoradiography, and the 60 nm sections were stained for electron microscopy. Individual neurons which had ceased protein synthesis were identified by autoradiography, and these cells were then evaluated electron microscopically in the adjacent thin section (Fig. 3).

Evaluation of cells that had ceased producing protein revealed that the earliest and most dramatic changes were in the ribosomes themselves—they appeared to be totally destroyed (6). In place of the large numbers of ribosomes that are present in normal cells, the affected cells had only a fine granular material in their cytoplasm (Figs. 3 and 4). The destruction of ribosomes was particularly apparent when evaluating stacks of rough endoplasmic reticulum (RER), which are normally studded with large numbers of ribosomes. These stacks of RER were totally bare in the most severely affected cells. A remarkable feature of the response is its rapidity. Signs of ribosome destruction could be detected 1 hour after removal of the cochlea (Fig. 4B), and ribosome destruction appeared complete in some neurons by 6 hours (Fig. 4D). Given the destruction of ribosomes, the cessation of protein synthesis and the eventual death of the cells is not surprising.

The mechanisms responsible for ribosome destruction must still be defined. However, there are some clues. The first clue is the selectivity of the effect. Ribosomes appear to be completely destroyed despite the fact that they are, from the biochemical standpoint, one of the more stable elements in the cytoplasm. In contrast, other organelles which are considered to be much more labile (microtubules, endoplasmic reticulum, and mitochondria) are preserved. The second clue is the rapidity of the effect. Because ribosomes normally turn over very slowly in cells (on the order of days), the disappearance of ribosomes cannot be a result of a change in ribosome biosynthesis. Because ribosome destruction begins within 1 hour and appears virtually complete by 6 hours, an active destructive process is strongly suggested (for a more complete discussion, see 6).

The rapidity and selectivity of the effect suggest an active process which leads to the rapid destruction or disassembly of the ribosomal particle (perhaps some sort of a suicide-factor which is held in check by normal afferent activity). One possibility is some suicide enzyme which is newly synthesized or activated in response to decreases in activity. The fine electron dense ribosome debris is strikingly similar to the debris observed in tissue treated with RNAse (7), so that the activation of a powerful RNAse is clearly one possibility.

A remarkable aspect of the ribosome destruction is that it does not necessarily lead to the death of the affected cells. TTX blockade of eighth nerve activity led to the same changes in ribosomes as destruction of the cochlea (6); however other studies have shown that restoration of activity after 6 hours of TTX blockade rescued cells which would otherwise die and in which ribosomes were presumably destroyed (2). Thus, neurons exhibiting complete ribosome destruction can apparently reassemble the machinery for protein synthesis (by reassembling ribosomes or synthesizing new ones) and resume normal metabolic functions.

Although ribosome destruction is the most dramatic change in NM neurons undergoing transneuronal degeneration, it is not the only change. There are also decreases

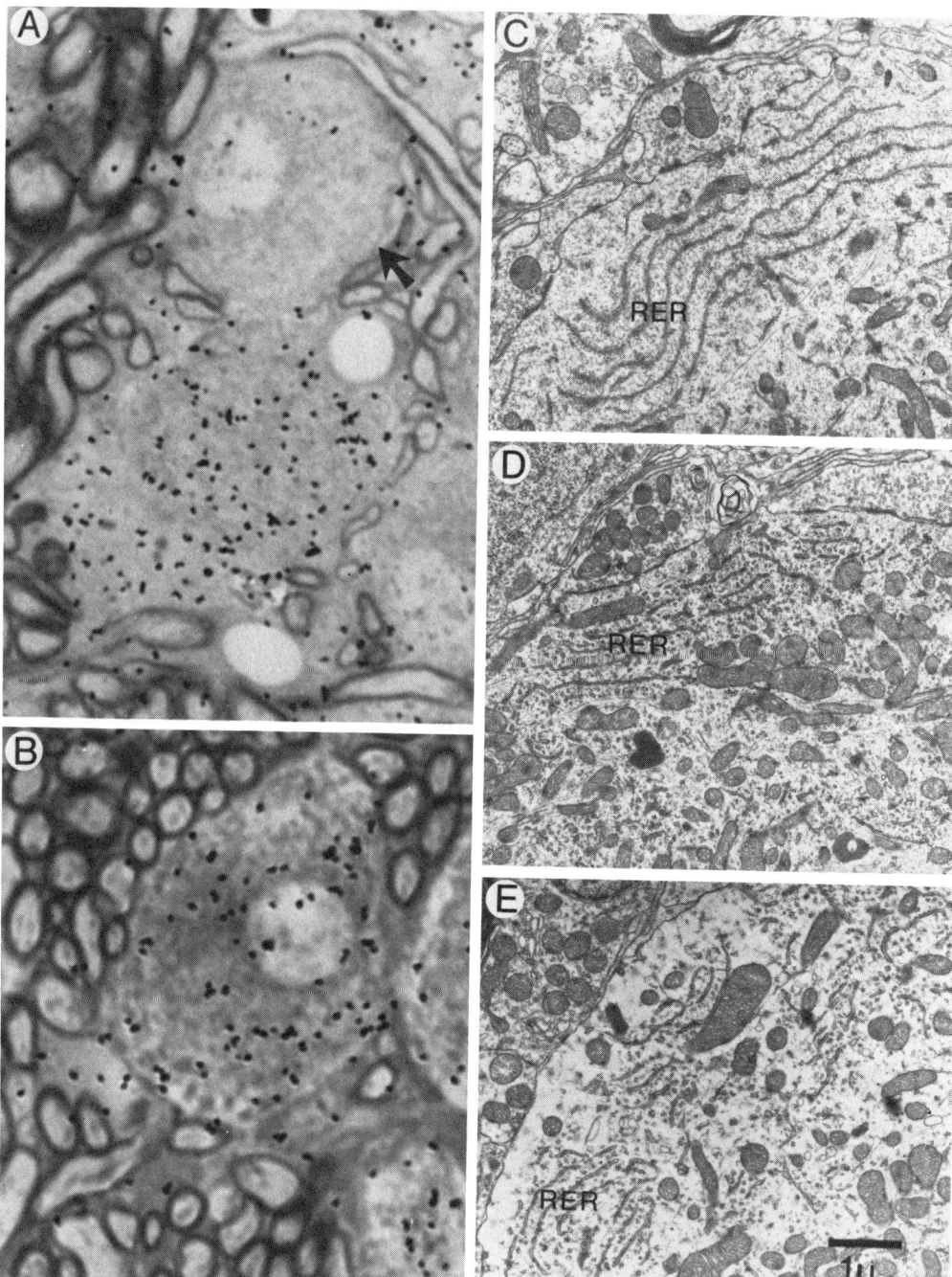

FIG. 3. *Destruction of ribosomes in neurons undergoing transneuronal degeneration.* The figure illustrates representative light microscope autoradiographs and electron micrographs of neurons in NM at 6 hours after cochlea removal. **A**: Autoradiographs of NM neurons ipsilateral to the cochlea removal. An unlabeled cell is evident in the upper portion of the field *(arrow)*, and a labeled cell is immediately adjacent. The ultrastructural appearance of the cytoplasm of these two cells is illustrated in **C** and **D**, respectively. Note the absence of ribosomes in the unlabeled cell (especially the absence of ribosomes from the stacks of endoplasmic reticulum) and the apparently normal appearance of ribosomes and rough endoplasmic reticulum *(RER)* in the labeled cell. Other cytoplasmic elements and synapses upon the unlabeled neuron appear normal. **B** and **E** illustrate a labeled NM neuron from the contralateral side of the same brain. From (6).

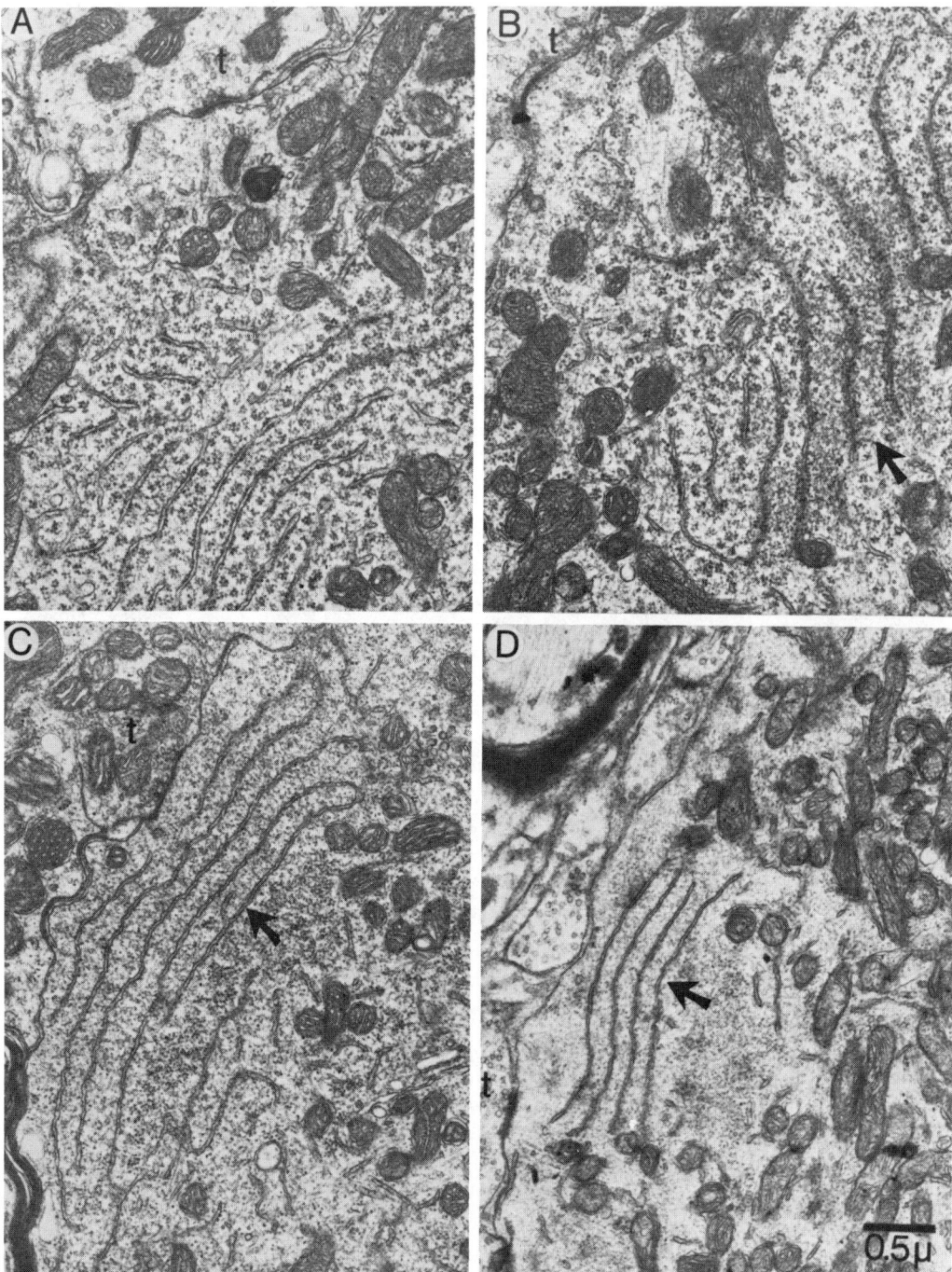

FIG. 4. *Time course of ribosome destruction in neurons undergoing transneuronal degeneration.* **A)** control side; **B)** 1 hr post cochlea removal; **C)** 3 hr post cochlea removal; **D)** 6 hr post cochlea removal. Note the progressive loss of ribosomes and the appearance of a fine electron-dense "dust," which we interpret as the debris from ribosomes. Apparently intact synaptic terminals can be seen contacting the NM neurons (*t*). From (6).

in immunostaining for various cytoskeletal proteins (including tubulin, actin, and the microtubule-associated protein MAP2), and changes in the activity of various Kreb's cycle enzymes. There are also changes in the distribution and number of mitochondria (for a more complete discussion, see 1). How all these changes are interrelated must still be defined. It is also unclear at this time whether the processes that occur in NM neurons are representative of the processes that occur in other neurons that die as a result of the loss of input. This latter question will be answerable only when the mechanisms of cell death in different populations of cells are defined.

Although numerous systems exhibit transneuronal degeneration (8), it is not invariably observed, even when the extent of degeneration is substantial. As noted above, transneuronal degeneration depends upon developmental age. Also, some cell types that are apparently denervated to approximately the same extent exhibit different responses. For example, the dorsal cochlear nucleus receives a substantial projection from the cochlea, yet does not degenerate along with the ventral cochlear nucleus (9). Some of the differences in the response of different neuron types may be a consequence of the fact that some neurons receive "sustaining" inputs from other sources. In fact, this may also explain some of the differences in the response to denervation in animals of different ages. Older animals may have a greater variety of inputs so that the removal of one would not remove as large a proportion of the total innervation as would occur earlier in development. This concept of alternate sustaining inputs is not likely to account for all of the differences, however, since the extent of denervation of neurons in the auditory brainstem appears to be comparable regardless of developmental age.

DENDRITIC ATROPHY FOLLOWING DENERVATION

When neurons survive denervation, there are usually adjustments in the neuron's receptive surface. Typically, denervation results in the disappearance of the portion of the postsynaptic cell that is denervated (transneuronal atrophy). For example, if a projection system terminates on dendritic spines, the removal of that input will usually lead to the disappearance of the denervated spines (10–13). If a particular afferent type provides the bulk of the innervation to a dendrite or part of a dendrite, elimination of that input may lead to a selective atrophy of the denervated segments. Atrophy of dendrites and spines may be permanent or transient, depending upon whether reinnervation occurs (see below).

One of the best-studied examples of dendritic atrophy following denervation is again provided by the auditory system. Neurons of the medial superior olive have bipolar dendritic trees that receive most of their input from the cochlear nucleus. One side of the bipolar dendritic arbor is innervated by the ipsilateral cochlear nucleus; the opposite arbor receives input from the contralateral cochlear nucleus. Selective destruction of the projections to one of these dendritic arbors (for example by cutting the crossing fibers at the midline) results in a rapid atrophy of the denervated dendrites (14).

This example of dendritic atrophy has been particularly well-studied in the chick. Nucleus laminaris (NL) is the avian homolog of the mammalian medial superior olive. The ventrally directed dendritic arbor of these cells receives input from the contralateral NM, whereas the dorsal arbor receives input from the ipsilateral NM (Fig. 1). The dorsal and ventral arbors of individual neurons are normally symmetrical; thus changes that occur following denervation can be easily documented by comparing the dorsal and ventral dendrites of individual neurons (Fig. 5). Transection of the crossing fibers leads to a very rapid atrophy of the ventrally directed dendritic arbor on which the fibers from the contralateral cochlear nucleus terminate. These changes have been studied using electron microscopy (15), Golgi techniques (16), and im-

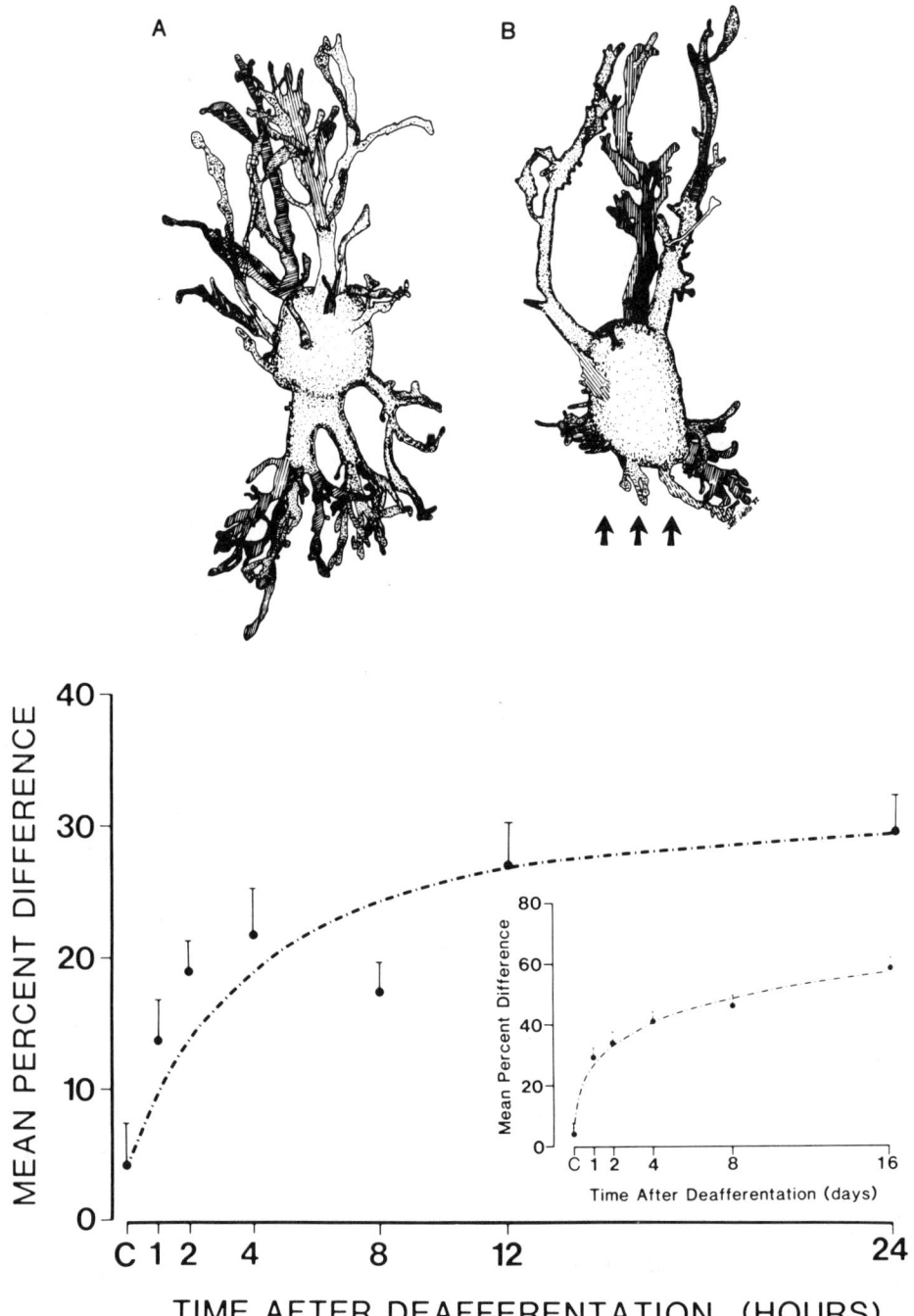

FIG. 5. *Selective atrophy of deafferented dendrites.* The drawings illustrate Golgi impregnated neurons from nucleus laminaris of a normal chick (**A**) and a chick in which the crossing fibers from the contralateral nucleus laminaris have been cut 16 days previously (**B**). The crossing fibers terminate selectively on the ventral dendrites. Note the disappearance of the denervated dendrites on the ventral side. The graph illustrates the time course of dendritic atrophy as revealed by quantitative Golgi analysis. The extent of the atrophy was estimated by calculating the percentage difference in the length of the dorsal and ventral dendrites of individual neurons. The *large graph* illustrates the change in dendrites over the first 24 hours after injury. The *inset* illustrates the change between 1 and 16 days. From (17).

munocytochemical markers for dendrite-specific cytoskeletal proteins (MAP2) (1). Decreases in the relative length of the denervated dendrites can be detected within hours of the injury, and dendrites continue to decrease in size for days. By 16 days after the injury, the denervated dendrites are about 60% shorter than their counterparts on the dorsal side of the nucleus. The changes are selective to the denervated dendrites, because there are no detectable changes in the dorsal dendrites that retain their normal innervation from the ipsilateral cochlear nucleus.

Ultrastructural studies that have sought to define the subcellular correlates of dendritic atrophy have revealed several changes (17). Within 4 hours after the injury, microtubule density at the base of the affected dendrites decreased. Microtubule density continued to decrease over time. By 12 hours, there was a similar decrease in neurofilament density at the base of the dendrites. Later, a lucent gap appeared at the base of the affected dendrites, and this became more pronounced over time. There was no evidence of fragmentation of the dendritic plasma membrane until 2 days following deafferentation. However, quantitative studies revealed an increase in the volume of the soma, suggesting a resorption of the dendritic membrane. Although these results provide hints about the cellular events underlying dendritic atrophy, the exact sequence of events is not clear. In particular, it is not known how the process of atrophy is set into motion and regulated.

There is evidence that indicates that because dendritic atrophy occurs rapidly in this cell type, reinnervation that might otherwise occur does not take place. One obvious source of fibers that seem optimally positioned to reinnervate the dendrites of NL neurons after partial removal of input from one NM are the fibers from the opposite NM. Thus, one might expect that destruction of the inputs to one set of dendrites might lead to a sprouting of fibers that are normally restricted to the opposite dendritic arbor. For example, after destruction of inputs to ventral dendrites, one might expect fibers from neurons in the ipsilateral NM to sprout into the ventral neuropil. However, studies of the distribution of ipsilateral projections of NM neurons after complete destruction of the crossing fibers revealed that such sprouting did not occur to any significant extent (Fig. 6). The most obvious interpretation of this outcome was that sprouting did not occur because the denervated dendrites disappeared before the sprouting could occur.

An experimental test of this hypothesis was made possible by taking advantage of the transneuronal degeneration of neurons in NM following cochlear removal. As noted above, cochlear removal results in the transneuronal degeneration of only some of the neurons in NM, leading to a partial denervation of the projections to neurons in nucleus laminaris. As might be expected, such partial denervation led to only a partial atrophy of the dendrites of nucleus laminaris neurons. Although some of the projections from the NM neurons without eighth nerve input were retained, they were presumably quiescent. To evaluate whether this partial denervation led to sprouting of projections from the opposite NM, the distribution of the crossing fibers was evaluated by cutting the fibers, and tracing their distribution with silver staining techniques (Fig. 7). In this situation, the inputs from the contralateral cochlear nucleus sprouted vigorously across the cell body laminae to reinnervate the partially denervated dendrites of NL neurons (18).

The results from the studies of sprouting in nucleus laminaris suggest several important conclusions. The first is that sprouting depends upon the presence of the postsynaptic cell. In situations where dendritic atrophy is pronounced, sprouting was not observed. It is an open question at this point whether sprouting occurs and the new sprouts are withdrawn because they find nothing to innervate, or whether sprouting does not occur in the first place. A second

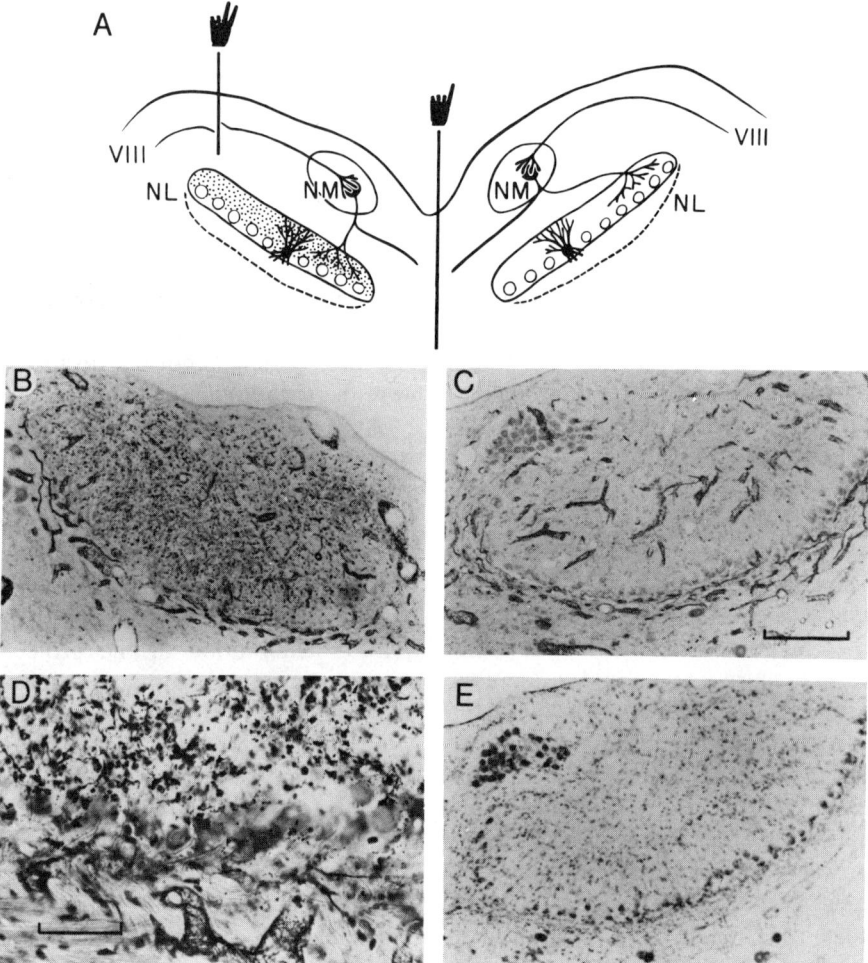

FIG. 6. *Absence of sprouting of NM axons after complete destruction of projections from the contralateral NM.* The crossed projections from one NM to the opposite NL were transected in young chicks, leading to the atrophy of ventral dendrites of neurons in NL. Several weeks later, the cochlea on the left side was removed in a second operation. Cochlea removal led to the degeneration of the axons of some NM neurons; the pattern of termination of these axons in NL could then be determined by Fink-Heimer staining. **A** is a diagrammatic illustration of the primary and secondary lesions. **B** and **D** illustrate the pattern of degeneration induced by the cochlea removal ipsilateral to the lesion. Note that degeneration debris is present only on the dorsal side of the cell body lamina. **C** and **E** illustrate a silver-stained section and Nissl-stained section, respectively, on the contralateral side. The absence of degeneration products in C indicates that all degeneration debris resulting from the primary lesion have been removed. The calibration bar in C = 0.2 mm; the bar in D = 50 μm. From (18).

implication is that the consequences of denervation apparently depend on the timing of atrophic and reconstructive processes. In the auditory system, dendritic atrophy begins very soon after denervation. If dendrites are at least partially preserved (for example following partial denervation) then the dendrites may be reinnervated as a result of sprouting.

Taken together, the results suggest two possibilities: 1) that the final extent of transneuronal atrophy may depend upon the tim-

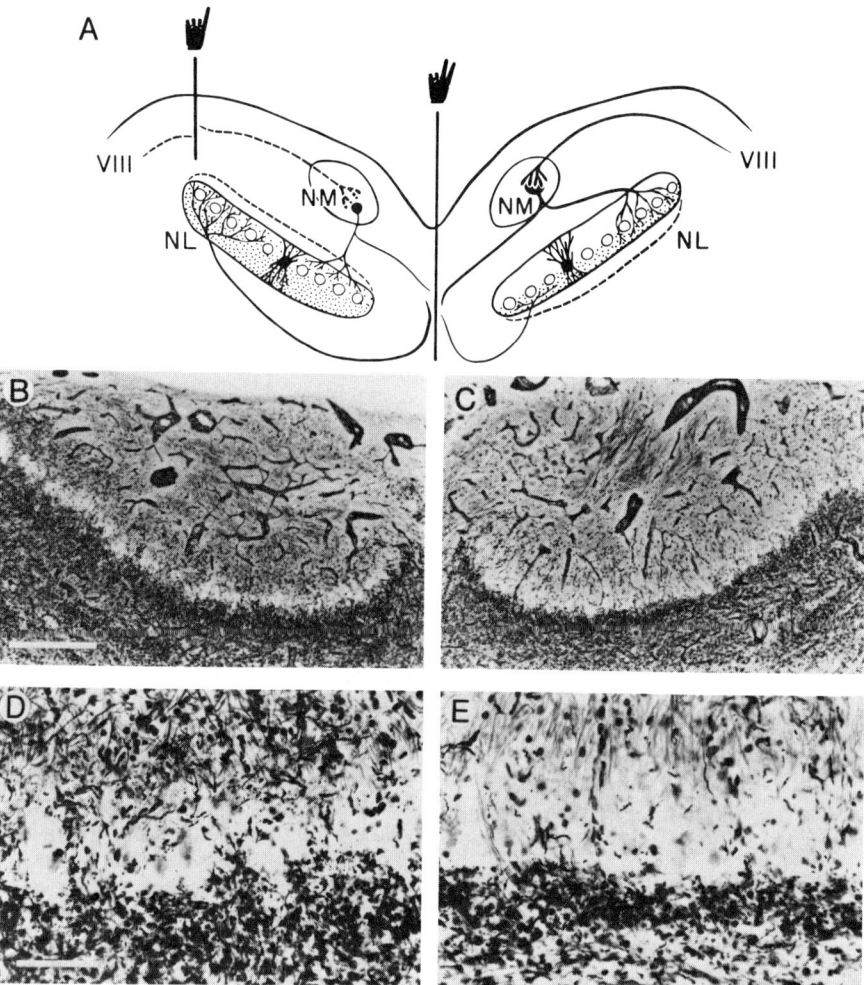

FIG. 7. *Sprouting of NM axons after partial denervation of NL dendrites.* NL dendrites were partially denervated by removing the cochlea, which leads to the transneuronal degeneration of some neurons in NM (the primary operation). Several weeks later, the crossing projections from the magnocellular nuclei on the experimental *(left)* and control *(right)* sides were traced by cutting the crossing fibers, and tracing the pattern of degeneration 4 days later using the Fink-Heimer technique. **A** is a diagrammatic representation of the experimental manipulations and the results. **B–E** illustrate the pattern of degeneration induced by the secondary lesions on the experimental (B and D) and control (C and E) sides. Note that on the experimental side, the degeneration debris is present in both the ventral and dorsal neuropil of NL (see D). On the control side, degeneration debris was present only in its normal location in the ventral neuropil. The calibration bar in B = 0.2 mm; the bar in D = 50 μm. From (18).

ing and extent of reinnervation; and 2) that the final extent of reinnervation may depend upon the timing and extent of the initial atrophy. The critical question is how these two regulatory interactions determine the final outcome. Once the events that lead to dendritic atrophy have begun, at what stage are they reversible? After atrophy has occurred, is it possible to regenerate some portion of the receptive surface to accept reinnervating fibers, or is the atrophy irreversible? Is the velocity of the atrophic process important? The answer to these questions will determine in part whether it is more appropriate to concentrate on intervention strategies that promote presynaptic growth or on strategies that prevent or delay transneuronal degeneration.

REMODELING THE POSTSYNAPTIC CELL'S RECEPTIVE SURFACE DURING REINNERVATION

The question of whether the postsynaptic surface of a denervated neuron can be restructured to accept reinnervating fibers can be answered at least in part in the case of the reinnervation that occurs in forebrain structures. Processes of postlesion growth that lead to reinnervation have now been reported in a variety of different brain regions (19–22). Indeed, there is now good reason to believe that reinnervation following injury is the rule rather than the exception. However, the best-studied example of reinnervation is clearly the one that occurs in the hippocampal dentate gyrus following destruction of input from the entorhinal cortex.

Quantitative electron microscopic studies have revealed that complete destruction of the entorhinal cortex leads to the degeneration of about 90% of the synapses upon distal dendrites of the dentate granule cells (23). Over time, these synapses are replaced as a result of the proliferation of a number of afferent systems that survive the lesion (24). Degenerating synapses are slowly phagocytosed by astrocytes, and new synapses begin to form on the denervated neurons at about 6 days postlesion (Fig. 8). The rate of synapse replacement is high between 6 and 12 days postlesion, and synapse formation continues at a slower rate after 12 days postlesion (23). These observations thus define the time frame in which to evaluate changes in dendrites.

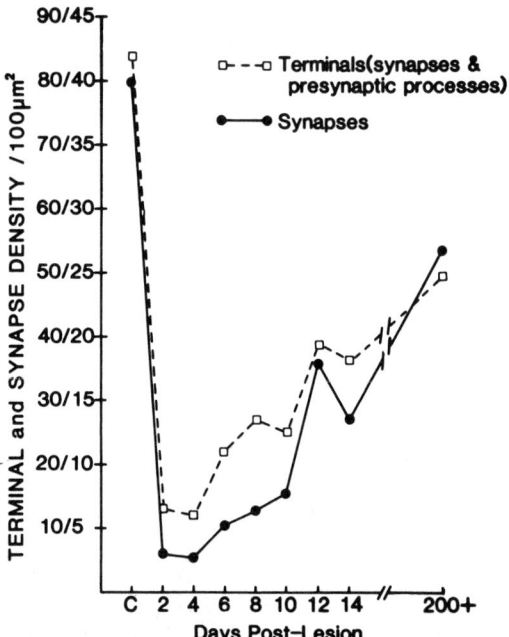

FIG. 8. *Time course of terminal proliferation and reactive synaptogenesis in the denervated dentate gyrus.* The graph illustrates terminal and synapse density in the middle molecular layer of the dentate gyrus at various times after unilateral lesions of the entorhinal cortex. The control value is the average from the contralateral sides of each animal. "Synapses" are vesicle-containing presynaptic processes that make a contact with a postsynaptic membrane specialization. "Terminals" include all presynaptic processes whether or not they form a contact. The two scales on the ordinate are for terminals and synapses, respectively. Terminal density is approximately twice as great as synapse density, as every presynaptic process that forms a synapse is also a terminal. From (23).

Loss and Reappearance of Dendritic Spines

The cycle of synapse loss and replacement in the dentate gyrus following lesions of the entorhinal cortex is accompanied by the disappearance and subsequent reappearance of spines on dentate granule cell dendrites (10,12). In general, the changes in spines on granule cell dendrites parallel the changes in synapses. At early postlesion intervals, when synapse numbers have been reduced by about 90%, total spine density on denervated dendritic segments decreased by about 50%. The long lollipop spines that are the predominant type on normal dendrites were particularly affected; these decreased by about 90% (see Fig. 9). Interestingly, the number of stubby spines actually increased. There were no detectable changes in complex spines.

Our interpretation of these observations is that the lollipop spines collapse into the dendrite. Some of the collapsed spines would then appear stubby, while others would be undetectable at the level of light microscopy. Electron microscopic observations strongly support the interpretation that spines collapse into the dendrite (23, 24). Overall, the spines that are observed in the denervated neuropil tend to be stubby and have unusual shapes. Many of these stubby spines would almost certainly not be visible at the light microscopic level.

After 10 days postlesion, total spine density recovered (Fig. 9). Initially, there was a further increase in stubby spines. Later, the number of lollipop spines increased, and the number of stubby spines decreased. Eventually, spine density and the relative proportions of different types of spines returned to control levels. The predominance of stubby spines during the period of reinnervation suggests that the reinnervating fibers terminate predominantly on such spines. Electron microscopic observations support this possibility; many of the nondegenerating synapses that are present early in the course of reinnervation terminate on stubby spines (23,24). Thus the regrowth of spines after reinnervation may involve a maturation of spines from a stubby type to the form characteristic of mature animals as a result of elongation of the spine and thinning of the spine neck.

An important implication of these results is that spine changes are a convenient indicator of the synaptic reorganization that is occurring. This conclusion is of considerable interest because of the substantial literature on spine changes in a variety of other situations in which changes in synapses have not been directly evaluated (25).

Taken together, the qualitative electron microscopic observations and the quantitative studies of spine changes suggest that synapse replacement on dendrites takes place via the sequence of events illustrated in Fig. 10. This sequence can occur only on dendrites that are preserved following denervation. Studies of the dendritic arbors of granule cells suggest that other processes must also be considered, since there appears to be a deterioration and regrowth of portions of the dendritic arbor.

Deterioration and Regrowth of Dendrites

Quantitative Golgi studies have revealed a deterioration of granule cell dendrites following denervation, followed by regrowth (10). During the early postlesion period, granule cell dendrites exhibited varicose swellings and irregularities in diameter that are typical of degenerating dendrites (Fig. 9). These are the same sorts of changes that have been interpreted as dendritic degeneration in pathological conditions (26) and following dendritic amputation and denervation (27). The changes suggestive of dendritic deterioration were most pronounced between 4 and 10 days postlesion, during the period of maximal spine loss. Some of the varicosities may result from the collapse of spines into the dendrites, because profiles that were suggestive of collapsed spines were often observed on the varicosities (Fig. 9). With the reappearance of spines, the varicose swellings and irregularities of dendritic diameter disappeared, and the dendrites assumed a more normal appearance (see Fig. 9).

Quantitative studies of dendritic field parameters have revealed a substantial reorganization of the dendritic arbor with denervation and reinnervation. For example, as synapses degenerate, there were decreases in the spread of the dendritic field of granule cells (dendritic field spread), the

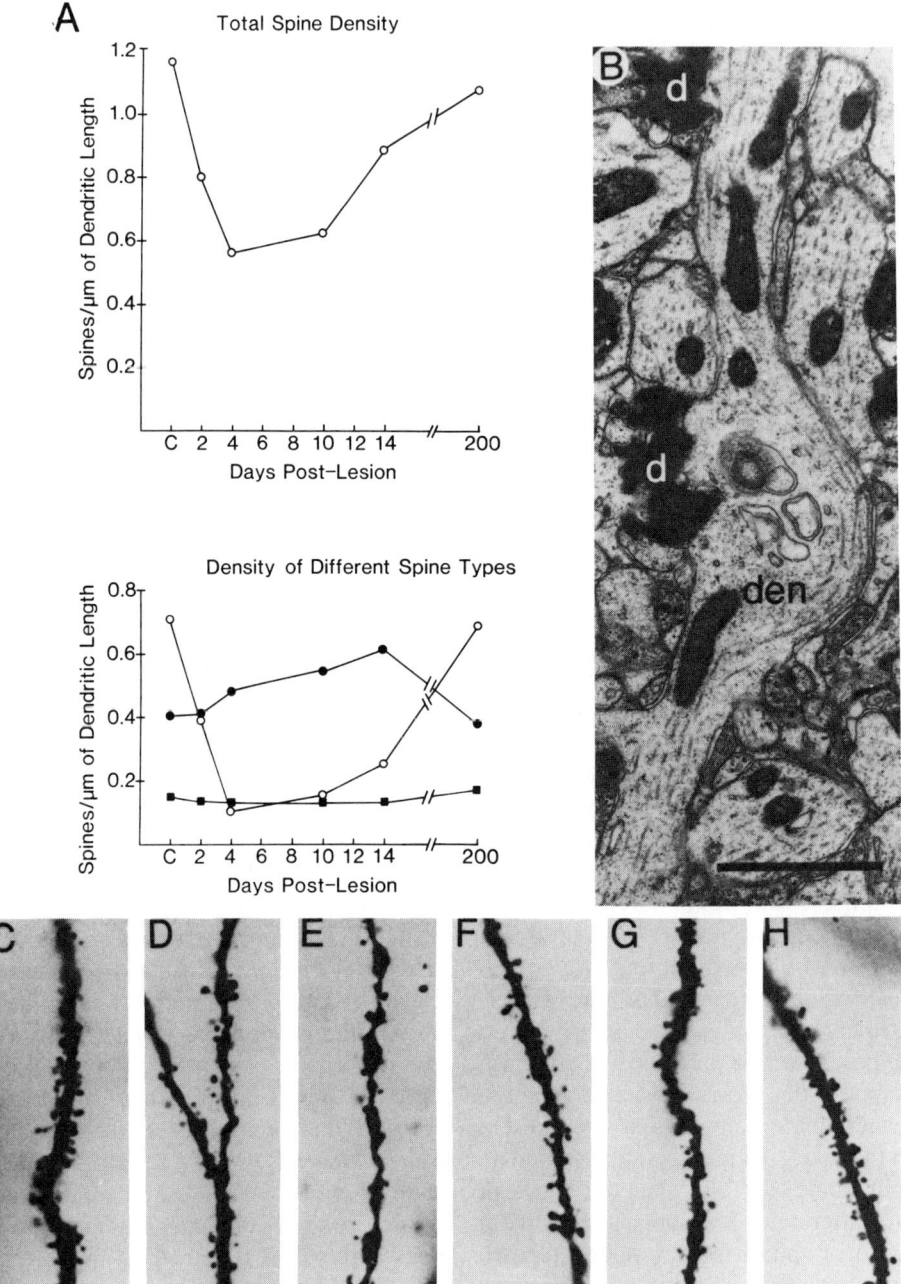

FIG. 9. *Deterioration and regrowth of spines with denervation and reinnervation.* **A**: The upper graph illustrates the time course of changes in total spine density on dendrites of dentate granule cells at various times after unilateral entorhinal cortical lesions. The counts are of the average total number of spines/1 μm length of dendrite. The lower graph illustrates counts of different types of spines. *Open circles,* lollipop spines; *solid circles,* stubby spines; *solid squares,* complex spines. **B**: An electron micrograph illustrating a varicose swelling on a dendrite of a denervated granule neuron. A degenerating synapse contacts the dendrite near the varicosity. The spine associated with this synapse is abnormally short, and appears to have collapsed into the dendrite. **C–H**: Examples of dendrites of granule cells at various postlesion intervals (Control, 2, 4, 10, 30, and 200 days postlesion, respectively). From (10).

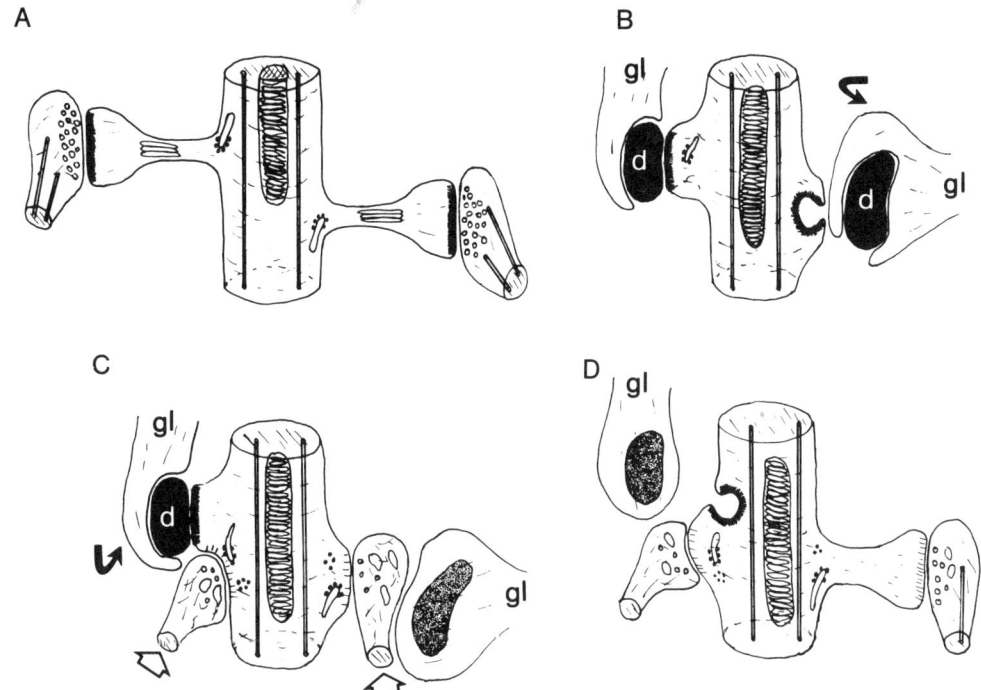

FIG. 10. *Schematic illustration of the sequence of events thought to occur during synapse replacement on dendritic segments that are preserved after denervation:* **A–D** illustrate the postulated sequence of events during the early phase of the reinnervation process. As terminals degenerate, they are removed by glia; the membrane specialization may be internalized in the dendrite. Either simultaneously *(left side of the dendrite)* or shortly thereafter *(right side of the dendrite)* a new synaptic site is constructed. Some of these new sites are at the base of existing spines. New synaptic sites often have underlying clusters of polyribosomes. From (36).

average total dendritic length, and the average number and length of dendritic segments. There was a recovery for each of the measures at longer postlesion intervals (30 days), suggesting a regrowth of dendrites with reinnervation. For example, Fig. 11 illustrates the changes in the average summed length of dendrites at different proximodistal locations. These data suggest that distal dendrites are particularly affected.

In addition to the decreases and later increases in each of the quantitative measures of the dendrites, there were dramatic changes in dendritic branching patterns. Dendritic branching was analyzed with a method that defines the probability that a given order of dendrite (first, second, third, etc., numbered centrifugally) will branch as a function of distance from the cell body (28). Normally, most of the branching of first through third order dendrites of dentate granule cells occurs very near the cell body laminae. In contrast, in the reinnervated dentate gyrus, dendrites had fewer branches near the cell body layer, and more branches distally in the molecular layer. The rearrangement of the dendritic tree can be seen clearly in graphs of the total number of branch points of first through fourth order dendrites at different proximodistal levels of the molecular layer (Fig. 12A). The changes in the branching patterns indicate a displacement of branch points into the outer molecular layer, indicating that dendrites extend further distally prior to branching. In fact, measurements of the length of first order dendrites (distance to

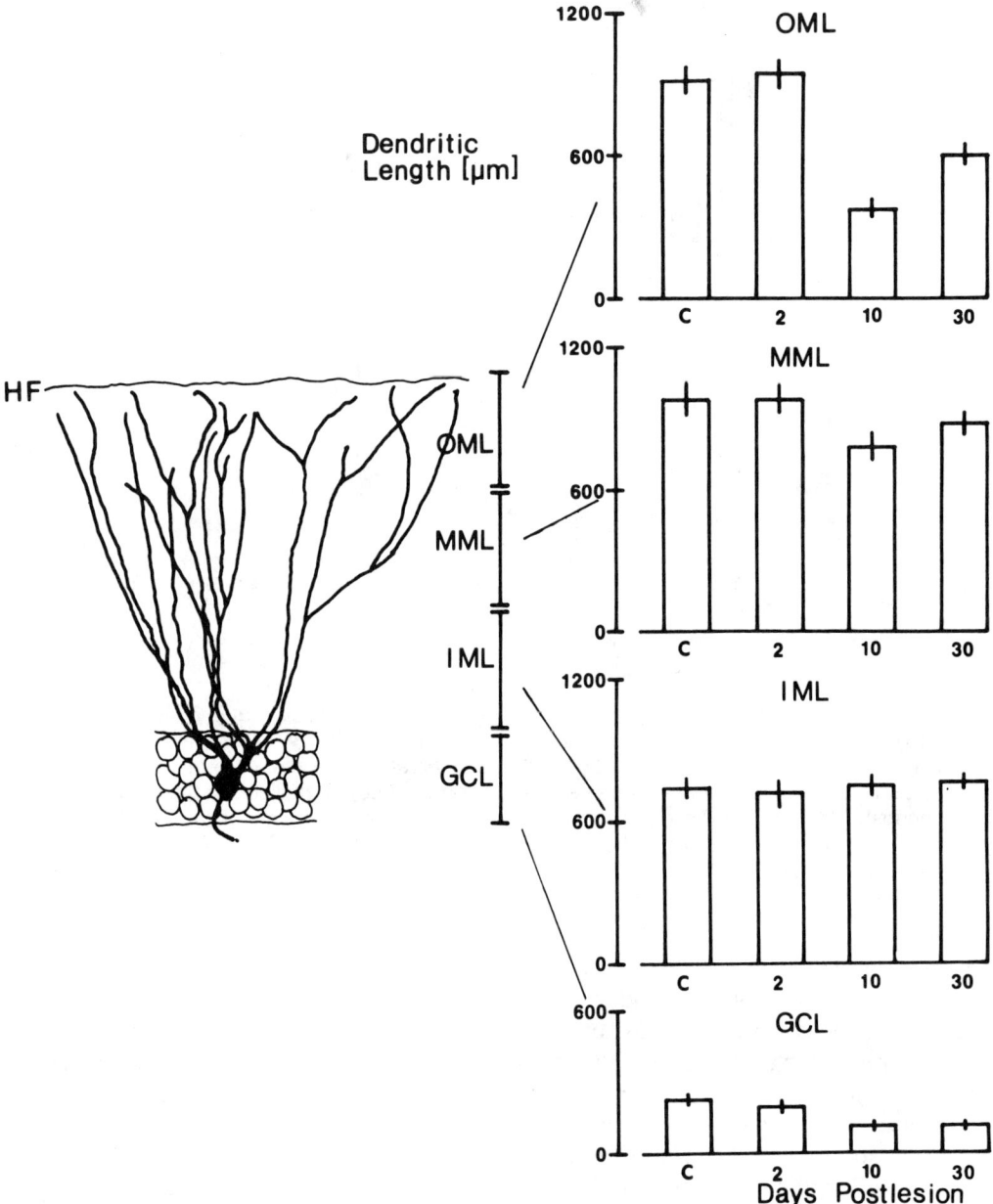

FIG. 11. *Deterioration and regrowth of dendrites with denervation and reinnervation.* The bar graphs indicate the average summed length of granule cell dendrites at four different proximodistal locations: *GCL,* granule cell body layer; *IML, MML,* and *OML,* inner, middle, and outer molecular layer, respectively. The denervation is restricted to MML and OML. There is a loss and reappearance of dendrites in the denervated zone, particularly the OML. The loss is not apparent at 2 days postlesion, is most pronounced at 10 days, and recovers somewhat by 30 days. From (10).

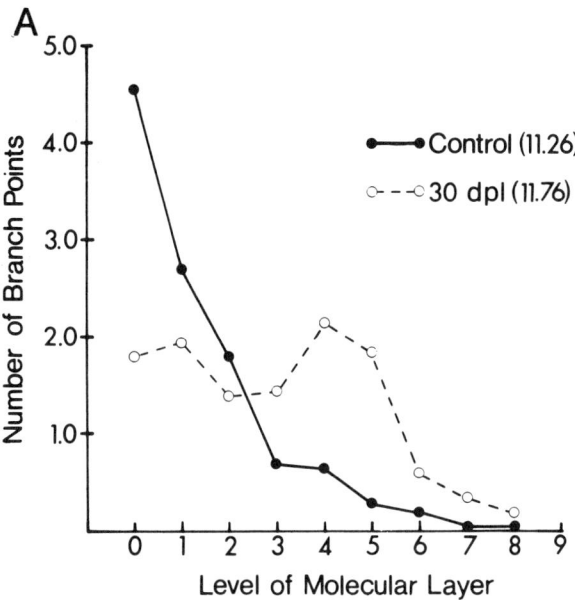
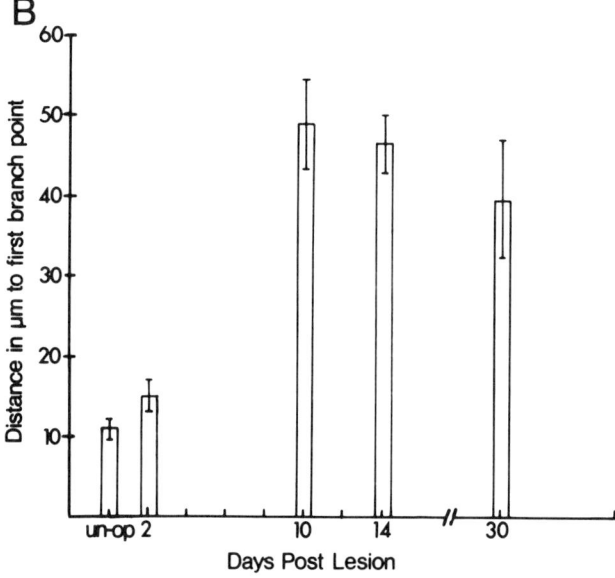

FIG. 12. *Changes in the branching patterns of dendrites with reinnervation.* **A** illustrates the number of branch points of first through fourth order dendrites of dentate granule cells from normal animals and at 30 days postlesion. In the case of dendrites from normal animals, most branching of first through fourth order dendrites occurs near the granule cell layer. At 30 days postlesion, there are fewer branch points proximally and more in the middle portions of the molecular layer. There are no differences in the total number of first through fourth order branch points, however (totals are indicated in the upper right of the graph). **B** illustrates the increases in the length of primary (first order) dendrites of granule cells at various postlesion intervals. From (10).

the first branch point) revealed that these were about threefold longer in the reinnervated dentate gyrus (Fig. 12B).

These results indicate that the overall change in the branching pattern involves 1) a loss and reappearance of dendrites in the denervated zone, and 2) a shift in branches from proximal to distal levels, which is accompanied by an increase in the length of the lower order dendrites. These changes could come about in two ways (see Fig. 13): 1) The elongation of lower order dendrites could result from the loss of higher order segments. If some branches disappeared, the next lowest order dendrite would extend for a greater distance before branching (Sequence A in Fig. 13). For this sort of change to account for the increase in the length of the first order dendrite, the loss would have to involve second order dendrites, and all higher segments originating from this second order stem. The increase in branches in the middle molecular layer would then have to come about as a consequence of a proliferation of branches within this zone. 2) Alternatively, there may be an actual elongation of the primary dendrite (involving intrasegmental growth). This would shift higher order branches distally into the molecular layer (Sequence B in Fig. 13). Elongation of the primary dendrites would account for the increased length of first order dendrites that can be observed by day 10; the reappearance of higher order dendrites in the denervated zone after day 10 would again come about as a consequence of a proliferation of branches within this zone.

On the basis of the available evidence, it is not possible to conclusively eliminate one or the other of these alternatives. The quantitative analyses reveal some loss of higher order branches, particularly fourth order through sixth order dendrites at the early postlesion intervals. This would be predicted by either sequence. There is no evidence, however, of a loss of first through third order segments, even during the period of maximal deterioration. This is important, since sequence A would predict a loss of second order segments (and all higher order segments originating from this second order stem) in order to account for the apparent increase in length of the first order segment. The lack of changes in the total number of first through third order branches is more consistent with the hypothesis that the increase in length of the first order dendrites comes about as a result of an actual intrasegmental growth. Even so, one must be cautious, since the loss of a branch of one order affects the ordering of attached dendrites both proximal and distal to the loss. For example, the distal segment of the dendrite on the right of the cell illustrated in Fig. 13 is normally a fifth order branch. During the period of maximal deterioration (sequence A), a more proximal branch is lost, making these fourth order dendrites. The addition of a proximal branch during regrowth makes these distal segments fifth order dendrites again.

Whichever sequence accounts for the reorganization of the granule cells' dendritic field, the data reveal a substantial remodeling of dendrites with reinnervation. An important conclusion is that the reorganization does not appear to be restricted to the denervated segments; there is a reorganization of the entire dendritic tree, which leads to the generation of a new branching pattern.

Lesion-Induced Growth: Coordinate Growth of Pre- and Postsynaptic Cells

The preceding data reveal that denervated granule cells are not passive participants in the growth response. Rather than simply being stripped of degeneration debris and reinnervated, these neurons actively remodel their receptive surface with reinnervation. This coordinate growth of pre- and postsynaptic processes during reinnervation is reminiscent of events which have been described in other systems. Indeed, in some systems, it has been suggested that mutual pre- and postsynaptic growth is necessary for the forma-

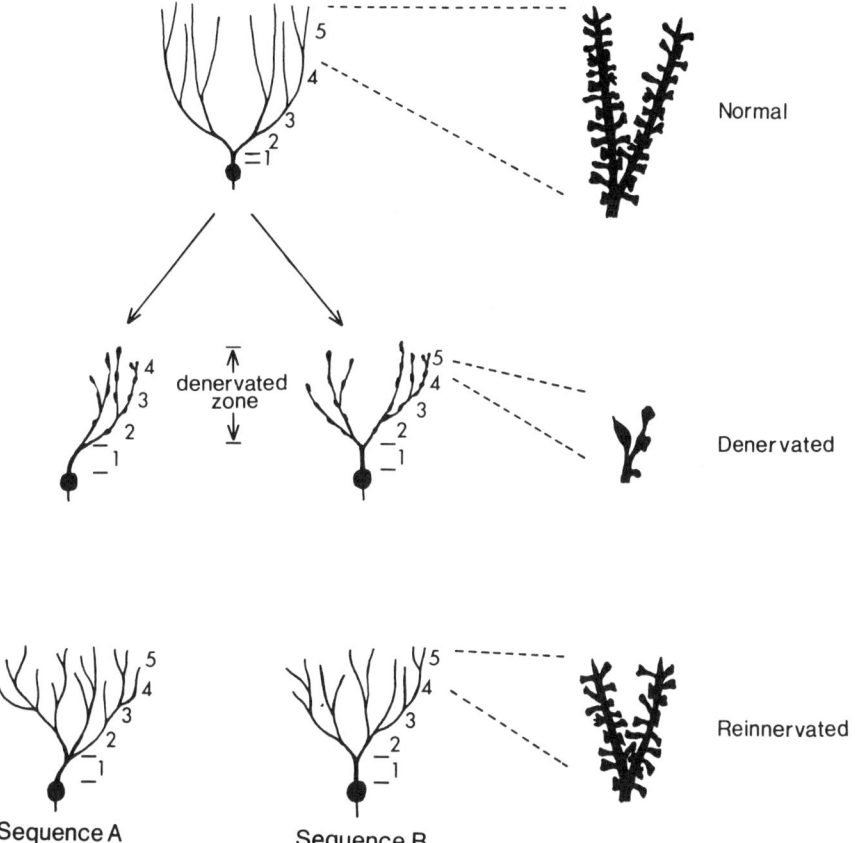

FIG. 13. *A schematic illustration of the possible nature of the reorganization of granule cell dendrites with denervation and reinnervation.* Two changes in the branching pattern of granule cell dendrites must be accounted for: the loss and reacquisition of dendrites in the denervated zone and the increase in length of the primary dendrites. These changes could come about in at least two ways. In one sequence (illustrated in the *left-hand portion* of the figure), denervation may lead to an extensive loss of dendrites, including some secondary dendrites, followed by a proliferation of dendrites in the denervated zone. The loss and regrowth would occur predominantly within the denervated zone, and the increase in the length of the primary dendrites would occur because of a loss of higher order branches. The second possible scheme is illustrated in the *middle portion* of the figure. Here, there is also a loss and regrowth of dendrites in the denervated zone, but there is also an intrasegmental growth of the primary dendrites. These possibilities are not mutually exclusive, and both processes may occur. The changes in spines and the deterioration and regrowth of distal dendrites are illustrated in the *right-hand portion* of the figure. From (24).

tion of some types of synaptic connections (29,30).

Not only the formation of the synapse, but also the presynaptic growth that precedes it may depend on the postsynaptic elements. The auditory system of the chick provides interesting evidence in this regard. As noted above, sprouting of axons can easily be documented at long survival intervals after partial denervation, but not after complete denervation. While it cannot be excluded that presynaptic growth occurred and later regressed after complete denervation, the final extent of the presynaptic growth depended on the preservation of the postsynaptic receptive element. Thus, at a minimum, events within denervated dendrites are likely to be permissive for the expression of presynaptic growth, and seem virtually certain to be important for regulating the final extent of reinnervation.

These observations reveal that the postsynaptic cell is a very active participant in the reinnervation process, substantially remodeling its receptive surface during reinnervation. The question then arises whether the postsynaptic changes are being induced by the reinnervating fibers, or whether the postsynaptic changes are regulated by the postsynaptic cell itself. At present, we favor the latter interpretation. The changes that we have described in the postsynaptic cell's receptive surface are accompanied by dramatic changes in cellular machinery within the dendrite. One of the most prominent of these involves an increase in the protein synthetic machinery that is selectively positioned beneath synaptic sites (7,31–33). This protein synthetic machinery is even more prominent beneath synapses during early development (32). Taken together, these data invite the speculation that synapse formation, either during normal development or during reinnervation, is regulated by processes within the postsynaptic cell. It remains to be determined exactly what these processes are, and how they may regulate the establishment of contact by the presynaptic elements.

CONCLUSIONS

The results summarized in this chapter suggest a number of conclusions regarding the possible fates of denervated neurons. One important conclusion is that the process that leads to cell death following deafferentation can be reversed for some period of time after the injury. This conclusion is based upon the studies of TTX-induced cell death in the auditory system. TTX initiates the process of transneuronal degeneration, but the process can be reversed if communication between afferents and the target is restored. Also, the process is dependent on synaptic communication, suggesting that "trophic" communication is coupled to the release of substances from the presynaptic cell (and thus potentially amenable to pharmacological intervention). Together, these results indicate that it may be possible to develop treatment strategies to prevent orthograde degeneration following CNS injury.

A second conclusion is that denervation may lead to selective atrophy of the portion of the postsynaptic cell that is denervated, and that this atrophy influences the extent to which the denervated neurons can subsequently be reinnervated. This conclusion has important implications for intervention strategies which seek to promote axon regeneration after injury. It will be important to determine whether postsynaptic neurons are available for reinnervation and to consider strategies to prevent or delay whatever transneuronal atrophy that would otherwise limit the final extent of reinnervation.

A third conclusion is that under some circumstances, transneuronal atrophy of dendrites and spines is reversible as a result of reinnervation. For the reasons noted above, it is important to determine the factors that allow such reconstruction. It may simply be a matter of timing—if transneuronal atrophy occurs slowly enough and/or reinnervation occurs rapidly enough, reconstruction may be favored. If atrophy occurs quickly, and reinnervation is slow, then these conditions may be unfavorable for reinnervation. These questions can be addressed experimentally through manipulations that alter the time course of one or the other process. Of course experimental manipulations may then suggest therapeutic intervention strategies that target the same processes.

ACKNOWLEDGMENTS

Thanks to Paula M. Falk for technical assistance. The author's research was supported by grants from the National Institutes of Health (NS12333) to O.S., D.C. 00395 to EWR, and a grant from the National Science Foundation BNS8818766 to O.S.

REFERENCES

1. Rubel EW, Hyson RL, Durham D. Afferent regulation of neurons in the brain stem auditory system. *J Neurobiol* 1989; 21(1): 169–196.
2. Born DE, Rubel EW. Afferent influences on brain stem auditory nuclei of the chicken: presynaptic action potentials regulate protein synthesis in nucleus magnocellularis neurons. *J Neurosci* 1988; 8: 901–919.
3. Born DE, Rubel EW. Afferent influences on brain stem auditory nuclei of the chicken: neuron number and size following cochlea removal. *J Comp Neurol* 1985; 231: 435–445.
4. Steward O, Rubel EW. Afferent influences on brain stem auditory nuclei of the chicken: cessation of amino acid incorporation as an antecedent to age-dependent transneuronal degeneration. *J Comp Neurol* 1985; 231: 385–395.
5. Hyson RL, Rubel EW. Transneuronal regulation of protein synthesis in the brain stem auditory system of the chick requires synaptic activation. *J Neurosci* 1989; 9: 2835–2845.
6. Rubel EW, Falk PM, Canady KS, Steward O. A cellular mechanism underlying activity-dependent transneuronal degeneration: rapid but reversible destruction of neuronal ribosomes. *Brain Dysfunction* 1991;55–74.
7. Steward O. Polyribosomes at the base of dendritic spines of CNS neurons: their possible role in synapse construction and modification. *Cold Spring Harbor Symp Quant Biol* 1983; 48: 745–759.
8. Cowan WM. Anterograde and retrograde transneuronal degeneration in the central and peripheral nervous system. In: Nauta WJH, Ebbesson SOE, ed. *Contemporary research methods in neuroanatomy.* New York: Springer-Verlag, 1970; 217–251.
9. Powell TPS, Erulkar SD. Transneuronal cell degeneration in the auditory relay nuclei of the cat. *J Anat (Lond)* 1962; 96: 249–268.
10. Caceres A, Steward O. Dendritic reorganization in the denervated dentate gyrus of the rat following entorhinal cortical lesions: a Golgi and electron microscopic analysis. *J Comp Neurol* 1983; 214: 387–403.
11. Colonnier M. Experimental degeneration in the cerebral cortex. *J Anat (Lond)* 1964; 98: 47–53.
12. Parnavelas J, Lynch G, Brecha N, Cotman C, Globus A. Spine loss and regrowth in the hippocampus following deafferentation. *Nature* 1974; 248: 71–73.
13. White LE, Westrum LE. Dendritic spine changes in prepyriform cortex following olfactory bulb lesions. *Anat Rec* 1964; 148: 410–411.
14. Liu CN, Liu CY. Role of afferents in maintenance of dendritic morphology. *Anat Rec* 1971; 169: 369.
15. Benes FM, Parks TN, Rubel EW. Rapid dendritic atrophy following deafferentation: an EM morphometric analysis. *Brain Res* 1977; 122: 1–13.
16. Deitch JS, Rubel EW. Afferent influences on brain stem auditory nuclei of the chicken: time course and specificity of dendritic atrophy following deafferentation. *J Comp Neurol* 1984; 229: 66–79.
17. Deitch JS, Rubel EW. Rapid changes in ultrastructure during deafferentation-induced dendritic atrophy. *J Comp Neurol* 1989; 281: 234–258.
18. Rubel EW, Smith ZDG, Steward O. Sprouting in the avian brainstem auditory pathway: dependence on dendritic integrity. *J Comp Neurol* 1981; 202: 397–414.
19. Bjorklund A, Stenevi U. Regeneration of monoaminergic and cholinergic neurons in the mammalian central nervous system. *Physiol Rev* 1979; 59: 62–100.
20. Cotman CW, Nieto-Sampedro M, Harris EW. Synapse replacement in the nervous system of adult vertebrates. *Physiol Rev* 1981; 61: 684–784.
21. Steward O, Jane JA. Repair and reorganization of neuronal connections following CNS trauma. In: Becker D, Gudeman S, ed. *Textbook of head injury.* Philadelphia: Saunders, 1989;466–506.
22. Steward O. Synapse replacement on cortical neurons following denervation. In: Jones E, Peters A, ed. *Cerebral cortex.* New York: Plenum, 1991;81–131.
23. Steward O, Vinsant SL. The process of reinnervation in the dentate of the adult rat: a quantitative electron microscopic analysis of terminal proliferation and reactive synaptogenesis. *J Comp Neurol* 1983; 214: 370–386.
24. Steward O. Making and modifying synapses in the mature CNS: towards a molecular biology of synapse growth and plasticity. In: Ruben J, ed. *The biology of change in otolaryngology.* Amsterdam: Excerpta Medica, 1986;235–254.
25. Globus A. Brain morphology as a function of presynaptic morphology and activity. In: Riesen A, ed. *Developmental neuropsychology of sensory deprivation.* New York: Academic Press, 1975;9–91.
26. Mihaly A. Early morphological changes of the apical dendrites of neocortical pyramidal cells in albino rats subjected to 3-aminopyridine seizures. In: Feher O, Joo F, eds. *Advances of physiological science.* Elmsford, NY: Pergamon Press, 1981;126–141.
27. Rutledge LT. Effects of cortical denervation and stimulation on axons, dendrites, and synapses. In: Cotman CW, ed. *Neuronal plasticity.* New York: Raven Press, 1978.
28. Desmond NL, Levy WB. A quantitative analysis of the dendritic field of the granule cell of the rat gyrus using a novel probabilistic method. *J Comp Neurol* 1982; 212: 131–145.

29. Hadley RD, Kater SB. Competence to form electrical connections is restricted to growing neurites in the snail, Heliosoma. *J Neurosci* 1983; 3: 924–932.
30. Hadley RD, Kater SB, Cohen CS. Electrical synapse formation depends on interaction of mutually growing neurites. *Science* 1983; 221: 466–468.
31. Steward O. Alterations in polyribosomes associated with dendritic spines during the reinnervation of the dentate gyrus of the adult rat. *J Neurosci* 1983; 3: 177–188.
32. Steward O, Falk PM. Protein synthetic machinery at postsynaptic sites during synaptogenesis; a quantitative study of the association between polyribosomes and developing synapses. *J Neurosci* 1986; 6: 412–423.
33. Steward O. Regulation of synaptogenesis through the local synthesis of protein at the postsynaptic site. *Prog Brain Res* 1986; 71: 267–279.
34. Steward O. Reorganization of neuronal connections following trauma: principles and experimental paradigms. *J Neurotrauma* 1989; 6: 99–152.
35. Steward O. *Principles of cellular, molecular, and developmental neuroscience*. New York: Springer-Verlag, 1989.
36. Steward O, Caceres AO, Reeves TM. Rebuilding synapses after injury: remodeling the postsynaptic cell's receptive surface during reinnervation. In: Petit T, Ivy G, eds. *Neural plasticity: a lifespan approach*. New York: Alan Liss, 1988; 143–158.

4

Supporting Cells

Central and Peripheral

Jean de Vellis

Departments of Anatomy and Cell Biology and Psychiatry, Mental Retardation Research Center, Brain Research Institute, Laboratory of Biomedical and Environmental Sciences, School of Medicine, University of California, Los Angeles, California 90024

Supporting cells of the central (CNS) and peripheral (PNS) nervous system greatly outnumber neurons, up to 10 to 1 in the CNS. The term neuroglia or "nerve glue" was coined by Rudolph Virchow who conceived of the neuroglia as an inactive interstitial CNS matrix holding neurons together. The staining techniques developed by Cajal and Rio-Hortega allowed these two great neurobiologists to distinguish in addition to the ependyma three types of supporting cells in the CNS: astrocytes, oligodendrocytes, and microglia. Astrocytes and oligodendrocytes, also termed macroglia, are derived from the neural tube like the neurons. The microglia were considered by Rio-Hortega (1) of mesodermal origin, an insight that has been proven correct. These cells are now considered CNS macrophages and constitute 5–10% of all the cells in the CNS (2). The supporting cells of the PNS, satellite cells around neuronal perikarya and Schwann cells ensheathing axons, derive from the neural crest, a part of the neuroectoderm that separates when the neural tube forms. In the CNS, connective tissue elements are largely kept on its external surface and along major blood vessels. However, in the PNS a totally different situation prevails. Connective tissue intimately intermingles with neural cells, contacting the basal lamina of each Schwann cell. The PNS has few macrophages, but they increase dramatically after various types of injuries. In this chapter the discussion of supporting cells will be limited to astrocytes, oligodendrocytes, microglia, and Schwann cells. Our knowledge of the biology of these cells has increased dramatically during the last two decades (3–5). It is now clear that central and peripheral glia play key roles in the physiology, development, and pathology of the nervous system. Glia are now viewed as forming a functional unit with neurons, interacting via complex active processes (3,6). The purpose of this chapter is to present a brief overview of the biology of glia to serve as a background for the discussion of the role of glia in neuroregeneration that will be presented in many chapters of this book.

MACROGLIA: ASTROCYTES AND OLIGODENDROCYTES

The Early Development of Macroglia

Neuroepithelium initially appears to contain only one population of stem cells. The stem cells are thought to give rise to an as yet undetermined number of progenitors that have more restricted potentialities to generate different types of neurons and glia. Regional heterogeneity of the types of progenitors for oligodendrocytes has been suggested. This is an important consideration when comparing studies using different regions of the CNS. Few progenitors have been characterized because of the lack of an adequate number of specific markers. To circumvent this problem, retrovirus vectors were used as lineage markers (7) because they provide a single cell marking. In this method a histochemical marker gene is transmitted and expressed by the retrovirus vector, thus providing the identification of all the progeny of the originally infected cell. This technique has provided evidence for the existence of a multipotential progenitor cell in the retina giving rise to various types of neurons and glia (8). Williams et al. (9) have recently reported that a small percentage of the colonies analyzed contain neurons and oligodendrocytes that seem to originate from a common precursor. Reynolds and Weiss (10) have obtained proliferating neuroepithelial cells from cultures established from adult mouse striatum that were treated with epidermal growth factor (EGF). These cells express nestin, an intermediate filament present in all neuroepithelial stem cells (11). Upon removal of EGF from the culture medium and addition of factors they differentiate into neurons and astrocytes. Another line of evidence for bipotential progenitors has been provided by the study of the phenotypes of cloned neural cell lines grown under different conditions. For instance, immortalization of neural cells via retrovirus-mediated oncogene transduction has given rise to cell lines with the potential of expressing either neuronal or glial markers (8) depending on the composition of the culture medium or the brain region in which they are transplanted (11). The developmental and phenotype plasticity of these cell lines offer new possibilities to consider in designing future strategies to accomplish functional neuroregeneration.

Later in development, during the postnatal period in the rat, when CNS cells are undergoing rapid differentiation many molecular markers are available to distinguish between cell types (Table 1). These markers have been very useful to study the differentiation of CNS cells both in vitro and in vivo.

The bipolar radial glia that span the thickness of the neural tube during neurogenesis and serve as scaffolding for neuronal migration are recognized as the cells that give rise to astrocytes (12,13). The suggestion (12) that radial glia give rise to oligodendrocytes has not been corroborated (13). Astrocytes may also originate directly from neuroepithelia stem cells in the germinal zone. This view is consistent with the results of lineage studies using retrovirus vectors.

Morphologists have long ago identified a pool of mitotic cells in the subventricular zone at E15 (14). By E18 as the generation of neuroblasts from the ventricular zone

TABLE 1. *Cell markers for identifying major CNS cell types*

Neuroepithelial stem cells
   Vimentin
   Nestin
Neurons
   Neurofilament proteins
   Enolase (γ, γ isozyme)
   Neurotransmitters—synthesizing enzymes
Astrocytes
   S-100 protein
   Glutamine synthetase
   Glial fibrillary acid protein (GFAP)
   Ran-2
Oligodendrocytes
   Galactocerebroside (GC)
   Myelin basic protein (MBP)
   Proteolipid protein (PLP)
   Myelin-associated glycoprotein (MAG)
   Cyclic nucleotide phosphohydrolase (CNP)
   Carbonic anhydrase II (CAII)
   Glycerol phosphate dehydrogenase (GPDH)
   Ganglioside G_{D3}
   O4
   Transferrin

subsides the number of proliferating cells in the subventricular zone exceeds that of the ventricular zone (15,16). The development of these glial precursors into oligodendrocytes in vivo has been mapped spatially and temporally using stage-specific markers (17,19). Most of the oligodendrocytes in the retina and brain seem to originate from the progenitors present in the subventricular zone. The work of Raff and his collaborators (20,21) on gliogenesis in rat optic nerve cultures has identified a biopotential glial progenitor. The oligodendrocyte-type 2 astrocyte progenitor cell (O2A cell) is a proliferating, highly motile bipolar cell whose dominant phenotypic markers are glycolipids stained by the A2B5 monoclonal antibody. Cultures of O2A cells, which are relatively homogenous, can be obtained with great purity. These cells when cultured in chemically defined media rapidly differentiate over a period of a few days into galactocerebroside (GC^+) $A2B5^-$ cells. O2A cells cultured in the presence of 10% fetal calf serum or ciliary neurotrophic factor (CNTF) become glial fibrillary acidic protein ($GFAP^+$) process bearing cells and remain $A2B5^+$. These cells were termed by Raff and colleagues type 2 astrocytes to distinguish them from the large flat polygonal astrocytes termed type 1 astrocytes that have a $GFAP^+/A2B5^-$ phenotype. Type 1 astrocytes and O2A cells represent distinct separate lineages that can be prepared on a large scale from rat cerebral neonatal cultures (22) and yield 95% enriched oligodendrocyte cultures in serum-free medium (23). Because the A2B5 monoclonal antibody is a poor marker in vivo it has not been possible to unequivocally identify the type 2 astrocyte in vivo (21). Other recent evidence is also not consistent with Raff's hypothesis. The morphological and immunocytochemical studies of mitotic cells in the rat optic nerve in vivo have shown that oligodendrocytes and astrocytes originate through separate lineages (24). Grafting of fluorescent labeled cultured O2A cells into postnatal cerebrum failed to show the generation of $GFAP^+$ cells from O2A cells (25). The expression of GFAP in immature oligodendrocytes in vivo has been observed (26). One interpretation is that GFAP may be only transiently expressed in the oligodendrocyte lineage during development. Another possibility worth exploring is to consider GFAP expression in the O2A cell lineage a response to some form of injury. Aspects of macroglia cell differentiation and function will now be briefly examined separately for oligodendrocytes and astrocytes.

Differentiation and Function of Oligodendrocytes

The O2A cell is not the only oligodendrocyte lineage cell capable of proliferation. The existence of its immediate precursor has been surmised by the elimination of O2A cells, preoligodendrocytes, and oligodendrocytes (see Fig. 1 for the phenotype of these 3 stages) from primary cultures of cerebral white matter cultures by antibody-mediated complement lysis. GC^+ oligodendrocytes were obtained from the treated cultures after addition of platelet-derived growth factor (PDGF) (27). The interpretation of the data depends on the total effectiveness of the complement lysis treatment. The positive identification of this precursor to the O2A cell has not been reported yet. A more differentiated progenitor cell than the O2A cell has been identified as an $O4^+/Tf^+/GD3^+/A2B5^-$ (Fig. 1), which we termed preoligodendrocyte because GC has been the standard marker to call a cell an oligodendrocyte. Noble (21) has called it the adult progenitor and characterized it as a more slowly proliferating and less motile cell than the O2A cell. In postnatal rat brain cultures (28) and in the adult brain (29) the preoligodendrocyte may be the major source for the generation of new oligodendrocytes, although mature myelinating oli-

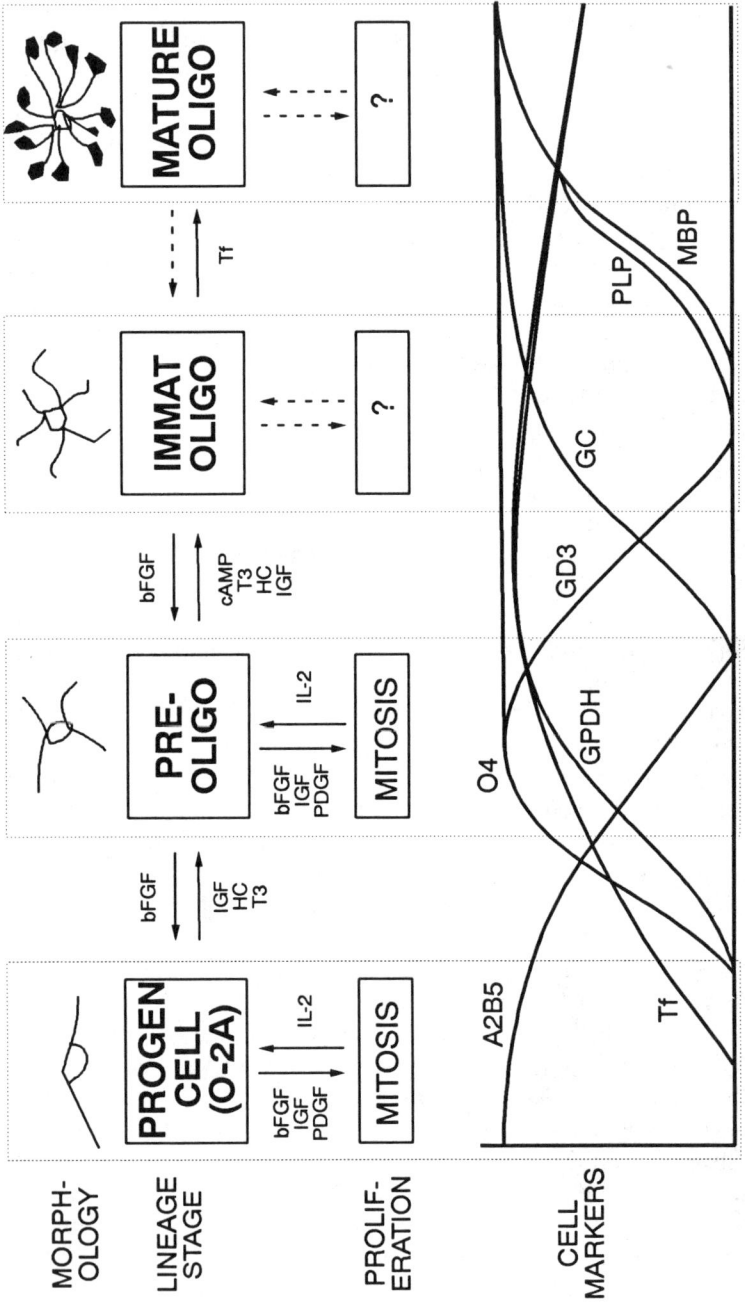

FIG. 1. The O2A lineage. The figure illustrates the characteristics that accompany the sequential differentiation of the O2A progenitor cells to mature oligodendrocytes in vitro. The various growth factors listed can regulate cell proliferation and/or differentiation. *Dashed arrows* indicate a particular direction may be possible but without solid proof. The time course of markers is shown at the bottom. Each stage has a unique antigen profile. Growth factors: IGF (insulin-like growth factor), bFGF (basic fibroblast growth factor), IL-2 (interleukin-2), T3 (triiodothyromine), HC (hydrocortisome, glucocorticoids), Tf (tranferrin). Cell markers: GPDH (glycerophosphate dehydrogenase), GC (galactocerebroside), PLP (proteolipid protein), MBP (myelin basic protein). (Modified from Arenander and de Vellis, ref. 6.)

godendrocytes may retain some potential for cell division (30). In our developmental scheme (Fig. 1) the mature oligodendrocyte is a cell that following the GC^+ stage expresses all the myelin proteins: myelin basic protein (MBP), myelin-associated glycoprotein (MAG), cyclic nucleotide phosphohydralase (CNP), and protcolipid protein (PLP). Additional markers have been reported but the ones indicated here have been the most commonly used.

The O2A cell lineage culture has been an excellent system to study the influence of growth factors on cell lineage development (20,23,31). PDGF and basic fibroblast growth factor (bFGF) are the most potent mitogens acting on the O2A cell in culture. In the presence of PDGF alone in a defined medium, the O2A progenitors undergo a fixed number of cell divisions and then differentiate into a GC^+ oligodendrocyte. PDGF receptor is down-regulated and therefore the O2A cell become unresponsive to additional challenge by PDGF. However, the simultaneous addition of PDGF and bFGF prevents differentiation of O2A cells, keeping them in a proliferative mode. bFGF appears to act by up-regulating the expression of the PDGF receptor (31). IGF-I seems to act as both a mitogen and a differentiation agent (32). Interleukin-2 (IL-2) inhibits the bFGF stimulation of O2A cell proliferation (33). Partially characterized mitogenic activities have been identified in brain extracts (34) and in CNS membranes (35). The membrane-associated mitogen stimulated the proliferation of Schwann cells but not astrocytes in culture.

The source of new oligodendrocytes needed for remyelination in the adult brain remains controversial (36). The presence of $O4^+$ cells suggests that these cells may act as progenitors like the $O4^+$ cells in the early postnatal period (29). However, Wood and Bunge (36) provide evidence that mature oligodendrocytes added to their dorsal root ganglion cultures proliferate and myelinate.

Unlike remyelination in the PNS, remyelination in the CNS is never fully realized after demyelination caused by disease, trauma, or experimental treatments (37). The extent of myelination decreases with repeated insult and becomes almost nil. The factors that contribute to this situation in the CNS have remained elusive. However, since many laboratories have now focused on this problem, much information will be rapidly forthcoming. Since fundamental aspects of the biology of myelin constitute an immense field and are so well covered in textbooks and reviews, this will not be further considered here, except that it is worth mentioning in addition to growth factors the effects of two types of hormones. Glucocorticoid treatment of developing oligodendrocytes (Fig. 1) transcriptionally activates glycerol phosphate dehydrogenase both in vivo and in vitro (for review, see ref. 38). Hydrocortisone also acts posttranscriptionally to increase MBP and PLP, mRNA levels as well as increase translational efficiency (for references, see ref. 39). Thus oligodendrocytes appear to be a major target for glucorticoid hormones. Thyroid hormones have been implicated in the regulation of myelination for over two decades, and a thyroid hormone-responsive element has recently been identified in the MBP promoter region (40).

The second major function of oligodendrocytes is the production of the iron transport glycoprotein transferrin. Oligodendrocytes are the major source of this protein in the brain. The choroid plexus epithelial cells are the secondary source. The role of transferrin in brain development and iron homeostasis has been recently reviewed (41). Transferrin has been shown to be essential for the survival of neurons in vitro. Oligodendrocytes and myelin accumulate large amounts of iron-ferritin complex. Demyelination and destruction of oligodendrocytes caused by injuries or diseases can lead to the liberation of free iron, which forms highly toxic free radicals. In addition to iron, transferrin can bind other metals but with much less affinity.

Myelin and transferrin are two examples of oligodendrocyte-neuron interactions that are essential for neuronal function and survival of the organism. However, the discovery that myelin and oligodendrocytes act as inhibitors of axonal outgrowth in the mammalian CNS has had a major impact on the field of neuroregeneration because it provides a possible reason for the lack of axonal regeneration in the CNS after injury (42). Two molecules have been characterized from oligodendroglial membranes. Neutralization of these antigens by antibodies restores axonal growth and permits elongation over the injury area and into the distal portion. Additions of the antigens to nervous tissue of lower species that are known to regenerate block the recovery after injury.

Differentiation and Functions of Astrocytes

The astrocytes are the most versatile and plastic cells in the CNS. Unlike neurons they do not undergo terminal differentiation nor are they as functionally specialized as the oligodendrocytes. Because of these properties the astrocytes are very heterogenous when they are examined at the same time across brain areas. These cells are easily identified by their microscopic morphology and ultrastructural features, particularly the large bundles of intermediate filaments made up of a specific protein, GFAP. GFAP is the most commonly used marker both in vivo and in vitro. GFAP content increases dramatically after injury, resulting in cellular hypertrophy. This process is called reactive gliosis (43). The subject of glial scarring is discussed in another chapter in this book. In spite of all the research done on astrocytes, including the generation of monoclonal antibodies against astrocyte antigens, few markers besides GFAP are currently in use. Glutamine synthetase and S-100 protein are the only other astrocyte markers that are frequently used (4). Glutamine synthetase is thought to participate in the glutamate/glutamine cycle between neurons and astrocytes. Glutamine synthetase is transcriptionally inducible by glucocorticoids (38) and is also regulated by neuronal astrocyte interactions (44). S-100 protein is a small acidic calcium-binding protein that is highly conserved whose role in the nervous system remains obscure. Interestingly it is secreted from astrocytes and acts as a neurite-promoting factor (for review, see ref. 45). The level of S-100 is increased in astrocytes after injury and it is elevated in Down syndrome brains as well as in senile plaques of Alzheimer brains. The S-100 protein is a good marker for tumors of neuroectodermal origin, e.g., Schwannoma, melanoma, and glioma. S-100 protein expression has been valuable in tumor diagnosis and in assessing the prognosis of patients.

During development, astrocytes and their embryonic precursors the radial glial cells assume many important functions (Table 2), serving as scaffolding for neuron migration and providing adhesion molecules (for review, see refs. 5,6,46). Astrocytes in cul-

TABLE 2. Functions of astrocytes

Developmental and morphogenic functions
   Axonal guidance
   Promotion of neurite outgrowth
   Guidance of neuronal migration (radial glia)
   Regulation of neuronal cytoarchitecture
   Secretion of extracellular matrix components
Metabolic and trophic functions
   Uptake and metabolism of neurotransmitters
   Urea detoxification
   Metabolism of hormones
   Glycogen storage
   Fatty acids and ketone bodies oxidation
   Production of growth factors and neuropeptides:
     bFGF, PDGF, S100 beta, CNTF, IGF-I, GMF, NGF, somatostatin, enkephalin, CCK, angiotensinogen
   Transfer of proteins to axons (invertebrate)
Regulation of the CNS internal milieu
   Induction of vascular endothelial blood-brain barrier
   Regulation of homeostasis potassium
   Regulation of extracellular space (astrocyte swelling)
   Regulation of blood supply
Pathological function
   Activation of neurotoxins
   Reactive gliosis, glial scar
   Majority of intracranial tumors

ture also produce a special form of laminin, s-laminin (47). As astrocytes grow they fence in neurons and oligodendrocytes. Astrocytes extend processes to cover all vascular capillaries and reach out to the CNS surface forming the glia limitans along the pia mater. In addition, the astrocytes selectively interact with areas of the neuronal surface. They extend processes to the node of Ranvier and the axon hillock, wrap processes around synapses, and ensheath neurites. Thus the astrocytes are strategically positioned to influence neuronal functions. Astrocytes express receptors for many neurotransmitters and neuromodulators (48) that are thought to be involved in coupling astrocytes functions to neuronal activity (49). An important function of astrocytes is the induction of the endothelial blood-brain barrier, which is essential for normal brain functions (50).

The presence of astrocyte processes at the synapse suggests that astrocytes are involved in neurotransmitter uptake, storage, and/or metabolism. This has been extensively documented for many neurotransmitters (see 4,5). Of special importance to neurogeneration is the production of neurotrophic growth factors by astrocytes. The production of the factors listed in Table 2 has been ascertained in rodent astrocyte cell culture. Few have been validated in vivo. However, with the technique of in situ hybridization it is now more directly feasible to identify the site of production of a growth factor.

A large number of mitogens induce a proliferative response in astrocytes in culture (49,51,52) (Table 3). These mitogens (51,52) as well as neurotransmitters (49) rapidly induce a large number of primary response genes that we refer to as early response genes (ERGs). Many of the ERGs code for transcriptional factors that can modulate in turn the expression of secondary genes. It is thought that some of these extracellular signals are active in vivo, but evidence is largely lacking. Astrocytes in normal adult brain are mitotically quiescent. However,

TABLE 3. *Growth factors and other mitogens active on astrocyte cultures*

Epidermal growth factor (EGF)
Basic fibroblast growth factor (bFGF)
Acidic fibroblast growth factor (aFGF)
Insulin-like growth factor (IGF-I)
Interleukin 1 (IL-1)
Interleukin-6 (IL-6)
Platelet-derived growth factor (PDGF)
Glial growth factor (GGF)
Nerve growth factor (NGF)
Glial maturation factor (GMF)
Plasminogen activator
Vasointestinal peptide (VIP)
Tumor neurosis factor (TNF)
Gamma-interferon (γ IF)
Endothelin

they proliferate rapidly during development and after trauma and several neurological disorders in the adult. Yong et al. (53,54) have shown that there are marked differences in the types of mitogens that are active in the young and adult brain. They also noted differences in the spectrum of mitogens that are active on rodent and human astrocytes. Astrocyte mitogen inhibitors have also been identified in brain extracts (46,55). These inhibitors may play a role in counteracting the action of mitogens to control astrocyte cell division in both the normal and injured CNS.

MICROGLIA

Rio-Hortega (1928; see ref. 1 for references to his earlier papers) was the first to discover and describe microglia and to deduce correctly their origin from circulating blood monocytes. Recent evidence has decided in favor of Rio-Hortega (1) over some who for the last 60 years have proposed a neuroepithelial origin of microglia. Rio-Hortega (1) described two forms of microglia, ameboid and ramified. During development ameboid microglia penetrate into brain parenchyma from the periphery as the blood-brain barrier begins to form (56). The ramified microglia with long processes appear after ameboid microglia take residence in the CNS. The mouse macrophage specific marker F4/80 has allowed researchers to follow monocytes entering the CNS and to follow their morphological transitions as they differentiate into ramified microglia (see 56). These cells are nonproliferative and are essentially resting inactive macrophages. Microglia constitute 5–10% of all neuroglia in the CNS. Their number can vary rapidly. Additional blood monocytes can invade the brain following temporary disruption of the blood-brain barrier caused by diseases or injury. Resident microglia can become activated, for instance, after injury, and become proliferative and phagocytic. Microglia are believed to be the main mediator of immunological responses in the CNS. As brain macrophages they act as antigen-presenting cells and immunoeffector cell secreting cytokines. The role of astrocytes as antigen-presenting cells (57) has not been demonstrated in vivo. Macrophage-related cells, such as vascular pericytes and microglia, can be MHCII positive, but not astrocytes. The antigens that are expressed when microglia become activated and/or phagocytic (Table 4) support the notion that microglia participate just like peripheral macrophages in immunological responses. The presence of the CD4 antigen on normal rat brain microglia coupled with the presence of HIV particles suggests that microglia are the CNS target for HIV (for review, see ref. 2).

The development of methods to culture pure populations of ameboid microglia from newborn rodent brain has greatly facilitated the study of the biology of these cells (58). The cells resemble peritoneal macrophages, but also have distinct markers and properties, suggesting that they are comparable to ameboid microglia in vivo. They can be transformed in vitro into process-bearing cells that look like resting microglia. Lipopolysaccharide (LPS) activation stimulates cultured rat microglia to make IL-1 alpha and beta as well as tumor necrosis factor (TNF) and nerve growth factor (NGF) (58–60). On the other hand the capability of astrocytes to synthesize IL-1 and TNF has recently come under strong attack and has been attributed to contamination of astrocyte cultures by microglia (58). The production of cytokines by microglia has led investigators (for review, see refs. 2,56,58) to make some provocative suggestions that bear on the response of CNS cells to various forms of injuries and neurodegenerative diseases. IL-1 and IL-6 may oppose each other in regulating astrocyte proliferation. IL-1 would stimulate (58) whereas IL-6 would inhibit proliferation. The cytokines released by microglia increase NGF and prostaglandin E release from astrocytes, generating trophic and inflammatory activities. TNF is a well-known angiogenic factor resulting in increased vascularization. In diseases that bring lymphocytic infiltration into brain parenchyma, IL-1 will stimulate T-lymphocyte proliferation, resulting in secretion of IL-2. The latter in turn regulates B-lymphocyte prolif-

TABLE 4. *Markers of rat microglia in various states of activity*

Antibody	Antigen recognized	Resting[a]	Activated[b]	Phagocytic
ox-42	CR3 complement receptor	+[c]	+ +	+ +
ox-18	MHC class I antigen	−/+	+	+
ox-6	MHC class II antigen	−	−/+	+
w3/25	CD4 antigen	−/+	−/+	+
Anti-vimentin	Vimentin	−	+	+
EDI	Monocyte antigen	−	−	−
Ki-M2R	Macrophage antigen	−	−	−

See Streit et al., ref. 2, for references.
[a]"Resting" refers to microglia in normal adult brain.
[b]"Activated" refers to proliferating nonphagocytic microglia.
[c]Code: −, absent; −/+, weak; +, distinctly positive; + +, strongly positive.

eration and hence production of antibodies. IL-2 acts on oligodendrocytes to down- or up-regulate their proliferation depending on the stage of oligodendroglial development (33).

The molecular characterization of the factors that mediate the injury response in microglia is still poorly understood. Giulian et al. (61) reported the partial characterization of two microglia mitogens that were purified from the brain of newborn rats and also after traumatic injury in the adult brain. These factors stimulate proliferation of ameboid microglia but not astroglia or oligodendroglia. One of the two factors showed macrophage colony-stimulating activity when applied to bone marrow progenitor cells.

SUPPORTING CELLS OF THE PERIPHERAL NERVOUS SYSTEM

The Cellular Organization of Nerves and Ganglia

In the peripheral nervous system both neurons and axons are ensheathed by a layer of cells. Classical histological nomenclature refers to cells encapsulating neuronal perikarya as *satellite cells* and those enfolding axons as *Schwann cells*. Satellite cells usually form a single cell covering over the neuronal perikarya, although like Schwann cells they possess the ability to form multilayered compacted myelin sheaths if presented to axons, suggesting that these two cell types are closely related and highly plastic. Schwann cells form two types of sheaths over axon. For axons of 1 μm or less in diameter, the Schwann cell can accommodate several axons individually invaginated into grooves in its cytoplasm. These axons are called *unmyelinated axons*. Schwann cells arranged in a line essentially form a continuous column containing multiple axons. The whole structure is surrounded by a *basal lamina* that is secreted by the Schwann cells. The basal lamina forms the boundary between the neural tissue and the thin connective tissue layer, called the endoneurium. The larger axons are ensheathed by a more complex membranous structure, the multilayered compact myelin. Each Schwann cell myelinates a single axon, forming a single segment or internode of myelin, separated from adjacent internodes by a bare axonal area, the node of Ranvier. The external surface of the myelinating Schwann cell is covered by a basal lamina. The cytological features that distinguish myelinating Schwann cells from oligodendrocytes include the presence of a basal lamina and of cytoplasmic channels in the compact myelin termed Schmidt-Lanterman clefts. Furthermore, unlike oligodendrocytes that can myelinate up to 50 axons, a Schwann cell myelinates a single axon. Generally a peripheral axon is either myelinated or unmyelinated over its entire length. Exceptions to this rule as well as to the general cytological organization described above are rare in mammals (14). This brief description of the histological organization of peripheral nerves is important to bear in mind when peripheral degenerating and regenerating events are considered. For instance, even in second-degree injuries where the distal portions of axons degenerate, the continuity of the endoneurial tube is usually preserved and the damaged axon grows along the same endoneurial tube. This kind of track controlling directionality of regenerating axons is absent from the adult CNS that unlike embryonic CNS lacks radial glia.

The Differentiation of Schwann Cells

During embryogenesis, at day 14–15 in the rat, Schwann cell precursors originating from the neural crest have been identified as rapidly proliferating cells over bundles of peripheral axons. As the number of Schwann cells increases, small groups of axons are individually engaged by a cell or two (62).

Progressively, the Schwann cell insinuates its cytoplasm around each axon and simultaneously on its external surface forms a basal lamina that comes in contact with the developing connective tissue, the endoneurium. Basal lamina components are essential for myelination. Inhibition of basal lamina formation inhibits myelination, whereas substances such as vitamin C that increase basal lamina assembly promote myelination (63). Interaction of the Schwann cell with the axon provides the major signal that regulates the proliferation of Schwann cells (64,65). The entire process of Schwann cell differentiation, from proliferation to myelination, can be reproduced in co-cultures of neurons and Schwann cells.

The molecular phenotype of the myelin- and non-myelin-forming Schwann cells differ greatly and has been extensively characterized by using a battery of antibodies (for review, see 66). The myelin-forming cells express myelin components: MBP, Po glycoprotein equivalent to PLP of central myelin, MAG, and P_2. Surprisingly PLP is expressed in the cytoplasm of Schwann cells, but not in its myelin sheath. The function of cytoplasmic PLP is not yet understood (67). The non-myelin-forming cells share some properties with astrocytes as exemplified by the expression of GFAP and Ran-2 (68,69). They also express the adhesion molecules N-CAM and L1 (70). An excellent marker for non-myelin-forming cells in developing and adult nerves as well as in Wallerian degeneration is the low affinity p75 NGF receptor (NGFR). This receptor is recognized by several antibodies, one of which, 217c, was used for a long time as a Schwann cell specific marker (71) but it was recently shown to be against p75NGFR (72). The antibody 217c was originally developed against a C6 glioma-associated antigen (73). In addition to rat and human glioma, NGFR is also expressed on melanoma and on Schwannoma (74). NGF treatment up-regulates p75 NGFR mRNA not only in Schwann cells, Schwannoma, and glioma but also in astrocytes (75). NGF treatment inhibits C6 glioma cell proliferation and induces c-fos and Jun B (72). Thus the function of NGFR in Schwann cells and glia may be important. The markers for non-myelin-forming Schwann cells that we have just discussed are not expressed by the peripheral myelin-forming cells. A third class of markers, such as vimentin and laminin, are expressed by both types of Schwann cells, myelinating and nonmyelinating. Surprisingly, this class also includes galactocerebroside (76) and lipid antigens (04), which in the central nervous system are expressed by oligodendrocytes, the myelin-forming cells, but not astrocytes. Finally, the astrocytic marker S-100 is a very good marker for all Schwann cells in vivo and in vitro, except for early Schwann cell precursors that migrate from the neural crest to take up residence in embryonic peripheral nerves.

Schwann cell precursors in embryonic nerves remain poorly characterized because of the lack of molecular markers. The first markers to appear as these cells progress along their developmental trajectory are S-100, 04, and then galactocerebroside (for review, see ref. 66). The axon-associated signals drive some of the galactocerebroside-positive cells to express myelin proteins while markers for nonmyelinating Schwann cells are down-regulated (77,78). The axon-associated signal that induces myelination remains to be fully characterized. Furthermore, the observation that small axons of less than 1 μM are not myelinated and that those greater than 1 μM are myelinated has not led yet to the identification of the molecules that determine whether precursor cells will myelinate or not.

The main function of the myelinating Schwann cell is its participation in saltatory conduction of the nerve impulse. Voltage-gated sodium channels clustering in the axon membrane at the node of Ranvier have been demonstrated immunocytochemically by using an antibody against rat brain sodium channels. The immunoreactivity is present in both Schwann cell cytoplasm and plasma membrane (79). Schwann cells and astrocytes in culture also express various types of sodium channels. Since both cell types project around the node of Ranvier, Ritchie et al. (79) have speculated that these glial cells might provide a supplemental source of sodium channels for transfer to axonal membrane at the node. Sodium channels have a short half-life, and the delivery of sodium channels synthesized in the neuronal perikaryon by axonal transport may not suffice. Other functions of Schwann cells are suggested by their molecular markers. As mentioned above interactions of Schwann cells with axons trigger the production of basal lamina components by Schwann cells. They include heparan sulfate proteoglycan, laminin, entactin, and collagen Types I, II, III, IV, and V (80). Some components of the extracellular matrix, such as fibronectin, are produced by fibroblasts of the endoneurium (81). Schwann cells and Schwannoma in culture secrete neurotrophic and neurite-promoting factors. Recently, glial nexin or protease nexin I, a neurite-promoting substance, has been identified after lesion of a peripheral nerve (82). The transfer of Schwann cell proteins (83) has been fairly well documented although it continues to have its skeptics.

Proliferation of Schwann Cells

Most Schwann cells are generated by proliferation after migration of neural crest precursors into embryonic nerves. Axonal contact appears to be the main signal that regulates Schwann cell proliferation. The pioneering studies of Wood and Bunge (84) elegantly demonstrated the phenomenon in Schwann cell cultures. In culture, agents that increase intracellular cyclic AMP induce the same program of differentiation as in vivo, i.e., expression of 04, myelin proteins mRNA (85) and the transcription factor (suppressed cyclic AMP induced protein) SCIP mRNA, a member of the POU gene family. The SCIP gene expression is associated with the proliferative stage of Schwann cells, a transitory stage between precursor or nonmyelinating Schwann cells and the myelinating Schwann cells (86). Cyclic AMP is not directly acting as a mitogen, but rather up-regulates the expression of platelet-derived growth factor receptor (87), which along with glial growth factor, transforming growth factor-beta, and fibroblast growth factor act as mitogens for rat Schwann cells in vitro (for references, see 88). Evidence for the in vivo role of an involvement of cyclic AMP in Schwann proliferation and differentiation remains an open question (66).

In the mature nerve Schwann cells stop proliferating. The reasons for this growth arrest are not known. However, they are not terminally differentiated cells. Nerve transection causes Schwann cells in the distal portion of the nerve to de-differentiate and recapitulate development. Myelin genes are down-regulated, NGFR is expressed (89,90), and the cells pass back transiently through the proliferative stage that correlates with SCIP gene expression.

In regenerating nerves, Schwann cells secrete NGF (91) and other growth factors (92) that are thought to replace target-derived growth factor necessary for axonal growth. The stimulus for NGF production by Schwann cells comes from IL-1 released by activated macrophages that have invaded the lesion (93). Inhibition of macrophage invasion into the lesioned nerve prevents degradation of myelin and blocks formation of NGF. To summarize, nerve lesions trigger the migration of macrophages into nerves. The phagocytosis of myelin by macrophages leads to synthesis and secretion of IL-1 by macrophages. The cytokine activates Schwann cells within 24 hours (94). Then Schwann cells express SCIP and rapidly proliferate. Thus both in normal development and after nerve transection SCIP is only expressed transiently during the period of rapid cell proliferation between the premyelinating and myelinating phases of Schwann cell differentiation. Transfection experiments (95) have shown that SCIP acts as a transcriptional repressor of myelin gene expression. Conversely, growth inhibition of Schwann cells has been proposed by Morgan et al. (96) as a permissive secondary signal for induction of myelination in quiescent cells by cyclic AMP. However, little is known about the factors and mechanisms that lead Schwann cells to become quiescent. Recent studies implicate Type I collagen and interferon gamma as potential growth inhibitors (97,98). Schwann cell culture conditioned medium may contain as yet uncharacterized growth inhibitor(s) (99). As in the case of CNS glia, investigators are now proposing that cell proliferation and its arrest result from the combinatorial control by multiple inhibitory and stimulatory substances.

ACKNOWLEDGMENTS

We thank Nancy Wainwright for assisting with the preparation of the manuscript. We also thank Sharon Belkin and Carol Gray of the MRRC Media Unit for assistance in preparing the illustrations. This work was supported by NIH grant HD-06576 and DOE contract DE-FC03-87-ER60615.

REFERENCES

1. Rio-Hortega P del. Tercera aportacion conocimiento morfologico e interpretacion functional de la oligodendroglia. *Mem Real Soc Esp Hist Nat* 1928; 14: 5–122.
2. Streit WJ, Graeber MB, Kreutzberg GW. Functional plasticity of microglia: a review. *Glia* 1988; 1: 301–307.
3. Arenander AT, de Vellis J. Frontiers of glial physiology. In: Rosenberg R, ed. *The clinical neurosciences.* New York: Churchill Livingston; 1983; 53–91.
4. Kimelberg HK, Norenberg MD. Astrocytes. *Sci Am* 1989; 260(4): 66–76.
5. Fedoroff S, Vernadakis A, eds. *Astrocytes.* New York: Academic Press; 1986.
6. Arenander AT, de Vellis J. Development of the nervous system. In: Siegel GJ et al. eds. *Basic neurochemistry: molecular, cellular, and medical aspects,* 4th ed. New York: Raven Press; 1989: 479–506.
7. Cepko C. Retrovirus vectors and their applications in neurobiology. *Neuron* 1988; 1: 345–353.
8. Cepko CL. Immortalization of neural cells via retrovirus-mediated oncogene transduction. *Annu Rev Neurosci* 1989; 12: 47–65.
9. Williams BP, Read J, Price J. The generation of neurons and oligodendrocytes from a common precursor cell. *Neuron* 1991; 7: 685–693.
10. Reynolds BA, Weiss S. Generation of neurons and astrocytes from isolated cells of the adult mammalian central nervous system. *Science* 1992; 255: 1707–1710.
11. Renfranz P, Cunningham M, McKay RDG. Region-specific differentiation of the hippocampal stem cell line HiB5 upon implantation into the developing mammalian brain. *Cell* 1991; 66: 713–729.
12. Choi BH, Kim RC, Lapham LW. Do radial glial give rise to both astroglial and oligodendroglial cells? *Dev Brain Res* 1983; 8: 119–130.
13. Misson J-P, Takahashi T, Caviness Jr, VS. Ontogeny of radial and other astroglial cells in murine cerebral cortex. *Glia* 1991; 4: 138–148.
14. Peters A, Palay SL, Webster H de F. *The fine structure of the nervous system,* 3rd ed. New York: Oxford University Press; 1991.
15. Mori S, Lebond CP. Electron microscopic identification of three classes of oligodendrocytes and a preliminary study of their proliferative activity in the corpus callosum of young rats. *J Comp Neurol* 1970; 139: 1–30.
16. Paterson J, Privat A, Ling EA, Leblond CP. Investigation of glial cells in semithin sections. III. Transformation of subependymal cells into glial cells, as shown by radioautography aft ^{3}H-thymidine injection into the lateral ventricle of the brain of young rats. *J Compar Neurol* 1973; 149: 83–103.
17. LeVine SM, Goldman J. Embryonic divergence of oligodendrocytes and astrocyte lineages in developing rat cerebrum. *J Neurosci* 1988a; 8(11): 3992–4006.
18. LeVine SM, Goldman J. Ultrastructural characteristics of GD3 ganglioside-positive glia in rat forebrain white matter. *J Comp Neurol* 1988b; 277: 456–464.
19. Hardy R, Reynolds R. Proliferation and differentiation potential of rat forebrain oligodendroglial progenitors both *in vitro* and *in vivo*. *Development* 1991; 111: 1061–1080.
20. Miller RH, ffrench-Constant C, Raff MC. The macroglial cells of the rat optic nerve. *Ann Rev* 1989; 12: 517–533.
21. Noble M. Points of controversy in the 0-2A lineage: clocks and type-2 astrocytes. *Glia* 1991; 4: 157–164.
22. McCarthy KD, de Vellis J. Preparation of separate astroglial and oligodendroglial cell cultures from rat cerebral tissue. *J Cell Biol* 1980; 85: 890–902.
23. Saneto RP, de Vellis J. Characterization of cultured rat oligodendrocytes proliferating in a serum-free, chemically defined medium. *Proc Natl Acad Sci USA* 1985b; 82: 3509–3513.
24. Skoff RP, Knapp PE. Division of astroblasts and

oligodendroblasts in postnatal rodent brain: evidence for separate astrocyte and oligodendrocyte lineages. *Glia* 1991; 4: 165–174.
25. Espinosa de los Monteros MA, Zhang M, de Vellis J. Transplantation of labelled cultured O2A and O4+ progenitors into postnatal rat brain: maturation into oligodendrocytes and absence of type 2 astrocytes. 1992; (submitted).
26. Choi BH, Kim RC. Expression of glial fibrillary acidic protein by immature oligodendroglia and its implications. *J Neuroimmunol* 1985; 8: 215–235.
27. Grinspan JB, Stern JL, Pustilnik SM, Pleasure D. Cerebral white matter contains PDGF-responsive precursors to 02A cells. *J Neurosci* 1990; 10: 1866–1873.
28. Gard AL, Pfeiffer SE. Two proliferative stages of the oligodendrocyte lineage (A2B5+O4− and O4+GalC−) under different mitogenic control. *Neuron* 1990; 5: 615–625.
29. Armstrong RC, Dorn HH, Kufta CV, Friedman E, Dubois-Dalcq ME. Pre-oligodendrocytes from adult human CNS. *J Neurosci* 1992; 12: 1538–1547.
30. Ludwin SK. Proliferation of mature oligodendrocytes after trauma to the central nervous system. *Nature* 1984; 308: 274–275.
31. McKinnon R, Matsui T, Dubois-Dalcq M, Aaronson SA. FGF modulates the PDGF-driven pathway of oligodendrocyte development. *Neuron* 1990; 5: 603–14.
32. Behar T, McMorris FA, Novotny EA, Barker JL, Dubois-Dalcq M. Growth and differentiation properties of O-2A progenitors purified from rat cerebral hemispheres. *J Neurosci Res* 1988; 21: 168–180.
33. Saneto RP, Altman A, Knobler RL, Johnson HM, de Vellis J. Interleukin 2 mediates the inhibition of oligodendrocyte progenitor cell proliferation in vitro. *Proc Natl Acad Sci USA* 1986; 83: 9221–9225.
34. Saneto RP, de Vellis J. Effect of mitogens in various organs and cell culture conditioned media on rat oligodendrocytes. *Dev Neurosci* 1985a; 7: 340–350.
35. Nordlund M, Hong D, Fei X, Ratner N. Schwann cells and cells in the oligodendrocyte lineage proliferate in response to a 50,000 dalton membrane-associated mitogen present in developing brain. *Glia* 1992; 5: 182–192.
36. Wood PM, Bunge RP. The origin of remyelinating cells in the adult central nervous system: the role of the mature oligodendrocyte. *Glia* 1991; 4: 225–232.
37. Ludwin SK. Remyelination in the central nervous system and the peripheral nervous system. In: Waxman SG, ed. *Advances in neurology, functional recovery in neurological disease*. New York: Raven Press; 1988: 215–254.
38. Kumar S, de Vellis J. Glucocorticoid-mediated functions in glial cells. In: Kimelberg H, ed. *Glial cell receptors*. New York: Raven Press; 1988: 243–264.
39. Kumar S, Cole R, Chiapelli F, de Vellis J. Differential regulation of oligodendrocyte markers by glucocorticoids: post-transcriptional regulation of both proteolipid protein and myelin basic protein and transcriptional regulation of glycerol phosphate dehydrogenase. *Proc Natl Acad Sci USA* 1989; 86: 6807–6811.
40. Farsetti A, Mitsuhashi T, Desvergne B, Robbins J, Nikodem VM. Molecular basis of thyroid hormone regulation of myelin basic protein gene expression in rodent brain. *J Biol Chem* 1991; 266: 23226–23232.
41. Espinosa de los Monteros A, Peña, de Vellis J. Does transferrin have a special role in the nervous system? *J Neurosci Res* 1989; 24: 125–136.
42. Caroni P, Schwab ME. Two membrane protein fractions from rat central myelin with inhibitory properties for neurite growth and fibroblast spreading. *J Cell Biol* 1988; 106: 1281–1288.
43. Duffy PE. *Astrocytes: normal, reactive and neoplastic*. New York: Raven Press; 1983.
44. Wu DK, Scully S, de Vellis J. Induction of glutamine synthetase in rat astrocytes by co-cultivation with embryonic chick neurons. *J Neurochem* 1988; 50: 929–935.
45. Kligman D, Hilt DC. The S100 protein family. *TIBS* 1988; 13: 437–443.
46. Hatten ME, Liem RKH, Shelanski ML, Mason CA. Astroglia in CNS injury. *Glia* 1991; 4: 233–243.
47. Chiu AY, Espinosa de los Monteros A, Cole RA, Loera S, de Vellis J. Laminin and s-Laminin are produced and released by astrocytes, Schwann cells, and Schwannomas in culture. *Glia* 1991; 4: 11–24.
48. Hamprecht B. Astroglia cells in culture: receptors and cyclic nucleotides. In: Federoff S, Vernadakis A, eds. *Astrocytes biochemistry, physiology, and pharmacology of astrocytes*, vol 2. New York: Academic Press; 1986: 77–106.
49. Arenander AT, de Vellis J, Herschman HR. Induction of c-fos and TIS genes in cultured rat astrocytes by neurotransmitters. *J Neurosci Res* 1989; 24: 107–114.
50. Janzer RC, Raff MC. Astrocytes induce blood-brain barrier properties in endothelial cells. *Nature* 1987; 325: 253–257.
51. Arenander AT, Lim RW, Varnum BC, Cole R, de Vellis J, Herschman HR. TIS gene expression in cultured rat astrocytes: induction by mitogens and stellation agents. *J Neurosci Res* 1989; 23: 247–256.
52. Arenander AT, Lim RW, Varnum BC, Cole R, de Vellis J, Herschman HR. TIS gene expression in cultured rat astrocytes: multiple pathways of induction of mitogens. *J Neurosci Res* 1989; 13: 257–265.
53. Yong VW, Kim SU, Pleasure DE. Growth factors for fetal and adult human astrocytes in culture. *Brain Res* 1988; 444: 59–66.
54. Yong VW, Tejada-Berges T, Antel JP, Yong FP. Differential proliferative response of adult human and neonatal mouse astrocytes to gamma-interferon and interleukin-1. *Glia* 1992; (in press).
55. Nieto-Sampedro M, Saneto RP, de Vellis J, Cotman CW. The control of glial populations in brain: changes in astrocyte mitogenic and mor-

phogenic factors in response to injury. *Brain Res* 1985; 343: 320–328.
56. Perry VH, Gordon S. Macrophages and microglia in the nervous system. *TINS* 1988; 44: 273–277.
57. Fontana A, Fierz W, Wekerle H. Astrocytes present myelin basic protein to encephalitogenic T-cell lines. *Nature* 1984; 307: 273–276.
58. Giulian D. Ameboid microglia as effectors of inflammation in the central nervous system. *J Neurosci Res* 1987; 18: 155–171.
59. Hetier E, Ayala J, Denèfle P, Bousseau A, Rouget P, Mallat M, Prochiantz A. Brain macrophages synthesize interleukine-1 and interleukine-1 nRNAs in vitro. *J Neurosci Res* 1988; 21: 391–397.
60. Mallat M, Houlgatte R, Brachet P, Prochiantz A. Lipopolysaccharide-stimulated brain macrophages release NGF in vitro. *Dev Biol* 1989; 133: 309–311.
61. Giulian D, Johnson B, Krebs JF, George JK, Tapscott M. Microglial mitogens are produced in the developing and injured mammalian brain. *J Cell Biol* 1991; 112: 323–333.
62. Webster H de F, Favilla JT. Development of peripheral nerve fibres. In: Dyck PJ, Thomas PK, Lambert EH, Bunge R, eds. *Peripheral neuropathy*. Philadelphia: W.B. Saunders; 1984: 329–359.
63. Eldridge GC, Bunge MB, Bunge MB, Wood PM. Differentiation of axon-related Schwann cells in vitro. I. Ascorbic acid regulates basal lamina assembly and myelin formation. *J Cell Biol* 1987; 105: 1023–1034.
64. Ratner N, Bunge RP, Glaser L. A neuronal heparan sulfate proteoglycan is required for dorsal root ganglion neuron stimulation of Schwann cell proliferation. *J Cell Biol* 1985; 101: 744–754.
65. Ratner N, Hong D, Lieberman MA, Bunge RP, Glaser L. The neuronal cell-surface molecule mitogenic for Schwann cells is a heparin binding protein. *Proc Natl Acad Sci USA* 1988; 85: 6992–6996.
66. Jessen KR, Mirsky R. Schwann cell precursors and their development. *Glia* 1991; 4: 185–194.
67. Puckett C, Hudson L, Ono K, Friedrich V, Benecke J, Dubois-Dalcq M, Lazzarini RA. Myelin-specific proteolipid protein is expressed in myelinating Schwann cells but is not incorporated into myelin sheaths. *J Neurosci Res* 1987; 18: 511–518.
68. Jessen KR, Thorpe R, Mirsky R. Molecular identity, distribution and heterogeneity of glial fibrillary acidic protein: an immunoblotting and immunohistochemical study of Schwann cells, satellite cells, enteric glia and astrocytes. *J Neurocytol* 1984; 13: 187–200.
69. Jessen KR, Mirsky R. Non-myelin-forming Schwann cells coexpress surface proteins and intermediate filaments not found in myelin forming cells: a study of Ran-2, A5E3 antigen and glial fibrillary acidic protein. *J Neurocytol* 1984; 13: 923–934.
70. Mirsky R, Jessen KR, Schachner M, Goridis C. Distribution of the adhesion molecules N-CAM and L1 on peripheral neurons and glia in adult rats. *J Neurocytol* 1986; 15: 799–815.
71. Fields KL, Dammerman M. A monoclonal antibody equivalent to anti-rat neural antigen-1 as a marker for Schwann cells. *Neuroscience* 1985; 15: 877–885.
72. Kumar S, Huber J, Pena LA, Perez-Polo JR, Werrbach-Perez K, de Vellis J. Characterization of functional nerve growth factor-receptors in a CNS glial cell line: monoclonal antibody 217c recognizes the nerve growth factor receptor on C6 glioma cells. *J Neurosci Res* 1990; 27: 56–70.
73. Peng WW, Bressler JP, Tiffany-Castiglioni E, de Vellis J. Development of a monoclonal antibody against a tumor-associated antigen. *Science* 1982; 215: 1102–1104.
74. Peacocke M, Yaar M, Mansur CP, Chao MV, Gilchrest BA. Induction of nerve growth factor receptors on cultured human melanocytes. *Proc Natl Acad Sci USA* 1988; 85: 5282–5286.
75. Kumar S, Pena L, de Vellis J. Expression of NGFR and trkB in normal and transformed glial cells. *Trans Am Soc* 1992; 23: 99.
76. Jessen KR, Mirsky R, Morgan L. Axonal signals regulate the differentiation of non-myelin forming Schwann cells: an immunohistochemical study of galactocerebroside in transected and regenerating nerves. *J Neurosci* 1987b; 7: 3362–3369.
77. Mirsky R, Winter J, Abney R, Pruss RM, Gavrilovic J, Raff MC. Myelin-specific proteins and glycolipids in rat Schwann cells and oligodendrocytes in culture. *J Cell Biol* 1980; 84: 483–494.
78. Jessen KR, Mirsky R, Morgan L. Myelinated, but not unmyelinated axons reversibly down-regulate N-CAM in Schwann cells. *J Neurocytol* 1987a; 16: 681–688.
79. Ritchie JM, Black JA, Waxman SG, Angelides KJ. Sodium channels in the cytoplasm of Schwann cells. *Proc Natl Acad Sci USA* 1990; 87: 9290–9294.
80. Bunge RP, Bunge MB, Eldridge CF. Linkage between axonal ensheathment and basal lamina production by Schwann cells. *Annu Rev Neurosci* 1986; 9: 305–328.
81. Sanes JR, Chiu AY. The basal lamina of the neuromuscular junction. *Cold Spring Harbor Symp Quant Biol* 1983; 48: 667–678.
82. Meier R, Spreyer P, Ortmann R, Harel A, Mondard D. Induction of glia-derived nexin after lesion of a peripheral nerve. *Nature* 1989; 342: 548–551.
83. Lasek RJ, Gainer H, Przybylski J. Transfer of newly synthesized proteins from Schwann cells to the squid giant axon. *Proc Natl Acad Sci USA* 1974; 71: 1188–1192.
84. Wood PM, Bunge RP. Evidence that sensory axons are mitogenic for Schwann cells. *Nature* 1975; 256: 662–664.
85. Lemke G, Chao M. Axons regulate Schwann cell expression of the major myelin and NGF receptor genes. *Development* 1988; 102: 499–504.

86. Monuki ES, Weinmaster G, Kuhn L, Lemke G. SCIP: a glial POU domain gene regulated by cyclic AMP. *Neuron* 1989; 3: 783–793.
87. Weinmaster G, Lemke G. Cell-specific cyclic AMP-mediated induction of the PDGF receptor. *EMBO J* 1990; 9: 915–920.
88. Davis JB, Stroobant P. Platelet-derived growth factors and fibroblast growth factors are mitogenic for rat Schwann cells. *J Cell Biol* 1990; 110: 1353–1360.
89. Taniuchi M, Clark HB, Johnson Jr, EM. Induction of nerve growth factor receptor in Schwann cells after axotomy. *Proc Natl Acad Sci USA* 1986; 83: 4094–4098.
90. Taniuchi M, Clark HB, Schweitzer JB, Johnson Jr, EM. Expression of nerve growth factor receptors by schwann cells of axotomized peripheral nerves: ultrastructural location, suppression by axonal contact, and binding properties. *J Neurosci* 1988; 8: 665–681.
91. Heumann R, Korsching S, Bandtlow C, Thoenen H. Changes of nerve growth factor synthesis in non-neuronal cells in response to sciatic nerve transection. *J Cell Biol* 1987a; 104: 1623–1631.
92. Bosch PE, Zhong W, Lim R. Axonal signals regulate expression of glial maturation factor beta in Schwann cells: an immunohistochemical study of injured sciatic nerves and cultured Schwann cells. *J Neurosci* 1989; 9: 3690–3698.
93. Heumann R, Lindholm D, Bandtlow C, et al. Differential regulation of mRNA encoding nerve growth factor and its receptor in rat sciatic nerve during development, degeneration and regeneration: role of macrophages. *Proc Natl Acad Sci USA* 1987b; 84: 8735–8739.
94. Le Beau JM, LaCorbiere M, Powell HC, Ellisman MH, Schubert D. Extracellular fluid conditioned during peripheral nerve regeneration stimulates Schwann cell adhesion, migration and proliferation. *Brain Res* 1988; 459: 93–104.
95. Monuki ES, Kuhn R, Weinmaster G, Trapp BD, Lemke G. Expression and activity of the POU transcription factor SCIP. *Science* 1990; 249: 1300–1303.
96. Morgan L, Jessen KR, Mirsky R. The effects of cAMP on differentiation of cultured Schwann cells: progression from an early phenotype (O4$^+$) to a myelin phenotype (P_0^+, GFAP$^-$, N-CAM$^-$, NGF-Receptor$^-$) depends on growth inhibition. *J Cell Biol* 1991; 112: 457–467.
97. Eccleston PA, Bannerman PGC, Pleasure DE, Winter J, Mirsky R, Jessen KR. Control of peripheral glial cell proliferation: enteric neurons exert an inhibitory influence on Schwann cell and enteric glial cell DNA synthesis in culture. *Development* 1989a; 107: 107–112.
98. Eccleston PA, Jessen KR, Mirsky R. Transforming growth factor-β and α-interferon have dual effects on growth of peripheral glia. *J Neurosci Res* 1989b; 24: 524–530.
99. Eccleston PA, Jessen KR, Mirsky R. Spontaneous Schwann cell immortalization in vitro: short-term cultures Schwann cells secrete growth inhibitory activity. *Development* 1991; (in press).

5

Adhesive Molecules of the Cell Surface and Extracellular Matrix in Neural Regeneration

Salvatore Carbonetto and Samuel David

Neuroscience Research Center, McGill University, Montreal General Hospital, Research Institute, Montreal, Quebec, H3G 1A4 Canada

During development retinal ganglion cells extend axons to the optic disc. The first axons to emerge from the retina into the optic nerve serve as pioneers for later arriving ones. At the optic chiasm axons make a critical choice, some crossing over to the opposite tectum and others turning back to grow toward the ipsilateral tectum. This choice appears to involve both repulsion at the chiasm and bundling of crossing axons with noncrossing ones from the contralateral eye. Once in the tract the axons grow near the surface of the brain and later into the tectum to form a topographical map.

In most vertebrates, after cutting of the optic nerve, recapitulation of the developmental events responsible for the original map is negligible and many neurons die (1). Even those cells that survive are normally unable to grow and reconnect with their targets, although they can regenerate axons and form synapses within the brain when connected by peripheral nerve grafts (2). This sequelae of abortive regeneration in the central nervous system (CNS) stands in stark contrast to that seen in the peripheral nervous system (PNS), where neurons that survive regenerate robustly to their targets after axotomy and reinnervate them with, at times, exquisite precision. At the myoneural junction this regeneration follows a template of extracellular matrix (ECM) proteins that control growth along the nerve (3) and reformation of both pre- and postsynaptic elements of the myoneural junction (4).

Many studies in vitro have implicated adhesive proteins in nerve fiber growth. Their function is fundamental to the motility of the growth cone, which must adhere to a substratum to generate the contractile forces that lead the extending axon. A detailed description of growth cone motility can be obtained from several recent reviews (e.g., 5). Briefly, the cellular events begin with extension of filopodia from the apex of the growth cone. Once extended, a filopodium may attach to either adhesive proteins of the cell surface or the extracellular matrix. The resulting ligand-receptor complexes associate or stabilize associations with cytoskeletal proteins, ultimately interacting with microfilaments and microtubules (6) to extend the main axon cylinder.

Studies over the past year have led to identification of several families of adhesive molecules that act together to mediate the chemoaffinities among neural cells postulated by Sperry (7) to be responsible for the specificity of connections in the CNS. These include three to four families of cell adhesion molecules (CAMs) as well as ECM adhesive proteins and their receptors. Our purpose here is to discuss these adhesive molecules in the context of neural regeneration. The reader can obtain a more comprehensive view of adhesion molecules from several excellent reviews discussing their structures and functions in neural and nonneural cells (8–15). In addition, we discuss the more recent notion that the CNS harbors molecules that are nonpermissive or actively inhibitory of nerve growth.

CELL ADHESION MOLECULES

The Immunoglobulin Superfamily

The molecules that belong to this superfamily all have structural motifs referred to as immunoglobulin (Ig) domains, each of which consists of about 100 amino acids looped by a disulfide bridge (16). The phylogenetically oldest and best-characterized member is neural cell adhesion molecule (N-CAM). Other members in the vertebrate nervous system include L1,Ng-CAM, contactin, F11/F3, Tag-1/axonin-1, MAG, P_0 (12,17), and two recently cloned molecules Nr-CAM (18) and SC1/DM-GRASP (19,20). Adhesion molecules with Ig-like domains have also been identified in the nervous system of invertebrates (21).

Neural Cell Adhesion Molecule

Multiple forms of membrane-associated N-CAM are derived from a single gene by alternative RNA splicing (16). In the rodent brain there are three isoforms with apparent molecular weights of 190, 135, and 115 kDa (22–24). The extracellular portions of these three isoforms are similar (25). The two larger isoforms possess membrane spanning and cytoplasmic domains, while the smallest isoform is anchored to the membrane via phosphatidylinositol (PI) (26,27). The two larger isoforms differ from each other in the length of their cytoplasmic carboxy terminal domains. Only the largest isoform is able to interact with cytoskeletal proteins (28,29), giving it less lateral mobility within the cell membrane, and implicating it in stabilization of cell contacts. The three forms are also distributed differentially amongst various cells, e.g., oligodendrocytes express mainly the 115 isoform (30), astrocytes express the 135 and 115 kDa isoforms (31), and neurons express mainly the 190 and 135 kDa isoforms of N-CAM (32). Soluble forms of N-CAM have also been identified in neural cell culture conditioned media, cerebrospinal fluid and blood. One of the soluble forms (115 kDa) appears to be the PI-linked N-CAM (26,33). In addition, a secreted form of N-CAM derived from a distinct mRNA has been identified in muscle and brain (34). The secreted forms of N-CAM can bind certain components of the extracellular matrix, and thus modulate N-CAM function. For example, N-CAM has been shown to bind to heparin and heparan sulfate (35,36), and may thus enhance or interfere with cell-matrix interactions. However, it is unlikely that soluble N-CAM competes with homophilic interactions of cellular N-CAM since its affinity is low.

N-CAM is highly glycosylated and contains side-chains of polysiliac acid residues (16). During development, N-CAM becomes less sialyated (37), less sulfated (24,38), and phosphorylated (38). Changes, particularly in polysialyation, influence the adhesive properties of N-CAM and are involved in the regulation of axonal growth during development (22,39,40). Moreover, Key and Akeson (41) have reported a uniquely glycosylated N-CAM in the olfactory system emphasizing the potential of carbohydrates on N-CAM in determining neural specificity. Antibodies against N-CAM have been shown to disrupt normal histogenesis of the retina in vitro (42,43). Injections of such antibodies into the developing eye in vivo resulted in disruption of the pattern of axon growth at the optic fissure and in the optic nerve (44,45). That N-CAM might influence other morphogenetic events was also suggested by the failure of the normal conversion of N-CAM from the embryonic to the adult form in the cerebellum of the staggerer mouse mutant (22). Antibodies against N-CAM have also been shown to partially inhibit the migration of cerebellar granule cells in explant cultures (43). This migration involves several adhesion molecules including astrotactin, tenascin, L1, laminin, and thrombospondin. Inhibition of any one of these molecules results in partial inhibition of the rate or distance of neuronal migration.

Neurite outgrowth on astrocyte monolayers is mediated via multiple adhesive systems including N-CAM (46). The degree of involvement of N-CAM varies among different neuronal cell types and with the age of the neurons (46). For example, N-CAM does not appear to contribute to the growth of ciliary neurons on astrocytes (47), but it does mediate growth from E11 (but not E7 chick) retinal neurons on astrocytes (48). Although purified N-CAM immobilized onto a nitrocellulose substrate was not found to promote neurite growth (49), growth is enhanced on monolayers of 3T3 cells transfected with N-CAM cDNA (50–53). In the latter experiments, the transmembrane and PI-linked isoforms of N-CAM were found to be potent promoters of neurite growth from postnatal day 7 cerebellar neurons, while 3T3 cell lines expressing the secreted form of N-CAM did not promote neurite growth (53). The adhesiveness of liposomes containing N-CAM is an exponential function of the amount of N-CAM in the liposomes. In cells, a threshold level of N-CAM is required before stimulation of neurite growth occurs, and small increases in N-CAM beyond this level result in large increases in neurite growth (51). Doherty et al. (53) have also reported a developmental loss in the ability of chick retinal neurons to extend neurites onto monolayers of 3T3 cells transfected with human N-CAM cDNA. E6 but not E11 chick retinal ganglion cells extend long neurites on transfected 3T3 cells. This loss in neurite outgrowth-promoting ability was attributed to changes in N-CAM polysialic acid (53).

Neurite growth from E6 chick retinal ganglion cells onto monolayers of 3T3 cells transfected with N-CAM cDNA can be inhibited by removal of α2-8-linked polysialic acid from the neuronal N-CAM (53). This observation might seem a bit surprising since reduction in polysialic acid increases the avidity of N-CAM-N-CAM interactions. However, neuronal attachment to adhesive substrata consisting of lectins (54), antibodies (55), or ECM proteins (56) does not correlate directly with neurite outgrowth. For example, growth cones adhere less well to laminin than to fibronectin but extend more vigorously on laminin (56). This discrepancy between adhesion and neurite growth may reflect the fact that adhesive contacts turnover as the axon advances. Quantitative assays of the kinetics of cell attachment (57) will help reveal the complexity of these interactions that must be adhesive enough to support growth cone attachment yet not so adhesive as to inhibit its advance.

During innervation of the developing chick hindlimb, decreases in polysialic acid results in increased axon-axon interaction and a decrease in branching of the nerves (58), possibly mediated via the adhesion molecule L1. Conversely, increases in polysialic acid produce increased axon-myotube interactions with increased branching of the nerves (40,58). In culture, Acheson et al. (59) showed that enzymatic removal of polysialic acid from a neuronal cell line augments cell-cell aggregation as well as cell-substrate attachment mediated via other adhesion molecules. Thus, the degree of sialyation of N-CAM may have an influence not only on N-CAM, but also on the effectiveness of other adhesion systems.

In the PNS, isoforms of N-CAM change in their expression and distribution in the nerve and muscle following nerve injury (60–63). N-CAM is also found at sites of contact between axons and Schwann cells and fibroblasts in the regenerating sciatic nerve (63), suggesting that N-CAM might play a role in axonal regeneration in the

PNS, as well as the reinnervation of muscle. The available evidence indicates that N-CAM is important in the genesis of nerve-muscle innervation but may contribute in a minor way to regeneration of peripheral nerves (64), although in the CNS of amphibians, antibodies to N-CAM substantially disrupt the reestablishment of the topographic projection of the retina onto the tectum (65).

L1, Ng-CAM

Another group of CAMs that belong to the Ig-superfamily include L1, which was identified in the mouse (66), and Ng-CAM (neuron-glial-CAM), identified in chicken (67). Unlike N-CAM, L1/Ng-CAM appears later in development, soon after neurons become postmitotic (68,69). It is found on neurons in the CNS and PNS, as well as on Schwann cells (69). Mouse L1 has immunochemical similarities to NILE (nerve growth factor inducible large external glycoprotein) in rat (70) and Ng-CAM in chicken (67). Recent studies, however, indicate only a 40% overall amino acid identity between Ng-CAM and L1 (71), suggesting that Ng-CAM is not merely the chick homologue of mouse L1. Comparison of mouse L1 with the partial amino acid sequence of rat and human NILE indicates more than 80% identity (70).

L1 is a glycoprotein that appears as three polypeptides of 200, 140, and 80 kDa (68, 72) produced by a single gene (73,74) with the 140 and 80 kDa proteins being derived from the 200 kDa protein (75). The same statements apply to Ng-CAM, which has forms of 210–190, 135, and 80 kDa (76). L1 and Ng-CAM are integral membrane glycoproteins, with six Ig-like domains, five fibronectin (FN) type III repeats (71,74), and potential phosphorylation sites on the cytoplasmic domain (71,74). There are, however, differences in the number and location of RGD (Arg-Gly-Asp) sequences (discussed below) in L1 and Ng-CAM. L1 has two RGD sequences in the sixth Ig-domain, while Ng-CAM has one such sequence in the second FN type III repeat. The 135 kDa polypeptide consists of the N-terminal region of the molecule with the six Ig-domains, while the 80 kDa polypeptide consists of part of the FN type III repeats and the transmembrane and cytoplasmic domains (71). Despite the poor overall amino acid identity between L1 and Ng-CAM, these molecules show many structural and functional similarities, suggesting that even if they are distinct molecules, they are closely related members of a family.

L1 and Ng-CAM appear to mediate axon-axon interactions, particularly, axon fasciculation. Its effects on axon fasciculation have been observed in explant cultures of the developing cerebellum (77) and peripheral dorsal root ganglia (43). Fasciculation is likely to be mediated via homophilic interactions, although heterophilic binding between Ng-CAM containing neuronal membrane vesicles and an as yet uncharacterized receptor on Ng-CAM-negative glial cells have also been demonstrated (67,78). L1-mediated interactions may also be involved in the migration of cerebellar granule cells from the external to the internal granule cell layer during development, which is inhibited in explant cultures by the presence of antibodies to L1/Ng-CAM (43,66). L1 and Ng-CAM probably function in the early stages of granule cell migration, and not the later stages, which involve interactions with Bergmann glia (79).

In addition, to its effects on axon fasciculation, L1 also mediates neurite growth, on other neurites (80), Schwann cells (81–83), Müller glia (84), and astrocytes (85). Purified L1 immobilized onto a nitrocellulose substrate is capable of promoting neurite outgrowth via a homophilic interaction (49). The growth on Müller glia and astrocytes must be via a heterophilic mechanism, since central glia do not express L1. Antibodies to L1 also have a profound inhibitory effect on the ensheathment of axons and neuronal cell bodies by Schwann cells (86). The blocking of ensheathment by anti-L1 is also accompanied by failure of Schwann cells to acquire other differentiation markers, such as the failure to express MAG or collagen or to form a basal lamina (86). Anti-N-CAM, however, has only a small effect on Schwann cell ensheathment, and no effect on the expression of the other differentiation markers (86). In the regenerating adult mouse sciatic nerve L1 is localized to the sites of contact between growing axons, and between axons and Schwann cells (63).

Nr-CAM

Recently, another cell adhesion molecule, Nr-CAM, has been identified which is related to Ng-CAM and belongs to the Ig-superfamily. Nr-CAM has a structure similar to Ng-CAM/L1 (18), i.e., six Ig-like domains, 5 FN type III repeats, a transmembrane, and short cytoplasmic domain. However, the identity of Nr-CAM to these CAMs is only about 40% (18). Nr-CAM specific antibodies recognize a glycoprotein of 145 kDa and a less prevalent protein of 170 kDa. Nr-CAM is localized to the cell surface of neurons, and increases during development of the brain up to embryonic day 12, followed by slightly lower levels (18).

SC1/DM-GRASP

Another member of the Ig-superfamily is SC1/DM-GRASP, which is an integral membrane glycoprotein with a Mr of 95–100 kDa found in embryonic chicken (19,20,87). This molecule has five Ig-like domains, a transmembrane, and a short cytoplasmic domain. SC1/DM-GRASP is expressed on spinal motor neurons, floor plate, and dorsal root ganglia of E5 chicks and disappears by E9 (19,20). The immunohistochemical labeling is distributed over neuronal cell bodies as well as axons. Experiments using an embryonic human kidney cell line expressing SC1 indicate that SC1 can mediate cell-cell adhesion (19). In vitro, antibodies to DM-GRASP inhibit neurite growth on axons, and purified DM-GRASP promotes neurite growth (20).

F3/F11, TAG-1/Axonin-1, Contactin

Another subclass of cell adhesion molecules that belong to the Ig-superfamily are those that are anchored to the cell membrane via phosphatidylinositol and that possess six Ig-like motifs and four FN type III repeats. These molecules include F3 (chick)/F11 (mouse) (88,89), TAG-1 (rat)/axonin-1 (chick) (90,91), and contactin (94). F3 and F11 show a 77% homology at the protein level, while TAG-1 and axonin-1 have a 76% sequence identity (93). The chick cell adhesion molecule contactin has a 64–79% amino acid identity with F3 in its extracellular portion (88). Contactin, however, differs from F3 in that it is an integral membrane glycoprotein with a transmembrane region and a cytoplasmic carboxy terminal region (94). These adhesion molecules have molecular weights of 130–135 kDa (89–92), and have been localized to the surface of neuronal cell bodies and axons, where they appear to mediate neurite and axon growth (90,95). In addition, these PI-linked adhesion molecules may also be released from the cell and could also mediate adhesion after being immobilized on to a suitable substrate (96). Recent evidence shows that similarly anchored cell surface proteins may form complexes with tyrosine kinases following binding of ligand or antibodies to the receptor (97). In the developing rat spinal cord, TAG-1 is found on the axons of commissural neurons before they cross the midline floor plate. After they cross the midline, these axons loose TAG-1 and acquire L1 on the contralateral portion (98). Thus, molecules such as TAG-1 might play a role at certain restricted times during the period of axon growth.

Cadherins

In contrast to the Ca^{++}-independent CAMs described above, the molecules that belong to the cadherin family mediate cell adhesion in a Ca^{++}-dependent manner (15). A number of cadherins have been identified (E, P, N, B, R, and T cadherins) and their cloned cDNAs indicate about 40–60% amino acid homology among them. N (neural), R (retinal), B (brain), and T (truncated) cadherins arc found in the CNS (99–101), and range in Mr between 120 and 127 kDa, expect for T-cadherin which has a Mr of 95 kDa. The various cadherins possess common structural features, such as four internally repeated extracellular domains, four conserved cysteine residues in the extracellular domain close to the membrane spanning region, and putative Ca^{++}-binding sites (102,103). All except T-cadherin, possess transmembrane and cytoplasmic domains (101). Cadherins interact with actin microfilaments, and cytoplasmic proteins called catenins (103). Unlike the other cadherins, T-cadherin is anchored to the membrane via phosphatidylinositol (101). The tripeptide HAV (His-Ala-Val), shown to be a cell adhesion recognition sequence, is conserved in all cadherins except T-cadherin, and is located in the first extracellular domain (104,105). Eight new cadherin cDNAs were recently isolated, which are expressed in the nervous system (106). Other members of the cadherin superfamily include the desmosomal glycoproteins, desmoglein and desmocollins. These have only a 30–35% homology with classic cadherins, such as N-cadherin (103).

Cadherins are expressed early in the developing nervous system (102). N-cadherin is expressed in the promordia of the CNS and PNS and is thought to play a role in the segregation of these cells from the E-cadherin-expressing ectoderm (102,107). In the chick retina, N-cadherin appears early (neuroepithelial stage) and gradually decreases before hatching, while R-cadherin appears later (E8) and persists (99). Ectopic expression of N-cadherin (107,108), or blocking of N-cadherin by antibodies (109), results in disruption of normal tissue histogenesis.

Cadherin-mediated adhesion is homophilic, i.e., one type of cadherin on one cell interacting with a like cadherin on another cell (102). Since cells may possess more than one type of cadherin, their intercellular recognition, sorting, and aggregation may depend upon the cadherin profile present on each cell type. The binding specificities of different cadherins have been localized to the N-terminal 113 amino acids, in particular the highly conserved HAV sequence and the nonconserved amino acids flanking this region (104,105). This region of the molecule has also been shown to mediate neurite outgrowth (52,85,105). Neurite growth on astrocytes and Schwann cells is mediated in part by N-cadherin (46), and the extent of its involvement in such growth differs with different types of neurons (47,48). Changes in the expression of cadherins in degeneration and regeneration in the nervous system have yet to be described.

THE EXTRACELLULAR MATRIX

The extracellular matrix (ECM) is organized into sheets of basement membrane beneath epithelia separating them from cells of mesenchymal origin and orienting the epithelium into basal and luminal aspects. In the nervous system basement membranes are found in endoneurial tubes (110) beneath the meninges (111), at the interface of capillary endothelium and processes of astroglia or ependymal tanycytes (112), and as part of the inner limiting membrane of the retina. Basement membranes also surround muscle cells and are specialized at myoneural junctions (113). Surrounding the basement membrane in peripheral nerves is a perineural space filled with a stroma of ECM that includes collagen fibrils oriented with the long axis of the nerve (114). Basement membranes are lacking among neural cells in the adult mammalian CNS, although densities of extracellular materials are commonly seen within synaptic clefts in electron micrographs of the CNS (111). The ECM of the adult CNS has a relatively large amount of proteoglycan (115,116) and is deficient in glycoproteins. In contrast, embryonic CNS contains laminin, fibronectin, thrombospondin, vitronectin, and cytotactin, all distributed diffusely outside basement membranes (117–123). Expression of laminin in neural tissues correlates with the ability to support nerve fiber growth in vivo and in vitro (124). Changes in both the amounts and distribution of ECM components alter the influence of the CNS milieu on neuronal development and regrowth.

Extracellular Matrix Glycoproteins

Molecular constituents of the ECM have been categorized broadly as collagens, noncollagenous glycoproteins, and proteoglycans. All of the ECM proteins in the nervous system were originally identified in nonneural tissues. More recent evidence indicates that there is an impressive variability of isoforms of these molecules that arise from multiple genes, alternative splicing, and combinatorial assembly of subunits. This molecular heterogeneity has functional consequences as evidenced by the neural specific expression of some forms within the nervous system. Several "unconventional" ECM proteins have been identified, including myelin-associated glycoprotein (63), N-CAM (62), agrin (4), as well as amyloid beta protein and its precursor (125), all of which have significant relationship to the nervous system.

Many, but not all of the functions of ECM proteins relate to their adhesive properties. Laminin has effects on cells that mimic those of EGF (126) and NGF (127). It also stimulates Schwann cell replication (128,129), neuronal survival (127,130), peripheral myelination (131), differentiation of pigmented epithelia into neurons (132), and induction of tyrosine hydroxylase (133). In addition to the endogenous growth factor activity of some ECM components, proteoglycans bind and/or regulate the activity of diffusible growth factors such as fibroblast growth factor (134,135) and transforming growth factor β (136) as well as proteases (137) and protease inhibitors (138).

The expanding data base of cloned and sequenced proteins together with details of their functions in cell adhesion and matrix assembly have brought into focus a variety of motifs within ECM proteins, their receptors, and CAMs. These motifs, which include EGF-like repeats, FN type III repeats, Ig domains, and lectin-binding regions, promise to simplify structure/function analyses of these otherwise varied and complex proteins. For example, FN type III repeats are found in tenascin, thrombospondin as well as the CAMs, N-CAM, L1, Ng-CAM, F3/F11, Tag-1/axonin-1, contactin, and Nr-CAM (discussed below). Recently, a gene coding for a secreted protein containing FN type III repeats has been implicated in Kallman's syndrome (139, 140), a genetic disorder in which a subset of hypothalamic neurons fails to migrate in from the olfactory epithelium (141,142).

Fibronectin has multiple sites for cell attachment that have been defined by proteolytic fragments and synthetic peptides that mimic regions within the native molecule as well as by mutated recombinant proteins. The first cell adhesion site identified included a key tripeptide sequence (RGD) (143) that is recognized by an integrin fibronectin receptor ($\alpha 5 \beta 1$) integrin. Proteolytic fragments of fibronectin encompassing this sequence mediate neurite outgrowth from dorsal root ganglion and sympathetic neurons (144). Nonoverlapping fragments closer to the carboxy terminus of fibronectin also mediate neurite growth (145). This latter domain contains a site that binds heparin as well as a distinct site (146) for cell attachment within the III CS region, an alternatively spliced domain within fibronectin (147,148). Neuronal adhesion and neurite outgrowth to the heparin-binding region is likely to be mediated through a cell-surface proteoglycan (149). Interestingly, a proteolytic fragment of fibronectin containing the carboxy terminal heparin-binding region and the III CS region, but not the RGD sequence mediates more neurite outgrowth from spinal cord neurons than does the RGD-containing fragment (145). Thus, integrins and proteoglycan receptors may be differentially expressed within the nervous system.

The identification of binding sites that are mimicked by short stretches of amino acids and the power of synthetic peptides that serve as antagonists in solution has generated great interest in extending this strategy to other ligands. A variety of sequences thought to mimic functional domains in laminin and fibronectin have been reported (150). RGD has a relatively widespread occurrence and is functional in a subset of ECM proteins, such as fibronectin, vitronectin, fibrinogen, and thrombospondin (151–153). However, the RGD sequence in laminin is nonfunctional in neurite growth. Indeed, denatured laminin has essentially no activity in neural adhesion, which is somewhat surprising since several synthetic peptides of laminin have been reported to mediate neurite outgrowth when immobilized on culture substrata (150,154).

Laminin, fibronectin, collagen and other ECM proteins are not individual molecules but multigene families. S-laminin, a B2 chain homologue that presumably assembles into a heterotrimer in vivo, is localized almost exclusively to the myoneural junction (155). Merosin, an A chain homologue (156) combined with a B1 and B2 subunit is found in the basal laminae surrounding Schwann-cells (157). S-laminin and merosin are encoded by genes distinct from their more conventional homologues. Substitution of A for M or S for B2 indicates that four distinct heterotrimers can be assembled, and it is likely that others will be discovered in the foreseeable future. The two A chain homologues (M, A) differ in the end of their long arms, a region implicated in receptor-mediated neurite outgrowth on laminin. However, initial studies indicate that the two isoforms behave similarly in cell adhesion (158) so that the regulation of their expression may be key to their functions in vivo.

The contribution of ECM molecules to peripheral nerve regeneration has been the subject of some controversy. In the PNS Schwann cells are the major cell type that interact with regenerating axons. Advancing growth cones are found in contact with basement membranes (159) as well as Schwann cells (160). Removal of Schwann cells by a variety of means substantially inhibits PNS regeneration (160). However, Schwann cells not only mediate growth via CAMs but also by the ECM proteins (81) they synthesize and assemble into a basement membrane. Depleting the nerve of Schwann cells to evaluate the contribution of cells versus ECM may alter the balance of adhesive systems normally sensed by growth cones. In peripheral nerves, laminin stimulates axon regeneration (161) and antibodies to laminin inhibit regeneration (3). In addition, an antibody to an integrin inhibits nerve regeneration (162). While the precise steps of nerve regeneration to which ECM proteins contribute have yet to be detailed, it seems clear that ECM proteins contribute to peripheral nerve regeneration.

Proteoglycans

There has been a great increase in information on proteoglycans in the nervous system (163) facilitated by new methods of analysis and molecular cloning of core proteins in nonneural tissues (14). Proteoglycans consist of a peptide backbone with glycosaminoglycan (GAG) side chains, in addition to N-linked carbohydrates. They have been classified by their major GAG component as heparan sulfate or chondroitin sulfate proteoglycans although it has long been recognized that there is considerable heterogeneity in their carbohydrate composition and core proteins. Proteoglycans can be extracellular matrix proteins, intracellular proteins associated with synaptic and secretory vesicles (164,165), or can be bound to the plasma membrane as transmembrane proteins (166). In neural cells, proteoglycans have been implicated in the localization of acetylcholine receptors (167) and acetylcholinesterase (168) at the myoneural junction, as well as in activity-dependent changes in central synapses (169). Proteoglycans interact with other molecules specifically by virtue of their GAG moieties or through their protein cores. As mentioned, cell surface proteoglycans mediate substratum adhesion and neurite outgrowth on thrombospondin (123) and fibronectin (146). In other instances, ECM proteoglycans inhibit neurite extension (discussed below). The fact that growth factors such as transforming growth factor beta (TGFβ) (170) and fibroblast growth factor (FGF) (170–172) bind avidly to basal lamina via heparan sulfate proteoglycans suggests that the ECM may serve as a reservoir of heparin-binding growth factors that could be released be proteases to act on neural cells. Moreover, FGF, which binds to a receptor tyrosine kinase, is first "activated" by binding to a cell surface heparan sulfate proteoglycan (172). Since FGF is a known neurotrophic agent these interactions with the ECM may affect its function in the nervous system.

Extracellular Matrix Receptors

Integrins

A wealth of data indicate that the major effectors of ECM proteins on cells are a multigene family of receptors called integrins. The name derives (173) from the transmembrane disposition of these receptors and their ability to integrate information from the ECM to the cytoplasm of the cells, as shown by their obvious involvement in cell shape and motility. Phylogenetically, the integrins arose before the split of multicellular organisms into vertebrates and invertebrates and have been implicated directly in *Drosophila* development by mutation analysis (reviewed in 21). There is ample evidence in vitro and in vivo that integrins are necessary for fundamental cellular events during neural development and regeneration. This of course does not rule out participation of other families of ECM receptors, especially when one considers the multifunctional properties of proteins such as laminin. Individual integrins are typically expressed in multiple tissues of the body (cf. 174) so that, like CAMs, their function in neural development may critically reflect the timing as well as distribution of their receptors and ligands during development and following trauma to the nervous system.

The ECM receptors within the integrin family belong largely, though not exclusively, to the β1 class. Other classes have either not been identified in neural cells or their functions are only beginning to be explored [α6β4 (175), αvβ3 (176)]. Although we emphasize here the function of integrins as ECM receptors, they can mediate cell-cell adhesion as well. For example, the α4β1 integrin binds not only to fibronectin but also with VCAM 1 (177), a member of the Ig super-family. A preliminary report implicates the α6β4 integrin in neuron astrocyte interactions (175). Moreover, expression of α8β1 heterodimer is restricted to the nervous system (174), where ECM adhesive proteins are sparse, which may be a clue that it is a CAM. Here, we limit our discussion primarily to the β1 class whose functions have been most well explored in neural cells. Integrins have been the subject of two recent reviews dealing with the nervous system (8,11).

Integrins are heterodimers of two noncovalently linked subunits (α and β). To date 18 α subunits and seven β subunits have been reported. Both α and β subunits can be alternatively spliced (178,179). Family members are classified by their β subunits since there is a tendency for an α subunit to associate with only a single type of β subunit. The receptor specificity is degenerate, e.g., the α1β1 integrin is both a laminin and collagen receptor and it is apparently redundant, e.g., there are at least five β1 receptors for laminin (α1β1, α2β1, α3β1, α6β1, α7β1). Although one cannot be certain whether novel ligands will be discovered that will distinguish these heterodimers, or whether their appearance in development and sites of expression may vary in vivo to minimize their redundancy, ligand specificity is determined by both subunits, which together form the ligand binding site (180,181). Interaction with cytoskeletal proteins (182) and the formation of cell substratum contacts (183) is similarly determined by the cytoplasmic domains of both subunits. Moreover, the same integrin may have distinct ligand-binding properties depending on the cell in which it is expressed (184). Although the details of this cell specific regulation are unclear, they are likely to involve posttranslational modification of the receptors. These and other mechanisms of integrin regulation may be of special significance to neural cells where they could contribute to the adhesive diversity among cells within the nervous system.

A number of studies have shown that integrins are involved in neurite outgrowth on fibronectin, collagen, laminin, thrombospondin, and vitronectin (46,185,186) by both peripheral and central neurons. On cellular rather than ECM substrates, integrins collaborate with CAMs to mediate neurite outgrowth. PC12 cells have two integrins that mediate neurite outgrowth on laminin, the α1β1 interacting with a site in the cross region of laminin and the α3β1 interacting with a site at the end of the long arm (187). However, the ligand specificity of the α1β1 integrin in peripheral neurons differs from that in PC12 cells. In primary neurons, the α1β1 integrin mediates axonal outgrowth on collagen, whereas laminin stimulates both dendritic and axonal outgrowth through as yet undefined integrins (188,189).

Many nonneural cell integrins are found in cell-substratum contacts, called focal contacts (183). Focal contacts are close appositions of the cell to its substratum containing an ECM protein linked via an integrin to accessory cytoskeletal proteins such as talin, vinculin, α-actinin, and actin (183). Primary neurons in culture do not make focal contacts (Wilson and Carbonetto, unpublished) and although growth cones have been reported to contain vinculin, talin, and α-actinin (189), these proteins are not obviously incorporated into their cell-substratum contacts.

During development integrins are functionally down-regulated, which may contribute to the reduced axonal regeneration seen in vivo as the nervous system matures. In the retina this regulation occurs at transcriptional and posttranslational levels. Cohen et al. (190–192) have shown that neurite outgrowth by embryonic retinal neurons in culture on laminin decreases from embryonic day 6 to a low point 3–4 days later. The same cells extend long neurites when cultured on astrocytes where growth is cadherin-mediated (48,190). For retinal ganglion cells this decrease in neurite growth correlates with transcriptional regulation of the α6 subunit, which is a subunit of the principle laminin receptor (α6β1) in ganglion neurons (193). The timing of this effect and its transcriptional regulation in ganglion, but not other retinal cells, suggests that the α6 mRNA is down-regulated as the axons of the ganglion cells reach the optic tectum. Consistent with this, removal of the tectum during development mitigates the functional down-regulation (192). However, this integrin and several others also show a developmental decrease in efficacy in nonganglion cells. Here, the regulation is posttranslational (192) since it can be reversed for some heterodimers by a novel antibody to the β1 subunit (194). Posttranslational modification of integrins is paralleled by a decrease in the polysialic content of N-CAM, which renders it a relatively weak mediator of nerve growth (53). N-Cadherin also declines in the developing retina but over a slower time course. Thus, several adhesive systems become functionally down-regulated as the nervous system matures.

Similar functional regulation of integrins to that in the retina occurs in peripheral neurons (195). However, in denervated peripheral nerves laminin and integrins are in part responsible for regeneration (3,162). In culture NGF has been shown to up-regulate integrin expression in PC12 cells (196), and although NGF is apparently not necessary for regeneration in the PNS it does mediate axonal sprouting (197). Conceivably, NGF acts to up-regulate integrins and enhance peripheral nerve sprouting while other growth factors (BDNF, NT3, etc.) use related mechanisms to stimulate nerve regeneration. In future studies, it will be important not only to catalog integrins and CAMs in the PNS and CNS, but to learn whether following trauma they are re-expressed or activated and whether these changes occur in the CNS as well as PNS.

Nonintegrin Receptors

A variety of protein receptors for ECM proteins that are not members of the integrin superfamily have been reported (198). These include cell-surface proteoglycans that recognize laminin, fibronectin and thrombospondin (discussed above) as well as several proteins that bind laminin or carbohydrates on ECM proteins. At least 2 of these have been implicated in neurite outgrowth (199,200) and several others have been identified within the nervous system. In some cases these molecules are referred to as ECM binding molecules since they may not be cell-surface receptors but ECM components themselves or perhaps intracellular molecules (201,202). This topic has been reviewed in detail recently (198). Here, we focus on non-integrin receptors that have been implicated in neural function.

High Affinity Laminin Receptors

A protein of 67 kDa that binds to laminin with a Kd of approximately 10^{-9} M (approximately 1,000 × higher than integrins) was reported in skeletal muscle and in a breast carcinoma cell line (203,204). A monoclonal antibody to this protein was found to inhibit the attachment of breast carcinoma cells to laminin, and the same antibody was used to molecularly clone a partial cDNA for the protein (204). However, subsequent full-length clones isolated by several laboratories were found to code for a protein of only 33 kDa that electrophoreses at 43 kDa (205–211). This protein had additional features inconsistent with it being a 67 kDa laminin receptor, including no putative signal sequence or membrane-spanning domain and an inability to bind laminin (209,211). Apparently the 43 kDa protein is an abundant one in many cells, and its cDNA has been cloned by groups interested in retinal development (207), tumor metastasis (208), protein translational regulation (210), and steroid receptors (Kelly et al., unpublished). Although it has been suggested that the 43 kDa protein is a metabolic precursor to the 67 kDa laminin receptor (212), the bulk of the data indicate that the two proteins are merely related immunologically.

Mecham and coworkers have identified a similar protein of 67 kDa that is an elastin receptor, involved in assembly of elastin fibrils, as well as a laminin receptor (213). This protein is apparently a peripheral membrane protein with a carbohydrate recognition site that alters the affinity of elastin binding. The site in laminin to which this protein binds is a pentapeptide, Isoleu-Lys-Val-Ala-Val (IKVAV) in the short arm region of the B1 chain that is distinct from the Tyr-Isoleu-Gly-Ser-Arg (YIGSR) sequence that has been reported by some laboratories to be the recognition site for the 67 kDa laminin receptor (214). In solution YIGSR has been reported to inhibit neurite outgrowth by some neural cell lines but is inactive on primary cultures of neurons (Carbonctto, unpublishcd). Molecular cloning of the elastin receptors will be of considerable importance in putting this family of receptor on firm footing as well as in resolving the relationship, if any, of the 43 kDa protein to the elastin/laminin receptor.

A surprising offshoot of work in this area is the observation by Drager and colleagues (207) that the 43 kDa protein, once thought to be a laminin receptor, has antigenic sites that are expressed in a dorsal-ventral gradient within the developing retina. The authors suggest that this protein may be involved in establishing the retinotropic projection in the visual system. The 43 kDa protein is also expressed in retinal ganglion cells in mature retinas (211) and in the cortical plate and ventricular zone during differentiation of the cerebral cortex (215). The function of this protein is unclear and speculation has shifted from its role as a laminin receptor to its possible involvement in the regulation of protein synthesis (210).

Smalheiser and Schwartz have reported a 110–120 kDa protein that binds laminin with a high affinity (Kd $<10^{-9}$ M) (216). Proteins of similar size and laminin-binding characteristics have been reported in brain (217) and NG-108 cells where antibodies to the protein inhibit neurite outgrowth by these cells (218). This receptor in primary neurons and a neural cell line has been reported to recognize a 19 amino acid synthetic peptide (219) whose sequence is derived from the laminin A chain. Immunocytochemical observations indicate that the 110 kDa protein increases following trauma to the rat CNS (220).

Lectin-Like Receptors

Shur and co-workers have identified a cell surface galactosyl-transferase that mediates adhesion of neural and other cells to laminin (221). The enzyme apparently binds to N-acetylglycosamine acceptor sites at the end of the long arm of laminin and, in the absence of UDP galactose, mediates cell adhesion. This receptor participates in neural crest migration in vitro as well as in neurite outgrowth in PC12 cells and primary neurons (199,222,223). Thus, while integrins appear to be the major adhesive systems for attachment of neural cells to laminin, the galactosyl transferase is a weaker, albeit significant, mediator of neurite outgrowth (223).

Other lectin-like molecules that bind to ECM proteins have been reported, including CBP-35/Mac 2 (224) and several low molecular weight lactose-binding lectins (225) that are immunologically related to the 67 kDa laminin/elastin receptor. Finally, selectins or LEC-CAMs (226) are a major family of cell surface receptors that mediate intercellular adhesion via recognition of carbohydrate residues on the cell surface. They have been described in most detail in the lymphatic system where they are responsible for targeting of lymphocytes to high endothelial venules for entry into the lymphatic system. As selectins have been recently discovered, their distribution in the nervous system is largely unknown except for one report identifying them in CNS glia and Schwann cells in vivo (227).

ANTI-ADHESIVE MOLECULES

There has been a great deal of interest recently in the identification of molecules that interfere with growth cone adhesion and neurite extension. The impetus has come from in vitro experiments on myelin-associated proteins, which have been shown to inhibit neurite outgrowth in culture and nerve regeneration in vivo.

In principle, inhibition of axonal growth can occur at many levels. Apart from defects in growth factor-related pathways, ECM molecules could be altered in amounts or activity or complexed with other molecules that mask their active sites. The level of expression and affinity of ECM receptors and CAMs can be similarly regulated. There is as yet no evidence for regulation of intracellular pathways following ligand receptor interactions primarily because the investigation of these pathways is in its infancy. Finally, and most interestingly, there is the possibility of parallel pathways including independent receptor systems that override adhesive systems on growth cones (discussed below).

Extracellular Matrix Inhibitory Molecules

Laminin (119) and fibronectin (120) are found within the ECM during development of the CNS. These proteins essentially disappear from the ECM as the CNS matures and become restricted only to basement membranes around blood vessels and at connective tissue interfaces. Instead a variety of proteoglycans (115) come to dominate the ECM of the CNS along with tenascin and thrombospondin (117,120). The loss of laminin appears to contribute to the reduced adhesiveness of the adult CNS tissues in cell cultures assays (124). However, upon denervation, laminin is expressed in the region of traumatized neurons most likely being produced by reactive astrocytes and leptomeningeal cells (228).

The function of proteoglycans vís a vís nerve growth is one of increasing interest. Unfortunately the types of proteoglycans in the CNS are only beginning to be identified and characterized (discussed above), a task which is complicated by the fact that the GAG side-chains may mediate or alter important biological activities of proteoglycans. As a result, it is premature to generalize about the function of proteoglycans in nerve regeneration. Nevertheless, several reports indicate that proteoglycans (229,230) and/or their GAG side-chains (144,231) are inhibitory of neurite outgrowth. This may explain why glycosaminoglycans are concentrated in regions such as the posterior half of developing somite or the roof plate of the spinal cord and midbrain (232) where developing axons are sparse. Or it may help explain why axons regenerating in the PNS fail to grow on the abaxonal surfaces of basement membranes (159) that have relatively high concentrations of heparan sulfate proteoglycan.

ECM proteoglycans may interfere with nerve growth as a result of their relatively high negative charge possibly adsorbing to and shielding active sites of ECM adhesive proteins, or they may bind specifically to active sites on the ECM proteins (147), competing with cell-surface proteoglycans that mediate adhesion (149). As mentioned above, proteoglycans also interact directly with N-CAM and with growth factors and growth factor receptors to modulate their activity. This plethora of possibilities may explain why some proteoglycans in culture stimulate neurite outgrowth (233). Systematic studies with well-defined proteoglycans and GAGs under physiologically relevant conditions will help sort out whether these molecules are likely to be inhibitory in vivo.

Tenascin is an interesting example of a molecule that is both adhesive and anti-adhesive (234). Tenascin has been implicated in the migration of granular cells in the cerebellum where it is expressed primarily in the molecular layer (235). It is also expressed in the developing somatosensory cortex of mice in barrel fields, where its distribution suggests that it may be important in restricting afferent inputs to these fields (236).

Studies by Lotz et al. (57) indicate that cells attach initially to tenascin but that this attachment weakens with time and temperature. Fragments of recombinant tenascin show that a distal region from the arms of this hexabrachion-shaped protein containing a FN type III repeat promotes cell adhesion whereas another region with EGF repeats inhibits cell attachment (234). In neural cells, tenascin has been reported to be nonpermissive for neurite outgrowth (237,238), possibly by inhibiting cell body attachment. However, when somata are allowed to attach, tenascin is a moderately good substratum for neurite outgrowth (239).

Tenascin in solution inhibits neurite outgrowth on laminin and fibronectin by a mechanism that does not appear to involve direct inhibition of ECM proteins or competition with them for fibronectin receptors (240). The RGD sequence in tenascin, which could, in principle, compete with fibronectin for its receptor seems to be nonfunctional (10). It has been speculated that tenascin may interact with an inhibitory receptor on the cell surface. Two candidate receptors have been reported for tenascin (241,242), but it is unknown whether either mediate cell adhesion or anti-adhesion.

In the distal segment of transected peripheral nerves, expression of tenascin increases but the protein is outside the endoneurial tube through which axons regenerate (243). In the first 2–3 weeks after a CNS lesion (244,245), increased tenascin immunolabeling is seen in leptomeningeal cells and in astrocytes that form the new glia limitans at the site of lesion (244). Tenascin may therefore participate in limiting the growth of axons across sites of CNS lesions in mammals.

Thrombospondin is another ECM glycoprotein with both adhesive and anti-adhesive effects on cells (10). Sparc, also a basement membrane glycoprotein, inhibits cell-substratum adhesion suggesting that the related molecule SC1 (not related to SC1/DM-GRASP), which is found in the brain (246), may be similarly anti-adhesive. J1/200 and J1/210 are immunochemically related molecules secreted by oligodendrocytes that reduce adhesion of astrocytes and cerebellar neurons (247). Finally, S-laminin, found at motor end-plates, appears to mediate neuron substratum attachment but not neurite outgrowth through a peptide (Lys-Arg-Ser) which may be a signal for the termination of axonal growth (248). The mechanism for termination of growth is unknown but may involve excessive adhesion from which the growth cone is unable to escape.

Myelin-Associated Inhibitory Molecules

Schwab and co-workers have identified on the surfaces of oligodendrocytes two immunologically related proteins that inhibit nerve growth in culture and in vivo. The observations are intriguing because they appear to involve a cell-surface receptor that, when activated by contact with oligodendrocytes, freezes growth cone activity or causes growth cones to retract. Several functional studies indicate that these proteins limit nerve regeneration in the adult CNS.

The two proteins of 35 and 250 kDa from CNS myelin inhibit neurite outgrowth in culture (249). IN-1, an antibody to these proteins, neutralizes the inhibition, allowing cell attachment and neurite outgrowth over previously inhibitory oligodendrocytes (249,250). In vivo, X-irradiation of newborn rats inhibits myelin formation, enhancing the regeneration of the transected corticospinal axons (251). Application of IN-1 antibody results in a similar level of regeneration in adult rats with normally myelinated corticospinal (252) tracts. However, in neither instance is the regeneration robust, emphasizing the involvement of additional barriers to CNS regeneration.

In time-lapse studies of neurites growing in culture, contact of growth cones with oligodendrocytes results in immotility or retraction of growth cones (249). This contact inhibition suggests involvement of a ligand-receptor interaction among the two cell types. Current thinking is that this interaction triggers some second messenger system that overrides the integrins and CAMs on these cells. Calcium influx, thought to be important in growth cone motility, seems a good candidate for this second messenger system, which might also explain how serotonin acts to inhibit growth cone motility (253). However, several recent observations suggest that neurite outgrowth does not require calcium (253–255). Regardless of the mechanism, the observation of anti-adhesive effects of these myelin proteins promises to be of fundamental importance not only for neurons but also for many other cell types whose adhesion is inhibited by these proteins.

Several other "collapsing" factors that cause similar effects on growth cones have been identified by three other groups (reviewed in 256). In one instance, this activity is localized within regions of the visual system (optic tectum) during development and may account in part for the topographic projection of retinal ganglion cells onto the tectum. At this point, the relationship of the various growth cone inhibitory molecules is unclear, as is their potential involvement in axonal regeneration.

CONCLUSIONS

Although there is compelling evidence that CAMs and ECM adhesive proteins participate in neural development, the details of their function in neural regeneration is relatively sparse. Even assuming that the major adhesive molecular systems that are functional in the nervous system have been identified, which is by no means certain, much groundwork will be necessary to identify their distribution and activities within neural pathways. This task will be hastened if adhesive molecules have conserved representations in pathways of different species. A major goal of research in this area is to devise means to stimulate axonal regeneration within the adult mammalian CNS. Our current state of knowledge does not allow us to discern which inhibitory systems should be inactivated or which facilitory systems bolstered to accomplish this task. Transgenic mice will be a tedious but valuable way to decipher this complexity. Mutant mice that overexpress an adhesive molecule or have their inhibitory systems disabled by homologous recombination or dominant negative mutations could be crossed with other mutants to generate strains in which regeneration of specific pathways can be assayed. They would also provide valuable models for assaying drugs, growth factors, and synthetic peptides that might regulate or mimic dysfunctional adhesive systems to increase regeneration.

ACKNOWLEDGMENTS

We thank our colleague Peter Richardson for his helpful comments on the text. Work for this review was supported by grants to S.C. and S.D. from the MRC of Canada. We are especially grateful to Gwen Peard for her help in preparing this manuscript.

REFERENCES

1. Ellis RE, Yuan J, Horvitz HR. Mechanisms and functions of cell death. *Annu Rev Cell Biol* 1991; 7: 663–698.
2. Vidal-Sanz M, Bray GM, Villegas-Perez MP, Aguayo AJ. Axonal regeneration and synapse formation in the superior colliculus by retinal ganglion cells in adult rat. *J Neurosci* 1987; 7: 2894–2907.
3. Sandrock WW, Matthew WD. An in vitro neurite promoting antigen functions in axonal regeneration in vivo. *Science* 1987; 237: 1605–1608.
4. McMahon UJ, Wallace BG. Molecules in basal lamina that direct the formation of synaptic specializations at neuro-muscular junctions. *Dev Neurosci* 1989; 11: 227–247.
5. Heidemann SR, Buxbaum RE. Growth cone motility. *Curr Opin Neurobiol* 1991; 1: 339–345.
6. Sabry JH, O'Connor TP, Evans L, Torosan-Raymond A, Kirschner M, Bentley D. Microtubule behavior during guidance of pioneer neuron growth cones in situ. *J Cell Biol* 1991; 151: 381–395.
7. Sperry RW. Chemoaffinity in the orderly growth of nerve fiber patterns and connections. *Proc Natl Acad Sci USA* 1963; 50: 73–77.
8. Reichardt LF, Tomaselli KJ. Extracellular ma-

trix molecules and their receptors: Functions in neural development. *Annu Rev Neurosci* 1991; 14: 531–510.
9. Schwarzburger JE. Fibronectin: From gene to protein. *Curr Opin Cell Biol* 1991; 3: 786–791.
10. Chiquet-Ehrismann R. Anti-adhesive molecules of the extracellular matrix. *Curr Opin Cell Biol* 1991; 3: 800–804.
11. deCurtis I. Neuronal interactions with the extracellular matrix. *Curr Opin Cell Biol* 1991; 3: 824–831.
12. Grumet M. Cell adhesion molecules and their subgroups in the nervous system. *Curr Opin Neurobiol* 1991; 3: 370–376.
13. Mecham RP. Laminin receptors. *Annu Rev Cell Biol* 1991; 7: 71–92.
14. Kjellen L, Lindahl U. Proteoglycans: structure and interactions. *Annu Rev Biochem* 1991; 60: 443–475.
15. Takeichi M. Cadherins: a molecular family important in selective cell-cell adhesion. *Annu Rev Biochem* 1990; 59: 237–252.
16. Cunningham BA, Hemperly JJ, Murray BA, Prediger EA, Brackenbury R, Edelman GM. Neural cell adhesion molecule: structure, immunoglobulin-like domains, cell surface modulations and alternative RNA splicing. *Science* 1987; 236: 799–806.
17. Rathjen FG. Neural cell contact and axonal growth. *Curr Opin Cell Biol* 1991; 3: 992–1000.
18. Grumet M, Mauro V, Burgoon MP, Edelman G, Cunningham BA. Structure of a new nervous system glycoprotein, NR-CAM, and its relationship to subgroups of neural cell adhesion molecules. *J Cell Biol* 1991; 113: 1399–1412.
19. Tanaka H, Matsui T, Agata A, Tomura M, Kubota I, McFarland KC, Kohr B, Lee A, Phillips HS, Shelton DL. Molecular cloning and expression of a novel adhesion molecule, SC1. *Neuron* 1991; 7: 535–545.
20. Burns FR, von Kannen S, Guy L, Raper JA, Kamholz J, Chang S. DM-GRASP, a novel immunoglobulin superfamily axonal surface protein that supports neurite extension. *Neuron* 1991; 7: 209–220.
21. Hortsch M, Goodman C. Cell and substrate molecules in Drosophila. *Annu Rev Cell Biol* 1991; 7: 505–557.
22. Edelman GM, Chuong C-M. Embryonic to adult conversion of neural cell adhesion molecules in normal and staggerer mice. *Proc Natl Acad Sci USA* 1982; 79: 7036–7040.
23. Hirn M, Ghandour MS, Degostini-Bazin H, et al. Molecular heterogeneity and structural evolution during cerebellar ontogeny detected by monoclonal antibody of the mouse cell surface antigen BSP-2. *Brain Res* 1983; 265: 87–100.
24. Lyles JM, Linnemann D, Bock E. Biosynthesis of the D2-cell adhesion molecule: post-translational modification, intracellular transport, and developmental changes. *J Cell Biol* 1984; 99: 2082–2091.
25. Owens GC, Edelman GM, Cunningham BA. Organization of the neural cell adhesion molecule (NCAM) gene: alternative exon usage as the basis for different membrane-associated domains. *Proc Natl Acad Sci USA* 1987; 84: 294–298.
26. He H-T, Baret J, Chaix JC, Goridis C. Phosphatidylinositol is involved in the membrane attachment of N-CAM-120, the smallest component of the neural cell adhesion molecule. *EMBO J* 1986; 5: 2489–2500.
27. Sadoul K, Meyer A, Low MG, Schachner M. Release of the 120 kDa component of the mouse cell adhesion molecule from the surfaces by phosphatidylinositol-specific phospholipase C. *Neurosci Lett* 1986; 72: 341–346.
28. Pollerberg EG, Schachner M, Davoust J. Differentiation-state dependent surface mobilities of two forms of the neural cell adhesion molecule. *Nature* 1986; 324: 462–465.
29. Pollerberg EG, Burridge K, Krebs KE, Goodman SR, Schachner M. The 180-kD component of the neural cell adhesion molecule NCAM is involved in cell-cell contacts and cytoskeleton-membrane interactions. *Cell Tissue Res* 1987; 240: 227–236.
30. Bhat S, Silberberg DH. Oligodendrocyte cell adhesion molecules are related to neural cell adhesion molecule (N-CAM). *J Neurosci* 1986; 6: 3348–3354.
31. Noble M, Albrechtsen M, Møller C, et al. Glial cells express N-CAM/D2-CAM like polypeptides in vitro. *Nature* 1985; 315: 725–728.
32. Nybroe O, Gibson A, Møller CJ, et al. Expression of N-CAM polypeptides in neurons. *Neurochem Int* 1986; 9: 539–544.
33. Nybroe O, Linnemann D, Bock E. Heterogeneity of soluble neural cell adhesion molecule. *J Neurochem* 1989; 53: 1372–1378.
34. Gower J, Barton CH, Elsom VL, Thompson J, Moore SE, Dickson G, Walsh FS. Alternative splicing generates a secreted form of N-CAM in muscle and brain. *Cell* 1988; 53: 955–964.
35. Cole GJ, Loewy A, Glaser L. Neuronal cell-cell adhesion depends on interactions of N-CAM with heparin-like molecules. *Nature* 1986; 230: 445–447.
36. Cole GJ, Akeson R. Identification of a heparin binding domain of the neural cell adhesion molecule N-CAM using synthetic peptides. *Neuron* 1989; 2: 1157–1165.
37. Rothbard JB, Brackenbury R, Cunningham BA, et al. Differences in the carbohydrate structures of neural cell-adhesion molecules from adult and embryonic chicken brains. *J Biol Chem* 1982; 257: 11064–11069.
38. Linnemann D, Lyles JM, Bock E. A developmental study of the biosynthesis of the neural cell adhesion molecule. *Dev Neurosci* 1985; 7: 230–238.
39. Hoffman S, Edelman GM. Kinetics of homophilic binding by embryonic and adult forms of the neural cell adhesion molecule. *Proc Natl Acad Sci USA* 1983; 80: 5762–5766.
40. Rutishauser U, Landmesser L. Polysialic acid

on the surface of axons regulates patterns of normal and activity-dependent innervation. *Trends Neurosci* 1991; 14: 528–532.
41. Key B, Akeson RA. Delineation of olfactory pathways in the frog nervous system by unique glycoconjugates and N-CAM glycoforms. *Neuron* 1991; 6: 381–396.
42. Buskirk DR, Thiery J-P, Rutishauser U, Edelman GM. Antibodies to a neural cell adhesion molecule disrupts histogenesis in cultured chick retinae. *Nature* 1980; 285: 488–489.
43. Hoffman S, Friedlander DR, Chuong C-M, Grumet M, Edelman GM. Differential contributions of Ng-CAM and N-CAM to cell adhesion in different neural regions. *J Cell Biol* 1986; 103: 145–158.
44. Thanos S, Bonhoeffer F, Rutishauser U. Fiber-fiber interaction and tectal cues influence the development of the chicken retinotectal projection. *Proc Natl Acad Sci USA* 1984; 81: 1906–1910.
45. Silver J, Rutishauser U. Guidance of optic axons in vivo by a preformed adhesive pathway on neuroepithelial endfeet. *Dev Biol* 1984; 106: 485–499.
46. Reichardt LF, Bixby JL, Hall DE, Ignatius MJ, Neugebauer KM, Tomaselli KJ. Integrins and cell adhesion molecules: neuronal receptors that regulate axon growth on extracellular matrices and cell surfaces. *Dev Neurosci* 1989; 11: 332–347.
47. Tomaselli KJ, Neugebauer KM, Bixby JL, Lilien J, Reichardt LF. N-cadherin and integrins: two receptor systems that mediate neuronal process outgrowth on astrocytes. *Neuron* 1988; 1: 33–43.
48. Neugebauer KM, Tomaselli KJ, Lilien J, Reichardt LF. N-cadherin, N-CAM and integrins promote retinal neurite outgrowth on astrocytes in vitro. *J Cell Biol* 1988; 107: 1177–1187.
49. Lemmon V, Farr KL, Lagenauer C. L1-mediated axon growth occurs via a homophilic binding mechanism. *Neuron* 1989; 2: 1597–1603.
50. Doherty P, Barton CH, Dickson G, Seaton P, Rowett LH, et al. Neuronal process outgrowth of human sensory neurons on monolayers of cells transfected with cDNAs for five human N-CAM isoforms. *J Cell Biol* 1988; 109: 789–798.
51. Doherty P, Fruns M, Seaton P, Dickson G, Barton CH, Sears TA, Walsh F. A threshold effect of the major isoform of NCAM on neurite outgrowth. *Nature* 1990; 343: 464–466.
52. Doherty P, Rowett LH, Moore SD, Mann DA, Walsh FS. Neurite outgrowth in response to transfected N-CAM and N-Cadherin reveals fundamental differences in neuronal responsiveness to CAMs. *Neuron* 1991; 6: 1–10.
53. Doherty P, Cohen J, Walsh FS. Neurite outgrowth in response to transfected NCAM changes during development and is modulated by polysialic acid. *Neuron* 1990; 5: 209–219.
54. DeGeorge JJ, Carbonetto S. Specificity and valency of concanavalin A in neuron-substratum adhesion and redistribution of cell surface receptors. *Dev Biol* 1987; 119: 45–58.
55. Hall D, Neugebauer K, Reichardt LF. Embryonic neural retina cell response to extracellular matrix proteins: developmental changes and effects of the cell substratum attachment antibody, CSAT. *J Cell Biol* 1987; 104: 623–634.
56. Gundersen RW. Response of sensory neurites and growth cones to patterned substrates of laminin and fibronectin in vitro. *Dev Biol* 1987; 121: 423–431.
57. Lotz MM, Berdsal CA, Erickson H, McClay DR. Cell adhesion to fibronectin and tenascin: quantitative measurements of initial binding and subsequent strengthening response. *J Cell Biol* 1989; 109: 1795–1805.
58. Landmesser L, Dahm L, Tang JC, Rutishauser U. Polysialic acid as a regulator of intramuscular nerve branching during embryonic development. *Neuron* 1990; 4: 655–667.
59. Acheson A, Sunshine JL, Rutishauser U. NCAM polysialic acid can regulate both cell-cell and cell-substrate interactions. *J Cell Biol* 1991; 114: 143–153.
60. Daniloff JK, Levi G, Grumet M, Rieger F, Edelman GM. Altered expression of neural cell adhesion molecules by nerve injury and repair. *J Cell Biol* 1986; 103: 929–945.
61. Covault J, Sanes J. Neural cell adhesion molecule (N-CAM) accumulates in denervated and paralysed skeletal muscle. *Proc Natl Acad Sci USA* 1985; 82: 4544–4548.
62. Sanes JR, Schachner M, Covault J. Expression of several adhesive macromolecules (N-CAM, L1, NILE, Uvomorulin, laminin, fibronectin, and a heparan sulfate proteoglycan) in embryonic, adult, and denervated adult skeletal muscle. *J Cell Biol* 1986; 102: 420–431.
63. Martini R, Schachner M. Immunoelectron microscopic localization of neural cell adhesion molecules (L1, N-CAM, and myelin-associated glycoprotein) in regenerating adult mouse sciatic nerve. *J Cell Biol* 1988; 106: 1735–1746.
64. Remsen LG, Strain GM, Newman MJ, Satterlee N, Daniloff JK. Antibodies to the neural cell adhesion molecule disrupt functional recovery in injured nerves. *Exp Neurol* 1990; 110: 268–273.
65. Fraser SE, Carhart MS, Murray BA, Chuong CM, Edelman G. Alterations in the Xenopus retinotectal projection by antibodies to Xenopus NCAM. *Dev Biol* 1988; 129: 217–230.
66. Lindner J, Rathjen FG, Schachner M. L1 mono and polyclonal antibodies modify cell migration in early postnatal mouse cerebellum. *Nature* 1983; 305: 427–430.
67. Grumet M, Edelman GM. Heterotypic binding between neuronal membrane vesicles and glial cells is mediated by a specific cell adhesion molecule. *J Cell Biol* 1984; 98: 1746–1756.
68. Rathjen FG, Schachner M. Immunocytological and biochemical characterization of a new neuronal cell surface component (L1 antigen)

which is involved in cell adhesion. *EMBO J* 1984; 3: 1–10.
69. Faissner A, Kruse J, Nieke J, et al. Expression of neural cell adhesion molecule L1 during development in neurological mutants and in the peripheral nervous system. *Dev Brain Res* 1984; 15: 69–82.
70. Harper JR, Prince JT, Healy PA, Stuart JK, Nauman SJ, Stallcup WB. Isolation and sequence of partial cDNA clones of human L1: homology of human and rodent L1 in the cytoplasmic region. *J Neurochem* 1991; 56: 797–804.
71. Burgoon M, Grumet M, Mauro V, Edelman GM, Cunningham BA. Structure of the chicken neuron-glia cell adhesion molecule, Ng-CAM: origin of the polypeptides and relation to the Ig superfamily. *J Cell Biol* 1991; 112: 1017–1029.
72. Linneman D, Bock E. Developmental study of the cell adhesion molecule L1. *Dev Neurosci* 1988; 10: 34–42.
73. Tacke R, Moos M, Teplow DB, et al. Identification of cDNA clones of the mouse cell adhesion molecule L1. *Neurosci Lett* 1987; 82: 89–94.
74. Moos M, Tacke R, Scherer H, et al. Neural adhesion molecule L1 as a member of the immunoglobulin superfamily with binding domains similar to fibronectin. *Nature* 1988; 334: 701–703.
75. Faissner A, Teplow DB, Kubler D, Keilhauer G, Kinzel V, Schachner M. Biosynthesis and membrane topography of the neural cell adhesion molecule L1. *EMBO J* 1985; 4: 3105–3113.
76. Grumet M, Hoffman S, Edelman GM. Two antigenically related neuronal cell adhesion molecules to different specificities mediate neuron-neuron and neuron-glia adhesion. *Proc Natl Acad Sci USA* 1984; 81: 267–271.
77. Fischer A, Kunemund V, Schachner M. Neurite outgrowth patterns in cerebellar microexplant cultures are affected by antibodies to the cell surface glycoprotein L1. *J Neurosci* 1986; 6: 605–612.
78. Grumet M, Hoffman S, Chuong C-M, Edelman GM. Polypeptide components and binding functions of neuron-glia cell adhesion molecules. *Proc Natl Acad Sci USA* 1984; 81: 7989–7993.
79. Hatten ME. Riding the glial monorail: a common mechanism for glial-guided neuronal migration in different regions of the developing mammalian brain. *Trends Neurosci* 1990; 13: 179–193.
80. Chang S, Rathjen FG, Raper JA. Extension of neurites on axons is impaired by antibodies against specific neural cells surface glycoproteins. *J Cell Biol* 1987; 104: 355–362.
81. Bixby JL, Lilien J, Reichardt LF. Identification of the major proteins that promote neuronal process outgrowth on Schwann cells in vitro. *J Cell Biol* 1988; 107: 353–362.
82. Kleitman N, Simon D, Schachner M, Bunge R. Growth on embryonic retinal neurites elicited by contact with Schwann cell surfaces is blocked by antibodies to L1. *Exp Neurol* 1988; 102: 298–306.
83. Seilheimer B, Schachner M. Studies of adhesion molecules mediating interactions between cells of peripheral nervous system indicate a major role for L1 in mediating sensory neuron growth on Schwann cells. *J Cell Biol* 1988; 107: 341–351.
84. Drazba J, Lemmon V. The role of cell adhesion molecules in neurite growth on Muller cells. *Dev Biol* 1990; 138: 82–93.
85. Chuah MI, David S, Blaschuk O. Differentiation and survival of rat olfactory epithelial neurons in dissociated cell culture. *Dev Brain Res* 1991; 60: 123–132.
86. Seilheimer B, Pershon E, Schachner M. Antibodies to L1 adhesion molecule inhibit Schwann cell ensheathment of neurons in vitro. *J Cell Biol* 1989; 109: 3095–3103.
87. Tanaka H, Obata K. Developmental changes in unique cell surface antigens of chick embryo spinal motor neurons and ganglion cells. *Dev Biol* 1984; 106: 26–37.
88. Gennarini G, Cibelli G, Rougon G, Mattei M-G, Goridis C. The mouse neuronal cell surface protein F3: a phosphatidylinositol-anchored membrane of the immunoglobulin superfamily related to chicken contactin. *J Cell Biol* 1989; 109: 775–788.
89. Brummendorf T, Wolff M, Frank R, Rathjen FC. Neural cell recognition molecule F11: homology with fibronectin type III and immunoglobulin type C domains. *Neuron* 1989; 2: 1351–1361.
90. Furley AJ, Morton SB, Manalo D, Karagogeos D, Dodd J, Jessell TM. The axonal glycoprotein TAG-1 is an immunoglobulin superfamily member with neurite outgrowth-promoting activity. *Cell* 1990; 61: 157–170.
91. Ruegg MA, Stoechli ET, Kuhn TB, Heller M, Zuellig R, Sonderegger P. Purification of axonin-1, a protein that is secreted from axons during neurogenesis. *EMBO J* 1988; 8: 55–63.
92. Ranscht B, Moss DJ, Thomas C. A neuronal surface glycoprotein associated with the cytoskeleton. *J Cell Biol* 1984; 99: 1803–1813.
93. Zuellig RA, Rader C, Schroeder A, Kalousek M, v Bohlen F, Fritz A, Stoeckli E, Hafen E, Affolter HU, Sonderegger P. cDNA cloning of the axon-associated adhesion molecule axonin-1. *Soc Neurosci Abstr* 1991; 17: 743.
94. Ranscht B. Sequence of contactin, a 130-kD glycoprotein concentrated in areas of interneuronal contact, defines a new member of the immunoglobulin supergene family in the nervous system. *J Cell Biol* 1988; 107: 1561–1573.
95. Gennarini G, Durbec P, Boned A, Rougon G, Goridis C. Transfected F3/F11 neuronal cell surface protein mediates intercellular adhesion and promotes neurite outgrowth. *Neuron* 1991; 6: 595–606.
96. Stoeckli E, Kuhn TB, Duc CO, Ruegg MA, Sonderegger P. The axonally secreted protein axonin-1 is a potent substratum for neurite growth. *J Cell Biol* 1991; 112: 1449–1455.

97. Stefanova I, Horejsi V, Ansotegui IJ, Knapp W, Stockinger H. GPI-anchored cell surface molecules complexed to protein tyrosine kinases. *Nature* 1991; 254: 1016–1019.
98. Dodd J, Morton SB, Karagogeos D, Yamamoto M, Jessell T. Spatial regulation of axonal glycoprotein expression on subsets of embryonic spinal neurons. *Neuron* 1988; 1: 105–116.
99. Inuzuka H, Miyatani S, Takeichi M. R-cadherin: a novel Ca^{2+}-dependent cell-cell adhesion molecule expressed in the retina. *Neuron* 1991; 7: 69–79.
100. Napolitano EW, Venstrom K, Wheeler EF, Reichardt LF. Molecular cloning and characterization of B-cadherin, a novel chick cadherin. *J Cell Biol* 1991; 113: 893–905.
101. Ranscht B, Dours-Zimmermann M. T-cadherin, a novel member of the cadherins in the nervous system lacks conserved cytoplasmic sequences. *Neuron* 1991; 7: 391–402.
102. Takeichi M. Cadherin cell adhesion receptors as a morphogenetic regulator. *Science* 1991; 251: 1451–1455.
103. McGee AI, Buxton RS. Transmembrane molecular assemblies regulated by the greater cadherin family. *Curr Opin Cell Biol* 1991; 3: 854–861.
104. Nose A, Tsuji K, Takeichi M. Localization of specificity determining sites in cadherin cell adhesion molecules. *Cell* 1990; 61: 147–155.
105. Blaschuk OW, Sullivan R, David S, Pouliot Y. Identification of a cadherin cell adhesion recognition sequence. *Dev Biol* 1990; 139: 227–229.
106. Suzuki S, Sano K, Tanihara H. Diversity of the cadherin family: evidence for eight new cadherins in nervous tissue. *Cell Regul* 1991; 97: 607–614.
107. Detrick RJ, Dickey D, Kintner CR. The effects of N-cadherin misexpression on morphogenesis in Xenopus embryos. *Neuron* 1990; 4: 493–506.
108. Fujimori T, Miyatani S, Takeichi M. Ectopic expression of N-cadherin perturbs histogenesis in Xenopus embryos. *Development* 1990; 110: 97–104.
109. Matsunaga M, Hatta K, Takeichi M. Role of N-cadherin cell adhesion molecules in the histogenesis of neural retina. *Neuron* 1988; 1: 289–295.
110. Bunge RP, Bunge MB, Eldridge CF. Linkage between axonal ensheathment and basal lamina production by Schwann cells. *Annu Rev Neurosci* 1986; 9: 305–328.
111. Peters A, Palay SL, Webster H. *The fine structure of the nervous system: the neurons and supporting cells.* Philadelphia: W.B. Saunders Company; 1991.
112. Fukuda T, Hashimoto PH. Distribution and fine structure of ependymal cells possessing intracellular cysts in the aqueductal wall of the rat brain. *Cell Tissue Res* 1987; 247: 555–564.
113. Chiu AY, Sanes JR. Development of basal lamina in synaptic and extrasynaptic portions of embryonic rat muscle. *Dev Biol* 1984; 103: 456–467.
114. Low FN. The perineurium and connective tissue of peripheral nerve. In: Landon DN, ed. *The peripheral nerve.* Salisbury, England: Chapman and Hall Ltd.; 1976: 159–187.
115. Aquino DA, Margolis RU, Margolis RK. Immunocytochemical localization of a chondroitin sulfate proteoglycan in nervous tissue. I. Adult brain, retina and peripheral nerve. *J Cell Biol* 1984; 99: 1117–1119.
116. Herndon ME, Lander AD. A diverse set of developmentally regulated proteoglycans is expressed in the rat central nervous system. *Neuron* 1990; 4: 949–961.
117. Crossin KL, Hoffman S, Grumet M, Thiery J-P, Edelman GM. Site-restricted expression of cytotactin during development of the chicken embryo. *J Cell Biol* 1986; 102: 1917–1930.
118. Stewart GR, Pearlman AL. Fibronectin-like immunoreactivity in the developing cerebral cortex. *J Neurosci* 1987; 7: 3325–3333.
119. Liesi P. Do neurons in the vertebrate CNS migrate on laminin? *EMBO J* 1985; 4: 1163–1170.
120. O'Shea KS, Reinheimer JST, Dixit VM. Deposition and role of thrombospondin in the histogenesis of the cerebellar cortex. *J Cell Biol* 1990; 110: 1275–1284.
121. Rogers SL, Edson KJ, Letourneau PC, McLoon SC. Distribution of laminin in the developing peripheral nervous system of the chick. *Dev Biol* 1986; 113: 429–435.
122. Riggott MJ, Moody SA. Distribution of laminin and fibronectin along peripheral trigeminal axon pathways in the developing chick. *J Comp Neurol* 1987; 258: 580–596.
123. Neugebauer KM, Emmett CJ, Venstrom KA, Reichardt LF. Vitronectin and thrombospondin promote retinal neurite outgrowth: developmental regulation and role of integrins. *Neuron* 1991; 6: 345–358.
124. Carbonetto S, Evans D, Cochard P. Nerve fiber growth in culture on tissue substrata from central and peripheral nervous systems. *J Neurosci* 1987; 7: 610–620.
125. Klier FG, Gole G, Stallcup W, Schubert D. Amyloid-β-protein precursor is associated with extracellular matrix. *Brain Res* 1990; 515: 336–342.
126. Panayotou G, End P, Aumailley M, Timpl R, Engel J. Domains of laminin with growth-factor activity. *Cell* 1989; 56: 93–101.
127. Edgar D, Timpl R, Theonen H. The heparin-binding domain of laminin is responsible for its effects on neurite outgrowth and neuronal survival. *EMBO J* 1984; 3: 1463–1468.
128. Kleinman HK, McGarvey ML, Hassell JR, Martin GR, Baron van Evercooren A, Dubois-Dalcq M. The role of laminin in basement membranes and in the growth, adhesion and differentiation of cells. In: Trelstad RL, ed. *The role of extracellular matrix in development.* New York: Alan R. Liss, Inc.; 1984: 123–143.
129. McCarthy JB, Palm SL, Furcht LT. Migration by haptotaxis of a Schwann cell tumor line to

the basement membrane glycoprotein laminin. *J Cell Biol* 1984; 97: 772–777.
130. Ernsberger U, Rohrer H. Neuronal precursor cells in chick dorsal root ganglia: differentiation and survival in vitro. *Dev Biol* 1988; 126: 420–32.
131. Wood PM, Schachner M, Bunge RP. Inhibition of Schwann cell myelination in vitro by antibody to the L1 adhesion molecule. *J Neurosci* 1990; 11: 3635–3645.
132. Reh TA, Nagy T, Gretton H. Retinal pigmented epithelial cells induced to transdifferentiate to neurons by laminin. *Nature* 1987; 330: 68–71.
133. Acheson A, Edgar D, Timpl R, Thoenen H. Laminin increases both levels and activity of tyrosine hydroxylase in calf adrenal chromaffin cells. *J Cell Biol* 1986; 102: 151–59.
134. Yayon A, Klagsbrun M, Esko JD, Leder P, Ornitz DM. Cell surface, heparin-like molecules are required for binding of basic fibroblast growth factor to its high affinity receptor. *Cell* 1991; 64: 841–848.
135. Rapraeger AC, Krufka A, Olwin BB. Requirement for heparan sulfate for bFGF-mediated fibroblast growth and myoblast differentiation. *Science* 1991; 252: 1705–1708.
136. McCaffrey TA, Falcone DJ, Brayton CF, Agarwal LA, Welt FGP, Weksler BB. Transforming growth factor-β activity is potentiated by heparin via dissociation of the transforming growth factor-β/α2-macroglobulin inactive complex. *J Cell Biol* 1989; 109: 441–448.
137. Silverstein RL, Harpel PC, Nachman RL. Tissue plasminogen activator and urokinase enhance the binding of plasminogen to thrombospondin. *J Biol Chem* 1986; 261: 9959–9965.
138. Narindrasorask S, Lowery D, Gonzalez-DeWhitt G, Dorrman RA, Greenberg B, Kisilevsky R. High affinity interactions between the Alzheimer's β-amyloid precursor protein and the basement membrane form of heparan sulfate proteoglycan. *J Biol Chem* 1991; 266: 12878–12883.
139. Franco BS, Guioli A, Pragliola B, et al. A gene deleted in Kallmann's syndrome shares homology with neural cell adhesion and axon-path finding molecules. *Nature* 1991; 353: 529–536.
140. Legouis R, Hardelin J-P, Levillers J, et al. The candidate gene for the X-linked Kallmann syndrome encodes a protein related to adhesion molecules. *Cell* 1991; 67: 423–435.
141. Schwanzel-Fakuda M, Pfaff DW. Origin of leutinizing hormone-releasing hormone neurons. *Nature* 1989; 338: 161–164.
142. Wray S, Grant P, Gainer H. Evidence that cells expressing leutinizing hormone-releasing hormone mRNA in the mouse are derived from progenitor cells in the olfactory placode. *Proc Natl Acad Sci USA* 1989; 86: 8132–8136.
143. Ruoslahti E, Pierschbacher MD. Arg-Gly-Asp: a versatile cell recognition signal. *Cell* 1986; 44: 517–518.
144. Carbonetto S, Gruver MM, Turner DC. Nerve fiber growth in culture on fibronectin, collagen and glycosaminoglycan substrates. *J Neurosci* 1983; 3: 2324–2335.
145. Rogers SL, Letourneau PC, Peterson BA, Furcht LT, McCarthy JB. Selective interaction of peripheral and central nervous system cells with two distinct cell-binding domains of fibronectin. *J Cell Biol* 1987; 105: 1435–42.
146. McCarthy JB, Skubitz APN, Zha Q, Yi X, Mickelson DJ, Klein DJ, Furcht LT. RGD-independent cell adhesion to the carboxy-terminal heparin-binding fragment of fibronectin involves heparin-dependent and independent activities. *J Cell Biol* 1990; 110: 777–787.
147. Humphries JM, Akiyama SK, Komoriya A, Olden K, Yamada KM. Identification of an alternatively spliced site in human plasma fibronectin that mediates cell type-specific adhesion. *J Cell Biol* 1986; 103: 2637–2647.
148. Humphries JM, Akiyama SK, Komoriya A, Olden K, Yamada KM. Neurite extension of chicken peripheral nervous system neurons on fibronectin: relative importance of specific adhesion sites in the central cell-binding domain and the alternatively spliced type III connecting segment. *J Cell Biol* 1988; 106: 1289–1298.
149. Saunders S, Bernfield M. Cell surface proteoglycan binds mouse mammary epithelial cells to fibronectin and behaves as a receptor for interstitial matrix. *J Cell Biol* 1988; 106: 423–430.
150. Yamada KM. Adhesive recognition sequences. *J Biol Chem* 1991; 266: 12809–12812.
151. Lawler J, Weinstein R, Hynes RO. Cell attachment to thrombospondin: the role of ARG-GLY-ASP, calcium and integrin receptors. *J Cell Biol* 1988; 107: 2341–2361.
152. Pytela R, Pierschbacher MD, Ruoslahti E. A 125/115 kDa cell surface receptor specific for vitronectin interacts with the arginine-glycine-aspartic acid adhesion sequence derived from fibronectin. *Proc Natl Acad Sci USA* 1985; 82: 5766–5770.
153. Pytela R, Pierschbacher M, Ginsburg M, Plow E, Ruoslahti E. Platelet membrane glycoprotein IIb/IIIa: a member of a family of ARG-GLY-ASP specific adhesion receptors. *Science* 1986; 231: 1559–1567.
154. Graf J, Ogle RC, Robey FA, Saskaki M, Martin GR, Yamada Y, Kleinman HK. A pentapeptide from the laminin B1 chain mediates cell adhesion and binds the 67,000 laminin receptor. *Biochemistry* 1987; 26: 6896–6900.
155. Hunter D, Shah V, Merlie J, Sanes J. A laminin-like adhesive protein concentrated in the synaptic cleft of the neuromuscular junction. *Nature* 1989; 338: 229–234.
156. Ehrig K, Leivo I, Argraves WS, Ruoslahti E, Engvall E. The tissue-specific basement membrane protein merosin is a laminin-like protein. *Proc Natl Acad Sci USA* 1990; 87: 3264–3268.
157. Sanes JR, Engvall E, Butkowski R, Hunter DD. Molecular heterogeneity of basal laminae: isoforms of laminin and collagen IV at the neuromuscular junction and elsewhere. *J Cell Biol* 1990; 111: 1685–1699.

158. Engvall E, Earwicker D, Day S, Muir D, Manthorpe M, Paulsson M. Merosin promotes cell attachment and neurite outgrowth and is a component of the neurite-promoting factor of RN22 Schwannoma cells. *Exp Cell Res* 1991; 198: 115–123.
159. Ide C, Tohyama K, Yokota R, Nitatori T, Onodera S. Schwann cell basal lamina and nerve regeneration. *Brain Res* 1983; 288: 61–75.
160. Hall SM. The effect of inhibiting Schwann cell mitosis on the re-innervation of acellular autografts in the peripheral nervous system of the mouse. *Neuropathol Appl Neurobiol* 1986; 12: 401–414.
161. Madison RD, Da Silva C, Dikkes P, Sidman RL and Chiu T-H. Peripheral nerve regeneration with entubulation repair: comparison of biodegradable nerve guides versus polyethylene tubes and the effects of a laminin-containing gel. *Exp Neurol* 1987; 95: 378–390.
162. Toyota B, Carbonetto S, David S. A dual laminin/collagen receptor acts in peripheral nerve regeneration. *Proc Natl Acad Sci USA* 1990; 87: 1319–1322.
163. Margolis RK, Margolis RV. Structure and localization of glycoproteins and proteoglycans, In Margolis RV and RK, eds.: *Neurology of glycoconjugates*. New York: Plenum Press; 1989: 85–126.
164. Carlson SS, Wight TN. Nerve terminal anchorage protein 1 (TAP-1) is a chondroitin sulfate proteoglycan: biochemical and electron microscopic characterization. *J Cell Biol* 1987; 105: 3075–86.
165. Benedum UM, Baeuerle PA, Konecki DS, Frank R, Powell J, Mallet J, Huttner WB. The primary structure of bovine chromogranin A: a representative of a class of acidic secretory proteins common to a variety of peptidergic cells. *EMBO J* 1986; 5: 1495–1502.
166. Saunders S, Jalkanen M, O'Farrell S, Bernfield M. Molecular cloning of syndecan, an integral membrane proteoglycan. *J Cell Biol* 1989; 108: 1547–1556.
167. Anderson MJ, Fambrough DM. Aggregates of acetylcholine receptors are associated with plaques of a basal lamina heparan sulfate proteoglycan on the surface of skeletal muscle fibers. *J Cell Biol* 1983; 97: 1396–1411.
168. Inestrosa NC, Perelman A. Association of acetylcholine-esterase with the cell surface. *J Membr Biol* 1990; 118: 1–9.
169. Kalb RG, Hockfield S. Induction of a neuronal proteoglycan by the NMDA receptor in the developing spinal cord. *Science* 1990; 250: 294–296.
170. Ruoslahti E, Yamaguchi Y. Proteoglycans as modulators of growth factor activities. *Cell* 1991; 64: 867–869.
171. Yayon A, Klagsbrun M, Esko JD, Leder P, Ornitz DM. Cell surface, heparin-like molecules are required for binding of basic fibroblast growth factor to its high affinity receptor. *Cell* 1991; 64: 841–848.
172. Klagsbrun M. The affinity of fibroblast growth factors (FGFs) for heparin; FGF-heparan sulfate interactions in cells and extracellular matrix. *Curr Opin Cell Biol* 1990; 2: 857–863.
173. Tamkun JW, DeSimone DW, Fonda D, Patel RS, Buck C, Horwitz AF, Hynes RO. Structure of integrin, a glycoprotein involved in the transmembrane linkage between fibronectin and actin. *Cell* 1986; 46: 271–282.
174. Bossy B, Bossy E, Reichardt LF. Characterization of the integrin $\alpha 8$ subunit: a new integrin $\beta 1$ associated subunit which is prominently expressed on axons and basal laminae in chick embryos. *EMBO J* 1991; 10: 2375–2385.
175. Weinstein DE, Marcantonio EE, Sonnenberg AK, Liem RKH. Inhibition of astrocyte proliferation requires the integrin $\alpha_6\beta_4$. *ASCB Abstr* 1991; 1151: 109a.
176. Tawil NJ, Carbonetto S. Immunocytochemical studies of integrin in type-2 astrocytes and oligodendrocytes. *ASCB Abstr* 1991; 115: 287a.
177. Elices MJ, Osborn L, Takada Y, Crouse C, Luhowskyj S, et al. VCAM-1 on activated endothelium interacts with the leukocyte integrin VKA-4 at a site distinct from the VKA-4/fibronectin binding site. *Cell* 1989; 60: 577–584.
178. van Kuppevelt TH, Languino LR, Gailit JO, Suzuki S, Ruoslahti E. An alternative cytoplasmic domain of the integrin beta 3 subunit. *Proc Natl Acad Sci USA* 1989; 86: 5415–18.
179. Brown NH, King DL, Wilcox M, Kafatos FC. Developmentally regulated alternative splicing of Drosophila integrin PS2 α transcripts. *Cell* 1989; 59: 185–95.
180. Smith JW, Cheresh DA. Integrin ($\alpha_v\beta_3$) ligand interaction: identification of a heterodimeric RGD binding site on the vitronectin receptor. *J Biol Chem* 1990; 265: 2168–2172.
181. D'Souza SE, Ginsberg MH, Burke TA, Lam SC-T, Plow EF. Localization of an Arg-Gly-Asp recognition site within an integrin adhesion receptor. *Science* 1988; 242: 91–93.
182. Horwitz A, Duggan K, Buck C, Berkerle M, Burridge K. Interaction of a plasma membrane fibronectin receptor with talin: a transmembrane linkage. *Nature* 1986; 320: 531–533.
183. Burridge J, Fath K, Kelly T, Nuckolls G, Turner C. Focal adhesion: transmembrane junctions between the extracellular matrix and the cytoskeleton. *Annu Rev Cell Biol* 1988; 4: 487–525.
184. Elices MJ, Hemler ME. The human integrin VLA-2 is a collagen receptor on some cells and a collagen/laminin receptor on others. *Proc Natl Acad Sci USA* 1989; 86: 9906–9910.
185. Bozyczko D, Horwitz AF. The participation of a putative cell surface receptor for laminin and fibronectin in peripheral neurite extension. *J Neurosci* 1986; 6: 1241–1251.
186. Turner DC, Flier LA, Carbonetto S. Identification of a cell-surface protein involved in PC12 cell-substratum adhesion and neurite growth on laminin and collagen. *J Neurosci* 1989; 9: 3287–96.
187. Tomaselli KJ, Hall DE, Flier LA, Gehlsen KR,

Turner DC, et al. A neuronal cell line (PC12) expresses two β_1-class integrins—$\alpha_1\beta_1$ and $\alpha_3\beta_1$—that recognize different neurite outgrowth-promoting domains in laminin. *Neuron* 1990; 5: 651–662.
188. Lein PJ, Higgins D, Turner DC, Flier LA, Terranova VP. The NC1 domain of type IV collagen promotes axonal growth in sympathetic neurons through interaction with the $\alpha_1\beta_1$ integrin. *J Cell Biol* 1991; 113: 417–428.
189. Letourneau PC, Shattuck TA. Distribution and possible interactions of actin-associated proteins and cell adhesion molecules of nerve growth cones. *Development* 1989; 105: 505–519.
190. Cohen J, Burne JF, Winter J, Bartlett P. Retinal ganglion cells lose response to laminin with maturation. *Nature* 1986; 322: 465–467.
191. Cohen J, Burne JF, McKinlay C, Winter J. The role of laminin and the laminin/fibronectin receptor complex in the outgrowth of retinal ganglion cell axons. *Dev Biol* 1987; 122: 407–418.
192. Cohen J, Nurcombe V, Jeffrey P, Edgar D. Developmental loss of functional laminin receptors on retinal ganglion cells is regulated by their target tissue, the optic tectum. *Development* 1989; 107: 381–387.
193. DeCurtis I, Quaranta V, Tamura RN, Reichardt LF. Laminin receptors in the retina: sequence analysis of the chick integrin α_6 subunit evidence for transcriptional and posttranslational regulation. *J Cell Biol* 1991; 113: 405–416.
194. Neugebauer KM, Reichardt LF. Cell surface regulation of β_1-integrin activity on developing retinal neurons. *Nature* 1991; 350: 68–71.
195. Tomaselli KJ, Reichardt LF. Peripheral motoneuron interactions with laminin and Schwann cells-derived neurite-promoting molecules: developmental regulation of laminin receptor function. *J Neurosci Res* 1988; 21: 275–285.
196. Rossino P, Gavazzi IF, Timpl R, Aumailley M, Abbadini M, Giancotti F, et al. Nerve growth factor induces increased expression of a laminin binding integrin in rat pheochromocytoma PC12 cells. *Exp Cell Res* 1990; 189: 100–108.
197. Diamond J, Coughlin M, MacIntyre L, Holmes M, Visheau B. Evidence that endogenous β nerve growth factor is responsible for the collateral sprouting, but not the regeneration, of nociceptive axons in adult rats. *Proc Natl Acad Sci USA* 1987; 84: 6596–6600.
198. Mecham RP. Laminin receptors. *Annu Rev Cell Biol* 1991; 7: 71–92.
199. Begovac PC, Hall DE, Shur BD. Laminin fragment E8 mediates PC12 cell neurite outgrowth by binding to cell surface beta 1,4 galactosyltransferase. *J Cell Biol* 1991; 113: 637–644.
200. Kleinman HK, Ogle RL, Cannon FB, Little CD, Sweeny TM, Luckenbill-Eggs L. Laminin receptors for neurite formation. *Proc Natl Acad Sci USA* 1988; 85: 1282–1286.
201. Clegg DO, Helder JC, Hann BC, Hall DE, Reichardt LF. Amino acid sequence and distribution of mRNA encoding a major skeletal muscle laminin binding protein: an extracellular matrix-associated protein with an unusual COOH-terminal polyaspartate domain. *J Cell Biol* 1988; 107: 699–705.
202. Yazaki PJ, Salvatori S, Dahms AS. Amino acid sequence of chicken calsequestrin deduced from cDNA: comparison of calsequestrin and aspartactin. *Biochem Biophys Res Commun* 1990; 170: 1089–95.
203. Lesot H, Kuhl U, von der Mark K. Isolation of a laminin-binding protein from muscle cell membranes. *EMBO J* 1983; 2: 861–865.
204. Wewer UM, Liotta LA, Jaye M, Ricca GA, Drohan WN, Claysmith AP, Rao CN, Wirth P, Coligan JE, Albrechtsen R, Mudryj M, Sobel ME. Altered levels of laminin receptor in various carcinoma cells that have different abilities to bind laminin. *Proc Natl Acad Sci USA* 1986; 83: 7137–7141.
205. Segui-Real B, Savagner P, Ogle RC, Huang T, Martin GR, Yamada Y. Unusual features of the laminin receptor predicted from the cDNA clones. *FASEB J* 1988; 2: A1551.
206. Segui-Real B, Rhodes C, Yamada Y. The human genome contains a pseudogene for the $M_r = 32,000$ laminin binding protein. *Nucleic Acids Res* 1989; 17: 1257.
207. Rabacchi SA, Neve RL, Drager UC. A positional marker for the dorsal embryonic retina is homologous to the high-affinity laminin receptor. *Development* 1990; 109: 521–531.
208. Yow H, Wong JM, Chen HS, Lee C, Steele GD Jr, Chen LB. Increased mRNA expression of a laminin-binding protein in human colon carcinoma: complete sequence of a full-length cDNA encoding the protein. *Proc Natl Acad Sci USA* 1988; 85: 6394–6398.
209. Grosso LE, Park PW, Mecham RP. Characterization of a putative cone for the 67-kDa elastin/laminin receptor suggests that it encodes a cytoplasmic protein rather than a cell surface receptor. *Biochemistry* 1991; 30: 3346–3350.
210. Makrides S, Chitpatima ST, Bandyopadhyay R, Brawerman G. Nucleotide sequence for a major messenger RNA for a 40 kilodalton polypeptide that is under translational control in mouse tumor cells. *Nucleic Acids Res* 1988; 16: 2349.
211. Yang G, Douvville P, Gee S, Carbonetto S. Non-integrin laminin receptors. *J Neurobiol* 1992; in press.
212. Rao CN, Castronovo V, Schmitt C, Wewer UM, Claysmith AP, Liotta LA, Sobel ME. Evidence for a precursor of the high-affinity metastasis-associated murine laminin receptor. *Biochemistry* 1989; 28: 7476–7486.
213. Mecham RP, Hinek A, Griffin GL, Senior RM, Liotta L. The elastin receptor shows structural and functional similarities to the 67-kDa tumor cell laminin receptor. *J Biol Chem* 1989; 264: 16652–16657.
214. Graf J, Ogle FC, Iwamoto Y, et al. Identification of an amino acid sequence in laminin mediating cell attachment, chemotaxis, and receptor binding. *Cell* 1987; 48: 989–996.

215. Laurie GW, Stone CM, Yamada Y. Elevated 32kDa LBP and low laminin mRNA expression in developing mouse cerebrum. *Different* 1991; 46: 173–179.
216. Smalheiser NR, Schwartz NB. Cranin: a laminin binding protein of cell membranes. *Proc Natl Acad Sci USA* 1987; 84: 6457–6461.
217. Douville PJ, Harvey WJ, Carbonetto S. Isolation and partial characterization of high affinity laminin receptors in neural cells. *J Biol Chem* 1988; 263: 14964–14969.
218. Kleinman HK, Weeks BS, Cannon FB, et al. Identifications of a 110kD non-integrin cell surface laminin-binding protein which recognizes an A chain neurite promoting peptide. *Arch Biochem Biophys* 1991; 290: 320–325.
219. Jucker M, Kleinman HK, Ingram DK. Fetal rat septal cells adhere to and extend processes on basement membrane laminin and a synthetic peptide from the laminin A chain sequence. *J Neurosci Res* 1991; 28: 507–517.
220. Jucker M, Kleinman HK, Höhmann CF, Ordy JM, Ingram DK. Distinct immunoreactivity to 110 kD LBP in normal and lesioned adult rat forebrain. *Brain Res* 1991; 555: 305–312.
221. Shur BD. Glycoconjugates as mediators of cellular interactions during development. *Curr Opin Cell Biol* 1989; 1: 905–912.
222. Runyan RB, Maxwell GD, Shur BD. Evidence for a novel enzymatic mechanism of neural crest cell migration on extracellular glycoconjugate matrices. *J Cell Biol* 1986; 102: 434–441.
223. Riopelle RJ, Dow KE. Neurite formation on laminin: effects of galactosyltransferase on primary sensory neurons. *Brain Res* 1991; 541: 265–272.
224. Woo H-J, Shaw LM, Messier JM, Mercurio AM. The major non-integrin laminin binding protein of macrophages is identical to carbohydrate binding protein 35(Mac-2). *J Biol Chem* 1990; 265: 7097–7099.
225. Barondes SH. Bifunctional properties of lectins: lectins redefined. *Trends Biochem Sci* 1988; 13: 480–482.
226. Springer TA. The sensation and regulation of interactions with the extracellular environment: the cell biology of lymphocyte adhesion receptors. *Annu Rev Cell Biol* 1990; 6: 359–402.
227. Picker LJ, Nakachi M, Butcher EC. Monoclonal antibodies to human lymphocyte homing receptors define a novel class of adhesion molecules on diverse cell types. *J Cell Biol* 1989; 109: 927–937.
228. Giftochristos N, David S. Laminin and heparan sulphate proteoglycan in the lesioned adult mammalian central nervous system and their possible relationship to axonal sprouting. *J Neurocytol* 1988; 17: 385–397.
229. Snow DM, Lemmon V, Currino CA, Caplan AI, Silver J. Sulfated proteoglycans in astroglial barriers inhibit neurite outgrowth in vitro. *Exp Neurol* 1990; 109: 111–130.
230. Oohira A, Matsui F, Katoh-Semba R. Inhibitory effects of brain chondroitin sulfate proteoglycans on neurite outgrowth from PC12D cells. *J Neurosci* 1991; 11: 822–827.
231. Akeson R, Warren SL. PC12 adhesion and neurite formation on selected substrates are inhibited by some glycosamino-glycans and a fibronectin-derived tetrapeptide. *Exp Cell Res* 1986; 162: 347–362.
232. Snow DM, Steindler DA, Siler J. Molecular and cellular characterization of the glial roof plate of the spinal cord and optic tectum: a possible role for a proteoglycan in the development of an axon barrier. *Dev Biol* 1990; 138: 359–376.
233. Riopelle RJ, Dow KE. Functional interactions of neuronal heparan sulphate proteoglycan with laminin. *Brain Res* 1990; 525: 92.
234. Spring J, Beck H, Chiquet-Ehrismann R. Two contrary functions of tenascin: dissection of the active sites by recombinant tenascin fragments. *Cell* 1989; 59: 325–34.
235. Chuong CM, Crossin KL, Edelman GM. Sequential expression and differential function of multiple adhesion molecules during the formation of cerebellar cortical layers. *J Cell Biol* 1987; 104: 331–342.
236. Steindler DA, Cooper NGF, Faissner A, Schachner M. Boundaries defined by adhesion molecules during development of the cerebral cortex: the J1/tenascin glycoprotein in the mouse somatosensory cortical barrel field. *Dev Biol* 1989; 131: 243–260.
237. Faissner A, Kruse J. J1/tenascin is a repulsive substrate for central nervous system neurons. *Neuron* 1990; 5: 627–637.
238. Lochter A, Vaughan L, Kaplony A, Prochiantz A, Schachner M, Faissner A. J1/tenascin in substrate-bound and soluble forms displays contrary effects on neurite outgrowth. *J Cell Biol* 1991; 113: 1159–1171.
239. Wehrle B, Chiquet M. Tenascin is accumulated along developing peripheral nerves and allows neurite outgrowth in vitro. *Development* 1990; 110: 401–415.
240. Faissner A, Kruse J, Kuhn, Schachner M. Binding of the J1 adhesion molecules to extracellular matrix constituents. *J Neurochem* 1990; 54: 1004–1015.
241. Bourdon MA, Ruoslahti E. Tenascin mediates cell attachment through an RGD-dependent receptor. *J Cell Biol* 1989; 108: 1149–1155.
242. Crossin KL, Prieto AL, Hoffman S, Jones FS, Friedlander DR. Expression of adhesion molecules and the establishment of boundaries during embryonic and neural development. *Exp Neurol* 1990; 109: 6–18.
243. Martini R, Schachner M, Faissner A. Enhanced expression of the extracellular matrix molecule J1/tenascin in the regenerating adult mouse sciatic nerve. *J Neurocytol* 1990; 19: 601–616.
244. Ajemian A, David S. Immunocytochemical detection of tenascin in the transected adult rat optic nerve. *Soc Neurosci Abstr* 1991; 17: 49.
245. Laywell ED, O'Brien TF, Harrington K, Steindler DA, Schachner M, Dorries U. In situ hy-

bridization studies of J1/tenascin reappearance following traumatic brain injury in mouse and human. *Soc Neurosci Abstr* 1991; 17: 49.
246. Johnston IG, Paladino T, Gurd JW, Brown JR. Molecular cloning of SC1: a putative brain extracellular matrix glycoprotein showing partial similarity to osteonectin/BM40/SPARC. *Neuron* 1990; 2: 165–176.
247. Morganti MC, Taylor J, Pesheva P, Schachner M. Oligodendrocyte-derived J1-160/180 extracellular matrix glycoproteins are adhesive or repulsive depending on the partner cell type and time of its interaction. *Exp Neurol* 1990; 109: 98–110.
248. Hunter DD, Porter BE, Bulock JW, Adams SP, Merlie JP, Sanes JR. Primary sequence of a motor neuron-selective adhesive site in the synaptic basal lamina protein S-laminin. *Cell* 1989; 59: 905–913.
249. Bandtlow C, Zachleder T, Schwab ME. Oligodendrocytes arrest neurite growth by contact inhibition. *J Neurosci* 1990; 101: 3837–3848.
250. Caroni P, Schwab ME. Two membrane protein fractions from rat central myelin with inhibitory properties for neurite growth and fibroblast spreading. *J Cell Biol* 1988; 106: 1281–1288.
251. Savio T, Schwab MR. Lesioned corticospinal tract axons regenerate in myelin-free rat spinal cord. *Proc Natl Acad Sci USA* 1990; 87: 4130–4133.
252. Schnell L, Schwab ME. Axonal regeneration in the rat spinal cord produced by an antibody against myelin-associated neurite growth inhibitors. *Nature* 1990; 343: 269–272.
253. Kater SR, Mills LR. Regulation of growth cone behaviour by calcium. *J Neurosci* 1991; 11: 891–897.
254. Campenot RB, Draker DD. Growth of sympathetic nerve fibers in culture does not require extracellular calcium. *Neuron* 1989; 3: 733–743.
255. Turner DC, Flier LA, Carbonetto S. Magnesium-dependent attachment and neurite outgrowth by PC12 cells on collagen and laminin substrata. *Dev Biol* 1987; 121: 510–525.
256. Walter J, Allsopp TE, Bonhoeffer F. A common denominator of growth cone guidance and collapse? *TINS* 1990; 13: 447–452.

6

Neurotrophic Function in Normal Nerve and in Peripheral Neuropathies

Bruce G. Gold and Peter S. Spencer

Center for Research on Occupational and Environmental Toxicology, Oregon Health Sciences University, Portland, Oregon 97201

The evolution of larger species of animals coincides with the development of neurons with long axonal processes, some of which extend over a meter in length. The axon is dependent upon the nerve cell body (soma) for a continued supply of materials essential for maintenance of axonal structure and function, since protein synthesis is largely restricted to the neuronal soma. To meet this requirement, nature has evolved an elaborate system—axonal transport—to deliver materials to the axon over long distances and return them from the axon to the soma. Although this system is incompletely defined, recent studies have greatly advanced understanding of the molecular mechanisms underlying the movement of materials through the axoplasm (for review, see 1). Fast anterograde (from soma to axon terminal) and retrograde (from axon terminal to soma) transport appears to utilize distinct adenosine triphosphate (ATP)-dependent protein motors for force generation, namely kinesin and dynein, respectively. Whether these proteins can be independently perturbed (by chemicals and in disease), and what the functional consequences are of a selective impairment of the associated cellular transport processes are important avenues for future research.

The polarized architecture of the neuron, with the soma and axon terminal at opposite ends, and the axon's dependency upon an energy-dependent transport system for supply and clearance of materials, are important contributors to the selective vulnerability of axons to numerous exogenous chemicals and abnormal metabolic states. A priori, the distal portion of the axon would be most vulnerable to a defect in axonal transport because it is most removed from the source of somal resupply of essential materials. This is the most commonly advanced explanation for the spatial-temporal pattern of nerve fiber degeneration—distal, retrograde ("dying-back") axonopathy—found in the large number of sensorimotor peripheral neuropathies associated with disparate chemical intoxications, as well as with various forms of spontaneous or inherited metabolic compromise. However, it has yet to be proven that a defect in axonal transport (fast or slow) underlies the development of axonal degeneration in any such situation (see below). In addition to the proposed defects of axonal transport in the development of peripheral neuropathies, axonal transport also appears to play an important role in recovery from nerve-fiber injury; the rate of axonal elongation from the damage site coinciding with the rate of slow axonal transport. Successful axonal regeneration is dependent upon the environment of the axonal sprout which provides a chemotropic pathway for the elongating axon.

This active process appears to influence the somal response to axonal injury.

This chapter examines recent advances in understanding the mechanisms underlying successful axonal regeneration in the peripheral nervous system (PNS). The major emphasis is on the role of nerve growth factor (NGF) in providing both neurotrophic (nourishment) and neurotropic (guidance) support to neurons in the adult PNS. We attempt to synthesize basic research with clinical observation by focusing upon the morphological alterations accompanying axonal degeneration and regeneration. This bridge of experimental and human studies is timely since, at the rate at which advances are currently taking place in the laboratory setting, clinical trials of many novel approaches for the enhancement of axonal regeneration appear imminent.

AXONAL TRANSPORT IN PERIPHERAL NEUROPATHIES

The most common type of peripheral neuropathy in humans is loss of the distal region of long and large-diameter axons with survival of most neuronal somata. These pathological changes are characteristically associated with a stocking-and-glove pattern of sensory loss, which is later accompanied by a similar distribution of motor weakness. Such changes are found in a number of vitamin-deficiency states, metabolic disorders such as diabetes mellitus, and in advanced age. These conditions are supplemented by a large number of localized mechanical nerve injuries that lead directly to distal axonal degeneration. A variety of chemical agents, such as thallium and arsenic salts, 2,5-hexanedione, and acrylamide, also elicit distal axonal degeneration in humans or animals, or both (see 2). The presence of axonal loss, together with the dependency of the axon on the neuronal soma, suggests that defects or interruptions in the delivery of materials via axonal transport are key to the pathogenesis of axonal degeneration in human axonopathies (see 3).

A defect in *slow* axonal transport has been demonstrated in a number of situations, including experimental acrylamide intoxication (4). Defects in slow axonal transport lead to changes in axonal caliber but not distal axonal degeneration. This has been best demonstrated in β,β'-iminodipropionitrile (IDPN) neuropathy where there is a selective defect of neurofilament transport (5–7). Neurofilaments (NFs) are transported along the axon at the rate of the slower component of slow axonal transport, i.e., the SCa phase (8,9). NFs (together with microtubules) form the cytoskeletal matrix of axons and are the major determinants of axonal caliber in large myelinated fibers (10,11). Alterations in axonal caliber (neurofilament content) are seen in experimental IDPN neuropathy, but this occurs in the absence of axonal degeneration (12). Changes in axonal caliber, with increased diameters proximally and decreases distally, are also associated with slow transport defects (SCa and SCb) in experimental diabetic neuropathy, whether induced by systemic streptozotocin treatment (13–15), as a spontaneously arising abnormality seen in BB rats (14,16–18), or in mutant mouse models of diabetes mellitus (19). Once again, changes in slow axonal transport appear to underlie axonal caliber changes in these animals (13–15, 20,21).

Whereas defects in slow axonal transport lead to changes in axon caliber, chemicals that reduce either the rate or amount of *fast* anterogradely transported materials appear to cause distal axonal degeneration (see 3). A decrease in the amount of fast anterogradely transported materials reaching the distal axon, as opposed to an alteration in transport rate (suggested by Carrington et al., 22), has been found early on (hours) following a single injection of either an organophosphate (22,23) or the nicotinamide analog Vacor (N-3-pryidylmethyl-N'-p-nitrophenlyurea) (24), agents which induce distal axonopathy following a single dose. A retardation in fast anterogradely transported proteins also has been suggested to occur 24 hours following a single, high-dose injection of acrylamide (25). However, these findings are not definitive since data were not normalized to the amount of radioactivity present in the injected dorsal root ganglia (DRG). We have recently re-examined this issue and were unable to confirm the observation. However, we found that a single systemic injection of acrylamide (50–100 mg/kg, i.p.) 24 hours prior to radiolabeling impaired outflow of glycoproteins in the sciatic nerve in a dose-dependent fashion (B.G. Gold, T. Storm-Dickerson, unpublished observations). Further transport and autoradiographic studies are needed to ascertain whether this defect is due to a decrease in materials delivered to the distal axon or to a reduction in the rate of fast anterograde transport.

Experimental (streptozotocin-induced) diabetic neuropathy is also associated with a reduced amount of fast anterogradely transported proteins but no overall change in transport rate (26). A defect in fast anterograde transport of specific receptors and neurotransmitter enzymes, as measured by their accumulation proximal to a nerve ligature, has been demonstrated in streptozotocin-induced diabetic neuropathy (27–29). Whether this decrease in amount of fast anterogradely transported materials results from a decreased delivery of SCb (microtubules) materials to the distal (see above) axon is an important question. A demonstration of this type would suggest that defective SCb transport, which maintains the microtubules on which fast transport depends (30–32), could lead secondarily to axonal degeneration (14).

Impairment in retrograde axonal transport, which occurs very early (hours) after systemic administration of chemicals, has been found to be associated with the subsequent (days) development of distal axonal degeneration. Miller and Spencer (33) found that acrylamide reduced the rate of retrograde axonal transport within hours, and the abnormality increased as a function of repeated dosing until axonal degeneration ensued. A progressive decrease in retrograde transport also has been observed after a single dose of an organophosphate capable of inducing axonal neuropathy (34). Decreased retrograde axonal transport of glycoproteins, measured by accumulation distal to a nerve ligature (35), has been found in experimental streptozotocin-induced diabetic neuropathy. Taken together, these data might suggest that an early defect in retrograde axonal transport underlies the development of axonal degeneration in these various axonopathies. However, recent evidence, presented below, indicates that a defect in retrograde axonal transport leads to a loss of target tissue-derived "trophic" support. This hypothesis appears to be consistent with the decrease in retrograde transport of NGF that has been observed in both diabetic (36,37) and acrylamide (38) neuropathies, two situations leading to very different patterns of axonal pathology. On the basis of the evidence presented below, it seems likely that a defect in retrograde axonal transport is unable to induce axonal degeneration but rather signals the neuronal soma to initiate regenerative changes comparable to those seen following axotomy (i.e., axotomy-like alterations).

FATE OF THE NEURONAL SOMA AND PROXIMAL AXON

How is the neuronal soma informed that it has lost its axon (either by direct mechanical injury or from a chemically induced axotomy)? This simple and fundamental question in neurobiology is unanswered. Despite recognition of the neuron somal response to injury (axon reaction) for more than a century, little is known about the mechanism by which the axon reaction is initiated. Studies of the response of the neuronal soma and proximal axon to axotomy provide valuable clues as to the mechanism underlying induction of the axon reaction.

The Axon Reaction

Transection of peripheral nerve fibers (axotomy) is associated with a series of structural, physiological, and biochemical changes in the soma (and proximal axon) of injured neurons, collectively termed the axon reaction (11,39–45; for review, see 46,47). From a teleological perspective, these changes may be envisioned as a generalized switch of the neuron from its normal state to a regenerative mode. For example, the neuron normally functions to transmit action potential spikes along its axon. Since conduction velocity is a function of axonal diameter (and myelination), the neuron (now disconnected from its target) is temporarily unconcerned with the transmission of electrical impulses but needs to regrow the lost portion of distal axon and thereby reconnect with the target tissue. Thus, the neuronal soma reduces synthesis of materials (NFs) important for the maintenance of axonal diameter (caliber) and increases production of those components (microtubules and microfilaments) needed for axon elongation. This corresponds, respectively, to a decrease in synthesis of the NF triplet proteins and an increased synthesis of tubulin and actin (48,49). The probable structural correlate of these somal biochemical events is the dispersion of compact Nissl bodies (ribosome-associated endoplasmic reticulum), an event known as chromatolysis (46,47, 50). Additionally, the nucleus is displaced from its normal centric location to the periphery of the soma (i.e., nuclear eccentricity). The chromatolytic response varies with the age of the animal, species, and the proximity of the transection to the neuronal soma (see 47).

The axon reaction is best studied by focusing attention on early and specific components of the process that can be readily recognized and quantified. NFs meet these requirements. Moreover, studies of these structural proteins are of particular interest since alterations involving NFs have been linked to certain human disorders, such as amyotrophic lateral sclerosis (ALS), where they are the principal ultrastructural constituents of giant axonal swellings (51–53). Although the specificity of these pathological changes has not been established, they are readily reproduced in laboratory animals following treatment with a number of substances known to induce neuropathy. These considerations led one of us (B.G.G.) to focus upon two components of the axon reaction, namely somatofugal axonal atrophy and aberrant NF phosphorylation.

Somatofugal Axonal Atrophy

One of the most readily quantifiable features of the axon reaction is a reduction in axonal caliber in the proximal stump. This structural change reflects a decrease in NF content in the axon (11,54). Following axotomy, somal synthesis of NF proteins is decreased, as indicated by the smaller amount of NF mRNA in neuronal somata (48,55–57). The amount of NF protein delivered to the proximal axon is consequently reduced (44), and NF content in proximal axons is decreased (11). This reduced delivery of NFs is associated with a marked reduction in axonal calibers, reflecting the linear relationship of the cross-sectional area of large axons to NF content (10,11). Axonal atrophy begins near the neuronal soma and proceeds in a somatofugal fashion along the nerve, advancing at the rate of slow axonal transport, hence the term, somatofugal axonal atrophy (SAA) (11,58–62). Return to normal caliber is dependent upon reconnection of the axon with its target tissue; if regeneration is prevented, axonal atrophy persists (62). This suggests that the target organ produces a "trophic" signal(s) that functions to regulate (increase) NF content of the axon, thereby increasing axonal caliber (see "Trophic Regulation of the Axon Reaction" below).

Phosphorylated Neurofilament Epitopes

Another component of the axon reaction of DRG is alteration in the expression of phosphorylated NF (pNF) epitopes in neuronal somata (63–65). Phosphorylation occurs primarily on the carboxy-terminal domain, and the extent of phosphorylation correlates with subunit length (66–70). Phosphorylated NF epitopes of the medium (NF-M) and heavy (NF-H) proteins are present at very low levels in normal neuronal somata (71) and are markedly enriched in axons (72–74). Aberrant expression of pNF epitopes appears to represent a component of the axon reaction in DRG neurons, whether as a consequence of axotomy or local nerve application of colchicine to block axonal transport (75). We have recently found (see "Trophic Regulation of the Axon Reaction" below) that this component of the axon reaction exhibits a target-dependency for "trophic" regulation similar to that observed for NF content and axonal caliber.

The significance of aberrant expression of pNF epitopes in the soma of neurons with ongoing distal axonal degeneration is unknown. For the axon, increased NF phosphorylation correlates with the formation of a stationary NF network in the axoplasm (74,76) and the attainment of a mature (adult) diameter during postnatal development (62). If, as suggested elsewhere (77), the carboxy-terminal tail domains of the NF-M and NF-H subunits form projection arms that interact with NF elements (67,78), phosphorylation at these sites might serve to stabilize the NF network, locally reduce NF movement, and thereby cause focal increases in axonal caliber. However, dephosphorylation of axonal NFs does not alter the ability of the carboxy-terminal tail projections to form cross-bridges in vitro (79). Aberrant NF phosphorylation in the neuronal soma has been proposed to represent a mechanism leading to retention of NFs (72). Phosphorylated NFs in the neuronal soma might (by way of negative-feedback mechanism) serve to reduce the synthesis of NFs in the cell body (80). However, the recent demonstration that aberrant expression of pNF epitopes is present in DRG of IDPN-intoxicated rats (81), where there is no alteration (decrease) in NF gene expression (82), does not lend support to this hypothesis (at least at the level of transcriptional control). Taken together, inappropriate NF phosphorylation in sensory neurons appears to correlate best with a reduced delivery of NFs to the axon and the production of SAA. This statement is supported by the recent demonstration (83) that dephosphorylated NFs bind to microtubules (which would produce NF movement; see 1), suggesting that phosphorylated NFs are stationary.

The observation that neuronal somal immunoreactivity to pNF epitopes is present in fresh frozen hippocampus (84) deserves comment. Whether pNF immunostaining can be obtained in normal but chemically unfixed DRG neurons is unknown. However, if this is demonstrated, it will then be important to determine why pNF epitopes from axotomized nerves are resistant to the effects of fixation and processing. Should chemical fixation prove to be the key factor dictating the detection of pNF epitopes, the issue at hand would change from one of aberrant expression after axotomy to their differential resistance to fixation-induced denaturation. Nevertheless, it appears clear that axotomy leads to an alteration in NF structure resulting in an increase in immunodetectable levels of phosphorylated epitopes.

Trophic Regulation of the Axon Reaction

Various components of the axon reaction appear to be dependent upon intercourse between the axon terminal and the target organ. This phenomenon is known as target control. The most compelling evidence for target control is the reversal of axotomy-induced SAA and the up-regulation and down-regulation in NF and tubulin synthesis, respectively, upon reconnection of the regenerating nerve fiber with the target tissue (11,48,49). However, some components (e.g., actin synthesis) appear to be independent of target control (56). More importantly, some components of the axon reaction can be produced in *intact* neurons, indicating that physical separation of axon and target organ is not required to induce the axon reaction. For example, systemic injection of botulinum toxin reproduces the axotomy-induced increase in somal RNA synthesis (85), electrophysiological alterations (86), and SAA (87) in hypoglossal neurons. Moreover, blockade of retrograde axonal transport by direct colchicine application to a nerve segment causes many axotomy-like alterations in vertebrate and invertebrate neurons; these include SAA (88), aberrant NF phosphorylation (75), electrophysiological properties (89–91), synaptic dysfunction (91,92), and regenerative capabilities (93). Taken together, these findings are consistent with the proposal that a target-derived retrogradely transported "trophic" signal regulates normal neuronal properties. Loss of this putative signal appears to be responsible for at least these components of the axon reaction (86,94). We have conducted experiments to determine whether the putative signal in adult animals is nerve growth factor.

Putative Role of Nerve Growth Factor

Nerve growth factor (NGF) is the best-characterized neurotrophic factor in the nervous system (for reviews, see 95,96). A continual supply of NGF is required during development for the survival and growth of sensory (DRG) and sympathetic neurons (97,98). Sensory neurons lose their dependence on NGF for survival during postnatal development (99–101); administration of NGF antiserum fails to produce detectable cell death in adult DRG (102,103). However, throughout life, NGF is still specifically taken up at both peripheral and central processes of sensory neurons (104) and transported retrogradely to the neuronal soma (105); approximately 40% of the neurons in the adult DRG display high-affinity NGF receptors (106–108; for review, see 109) which appear to be necessary for transport of NGF to the neuronal soma. Whether the trk proto-oncogene product, a component of the NGF receptor that is required for production of high-affinity NGF binding (110–114), actively participates in the retrograde transport of NGF is unknown. Moreover, NGF receptors are present in DRG neuronal somata of all sizes, suggesting a role for NGF beyond merely promoting survival of small sensory neurons; the majority of NGF receptors in neuronal somata are not inserted into the plasmalemma and are either awaiting anterograde axonal transport or have been retrogradely transported with NGF from the periphery (115).

The function of NGF in adult sensory DRG neurons is unknown. Studies by others, however, suggest that NGF can regulate certain functional aspects of mature sensory neurons. For example, continuous infusion of NGF to the cut end of the proximal stump of a transected sciatic nerve prevents some of the morphological, biochemical, and electrophysiological alterations in axotomized DRG neuronal somata (103,116–118). Furthermore, NGF regulates gene expression and content of substance P and calcitonin gene-related peptide in DRG neurons (107,119,120); NGF deprivation results in marked reductions in substance P levels in DRG (103) and atrophy of DRG neuronal somata (117). In addition, the reduction (80%) in high-affinity NGF receptor binding on sensory neurons following axotomy fails to occur if NGF is applied to the cut end of a proximal nerve stump (107). Taken together, these findings suggest a continued, albeit undefined, role for NGF in adult (mature) sensory neurons.

Recent studies (80,94,121) indicate that NGF loss in adult sensory DRG neurons is responsible for production of at least three components of the axon reaction: 1) somatofugal axonal atrophy, which is the reduction in axonal caliber beginning in the proximal axon resulting from a decrease in NF synthesis; 2) nuclear eccentricity; and 3) aberrant expression of pNF epitopes in neuronal soma. Together, these observations suggest that NGF influences axonal size while serving in the broader capacity of a more generalized "trophic" (nourishment) factor which regulates the functional status of mature sensory neurons. It is unclear how NGF increases NF synthesis in mature DRG neurons. It appears to increase mRNA levels for NF-M (80) but not the light (NF-L) subunit (122) in DRG neurons. The lack of increase in mRNA levels for NF-L does not rule out an effect of NGF on NF synthesis since increased synthesis can occur by other means, namely increased translation of the mRNAs. However, the reason for failure to observe an effect of NGF on mRNA levels for the NF-L polypeptide (122) is unclear, particularly in view of the parallel NGF-induced increase in mRNA levels for these two NF polypeptides in PC12 cells (123) and the similar reductions in mRNA levels for the NF triplet proteins observed in axotomized nerves (56,124). However, it should be emphasized that changes in mRNA levels do not necessarily correlate directly with changes in NF synthesis. Our studies supplement these observations because they show that NGF promotes a functional increase in axonal NFs, supporting an effect on NF synthesis (80).

Role of Schwann Cell-Derived NGF

NGF is also produced by Schwann cells in the distal stump following axotomy (125). Schwann cell-derived NGF primarily appears to act locally to promote axonal regeneration (126), although some NGF from the distal stump is retrogradely transported to neuronal somata (127). However, Schwann cell-derived NGF is unlikely to compensate for the loss of target tissue-derived NGF since the amount transported to neuronal somata in axotomized nerves is markedly reduced (by approximately 2/3) from that in intact neurons (128,129). In distal lesions, neurons may remain relatively unresponsive to NGF (129) because axotomy results in loss of high-affinity NGF receptors (107,108; for review, see 109). NGF, albeit low amounts, may still be transported to the neuronal soma (127,129) where it might prevent cell death following axotomy (130); this could explain why very proximal (spinal root) transections produce both a robust axotomy-response (loss of NGF from target) and neuronal degeneration (loss of NGF from distal stump). Schwann cell-derived NGF acting on neuronal somata may also explain why NF synthesis begins to return to normal prior to reconnection of regenerating axons with the target tissue (56). Support for this hypothesis may be found in the observation that NF synthesis is not reduced to zero after axotomy (80,131). Furthermore, initial studies (B.G. Gold, D.R. Austin, and W.C. Mobley, unpublished observation) indicate that removal of NGF from the distal stump of a crushed nerve (by injection of NGF antiserum) increases the degree of axonal atrophy in the DRG.

Triggering the Axon Reaction

Does loss of target-derived NGF serve to initiate the axon reaction in DRG neurons? Resolution of this question would address the hypothesis of Cragg (132) that loss of a retrogradely transported "trophic" signal initiates the neuron somal response to injury (chromatolysis). While the veracity of this idea is unknown, there is evidence suggesting a broader role for NGF in the regulation of somal function. For example, axotomy-induced chromatolysis of sympathetic ganglion neurons in vitro is blocked by application of NGF (133,134). Furthermore, axotomy-induced changes in neurophysiological properties of sympathetic neurons are prevented or induced by treatment with either NGF or NGF antisera, respectively (133). Moreover, preliminary studies in our laboratory indicate that systemic NGF antiserum injections for 4 weeks produce early chromatolytic-like changes (displacement of the rough endoplasmic reticulum to the periphery of the neuronal soma) and aberrant expression of pNF epitopes in rat DRG neurons (121). Furthermore, we have also found that continuous infusion of NGF into the subarachnoid space of the lumbar spinal cord reduces the degree of expression of pNF epitopes in DRG neuronal somata (B.G. Gold, D.R. Austin, W.C. Mobley, and T. Storm-Dickerson, unpublished observation). Presumably, therefore, loss of NGF leads to aberrant expression of pNF epitopes only in those NGF-responsive neurons that demonstrate pNFs epitopes in their neuronal soma following axotomy. This suggests that another "trophic" factor (brain-derived neurotrophic factor [BDNF], neurotrophin-3 [NT-3] ?) is responsible for induction of this alteration in non-NGF responsive (those lacking high-affinity NGF receptors) neurons. Furthermore, we observed an accumulation of lysosomes and lipofuscin granules in DRG neuronal somata; similar accumulations occur with age (135,136) and may arise following axotomy from an alteration in the balance between synthesis and degradation (40,46).

Taken together, these findings indicate that NGF plays an important role in the maintenance of normal (phenotypic) neuronal properties in adult DRG neurons and its loss may be responsible for induction of the axon reaction in NGF-responsive neurons. It has also been suggested (80,131) that NGF plays a secondary (permissive) role by allowing another unidentified factor to regulate neuronal somal function. However, the observation that delivery of NGF alone to a transected nerve prevents the reduction in NF mRNA levels (80) and axonal caliber (121) argues that loss of NGF alone is sufficient to account for the production of these axotomy-like changes. In sum, loss of retrogradely transported NGF leads to a "switch" in the functional status of the neuronal soma, which appears to be analogous to the regenerative state observed following surgical (mechanical) axotomy (see also 129).

TROPHIC REGULATION IN CHEMICAL-INDUCED AXONOPATHIES

The preceding section examines the possibility that loss of target tissue-derived "trophic" support is responsible for induction of the axon reaction. Since NGF (and, presumably, other putative trophic factors active on non-sensory neurons) is delivered to the neuronal soma by retrograde axonal transport, perturbation of this transport system would predictably trigger regenerative (axotomy-like) changes in the neuronal soma (see Fig. 1). As discussed before, systemic treatment with neuropathy-inducing chemicals (such as acrylamide or organophosphates) leads to very early decrements in retrograde axonal transport and eventuates in distal axonal degeneration (33,34). While the mechanism underlying the chemical blockade of retrograde transport is not understood, the effect would predictably result in a reduction of target tissue-derived "trophic" support (NGF and other factors acting on motor neurons) for affected nerve cells and the consequent induction of axotomy-like somatic alterations in DRG neurons and anterior horn cells.

An attractive possibility is that chemical interference with retrograde transport of trophic factors required for maintenance of neuronal stability represents a common mechanism whereby axonal toxins trigger

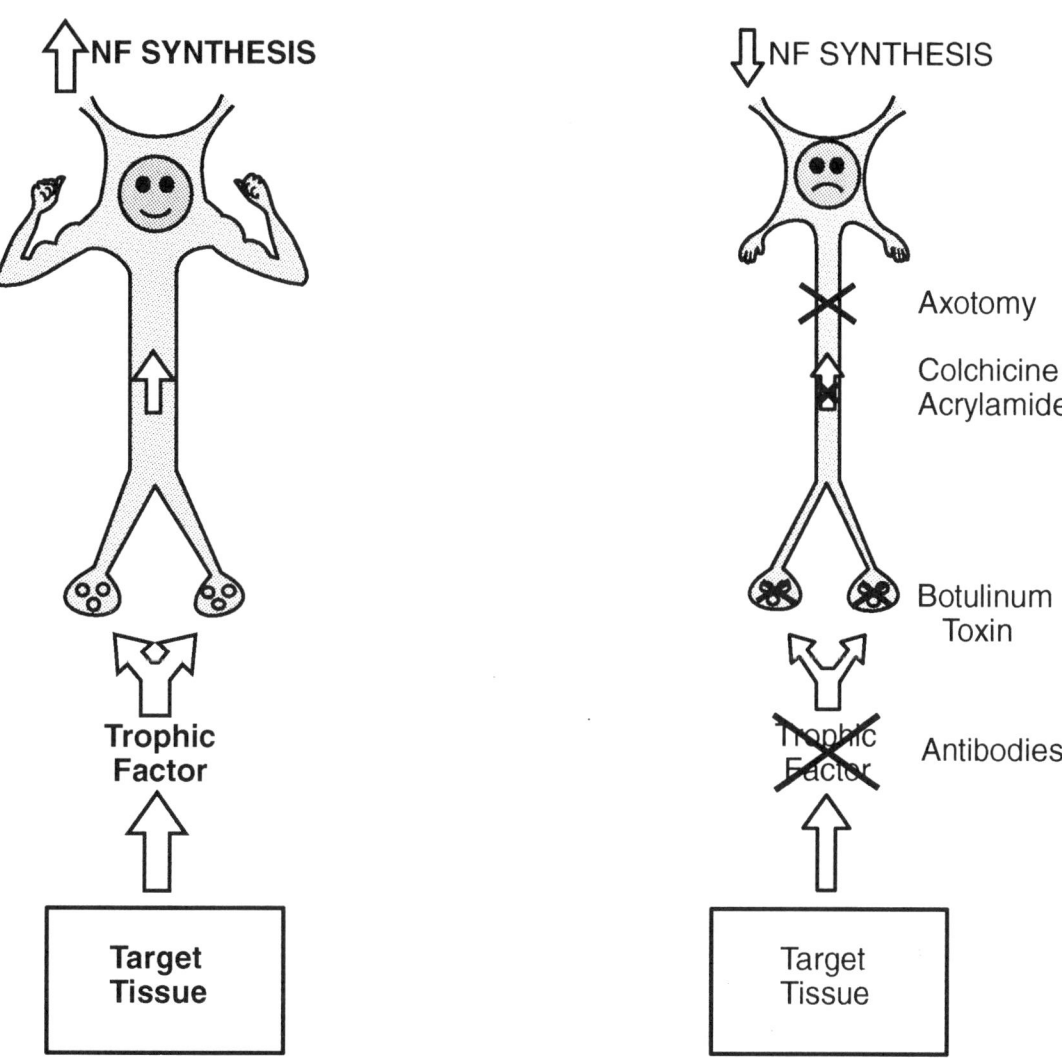

FIG. 1. Model showing consequence for the neuron of a defect in retrograde axonal transport and consequent loss of trophic support. In normal adult peripheral neurons *(left)*, a target-derived "trophic" factor is retrogradely transported to the neuronal soma where it acts to upregulate neurofilament synthesis *(arrows)* and subsequently, increase axonal caliber. This model is based upon the finding that the axotomy-induced reduction in neurofilament synthesis and axonal caliber can be produced in intact nerve fibers by a variety of experimental manipulations *(right)*: blockade of retrograde axonal transport (colchicine), prevention of vesicular neurotransmitter release (botulinum toxin), and removal of target tissue-derived "trophic" factor (NGF antiserum). Shown also are the axotomy-induced dendritic retraction, reduction (early on) in cell body size, and nuclear eccentricity, which may also be regulated by target-derived factors. Thus, a defect in retrograde axonal transport (e.g., by acrylamide) leads to axotomy-like (regenerative) changes in the neuronal soma and not axonal degeneration (see text).

axotomy-like alterations in the neuronal soma. For acrylamide, this hypothesis is supported by the production of axotomy-like alterations in acrylamide axonopathy (4,137,138), which markedly impairs the retrograde transport of NGF following a single injection (38). This mechanism can also account for the generation of axotomy-like changes in the neuronal soma either prior to (139) or without (86,140) the development of axonal loss.

FATE OF THE DISTAL STUMP

Wallerian Degeneration

Axotomy results in Wallerian degeneration of nerve fibers distal to the injury site, proliferation of associated Schwann cells inside their distal tubes of basal lamina (bands of Büngner), and denervation of postsynaptic cells. Ultimately, functional (clinical) recovery is dependent upon the ability of injured axons to regenerate and reach their appropriate targets. This is largely determined by the distal stump, which serves to support and guide the longitudinal growth of axon sprouts emerging from the proximal stump of damaged nerve fibers. Under conditions that are optimal for recovery (such as a focal nerve crush injury), these sprouts enter the bands of Büngner and develop intimate cellular relationships with the associated Schwann cells. In the event that the distal stump is misaligned with regenerating axons (as in a nerve transection), some axons may fail to enter a Schwann cell tube. Surviving axons that are destined to become myelinated—a property apparently determined by the neuronal soma and proximal axon (141–143)—develop unitary associations with Schwann cells at repeated intervals (future internodes) along the regenerating nerve. Other axons remain small, share individual Schwann cells, and acquire the characteristics of unmyelinated nerve fibers. The local factors that control interactions between the regenerating axonal sprouts and bipolar daughter Schwann cells in distal stumps have yet to be defined, but it is likely that understanding these events will shed light on how to promote regeneration of CNS fibers. Ultimately, the longitudinal columns of Schwann cells guide the regenerating axons to their appropriate end-organ sites.

The process by which the distal stump prepares to receive regenerating axons has been extensively studied and is not reviewed here. In general, however, nerve-fiber degeneration proceeds in a proximal-distal fashion along the nerve (144). Schwann cells divide following loss of axonal contact and develop into de-differentiated bipolar cells (145). Schwann cell division spreads in a somatofugal direction at a rate comparable to that of fast axonal transport (146). This suggests that Schwann cell mitosis is activated by the loss of an axonal (plasmalemmal?) signal (147) coincident with the onset of axon degeneration (see, however, 148). The synthesis of myelin proteins (e.g., myelin-associated glycoprotein) is down-regulated (149), while other proteins (such as NGF) show increased production. Recently, an adhesion molecule (P30) has been demonstrated to increase in Schwann cells following loss of axonal contact (150).

The function of NGF synthesized by Schwann cells in the distal stump is unknown. Schwann cells in the axotomized distal stump increase both NGF synthesis and the number of their low-affinity NGF receptors (125,126,128,151). Axonal contact during regeneration appears to down-regulate these changes (125,152,153). NGF and its low-affinity receptor on Schwann cells might play a role in axonal elongation either directly by serving as a substratum for axonal sprouts (125,152) or indirectly via an autocrine regulation of Schwann cells (129). NGF has been shown to serve as a classical chemoattractive agent for sensory neurites in vitro (154). That NGF has a neurotropic (guidance) role in axonal elongation in vivo may be supported by the concurrent lack of regeneration of sensory axons (155) and NGF production in (mutant) C57BL/Ola mice (130). Furthermore, the axotomy-triggered synthesis in motor neuron somata of low-affinity NGF receptors (156–158) may serve to supply axonal sprouts with these receptors to hold NGF to homologous NGF receptors on Schwann cells (125). In this context, axons from a variety of neuronal types have been shown to regulate NGF receptor synthesis in Schwann cells (153). However, the function of low-affinity NGF receptors in motor neurons may be different from that in sensory neurons since motor axons regenerate normally in C57BL/Ola mice (159) despite a lack of synthesis of NGF and its receptor in the distal stump (130). One possibility is that motor neurons normally synthesize a high-affinity receptor to a yet-unidentified, NGF-like (homologous) "trophic" substance, which is interpreted to be a "low-affinity NGF receptor" in axotomized motor neurons based upon its ability to crossreact with NGF. This is suggested by the recent finding that low-affinity NGF receptors cannot distinguish between NGF and homologous molecules (e.g., BDNF) (160). However, since the role of the low-affinity receptor in high-affinity binding is unresolved (109–113), the possibility exists that expression of low-affinity NGF receptors conveys NGF-responsiveness (110,112) mediating an unknown function in injured motor neurons.

Macrophages play an essential role in the removal of debris from the distal stump and in subsequent regeneration. The importance of blood-borne macrophages in Wallerian degeneration was first established in the elegant experiments of Beuche and Friede (161). These studies demonstrated that Schwann cells fail to divide, and that myelin debris remains undigested, when leukocytes and monocytes are prevented from entering the nerve. This work has been extended through studies of C57BL/Ola mice, a mutant substrain that demonstrates a marked retardation in the rate of Wallerian degeneration (sciatic nerve) owing to a failure of recruitment of circulating monocytes following axotomy (159). This has been shown to result from a defect inherent in the nerve as opposed to an inability of the macrophages from this species to respond to the damaged tissue, although these studies do not rule out a defect in resident macrophages (162). Both macrophages and Schwann cells appear to be involved in phagocytosis (163), but the mechanism by which macrophages stimulate Schwann cells to digest myelin and other cellular debris is unclear. Recruitment of macrophages into peripheral nerve may require expression of Ia antigen by Schwann cells (163). Furthermore, macrophages appear to stimulate Schwann cells to synthesize and secrete NGF (127) via the release of IL-1 (151) following injury. Interestingly, Schwann cells from C57BL/Ola mice do not demonstrate an increase in NGF and NGF-receptor synthesis following axotomy (130,162), presumably due to a lack of macrophage infiltration and activation of Schwann cells.

Glucocorticoids block the increase in NGF synthesis in the distal stump of the sciatic nerve following axotomy (164). This appears to result from both a direct effect on cells (at least fibroblasts) in the nerve (164) and a blockade of the release of IL-1 by macrophages (165). Whether there is a direct effect on NGF transcription in Schwann cells is unknown. However, these findings suggest that glucocorticoid treatment might impair nerve regeneration in patients with peripheral nerve lesions.

Axon Regeneration

Functional recovery following nerve injury is dependent upon the restoration of target contact and function. If the Schwann cell basal lamina remains intact (i.e., following a crush injury), recovery may be largely complete. However, if the nerve itself is transected (severed nerves), full functional recovery rarely occurs. This is primarily due to a failure of regenerating axons to reach their targets and a mismatch between neuronal type and target tissue (reinnervation of muscle spindle afferents by fibers normally innervating tendon organs) (for review, see 166). Some evidence (167) exists in support of the neurotropic theory of Cajal (168), i.e., that there exist diffusible factors that serve to attract the growing sprouts toward their targets. However, recent studies (169) suggest that neurotrophism ultimately becomes more important for determination of directionality between sensory and motor axons during nerve repair (see 166). Sensory and motor neurites initially enter the distal stump of a transected nerve randomly, inappropriate axonal sprouts being eliminated by lack of trophic support (169). This preferential reinnervation by motor and sensory axons for their appropriate nerves (170) indicates that factors in addition to NGF (125) are involved, despite the presence of low-affinity NGF-receptors in motor neurons following axotomy (see above) (156–158). Logically, it would seem that this support is provided locally (i.e., at the level of the growing sprouts) in order for individual neurites to be selectively eliminated from a given neuron. Thus, it may be misleading to refer to these as "trophic" factors in the classical sense of providing nutritive support to the entire nerve cell. Nevertheless, identification of these supportive neuritic factors may enable development of pharmacological strategies to improve the directional growth of sensory and motor fibers. However, it is important to emphasize that in severed nerves only a relative preference of motor and sensory neurons for their respective nerve sheaths has been demonstrated (170).

INFLUENCE OF THE DISTAL STUMP ON THE NEURONAL RESPONSE TO INJURY

It is well established that the neuronal soma influences the growth of axonal sprouts in the distal stump via the synthesis and delivery of materials needed for axonal elongation (44,171–174). However, less well characterized is the dependency of the regenerative response of the neuronal soma on events occurring in the distal stump during nerve regeneration. Evidence (175,176) exists to support the presence of such a positive signal in the regulation of the axon reaction. Singer and co-workers (175) have shown that chromatolysis and increased uptake of 2-deoxyglucose by DRG are delayed by focal application of colchicine to a severed nerve proximal to the axotomy site. These data have been interpreted (175) to indicate that induction of the axon reaction is initiated by a retrogradely transported positive signal produced at the site of injury, a signal that is prevented from reaching the neuronal soma when retrograde transport is blocked by colchicine. However, structural interruption of the nerve and its target are not required to induce an injury response in the neuronal soma, as demonstrated by our findings (138,177) and those of others (85,86), that some components of the axon reaction (e.g., axonal caliber) can be elicited in *intact* nerve fibers (see "Trophic Regulation of the Axon Reaction" above). This position is supported by the observation that colchicine *induces* chromatolysis when applied locally to the intact hypoglossal nerve (178). Additionally, colchicine application to the sciatic nerve induces somatofugal axonal atrophy (88) and aberrant expression of pNF epitopes in DRG neuronal somata (75). Taken together, these findings argue against a role for a positive signal in the induction of the axon reaction.

The apparent paradox between the findings reported by Gold and colleagues and those of Singer and co-workers (175) may be resolved by studies showing a role for continued axonal elongation in the maintenance of the axon reaction. Specifically, aberrant expression of pNF epitopes in neuronal somata is not maintained when axonal elongation is prevented in the distal stump either by mechanical means (64) or by injection of the axonal toxin acrylamide (177). This situation differs from that demonstrated for the regulation of NF synthesis and axonal caliber, which remain reduced in nerves in which regeneration is prevented (11,48). Taken together, these findings suggest that another "trophic" factor (i.e., not NGF) serves as a positive signal (i.e., one induced by nerve transection) for the *maintenance* of at least one component (i.e., aberrant expression of pNF epitopes) of the axon reaction; this hypothesis is not inconsonant with the evidence presented above (see "Trophic Regulation of the Axon Reaction" above) that these alterations are initiated via a common mechanism (i.e., loss of NGF). There may be an analogous situation in CNS regeneration: In some CNS neurons, the neuronal soma initially demonstrates alteration in synthesis similar to that observed in PNS neurons, but these responses are not maintained unless the nerve is provided with a PNS graft (179). These findings stress the importance of the local environment of regenerating sprouts in the control of the neuron somal response to injury and the ultimate success of axonal regeneration (180).

CONTROL OF MYELINATION

As regenerating axons from myelinated fibers grow into the distal stump and increase their caliber, Schwann cells establish longitudinal territories (future internodes) and commence myelination (141). The axons appear to provide the signal to upregulate basal expression of myelin-synthesizing enzymes, or myelin-specific proteins and lipids, to levels required for myelin assembly (181). Detectable expression of increased synthesis of P_1 and P_2 myelin proteins precedes that of P_0, and increased production of all myelin proteins is demonstrable before myelin formation is seen morphologically (167). The internodal length of the regenerated nerve fiber is shorter than that of the proximal uninterrupted portion of the nerve fiber, probably because of cellular competition and the lack of limb growth in adult animals (182). The myelin sheath thickness therefore remains relatively thin for axonal caliber, although sheath size is correct for internodal length (183,184). Consequently, conduction velocity never returns to normal values, although this has little clinical consequence (for a complete description of the electrophysiological changes accompanying demyelination, see 185). At later times, there is extensive remodeling of the myelin sheath (e.g., nodal migration, myelin sheath breakdown, and elimination of redundant Schwann cells) owing to longitudinal crowding (186). Furthermore, if axons do not invade the distal stump, the Schwann cell columns disappear and the endoneurium is replaced with connective tissue (142; see, however, 148).

TREATMENT OF AXONAL NEUROPATHIES

Development of therapeutic regimens for the treatment of axonal neuropathies centers on either the prevention of axonal degeneration or the enhancement of axonal elongation. Gangliosides, such as G_{M1}, have been reported (187–196) to stimulate axonal sprouting and to enhance neuronal outgrowth. To date, however, only modest increases in overall rate of outgrowth have been demonstrated. This may be understood by their ubiquitousness in cell membranes. Gangliosides are concentrated in growth cones (197) where they appear to play a role in cell-cell recognition and adhesion (198); although antibodies to G_{M1} inhibit NGF-induced neuritic outgrowth (103) in vitro, this does not appear to be due to an effect on the NGF receptor (199). Thus, gangliosides may be effective in enhancing the rate of axonal elongation but their value in aiding regeneration over long distances, where reconnection of axonal sprouts with their appropriate targets is a persistent problem (see above), may be limited.

A recent exciting advance in the potential development of therapeutic means to prevent peripheral neuropathies is the demonstration that NGF administration prevents early on (days) some aspects (i.e., decreased size of the compound action potential in the tail nerve, decreased substance P levels in the DRG, increased pain threshold) of the development of experimental taxol neuropathy (200). Prevention by NGF of the reduction in spike amplitude in taxol neuropathy indicates an effect at the level of the tail nerve. However, this result does not necessarily indicate an axonal effect since an alteration in the morphology of the myelin sheath (201) or some aspect of electrical activity at the node cannot be ruled out; in this context, it is unfortunate that the authors did not examine the morphological correlate(s) of the alterations of spike amplitude. In contrast to these direct (local) effects, the ability of NGF to increase substance P levels and reduce pain sensation in taxol neuropathy is most likely explained by replacement of lost retrogradely transported NGF owing to the ability of taxol to impair microtubule function and promote assembly (202). Since NGF is responsible for the developmental increase in substance P levels, and NGF administration prevents the axotomy-induced reduction in substance P levels in DRG neurons (122), it is, therefore, not surprising that NGF administration reverses these alterations in phenotypic expression. Reduction in NGF levels in DRG neurons may also be responsible for the development of decreased neurotransmitter (catecholaminergic) synthesis in diabetic neuropathy (203). However, the important issue that remains unanswered is whether NGF administration can prevent somal loss or axonal degeneration in any situation. It seems premature, therefore, to propose (204) the onset of clinical trials in patients with these peripheral neuropathies. Nevertheless, together with our results, these studies indicate that NGF antiserum may be useful, in a general sense, for the treatment/management of peripheral neuropathies, for example, in the management of chronic pain via its ability to reduce substance P levels in the DRG (see 205). However, systematically administered NGF acting at the level of the DRG neuronal soma (see "Trophic Regulation of the Axon Reaction" above) may counteract the effects of NGF on axonal regrowth by reversing the somal component of the regenerative response, thereby reducing the supply of materials (conveyed by both fast and slow axonal transport) to the growing tips of axons necessary for axonal elongation.

How could NGF act to aid axonal elongation while its loss leads to induction of the axon reaction? These appear to be contradictory properties. The apparent paradox might be explained by restricted effects (under different circumstances) of NGF at the level the axon (local action) and neuronal soma (remote action) (94). According to this model, loss of high-affinity NGF receptors on the neuronal soma following axotomy (107) would serve to restrict the action of NGF produced in the distal stump to the growing tips of axons where it would act directly to promote axonal elongation (206). Thus, the ability of NGF to promote axonal elongation may be explained by an action on Schwann cells (125,207–209) and *not* the neuronal soma (129). The apparent paradox is therefore resolved since loss of retrogradely transported NGF would act in concert to promote regeneration by initiating an axon reaction in the neuronal soma. Delivery of NGF to the proximal stump may serve to maintain normal levels of high-affinity NGF receptors in DRG neurons

(107), thereby preventing the axotomy-induced reduction in NF synthesis (80) and axonal caliber (94).

The use of neurotrophins (e.g., NGF, BDNF, ciliary-derived neurotrophic factor [CNTF], NT-3) in the treatment of experimental models of human PNS and CNS neurodegenerative diseases will be an important new area of research during the next few years. A priori, it may be predicted that treatment with the appropriate (neuron-specific) neurotrophin, if given early enough, will prevent early neuronal cell death in the central nervous system (CNS). Such an effect has recently been demonstrated in vitro for mescencephalic dopaminergic neurons which can be rescued from the toxic effects of methylphenylpyridinium ion (MPP^+) (the neurotoxic metabolite of methylphenyltetrahydropyridine [MPTP]) by BDNF (210). In a similar vein, application of CTNF to the proximal stump of the facial nerve of newborn rats prevents the degeneration of corresponding motor neurons (211). However, it will be necessary to determine whether such an approach will be effective in the long term (i.e., in animal models), especially in situations where loss of "trophic" support may not underlie the pathogenesis of the neuronal somal degeneration.

CONCLUDING REMARKS

Perturbations of fast axonal transport are likely candidates for the pathogenesis of some peripheral neuropathies (e.g., Vacor neuropathy). It will be important to test selectively whether the independent impairment of fast anterograde and retrograde axonal transport leads, respectively, to axonal loss and the axon reaction. This may be possible by direct inhibition of kinesin and dynein, perhaps using DNA antisense probes, if these can be modified to access mammalian axoplasm.

NGF may have two separate functions in neuronal injury, namely, regulation of the axonal reaction in the neuronal soma and elongation of axonal sprouts in the distal stump. NGF is an important candidate agent for therapeutic trials in the treatment of various PNS and CNS neurodegenerative disorders. Although evidence indicates that NGF may aid axonal regeneration in peripheral neuropathies, NGF reaching DRG neuronal somata could also act to impair sensory nerve regeneration by reducing the synthesis and delivery to the axon of materials necessary for regeneration (i.e., GAP-43). Thus, future strategies for the clinical use of NGF may require the development of novel approaches aimed at directing NGF toward the axon (local effects) without eliciting the opposing somal (remote) actions of NGF in injured neurons.

ACKNOWLEDGMENTS

The authors thank Monica Fenton for copyediting the manuscript and Ms. Toni Storm-Dickerson for preparation of the figure. This work was supported in part by NIH grants NS 26265 (B.G.G.) and NS 19611 (P.S.S.).

REFERENCES

1. Vallee RB, Bloom GS. Mechanisms of fast and slow axonal transport. *Annu Rev Neurosci* 1991; 14: 59–92.
2. Schaumburg HH, Spencer PS, Thomas PK. *Disorders of peripheral nerves*. Philadelphia: F.A. Davis, 1983.
3. Griffin JW, Watson DF. Axonal transport in neurological disease. *Ann Neurol* 1988; 23: 3–13.
4. Gold BG, Griffin JW, Price DL. Slow axonal transport in acrylamide neuropathy: different abnormalities produced by single-dose and continuous administration. *J Neurosci* 1985; 5: 1755–1768.
5. Griffin JW, Hoffman PN, Clark AW, Carroll PT, Price DL. Slow axonal transport of neurofilament proteins: impairment of β,β'-iminodipropionitrile administration. *Science* 1978; 202: 633–635.
6. Griffin JW, Anthony DC, Fahnestock KE, Hoffman PN, Graham DG. 3,4-Dimethyl-2,5-hexanedione impairs the axonal transport of

neurofilament proteins. *J Neurosci* 1984; 4: 1516–1526.
7. Yokoyama K, Tsukita S, Ishikawa H, Kurokawa M. Early changes in the neuronal skeleton caused by β,β'-iminodipropionitrile: selective impairment of neurofilament polypeptides. *Biomed Res* 1980; 1: 537–547.
8. Hoffman PN, Lasek RJ. The slow component of axonal transport. Identification of major structural polypeptides of the axon and their generality among mammalian neurons. *J Cell Biol* 1975; 66: 351–366.
9. Lasek RJ, Hoffman PN. The neuronal cytoskeleton, axonal transport and axonal growth. Cold Spring Harbor Conferences on Cell Proliferation. *Cell Motil* 1976; 3:1021–1049.
10. Friede RI, Samorajski T. Axon caliber related to neurofilaments and microtubules in sciatic nerve fibers of rats and mice. *Anat Rec* 1970; 176: 379–388.
11. Hoffman PN, Griffin JW, Price DL. Control of axonal caliber by neurofilament transport. *J Cell Biol* 1984; 99: 705–714.
12. Griffin JW, Price DL. Proximal axonopathies induced by toxic chemicals. In: Spencer PS, Schaumburg HH, eds. *Experimental and clinical neurotoxicology*. Baltimore: Williams & Wilkins, 1980: 161–178.
13. Macioce P, Filliatreau G, Figliomeni B, et al. Slow axonal transport impairment of cytoskeletal proteins in streptozotocin-induced diabetic neuropathy. *J Neurochem* 1989; 53: 1261–1267.
14. Medori R, Jenich H, Autilio-Gambetti L, Gambetti P. Experimental diabetic neuropathy: similar changes of slow axonal transport and axonal size in different animal models. *J Neurosci* 1988; 8: 1814–1821.
15. Larsen JR, Sidenius P. Slow axonal transport of structural polypeptides in rat, early changes in streptozotocin diabetes, and effect of insulin treatment. *J Neurochem* 1989; 52: 390–401.
16. Bisby MA. Axonal transport of labeled protein and regeneration rate of nerves of streptozotocin diabetic rats. *Exp Neurol* 1980; 69: 74–84.
17. Jakobsen J, Sidenius P. Decreased axonal transport of structural proteins in streptozotocin diabetic rats. *J Clin Invest* 1980; 66: 292–297.
18. Brimijoin WS. Abnormalities of axonal transport: Are they a cause of peripheral nerve disease? *Mayo Clin Proc* 1982; 57: 707–714.
19. Vitadello M, Filliatreau G, Dupont JL, Hassig R, Gorio A, Di Giamberardino L. Altered axonal transport of cytoskeletal proteins in the mutant diabetic mouse. *J Neurochem* 1985; 45: 860–868.
20. Medori R, Autilio-Gambetti L, Jenich H, Gambetti P. Changes in axon size and slow axonal transport are related in experimental diabetic neuropathy. *Neurology* 1988; 38: 597–601.
21. Sima AAF, Bouchier M, Christensen H. Axonal atrophy in sensory nerves of the diabetic BB-Wistar rat: a possible early correlate of human diabetic neuropathy. *Ann Neurol* 1983; 13: 264–272.
22. Carrington CD, Lapadula DM, Abou-Donia MB. Acceleration of anterograde axonal transport in cat sciatic nerve by diisopropyl phosphorofluoridate. *Brain Res* 1989; 476: 179–182.
23. Reichert BL, Abou-Donia MB. Inhibition of fast axoplasmic transport by delayed neurotoxic organophosphorous esters: a possible mode of action. *Mol Pharmacol* 1980; 17: 56–60.
24. Watson DF, Griffin JW. Vacor neuropathy: ultrastructural and axonal transport studies. *J Neuropathol Exp Neurol* 1987; 46: 96–108.
25. Sickles DW. Toxic neurofilamentous axonopathies and fast anterograde axonal transport. I. The effects of single doses of acrylamide on the rate and capacity of transport. *Neurotoxicology* 1989; 10: 91–102.
26. Sidenius P, Jakobsen J. Anterograde fast component of axonal transport during insulin-induced hypoglycemia in nondiabetic and diabetic rats. *Diabetes* 1987; 36: 853–858.
27. Schmidt RE, Matschinsky FM, Godfrey DA, Williams AD, McDougal DB. Fast and slow axoplasmic flow in sciatic nerve of diabetic rats. *Diabetes* 1974; 24: 1081–1085.
28. Laduron PM, Janssen PFM. Impaired axonal transport of opiate and muscarinic receptors in streptozotocin-diabetic rats. *Brain Res* 1986; 380: 359–362.
29. Macioce P, Hässig R, Tavitian B, Di Giamberardino L. Axonal transport of the molecular forms of acetylcholinesterase in rats at the onset of diabetes induced by streptozotocin. *Brain Res* 1988; 438: 291–294.
30. Allen RD, Weiss DG, Hayden JH, Brown DT, Fujiwake H, Simpson M. Gliding movement of and bidirectional transport along single native microtubules from squid axoplasm: evidence for an active role of microtubules in cytoplasmic transport. *J Cell Biol* 1985; 100: 1736–1752.
31. Schnapp BJ, Vale RD, Sheetz MP, Reese TS. Single microtubules from squid axoplasm support bidirectional movement of organelles. *Cell* 1985; 40: 455–462.
32. Vale RD. Intracellular transport using microtubule-based motors. *Annu Rev Cell Biol* 1987; 3: 347–378.
33. Miller MS, Spencer PS. Single doses of acrylamide reduce retrograde transport velocity. *J Neurochem* 1984; 43: 1401–1408.
34. Moretto A, Lotti M, Sabri MI, Spencer PS. Progressive deficit of retrograde axonal transport is associated with the pathogenesis of di-n-butyl dichlorvos axonopathy. *J Neurochem* 1987; 49: 1515–1522.
35. Jakobsen J, Brimijoin S, Skau K, Sidenius P, Wells D. Retrograde axonal transport of transmitter enzymes, fucose-labeled protein, and nerve growth factor in streptozotocin-diabetic rats. *Diabetes* 1981; 30: 797–803.
36. Jakobsen J, Sidenius P. Decreased axonal flux of retrogradely transported glycoproteins in early experimental diabetes. *J Neurochem* 1979; 33: 1055–1060.
37. Schmidt RE, Modert CW, Yip HK, Johnson Jr

EM. Retrograde axonal transport of intravenously administered ^{125}I-nerve growth factor in rats with streptozotocin-induced diabetes. *Diabetes* 1983; 32: 654–663.
38. Miller MS, Miller MJ, Burks TF, Sipes IG. Altered retrograde axonal transport of nerve growth factor after single and repeated doses of acrylamide in the rat. *Toxicol Appl Pharmacol* 1983; 69: 96–101.
39. Eccles JC, Libet B, Young RR. The behavior of chromatolyzed motoneurons studied by intracellular recording. *J Physiol (Lond)* 1958; 143: 11–40.
40. Watson WE. Observations on the nucleolar and total cell body nucleic acid of injured nerve cells. *J Physiol (Lond)* 1968; 196: 655–676.
41. Kuno M, Llinas R. Enhancement of synaptic transmission by dendritic potentials in chromatolyzed motoneurons of the cat. *J Physiol (Lond)* 1970; 210: 807–821.
42. Kuno M, Llinas R. Alterations of synaptic action in chromatolyzed motoneurons of the cat. *J Physiol (Lond)* 1970; 210: 823–838.
43. Price DL, Porter KR. The response of ventral horn neurons to axonal transection. *J Cell Biol* 1972; 53: 24–37.
44. Hoffman PN, Lasek RJ. Axonal transport of the cytoskeleton in regenerating neurons: constancy and change. *Brain Res* 1980; 202: 317–333.
45. Kreutzberg GW, Emmert H. Glucose utilization of motor nuclei during regeneration: a [^{14}C]2-deoxyglucose study. *Exp Neurol* 1980; 70: 712–716.
46. Lieberman AR. The axon reaction: a review of the principal features of perikaryal responses to axon injury. In: Pfeiffer CC, Smythies JR, eds. *International review of neurobiology*, vol 14. New York: Academic Press; 1971: 49–124.
47. Price DL, Griffin JW, Hoffman PN, Cork LC, Spencer PS. The response of motor neurons to injury and disease. In: Dyck PJ, Thomas PK, Lambert EH, Bunge R, eds. *Peripheral neuropathy*, vol 1. Philadelphia: W.B. Saunders; 1984: 732–759.
48. Hoffman PN, Cleveland DW, Griffin JW, Landes PW, Cowan NJ, Price DL. Neurofilament gene expression: a major determinant of axonal caliber. *Proc Natl Acad Sci USA* 1987; 84: 3472–3476.
49. Hoffman PN, Cleveland DW. Neurofilament and tubulin expression recapitulates the developmental program during axonal regeneration: induction of a specific β-tubulin isotope. *Proc Natl Acad Sci USA* 1988; 85: 4530–4533.
50. Grafstein B, McQuarrie IG. Role of the nerve cell body in axonal regeneration. In: Cotman CW, ed. *Neuronal plasticity*. New York: Raven Press; 1978: 155–196.
51. Carpenter S. Proximal axonal enlargement in motor neuron disease. *Neurology* 1968; 18: 841–851.
52. Inoue K, Hirano A. Early pathological changes in amyotrophic lateral sclerosis: autopsy findings of a case of 10 months' duration. *Neurol Med Chir* (Tokyo) 1979; 11: 448–455.
53. Chou S-M, Kuzuhara S, Gibbs Jr CJ, Gajdusek DC. Giant axonal spheroids along corticospinal tracts in a case of Guamanian ALS. *J Neuropathol Exp Neurol* 1980; 39: 345.
54. Pfeiffer G, Friede RL. A morphometric study of nerve fiber atrophy in rat spinal roots. *J Neuropathol Exp Neurol* 1985; 44: 546–558.
55. Wong J, Oblinger MM. Changes in neurofilament gene expression occur after axotomy of dorsal root ganglion neurons: an *in situ* hybridization study. *Met Brain Dis* 1987; 2: 291–303.
56. Tetzlaff W, Bisby MA, Kreutzberg GW. Changes in cytoskeletal proteins in the rat facial nucleus following axotomy. *J Neurosci* 1988; 8: 3131–3189.
57. Goldstein ME, Weiss SR, Lassarini RA, Shneidman PS, Lees JF, Schlaepfer WW. mRNA levels of all three neurofilament proteins decline following nerve transection. *Mol Brain Res* 1988; 3: 287–292.
58. Cragg BG, Thomas PK. Changes in conduction velocity and fibre size proximal to peripheral nerve lesions. *J Physiol (Lond)* 1961; 157: 315–327.
59. Aitkin JT, Thomas PK. Retrograde changes in fibre size following nerve section. *J Anat* 1962; 96: 121–129.
60. Kreutzberg GW, Schubert P. Volume changes in the axon during regeneration. *Acta Neuropathol (Berl)* 1971; 17: 220–226.
61. Carlson J, Lais AC, Dyck PJ. Axonal atrophy from permanent peripheral axotomy in the adult cat. *J Neuropathol Exp Neurol* 1979; 38: 579–585.
62. Hoffman PN, Thompson GW, Griffin JW, Price DL. Changes in neurofilament transport coincide temporally with alterations in the caliber of axons in regenerating motor fibers. *J Cell Biol* 1985; 101: 1332–1340.
63. Moss TH, Lewkowicz SJ. The axon reaction in motor and sensory neurones of mice studied by a monoclonal antibody marker of neurofilament protein. *J Neurol Sci* 1983; 60: 267–280.
64. Rosenfeld J, Dorman ME, Griffin JW, Gold BG, Sternberger LA, Sternberger NH, Price DL. Distribution of neurofilament antigens after axonal injury. *J Neuropathol Exp Neurol* 1987; 40: 269–282.
65. Goldstein ME, Copper HS, Bruce J, Carden MJ, Lee VM-Y, Schlaepfer WW. Phosphorylation of neurofilament proteins and chromatolysis following transection of rat sciatic nerve. *J Neurosci* 1987; 7: 1586–1594.
66. Jones SM, Williams Jr RC. Phosphate content of mammalian neurofilaments. *J Biol Chem* 1982; 257: 9902–9905.
67. Julien J-P, Mushynski WE. The distribution of phosphorylation sites among identified proteolytic fragments of mammalian neurofilaments. *J Biol Chem* 1983; 258: 4019–4025.
68. Wong J, Hutchison SB, Liem HK. An isoelectric variant of the 150,000-dalton neurofilament polypeptide. Evidence that phosphorylation af-

fects are associated with the filament. *J Biol Chem* 1984; 259: 10867–10874.
69. Carden MJ, Schlaepfer WW, Lee VM. The structure, biochemical properties, and immunogenicity of neurofilament peripheral regions are determined by phosphorylation state. *J Biol Chem* 1985; 260: 9805–9817.
70. Ksiezak-Reding H, Yen SH. Two monoclonal antibodies recognize Alzheimer's neurofibrillary tangles, neurofilaments, and microtubule-associated proteins. *J Neurochem* 1987; 48: 455–462.
71. Lee VM-Y, Carden MJ, Schlaepfer WW, Trojanowski JQ. Monoclonal antibodies distinguish several differentially phosphorylated states of the two largest rat neurofilament subunits (NF-H and NF-M) and demonstrate their existence in the normal nervous system of adult rats. *J Neurosci* 1987; 7: 3474–3488.
72. Sternberger LA, Sternberger NH. Monoclonal antibodies distinguish phosphorylated and nonphosphorylated forms of neurofilaments *in situ*. *Proc Natl Acad Sci USA* 1983; 80: 6126–6130.
73. Bennett GS, Tapscott SJ, DiLullo C, Holtzer H. Differential binding of antibodies against the neurofilament triplet proteins in different avian neurons. *Brain Res* 1984; 304: 291–302.
74. Nixon RA, Lewis SE, Marotta CA. Posttranslational modification of neurofilament proteins by phosphate during axoplasmic transport in retinal ganglion cell neurons. *J Neurosci* 1987; 7: 1145–1158.
75. Gold BG, Austin DR. Regulation of aberrant neurofilament phosphorylation in neuronal perikarya I. Production following colchicine application to the sciatic nerve. *J Neuropathol Exp Neurol* 1991; 50: 615–626.
76. Nixon RA, Logvinenko KB. Multiple fates of newly synthesized neurofilament proteins: Evidence for a stationary neurofilament network distributed nonuniformly along axons of retinal ganglion cell neurons. *J Cell Biol* 1986; 102: 647–659.
77. Nixon RA, Sihag RK. Neurofilament phosphorylation: a new look at regulation and function. *Trends Neurosci* 1991; 14: 501–506.
78. Geisler N, Kaufmann E, Fischer S, Plessmann U, Weber K. Neurofilament architecture combines structural principles of intermediate filaments with carboxy-terminal extensions increasing in size between triplet proteins. *EMBO J* 1983; 2: 1295–1302.
79. Hisanaga S, Hirokawa N. The effects of dephosphorylation on the structure of the projections of neurofilament. *J Neurosci* 1989; 9: 959–966.
80. Verge VMK, Tetzlaff W, Bisby MA, Richardson PM. Influence of nerve growth factor on neurofilament gene expression in mature primary sensory neurons. *J Neurosci* 1990; 10: 2018–2025.
81. Gold BG, Austin DR. Regulation of aberrant neurofilament phosphorylation in neuronal perikarya. III. Alterations following single and continuous β,β'-iminodipropionitrile administrations. *Brain Res* 1991; 563: 151–162.
82. Parhad IM, Swedberg EA, Hoar DI, Krekoski CA, Clark AW. Neurofilament gene expression following β,β'-iminodipropionitrile (IDPN) intoxication. *Mol Brain Res* 1988; 4: 293–301.
83. Hisanaga S, Hirokawa N. Dephosphorylation-induced interactions of neurofilaments with microtubules. *J Biol Chem* 1990; 265: 21852–21858.
84. Poltorak M, Freed WJ. Immunoreactive phosphorylated epitopes on neurofilaments in neuronal perikarya may be obscured by tissue pre-processing. *Brain Res* 1989; 480: 349–354.
85. Watson WE. The response of motoneurones to intramuscularly injected botulinum toxin. *J Physiol (Lond)* 1969; 202: 611–630.
86. Pinter MJ, Noven SV, Muccio D, Wallace N. Axotomy-like changes in cat motoneuron electrical properties elicited by botulinum toxin depend on the complete elimination of neuromuscular transmission. *J Neurosci* 1991; 11: 657–666.
87. Gold BG, Griffin JW, Pestronk A, Hoffman PN, Stanley EF, Price DL. Somatofugal axonal atrophy produced by botulinum toxin. *Soc Neurosci Abstr* 1986; 12: 1108.
88. Gold BG, Dark C. Somatofugal axonal atrophy produced by colchicine application to the sciatic nerve. First annual meeting of the Society for Experimental Neuropathology. Oct. 1, 1988, Philadelphia, PA. *Ann Neurol* 1988; 24: 481.
89. Pitman RM, Tweedle CD, Cohen MJ. Electrical responses of insect central neurons: augmentation by nerve section of colchicine. *Science* 1972; 78: 507–509.
90. Pilar G, Landmesser L. Axotomy mimicked by localized colchicine application. *Science* 1972; 177: 1116–1118.
91. Purves D. Functional and structural changes in mammalian sympathetic neurons following colchicine application to post-ganglionic nerves. *J Physiol (Lond)* 1976; 259: 159–175.
92. Cull RE. Role of axonal transport in maintaining central synaptic connections. *Exp Brain Res* 1975; 24: 97–101.
93. Richardson PM, Verge VMK. The induction of a regenerative propensity in sensory neurons following peripheral axonal injury. *J Neurocytol* 1986; 15: 585–594.
94. Gold BG, Mobley WC, Matheson SF. Regulation of axonal caliber, neurofilament content and nuclear localization in mature sensory neurons by nerve growth factor. *J Neurosci* 1991; 11: 943–955.
95. Thoenen H, Barde Y-A. Physiology of nerve growth factor. *Physiol Rev* 1980; 60: 1284–1335.
96. Purves D. *Body and brain: A trophic theory of neural connections*. Cambridge, MA: Harvard University Press; 1988.
97. Gorin PD, Johnson EM, Jr. Experimental autoimmune model of nerve growth factor deprivation: effects on developing peripheral sym-

pathetic and sensory neurons. *Proc Natl Acad Sci USA* 1979; 76: 5382–5386.
98. Johnson Jr EM, Gorin PD, Brandeis LD, Pearson J. Dorsal root ganglion neurons are destroyed by exposure *in utero* to maternal antibody to nerve growth factor. *Science* 1980; 210: 916–918.
99. Bondok AA, Sansone FM. Retrograde and transganglionic degeneration of sensory neurons after a peripheral nerve lesion at birth. *Exp Neurol* 1984; 86: 322–330.
100. Yip HK, Rich KM, Lampe PA, Johnson Jr EM. The effects of nerve growth factor and its antiserum on the postnatal development and survival after injury of sensory neurons in rat dorsal root ganglia. *J Neurosci* 1984; 4: 2986–2992.
101. Miyata Y, Kashihara Y, Homma S, Kuno M. Effects of nerve growth factor on the survival of synaptic function of Ia sensory neurons axotomized in neonatal rats. *J Neurosci* 1986; 6: 2012–2018.
102. Gorin PD, Johnson Jr EM. Effects of long-term nerve growth factor deprivation on the nervous system of the adult rat: an experimental autoimmune approach. *Brain Res* 1980; 198: 27–42.
103. Schwartz M, Spirman M. Sprouting from chicken embryo dorsal root ganglia induced by nerve growth factors is specifically inhibited by affinity-purified antiganglioside antibodies. *Proc Natl Acad Sci USA* 1982; 79: 6080–6083.
104. Richardson PM, Riopelle RJ. Uptake of nerve growth factor along peripheral and spinal axons of primary sensory neurons. *J Neurosci* 1984; 4: 1683–1689.
105. Stockel K, Schwab M, Thoenen H. Specificity of retrograde transport of nerve growth factor (NGF) in sensory neurons: a biochemical and morphological study. *Brain Res* 1975; 89: 1–14.
106. Richardson PM, Verge Issa VMK, Riopelle RJ. Distribution of neuronal receptors for nerve growth factor in the rat. *J Neurosci* 1986; 6: 2312–2321.
107. Verge VMK, Riopelle RJ, Richardson PM. Nerve growth factor receptors on normal and injured sensory neurons. *J Neurosci* 1989; 8: 914–922.
108. Verge VMK, Grondin J, Riopelle RJ, Richardson PM. Receptor radioautography and *in situ* hybridization for NGF receptors in primary sensory neurons. *Soc Neurosci Abstr* 1991; 17: 1498.
109. Richardson PM. Neurotrophic factors in regeneration. *Curr Opin Neurobiol* 1991; 1: 401–406.
110. Heamstead BI, Martin-Zanca D, Kaplan DR, Parada LF, Chao MV. High-affinity NGF binding requires coexpression of the trk proto-oncogene and the low-affinity NGF receptor. *Nature* 1991; 350: 678–683.
111. Kaplan DR, Hempstead BL, Martin-Zanca D, Chao MV, Parada LF. The trk proto-oncogene product: a signal transducing receptor for nerve growth factor. *Science* 1991; 252: 554–558.
112. Klein R, Jing S, Nanduri V, O'Rourke E, Barbacid M. The trk proto-oncogene encodes a receptor for nerve growth factor. *Cell* 1991; 65: 189–197.
113. Nebreda AR, Martin-Zanca D, Kaplan DR, Parada LF, Santos E. Induction by NGF of meiotic maturation of *Xenopus* oocytes expressing the trk proto-oncogene product. *Science* 1991; 252: 558–561.
114. Radeke MJ, Feinstein SC. Analytical purification of the slow, high affinity NGF receptor: identification of a novel 135 kd polypeptide. *Neuron* 1991; 7: 141–150.
115. Raivich G, Kreutzberg GW. Expression of growth factor receptors in injured nervous tissue. I. Axotomy leads to a shift in the cellular distribution of specific β-nerve growth factor binding in the injured and regenerating PNS. *J Neurocytol* 1987; 16: 261–268.
116. Fitzgerald MP, Wall D, Goedert M, Emson PC. Nerve growth factor counteracts the neurophysiological and neurochemical effects of chronic sciatic nerve section. *Brain Res* 1985; 332: 131–141.
117. Rich KM, Luszczinski JR, Osborne PA, Johnson EM, Jr. Nerve growth factor protects adult sensory neurons from cell death and atrophy caused by nerve injury. *J Neurocytol* 1987; 16: 261–268.
118. Otto D, Unsicker K, Grothe C. Pharmacological effects of nerve growth factor and fibroblast growth factor applied to the transected sciatic nerve on neuron death in adult rat dorsal root ganglia. *Neurosci Lett* 1987; 83: 156–160.
119. Lindsay RM, Harmar AJ. Nerve growth factor regulates expression of neuropeptide genes in adult sensory neurons. *Nature* 1989; 337: 362–364.
120. Verge VMK, Richardson PM, Benoit R, Riopelle RJ. Histochemical characterization of sensory neurons with high-affinity receptors for nerve growth factor. *J Neurocytol* 1989; 18: 583–591.
121. Gold BG, Austin DR, Mobley WC, Storm-Dickerson T. Chromatolytic-like alterations and aberrant neurofilament phosphorylation in neuronal perikarya following NGF antiserum injection. *Soc Neurosci Abstr* 1991; 17: 1497.
122. Wong J, Oblinger MM. NGF rescues substance P expression but not neurofilament or tubulin gene expression in axotomized sensory neurons. *J Neurosci* 1991; 11: 543–552.
123. Lindenbaum MH, Carbonetto S, Grosveld F, Flavell D, Mushynski WE. Transcriptional and post-transcriptional effects of nerve growth factor on expression of the three neurofilament subunits in PC-12 cells. *J Biol Chem* 1988; 263: 5662–5667.
124. Muma NA, Hoffman PN, Slunt HH, Applegate MD, Lieberburg I, Price DL. Alterations in levels of mRNAs coding for neurofilament protein subunits during regeneration. *Exp Neurol* 1990; 107: 230–235.
125. Taniuchi M, Clark HB, Schweitzer JB, Johnson Jr EM. Expression of nerve growth factor receptors by Schwann cells of axotomized peripheral nerves: ultrastructural location, suppression by axonal contact, and binding properties. *J Neurosci* 1988; 8: 664–681.

126. Taniuchi M, Clark HB, Johnson EM, Jr. Induction of nerve growth factor receptor in Schwann cells after axotomy. *Proc Natl Acad Sci USA* 1986; 83: 4054–4098.
127. Heumann R, Lindholm D, Brandtlow C, et al. Differential regulation of mRNA encoding nerve growth factor and its receptor in rat sciatic nerve during development, degeneration, and regeneration: role of macrophage. *Proc Natl Acad Sci USA* 1987; 84: 8735–8739.
128. Heumann R, Korsching S, Brandtlow C, Thoenen H. Changes of nerve growth factor synthesis in non-neuronal cells in response to sciatic nerve transection. *J Cell Biol* 1987; 104: 1623–1631.
129. Raivich G, Hellweg R, Kreutzberg GW. NGF receptor-mediated reduction in axonal NGF uptake and retrograde transport following sciatic nerve injury and during regeneration. *Neuron* 1991; 7: 151–164.
130. Brown MC, Perry VH, Lunn ER, Gordon S, Heumann R. Macrophage dependence of peripheral sensory nerve regeneration: possible involvement of nerve growth factor. *Neuron* 1991; 6: 359–370.
131. Verge VMK, Tetzlaff W, Richardson PM, Bisby MA. Correlation between GAP43 and nerve growth factor receptors in rat sensory neurons. *J Neurosci* 1990; 10: 926–934.
132. Cragg BG. What is the signal for chromatolysis? *Brain Res* 1970; 23: 1–21.
133. Nja A, Purves D. The effects of nerve growth factor and its antiserum on synapses in the superior cervical ganglion of the guinea-pig. *J Physiol (Lond)* 1978; 277: 53–75.
134. West NR, Bunge RP. Prevention of the chromatolytic response in rat superior cervical ganglion cells by nerve growth factor. *Neuroscience* 1976; 2: 1038 (Abstr).
135. Porta EA. Role of oxidative damage in the aging process. In: Chow CK, ed. *Cellular antioxidant defense mechanisms,* vol III. New York: CRC Press; 1988: 1–52.
136. LeBel CP, Bondy SC. Persistent protein damage despite reduced oxygen radical formation in the aging rat brain. *Int J Dev Neurosci* 1991; 9: 139–146.
137. Bisby M, Redshaw JD. Acrylamide neuropathy: changes in the composition of proteins of fast axonal transport resemble those observed in regenerating axons. *J Neurochem* 1987; 48: 924–928.
138. Gold BG, Price DL, Griffin JW, Rosenfeld J, Hoffman PN, Sternberger NH, Sternberger LA. Neurofilament antigens in acrylamide neuropathy. *J Neuropathol Exp Neurol* 1988; 47: 145–157.
139. Gold BG, Griffin JW, Price DL. Somatofugal axonal atrophy precedes development of axonal degeneration in acrylamide neuropathy. *Arch Toxicol* 1992; 66: 57–66.
140. Griffin JW, Drucker N, Gold BG, et al. Schwann cell proliferation and migration during paranodal demyelination. *J Neurosci* 1987; 7: 682–699.
141. Weinberg HJ, Spencer PS. Studies on the control of myelinogenesis. I. Myelination of regenerating axons after entry into a foreign unmyelinated nerve. *J Neurocytol* 1975; 4: 395–418.
142. Weinberg HJ, Spencer PS. The fate of Schwann cells isolated from axonal contact. *J Neurocytol* 1978; 7: 555–569.
143. Weinberg HJ, Spencer PS. Studies on the control of myelinogenesis. II. Evidence for neuronal regulation of myelin production. *Brain Res* 1976; 113: 363–378.
144. Lubinska L. Patterns of Wallerian degeneration of myelinated fibres in short and long peripheral stumps and in isolated segments of rat phrenic nerve. Interpretation of the role of axoplasmic flow of the trophic factor. *Brain Res* 1982; 233: 227–240.
145. Pellegrino RG, Politis MJ, Ritchie JM, Spencer PS. Events in degenerating cat peripheral nerve, induction of Schwann cell S phase and its relation to nerve fiber degeneration. *J Neurocytol* 1986; 15: 17–28.
146. Oaklander AL, Miller MS, Spencer PS. Rapid anterograde spread of premitotic activity along degenerating cat sciatic nerve. *J Neurochem* 1987; 48: 111–114.
147. Oaklander AL, Spencer PS. Cold blockade of axonal transport activated premitotic activity of Schwann cells and Wallerian degeneration. *J Neurochem* 1988; 50: 490–496.
148. Kidd GJ, Health JW. Myelin sheath survival following axonal degeneration in doubly myelinated nerve fibers. *J Neurosci* 1991; 11: 4003–4014.
149. Willison HJ, Trapp BD, Bacher JT, Quarles RH. The expression of myelin-associated glycoprotein in regenerating cat sciatic nerve. *Brain Res* 1988; 444: 10–16.
150. Daston MM, Ratner N. Expression of P30, a protein with adhesive properties, in Schwann cells and neurons of the developing and regenerating peripheral nerve. *J Cell Biol* 1991; 112: 1229–1239.
151. Lindholm D, Heumann R, Meyer M, Thoenen H. Interleukin 1 regulates synthesis of nerve growth factor in non-neuronal cells of rat sciatic nerve. *Nature* 1987; 330: 658–659.
152. Johnson EM, Taniuchi M, DiStefano PS. Expression and possible function of nerve growth factor receptors on Schwann cells. *Trends Neurosci* 1988; 11: 299–304.
153. DiStefano PS, Chelsea DM. Regulation of Schwann cell surface and truncated nerve growth factor receptors *in vitro* by axonal components. *Brain Res* 1990; 534: 340–344.
154. Gunderson RW, Barrett JN. Neuronal chemotaxis: Chick dorsal root axons turn toward high concentrations of nerve growth factor. *Science* 1979; 206: 1079–1080.
155. Bisby MA, Chen S. Delayed Wallerian degeneration in sciatic nerves of C57BL/Ola mice is associated with impaired regeneration of sensory axons. *Brain Res* 1990; 530: 117–120.
156. Enfors P, Henschen A, Olson L, Persson H. Expression of nerve growth factor receptor

mRNA is developmentally regulated and increased after axotomy in rat spinal cord motoneurons. *Neuron* 1989; 2: 1605–1613.
157. Saika T, Senba E, Noguchi K, Sato M, Yoshida S, Kubo T, Matsunaga T, Tohyama. Effects of nerve crush and transection on mRNA levels for nerve growth factor receptor in the rat facial motoneurons. *Mol Brain Res* 1991; 9: 157–160.
158. Armstrong DM, Brady R, Hersh LB, Hayes RC, Wiley RG. Expression of choline acetyltransferase and nerve growth factor receptor within hypoglossal motoneurons following nerve injury. *J Comp Neurol* 1991; 304: 596–607.
159. Lunn ER, Perry VH, Brown MC, Rosen H, Gordon S. Absence of Wallerian degeneration does not hinder regeneration in peripheral nerve. *Eur J Neurosci* 1989; 1: 27–33.
160. Rodriguez-Tébar A, Dechant G, Yves-Alain B. Binding of brain-derived neurotrophic factor to the nerve growth factor receptor. *Neuron* 1990; 4: 487–492.
161. Beuche W, Friede RL. The role of non-resident cells in Wallerian degeneration. *J Neurocytol* 1984; 13: 767–796.
162. Perry VH, Brown MC, Lunn ER, Tree P, Gordon S. Evidence that very slow Wallerian degeneration in C57BL/Ola mice is an intrinsic property of the peripheral nerve. *Eur J Neurosci* 1990; 2: 802–808.
163. Stoll G, Griffin JW, Li CY, Trapp BD. Wallerian degeneration in the peripheral nervous system: participation of both Schwann cells and macrophages in myelin degradation. *J Neurocytol* 1989; 18: 671–683.
164. Lindholm D, Hengerer B, Heumann R, Carroll P, Thoenen H. Glucocorticoid hormones negatively regulate nerve growth factor expression *in vivo* in cultured rat fibroblasts. *Eur J Neurosci* 1990; 2: 795–801.
165. Lindholm D, Heumann R, Hengerer B, Thoenen H. Interleukin 1 increases stability and transcription of mRNA encoding nerve growth factor in cultured rat fibroblasts. *J Biol Chem* 1988; 263: 16348–16351.
166. Brushart TME. The mechanical and humoral control of specificity in nerve repair. In: Gelberman RH, ed. *Operative nerve repair and reconstruction,* vol I. Philadelphia: J.B. Lippincott; 1991: 215–230.
167. Politis MJ, Sternberger N, Ederle K, Spencer PS. Studies on the control of myelinogenesis. IV. Neuronal induction of Schwann cell myelin-specific protein synthesis during nerve fiber regeneration. *J Neurosci* 1982; 2: 1252–1266.
168. Ramón y Cajal S. *Degeneration and regeneration of the nervous system* (translated by May, R.). London: Oxford University Press; 1928.
169. Brushart TME. Preferential motor reinnervation: a sequential double-labeling study. *Restor Neurol Neurosci* 1990; 1: 281–287.
170. Brushart TM. Preferential reinnervation of motor nerves by regenerating motor axons. *J Neurosci* 1988; 8: 1026–1031.

171. Skene JHP, Willard MJ. Changes in axonally transported proteins during axon regeneration in toad retinal ganglion cells. *J Cell Biol* 1981; 89: 86–95.
172. Skene JHP, Willard MJ. Axonally transported proteins associated with growth in rabbit central and peripheral nervous system. *J Cell Biol* 1981; 89: 96–103.
173. McQuarrie IG. Role of axonal cytoskeleton in the regenerating nervous system. In: Seil FJ, ed. *Nerve, organ, and tissue regeneration: research perspectives.* New York: Academic Press; 1983: 51–88.
174. McQuarrie IG. Effect of a conditioning lesion on axonal transport during regeneration: the role of slow transport. *Adv Neurochem* 1984; 6: 185–209.
175. Singer PA, Mehler S, Fernandez HL. Blockade of retrograde axonal transport delays the onset of metabolic and morphological changes induced by axotomy. *J Neurosci* 1982; 2: 1299–1306.
176. Singer PA, Mehler S, Fernandez HL. Effect of extracts of injured nerve on initiating the regenerative response in the hypoglossal nucleus in the rat. *Neurosci Lett* 1988; 84: 155–160.
177. Gold BG, Austin D, Griffin JW. Regulation of aberrant neurofilament phosphorylation in neuronal perikarya. II. Correlation with continued axonal elongation following axotomy. *J Neuropathol Exp Neurol* 1991; 50: 627–648.
178. Aldkogius H, Svensson M. Effect on the rat hypoglossal nucleus of vinblastine and colchicine applied to the intact or transected hypoglossal nerve. *Exp Neurol* 1988; 99: 461–473.
179. Tetzlaff W, Tsui BJ, Balfour JK. Rubrospinal neurons increase GAP43 and tubulin mRNA after cervical but not after thoracic axotomy. *Soc Neurosci Abstr* 1990; 16: 3381.
180. Benfey M, Aguayo AJ. Extensive elongation of axons from rat brain into peripheral nerve grafts. *Nature* 1982; 296: 150–152.
181. Poduslo JF, Berg CT, Ross SM, Spencer PS. Regulation of myelination: axons not required for the biosynthesis of basal levels of the major myelin glycoprotein by Schwann cells in denervated distal segments of the adult cat sciatic nerve. *J Neurosci Res* 1985; 14: 177–185.
182. Friede RL, Bischhausen R. How are sheath dimensions affected by axon caliber and internode length? *Brain Res* 1982; 235: 335–350.
183. Smith KJ, Blakemore WF, Murray JA, Patterson RC. Internodal myelin volume and axon surface area. A relationship determining myelin thickness? *J Neurol Sci* 1982; 55: 231–246.
184. Beuche W, Friede RL. A new approach toward analyzing peripheral nerve fiber populations. II. Foreshortening of regenerated internodes corresponds to reduced sheath thickness. *J Neuropathol Exp Neurol* 1985; 44: 73–84.
185. Waxman SG. Normal and abnormal axonal properties. In: Asbury AK, McKhann GM, McDonald WI, eds. *Diseases of the nervous system: clinical neurobiology,* vol 1. Philadelphia: W.B. Saunders Co; 1986: 36–56.

186. Hildebrand C, Kocsis JD, Berglund S, Waxman SG. Myelin sheath remodelling in regenerated rat sciatic nerve. *Brain Res* 1985; 358: 163–170.
187. Moroni M, Colombi A, Gilioli R, et al. Effect of ganglioside therapy on experimental CS2 neuropathy. In: Manzo L, ed. *Advances in neurotoxicology: proceedings of the international congress on neurotoxicology.* Varese, Italy, September 27–30, 1979. Oxford: Pergamon Press; 1980.
188. Roisen FJ, Bartfeld H, Nagele L, Yorke G. Ganglioside stimulation of axonal sprouting *in vitro. Science* 1981; 214: 577–578.
189. Sparrow JR, Grafstein B. Sciatic nerve regeneration in ganglioside-treated rats. *Exp Neurol* 1982; 77: 230–235.
190. Rybak S, Ginzburg I, Yavin E. Gangliosides stimulate neurite outgrowth and induce tubulin mRNA accumulation in neural cells. *Biochem Biophys Res Commun* 1983; 116: 974–980.
191. Toffano G, Savoini G, Moroni F, Lombardi G, Calza L, Agnati LF. GM1 ganglioside stimulates the regeneration of dopaminergic neurons in the central nervous system. *Brain Res* 1983; 261: 163–168.
192. Gorio A, Carmignoto G, Ferrari G. Axon sprouting stimulated by gangliosides; a new model for elongation and sprouting. In: Rapport MM, Gorio A, eds. *Gangliosides in neurological and neuromuscular function, development and repair.* New York: Raven Press; 1981: 177–195.
193. Gorio A, Marini P, Zanoni R. Motor neuron sprouting capacity enhancement by exogenous gangliosides. *Neuroscience* 1983; 8: 417–429.
194. Facci L, Leon A, Toffano G, Sonnino S, Ghidoni R, Tettamanti G. Promotion of neuritogenesis in mouse neuroblastoma cells by exogenous gangliosides. Relationship between the effect and the cell association of ganglioside GM1. *J Neurochem* 1984;42: 299–305.
195. Doherty P, Dickson JG, Flanigan TP, Walsh FS. Ganglioside GM1 does not initiate, but enhances neurite regeneration of nerve growth factor dependent sensory neurons. *J Neurochem* 1985; 44: 1259–1265.
196. Doherty P, Dickson JG, Flanigan TP, Leon A, Toffano G, Walsh FS. Molecular specificity of ganglioside effects on neurite regeneration of sensory neurons *in vitro. Neurosci Lett* 1985; 62: 193–198.
197. Ledeen RW. Ganglioside structures and distribution: Are they localized at the nerve ending? *J Supramol Struct* 1978; 8: 1–17.
198. Gorio A, Haber B, eds. *Neurobiology of gangliosides.* New York: Alan R. Liss, Inc.; 1984.
199. Doherty P, Walsh FS. Ganglioside G_{M1} antibodies and β-cholera toxin bind specifically to embryonic chick dorsal root ganglion neurons but do not modulate neurite regeneration. *J Neurochem* 1987; 48: 1237–1244.
200. Apfel SC, Lipton RB, Arezzo JC, Kessler JA. Nerve growth factor prevents toxic neuropathy in mice. *Ann Neurol* 1991; 29: 87–90.
201. Hulsebosch CE, Perez-Polo JR, Coggeshall RE. *In vivo* anti-NGF induces sprouting of sensory axons in dorsal roots. *J Comp Neurol* 1987; 259: 445–451.
202. Roytta M, Horwitz SB, Raine CS. Taxol-induced neuropathy: short term effects of local injection. *J Neurocytol* 1984; 13: 685–701.
203. Hellweg R, Hartung HD. Endogenous levels of nerve growth factor (NGF) are altered in experimental diabetes mellitus: a possible role for NGF in the pathogenesis of diabetic neuropathy. *J Neurosci Res* 1990; 26: 258–267.
204. Moran E, Apfel SC, Arezzo JC, Kessler JA. Nerve growth factor prevents toxic neuropathy. *Soc Neurosci Abstr* 1991; 17: 1497.
205. Cheshire WP, Snyder CR. Treatment of reflex sympathetic dystrophy with topical capsaicin. Case report. *Pain* 1990; 42: 307–311.
206. Horie H, Bando Y, Chi H, Takenaka T. NGF enhances neurite regeneration from nerve-transected terminals of young adult and aged mouse dorsal root ganglia *in vitro. Neurosci Lett* 1991; 121: 125–128.
207. Ard MD, Bunge RP, Bunge MB. Comparison of the Schwann cell surface and Schwann cell extracellular matrix as promoters of neurite growth. *J Neurocytol* 1987; 16: 539–555.
208. Bunge MB, Johnson MI, Ard MD, Kleitman N. Factors influence the growth of regenerating nerve fibers in culture. *Prog Brain Res* 1987; 71: 61–74.
209. DiStefano PS, Johnson Jr EM. Nerve growth factor receptors on cultured rat Schwann cells. *J Neurosci* 1988; 8: 231–241.
210. Hyman C, Hofer M, Yves-Alain B, Juhasz M, Yancopoulos GD, Squinto SP, Lindsay RM. BDNF is a neurotrophic factor for dopaminergic neurons of the substantia nigra. *Nature* 1991; 350: 230–232.
211. Sendtner M, Kreutzberg GW, Thoenen H. Ciliary neurotophic factor prevents degeneration of motor neurons after axotomy. *Nature* 1990; 345: 440–441.

7

Human Schwann Cells in Culture

Recent Advances and Relevance to Nerve Pathology

Elio Scarpini, Pierluigi Baron, and Guglielmo Scarlato

Institute of Neurology, Dino Ferrari Center for Neuromuscular Diseases, University of Milan, 20122 Milan, Italy

Despite the major advances that have been made in the recent years, many important questions still remain unanswered about the cellular and molecular control of myelination in the peripheral nervous system. Some of the issues that remain to be addressed are relevant to the understanding of peripheral neuropathies, which do not represent a minor aspect in the clinical practice of a neurologist.

A fundamental role in the process of myelination is played by the Schwann cell. The developmental, proliferative, and differentiative characteristics of this cell have been extensively studied in the past years by several authors, using "in situ" techniques and tissue cultures with and without dissociated dorsal root ganglion neurons. Most studies were performed employing Schwann cells obtained from experimental animals, i.e., mice, rats, and rabbits, mainly at embryonic stage. However, very few reports, describing the behavior of Schwann cells obtained from human nerves, are so far available. According to some authors, differences among species are present. For instance, rat Schwann cells have only 7% of the plasmalemmal Na+ channels and much less saxitoxin binding than rabbit Schwann cells (1). Moreover, differences between embryonic/neonatal and adult Schwann cells have been described, involving the expression of some antigens and the response to growth factors and cytokines. Recently, Jessen et al. (2) described precursors of glial cells, which display specific characteristics different from mature cells. They are present in hindlimb nerves of 14–15 day old rat embryos and lack two fundamental properties of cells from older nerves, i.e., the ability to survive in vitro in routine serum containing media, and expression of the Schwann cell marker S-100 protein. These cells leave a characteristic flattened morphology in vitro and already express most of the same properties that characterize non-myelin-forming Schwann cells in adult nerves. In culture these cells can be distinguished from fibroblastic cells by antibodies against nerve growth factor (NGF) receptor, which has been previously established as a marker for cultured Schwann cells. So, the availability of Schwann cells from both adult and fetal subjects, and possibly from human nerves, has been proved extremely useful in understanding the influences that regulate their proliferation and differentiation and for the screening of the several possible growth factors so far available, giving a substantial contribution to our knowledge of mechanisms involved in nerve regeneration.

DEVELOPMENT AND FUNCTION OF THE SCHWANN CELLS

The development and function of rat Schwann cells has been extensively studied by several authors. Essential contributions were made by R.P. Bunge and coworkers (see 3 for review). The most recent advances in this field are the morphologic and biochemical changes in the Schwann cell during the transition from the premyelinating to the myelinating state. For these studies, neuron/Schwann cell cultures are currently used. Dissociated dorsal root ganglion neurons are purified during the initial culture period by treatment with antimitotic drugs such as fluorodeoxyuridine and then combined with pure Schwann cell from newborn rat sciatic cells (4–7). In these cultures, Schwann cell development demonstrates several parallels with Schwann cell development "in vivo," and advanced maturation of the cells can be observed. This technique has proved to be a good opportunity for studying both the initiation of myelination and the maintenance of myelin sheaths. Serum and abscorbic acid must be added to the medium in order to allow the initiation of myelin formation. In Table 1, the effects on rat Schwann cell functions of serum/ascorbated addition in neuron/Schwann cultures are summarized. Cell proliferation is decreased, whereas elongation begins and extensive myelination appears. Cultured Schwann cells, when presented with an axon, adhere to the axon, which in turn elicits a transient burst of Schwann cell proliferation (8,9) and induces a new basal lamina formation (10,11) and the reappearance of galactocerebroside of the Schwann cells surface (12), while diminishing Schwann cell expression of N-CAM (13) and of NGF receptor (14,15).

If the axon contacted is of sufficient caliber (>1 μm in diameter), synthesis of myelin-specific proteins and unsheathment of the axon by myelin lamellae also occur (12,13,16–18). Thus, using reconstituted coculture techniques the process by which Schwann cells interact with axons to form myelin can be analyzed and followed in details. Moreover, methods for depletion of satellite cells from dorsal root ganglion (DRG) cultures, yielding naked neuron cultures, appear ideal as testing systems for exogenous Schwann cells. In fact, to our way of thinking, the capacity to pass through the developmental sequence described above can be considered the ultimate test of Schwann cell "normality."

CELL TYPE SPECIFIC MARKERS FOR SCHWANN CELLS

In the past the identification of Schwann cells in culture has been dependent primarily upon morphological criteria, using phase contrast microscopy, which can be inaccurate and confusing. Recently, immunochemical methods using cell type specific markers have become a useful solution for this problem and now are available for identifying major cell types in PNS cultures (Table 2).

Since the first report by Ross et al. (19) demonstrating a positive immunostaining of human Schwann cells by mouse anti-human NGF receptor (NGFR) serum, antibody directed against the receptor for the NGF has been the most reliable and commonly ap-

TABLE 1. Regulation of Schwann cell (SC) function in neuron-SC cultures by serum-ascorbate (3)

	Serum	
SC function	Ascorbate-free	Ascorbate-rich
Adhesion to axons	Strong	Strong
Proliferation	Sustained	Decreases
Basal lamina formation	None	Variable
Elongation	Round/short	Elongated
Process extension/axon sorting	Some	Some
1:1 relationship	None	Many
Myelination	None	Extensive
Nonmyelinating ensheathment	None	Some

TABLE 2. Effects of serum/ascorbate on immunocytochemical phenotype expressed by Schwann cells (SC) in neuron-SC cultures (3)

SC molecules	Serum/ascorbate-free	Serum/ascorbate-rich
A. 217C	Most SC	Nonmyelinating SC
B. C4	Most SC	Nonmyelinating SC
C. Cell adhesion		
L1	Weak on many	Absent on myelinating SC
NCAM	Most SC	Nonmyelinating SC
J1	ND	Most SC
D. ECM		
laminin	Weak, punctate	Bright, continuous
Type 4 collagene	Not detectable	Bright, continuous
Heparan sulfate	Weak, punctate	Bright, continuous
E. Myelin		
GalC	Most SC, smooth/punctate	Myelinating SC only
MAG	Most SC, punctate	Myelinating SC only
P0	Not detectable	Compact myelin
MBP	Not detectable	Compact myelin

plied cell type specific marker for Schwann cell in culture. Its usefulness is also evident in tissue sections because of possibility preserving surface antigens of Schwann cell body and processes in sections (14). Thus, NGFR immunostaining can be detected only in cell membrane of axotomized Schwann cells and is not seen with other neural cell types.

Other specific cell markers for Schwann cells include several major components of the myelin sheath. PNS myelin is very rich in lipids and the rest is made up of proteins. The principal myelin lipids considered specific markers for Schwann cells by biochemical and immunocytochemical criteria are galactocerebroside (Galc) and sulfatide (20,21). The myelin proteins consist mainly of P_0 glycoprotein, which comprises 50% of total protein content (22). Other glycoproteins include myelin-associated glycoprotein MAG, a minor component of the myelin sheath (<1%) (23) and $P_{170}K$, a relatively abundant (<5%) PNS myelin-specific glycoprotein (24). Two structurally similar basic proteins, myelin basic protein (MBP) and P_2, account for approximately 15% of total myelin protein content (25). Antisera or antibodies specific for these major myelin proteins naturally become excellent candidates for the cell type specific markers for Schwann cells.

These markers have been used mostly in rat or mouse cells. Studies using developing or regenerating peripheral nerves have demonstrated immunohistochemically the sequential appearance of P_O, MBP, and P_2 within the compact portion of developing myelin sheaths (26). Interestingly, a similar situation pertains in the CNS where oligodendrocytes rather than Schwann cells are responsible for myelination. Oligodendrocytes first express GalC which is followed sequentially by MBP, MAG, and finally proteolipid protein (PLP), the major structural protein of CNS myelin (27). The mechanism for this nonsimultaneous expression of elements comprising compact myelin in both the CNS and the PNS is not understood. Presumably, myelination is not a one-step process but requires the orderly construction of an organelle which has a distinctive spatial organization.

Recently PLP, the principal structural protein of CNS myelin, has been found in human tumors of Schwann cell origin, as well as in sciatic nerve from a number of species (28). PLP protein was localized to the Schwann cells, but was not found in PNS myelin. In contrast to oligodendrocytes, PLP immunoreactivity could not be detected in the plasma membrane of Schwann cells cultured without neurons, suggesting that the sustained expression of

PLP, like that of the major PNS myelin proteins, appears to depend on neuronal signals (29,30).

MODULATION OF ANTIGENIC EXPRESSION BY SCHWANN CELLS

The factors that translate axon-Schwann cell interaction into Schwann cell differentiation have not been delineated. Myelin in the PNS is the product of differentiated Schwann cell associated with axons of the appropriate caliber and suitable collagen-containing ground substance. With establishment of axon-Schwann cell contact during development or regeneration of vertebrate peripheral nerves, Schwann cells are transformed from a quiescent to a metabolically active state, first exhibiting high mitotic rates than the synthesis of proteins and lipids typical of the differentiating cell (26–35). These Schwann cells are targeted for the myelin sheath where they probably serve to organize its complex multilamellar membraneous structure. Evidence from a number of sources suggests that myelination is controlled by a multifactorial regulatory system. Studies with Schwann cell cultures have indicated that cyclic adenosine 3',5'-monophosphate (cAMP) plays a role in this system. Schwann cells cultured in the absence of axons transiently express the major myelin proteins. After a week in culture, little or no P_0 or MBP proteins or their mRNAs can be detected, and NGFR expression is induced (21,36). Exposure of purified Schwann cell cultures to cAMP analogues or the adenylate cyclase activator, forskolin, either stimulates mitosis or, at higher concentrations, induces the synthesis of galactocerebroside (37) and the major components of the myelin sheath (38) normally absent from quiescent Schwann cells. Recently it has been demonstrated that the expression of immunoreactive PLP in cultured rat Schwann cells is dependent on external, presumably axonal signals (29–31).

Expression of PLP in Schwann cells can be induced by culturing the cells in the presence of dibutyryl cyclic AMP (dBcAMP) (30,31). However, unlike the induction of the major myelin proteins P_0 and MBP, dBcAMP induction of PLP is not accompanied by changes in the steady-state level of PLP mRNA, suggesting that regulation of PLP induction occurs at a posttranscriptional level (31).

In contrast to reinduction of the major myelin constituents, NGFR synthesis is repressed by raising Schwann cell intracellular cAMP (39). The down regulation of NGF receptor by elevation in Schwann cell cAMP metabolism is consistent with previous observation of the effect of the phosphodiesterase inhibitor theophylline, which was noted to decrease the expression of NGF receptor by melanoma cells (40), though not by PC12 pheochromocytoma cells (41).

In conclusion, it is apparent that beyond the initial requirement of axonal contact, myelin induction and myelin maintenance are under the control of multiple and interdependent regulatory steps. Although little is known about the in vivo regulation of myelination, the in vitro data indicate that Schwann cells intracellular cAMP may be one participant in this complex regulatory process.

SCHWANN CELL MITOGENS

The rate of proliferation of cultured Schwann cell is quite low and insufficient to compensate for Schwann cell losses from the monolayer, and therefore the number of Schwann cells in culture diminishes with time. Several factors, including composition of the culture medium (42,43), laminin and fibronectin (44,45), glial growth factor (GGF) (46–48), products of activated blood mononuclear-cells (49), axolemma fragments (50,51), and cAMP analogues or forskolin (46,50), have shown their influence on the rate of mitosis of cultured

TABLE 3. *Neurofibroma Schwann-like cells (SLC), adult human Schwann cells, and neonatal rat Schwann cells: comparison of phenotypic and proliferative properties (96)*

	SLC	Adult human Schwann cells	Neonatal rat Schwann cells
Elongated and bipolar or multipolar	Yes	Yes	Yes
Surface laminin	Yes	Yes	Yes
Surface NGF receptor	Yes	Yes	Yes
Surface fibronectin	No	No	No
Baseline proliferative rate in culture	Slow	Slow	Slow
Mitogenic response to axolemmal fragments	+++ or 0	+	+++
Mitogenic response to cAMP analogues	Inhibitory	?	++
Mitogenic response to GGF	++	++	++

Schwann cells. Since the first report on enhancement of Schwann cell proliferation using GGF associated with adenylate cyclase activator cholera toxin (42,46,52), several studies have shown that combined application of cAMP and polypeptide growth factors such as platelet-derived growth factor (PDGF), epidermal growth factor (EGF), fibroblast growth factor (FGF), or insulin, typically promotes a synergistic stimulation of cell proliferation (46,53–56). An explanation for this widely observed cooperativity has been proposed by Weinmaster and Lemke (57) who have demonstrated that although PDGF is a very poor mitogen when assayed alone, it is capable of strongly stimulating Schwann cell proliferation when assayed in the presence of forskolin. This cAMP-dependent PDGF stimulation is accompanied by a corresponding cAMP induction of mRNA encoding the PDGF receptor. These results indicate that the synergistic proliferative effect obtained from the combination of cAMP and polypeptide growth factors may result from the cAMP-mediated induction of growth factor receptors. Induction of these receptors may further account for the widely observed mitogenicity of cAMP alone, since in vitro proliferation assays are typically conducted in the presence of serum, which contains low concentrations of PDGF and other polypeptide growth factors. In this regard, it has been previously noted that elevation of intracellular cAMP does not trigger Schwann cell division if these cells are cultured in medium containing very low concentrations of serum (46).

Unlike rat Schwann cells, only few data are available on human Schwann cell mitogens (Table 3). In view of the well-known proliferation of Schwann cells following the contact with regenerating axons, it has been shown that the rate of proliferation of cultured human Schwann cells is considerably accelerated by addition of fragments of human axonal plasma membrane to the medium (51). In this respect, human Schwann cells resemble rat Schwann cells. However, these observations suggest, but do not prove, that human Schwann cells proliferate in response to the other known mitogens effective on rodent Schwann cells. Further studies are needed to expand human Schwann cells in vitro. The ability to produce large numbers of human glial cells from nerve biopsy and to analyze not only their morphological and immunologic but also biochemical and molecular properties would be of enormous value in identifying the cellular abnormalities that result in demyelinating disease.

TRANSCRIPTIONAL AND POSTTRANSCRIPTIONAL CONTROL OF MYELIN PROTEIN GENES

Myelin production depends on the coordinately regulated expression of a set of genes encoding specific structural cell components during the differentiation of myelinating glia in both the central and the peripheral nervous system. Some of these genes have been extensively studied, including those encoding the MAG (58), PLP (59), protein zero (P_0) (60), and MBP (61,62). Schwann cells require contact with axons for initial induction of myelin-specific proteins. The same requirement has been demonstrated for the induction and the maintained expression of the corresponding genes (63). The axonal regulation of P_0 and MBP genes has been recently studied both in vivo and in vitro using in situ hybridization and RNA blot hybridization methods (64). Signals for mRNAs encoding those genes fall dramatically in axon-deprived cells and in Schwann cells dissociated from the sciatic nerve and cultured for several days in the absence of axons. According to the authors, this axonal dependence of gene expression observed in vivo and in vitro will most likely reflect changes in the instantaneous rate of transcription of the major myelin genes, rather than alteration in the turnover rate of the mRNAs transcribed from them. The requirement for continuous axonal contact can be significantly overcome by any experimental condition that increases the level of intracellular cAMP. In cultured Schwann cells the addition of cAMP analogues such as cholera toxin and forskolin induces major myelin genes (65), and the same effect is shown by a novel glial transcription factor ("suppressed cAMP inducible POU") (64). However, besides the factors that regulate the developmental expression of the myelin protein genes at the transcriptional level, a number of posttranscriptional events, which might serve as potential regulatory points in the production of the myelin proteins and their assembly into the membrane, can be also involved. In the CNS, one such event in the expression of the MBP gene is the translocation of MBP mRNA from oligodendrocyte cell bodies to their processes. This translocation has been observed "in vivo" and in primary mixed glial cell cultures using "in situ" hybridization histochemistry by Campagnoni et al. (66). According to the authors, the conception of MBP mRNA translocation within the oligodendrocyte is as follow: The myelin membrane is surrounded by and infiltrated by cytoplasmic channels, called the outer/lateral loops, and longitudinal incisures, respectively. The vast majority of available evidence suggests that MBP mRNA can be translocated from its site of synthesis within the oligodendrocyte somas to the myelin membrane via these cytoplasmic channels. The transport of the MBP mRNA might occur on polyribosomes, although no direct evidence exists that this is the form in which the message is translocated. Synthesis of MBP can occur both within the cell body as well as in the processes, but it is unclear whether MBP synthesized in the soma can be transported independently to the myelin sheath or whether it simply turns over. Presumably, MBP synthesized within the oligodendrocyte processes and myelin channels is incorporated into the myelin sheath. An apparent failure of translocation may account for the lack of incorporation of newly synthesized MBP into jimpy myelin, whereas in quaking myelin, where MBP assembly is also defective, translocation appears to be normal, suggesting that incorporation of MBP into the membrane also is regulated posttranslationally. Among the possible factors influencing the pattern of translational regulation, glucocorticoids have been shown to be capable of stimulating the translation of MBP and PLP mRNAs and inhibiting the translation of CNP in cell-free systems (66).

STUDY OF PNS GLIA USING IMMORTALIZED SCHWANN CELL LINES

Many of the recent advances in the understanding of Schwann cell biology have resulted from "in vitro" studies, given the advantages of studying isolated cells in a controlled environment. Most studies were done on rodent Schwann cells because of the ease with which neonatal rat cells can be cultured. However, the isolation of Schwann cells from neonatal rat sciatic nerves is laborious, the number of cells obtained from each preparation is variable and often insufficient for biochemical and molecular studies, and the acquisition of large numbers of cells is time consuming as Schwann cells in culture replicate slowly with a doubling time of 7 days. A larger amount of cells can be obtained by the use of mitogen agents, such as cholera toxin, forskolin, and glial growth factor (46). Although this allows for the rapid expansion of cell numbers, the phenotypic properties of secondary Schwann cells change during passage in culture, and therefore, results obtained with cells passaged for various times may differ (67). An alternative can be represented by the immortalization and the availability of permanent cell lines. Peden et al. (67) have obtained immortalized Schwann cell lines using SV40 large T antigen under the control of the inducible mouse metallothionein-I promoter. These cells have many properties of untransfected Schwann cells in culture, including their ability to form myelin "in vitro" and can be useful in understanding the processes of myelination and demyelination.

TISSUE CULTURE OF HUMAN SCHWANN CELLS

Many techniques have been described to obtain pure populations of nonhuman Schwann cells that permit studies of cellular antigens and proliferative response. Only a few studies have been reported describing techniques for obtaining human Schwann cells, usually obtained from diagnostic peripheral nerve biopsies and autopsy material. A technique for the preparation of highly purified populations of Schwann cells from human fetal nerves has been described (68). Cultures are prepared by chemical and mechanical dissociation of human fetal sciatic nerves by a modification of the method previously described for newborn rat nerve (69). These cultures were compared with cultures obtained with the method of Askanas et al. (70) which results in enriched Schwann cell cultures by utilizing several successive re-explantations of the nerve explant. This method has been widely employed for human adult Schwann cell isolation, but the procedure is time consuming and the yield is not very high. The Schwann cell isolation by enzyme treatment has been proved effective for human autopsy material (71). The method of human fetal Schwann cell isolation by mechanical and enzymatic dissociation offers the advantages of speed, high yield, and simplicity, avoids the exposure of cells to antisera, complement, and cytotoxic drugs, and does not give the variations in yield and homogeneity observed with differential adhesion. Enriched populations of human Schwann cells cultured for at least 4 weeks are provided. After 7 days, about 80% of the cells are bipolar and S-100 positive, and this percentage remains relatively stable for approximately 14 days (Fig. 1). This method exploits the higher proliferation rate of fetal Schwann cells compared to the adult Schwann cells to reduce the number of contaminating fibroblasts. This fact is consistent with the observation of Moretto et al. (71), who found that the younger the donor age, the better the results of Schwann cell isolation. The cells obtained by this method display the typical morphological and immunological characteristics described in human fetal and adult Schwann cells obtained with the explantation-re-explantation method: they express surface laminin and NGF receptors, whereas surface fibronectin (FN) is absent (Figs. 2,3).

This method yields preparations from which cells attach readily to glass or plastic surface, providing normal human Schwann cells in quantities sufficient for a) morphological, biochemical, and immunological characterization during different stages of maturation, also of myelin- or axon-associ-

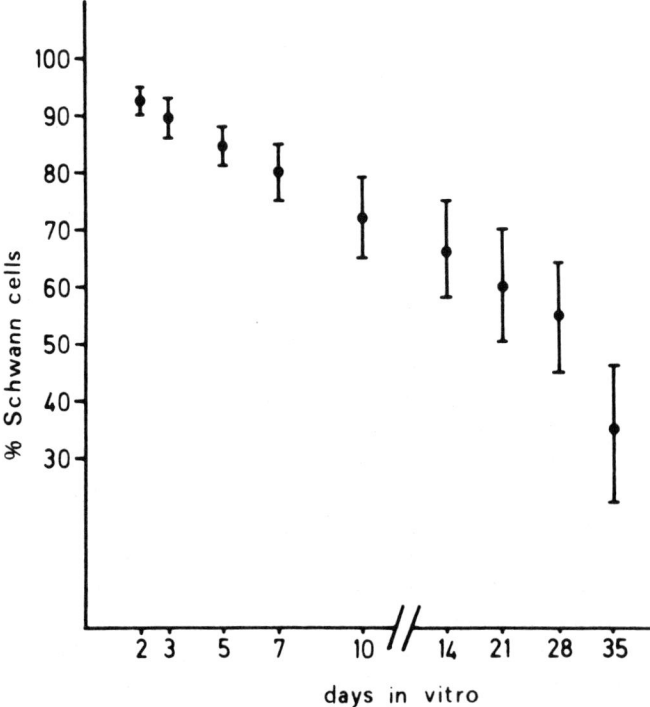

FIG. 1. Percentage of SCs in dissociated cultures from human fetal nerves as a function of time in culture. SCs were identified by their expression of the intracellular protein S-100 using immunoperoxidase. Each point represents the mean value of at least ten fields per coverslip; three coverslips per experiment were counted in each of the 12 experiments performed. Vertical lines denote S.E.M. ($p < .01$).

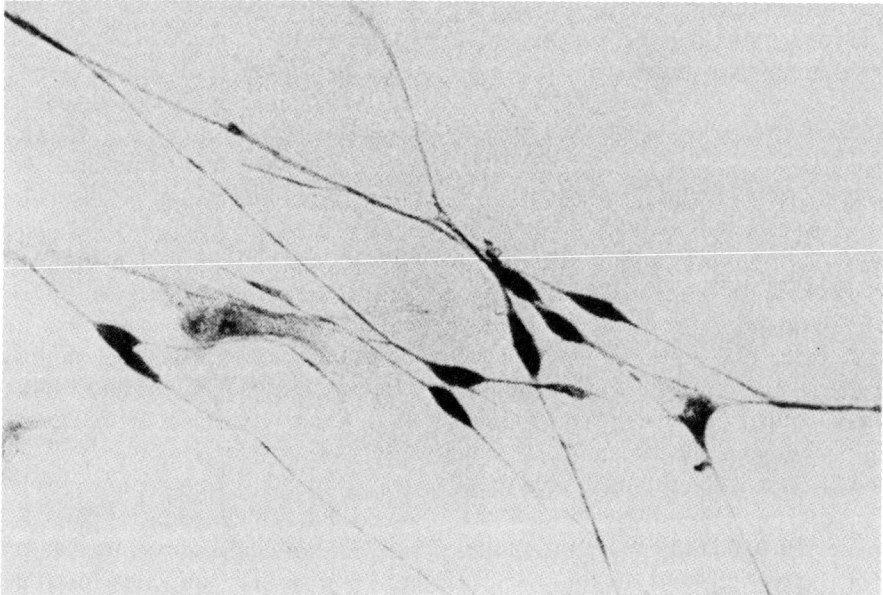

FIG. 2. S-100 protein immunostaining of human Schwann cells from dissociated fetal nerves. Strong positivity in contrast to fibroblast complete negativity; fetal nerve at 19 weeks of gestation counterstained with hematoxylin at 7 days in vitro. ×250.

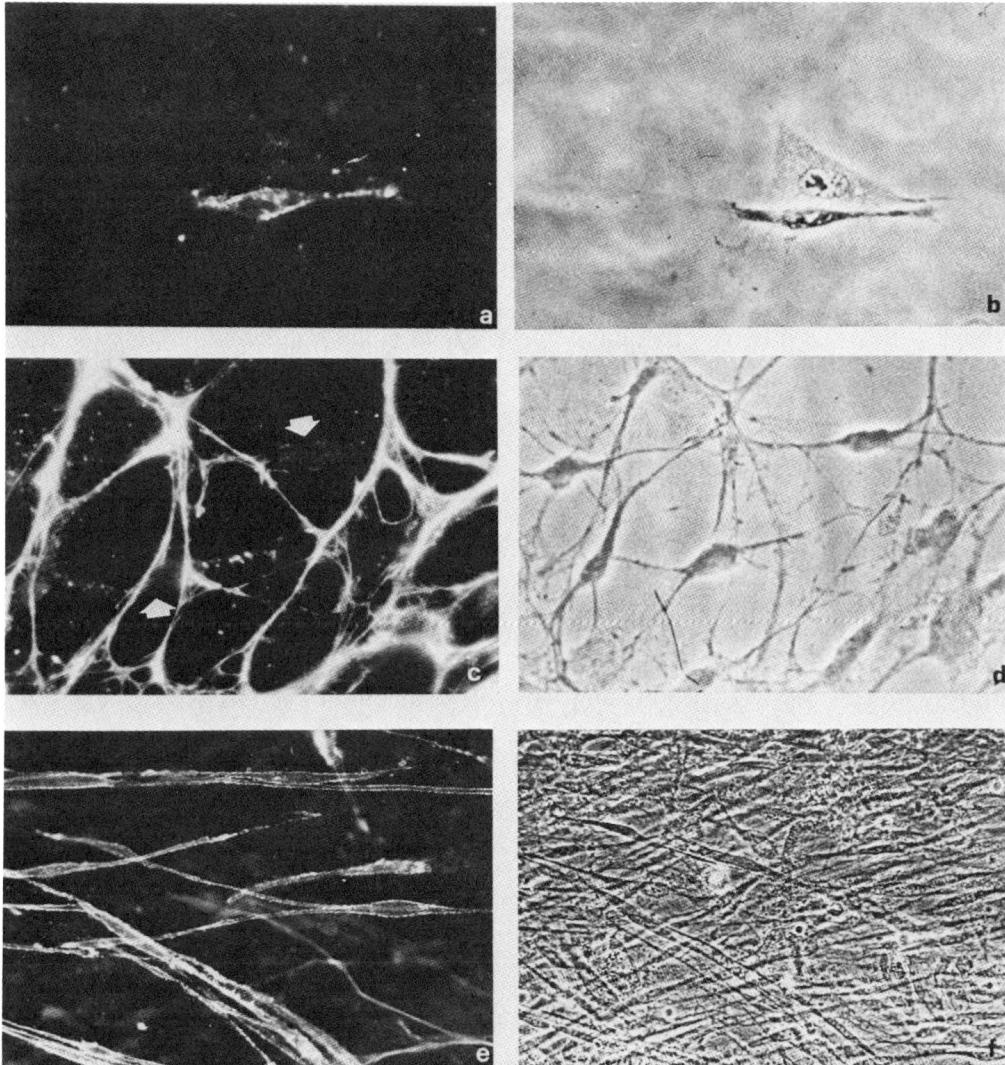

FIG. 3. Immunocytochemical characteristics of human Schwann cells cultured from dissociated fetal nerves. **A:** Anti-laminin immunofluorescence: a spindle-shaped Schwann cell is strongly positive for surface laminin (unfixed culture). **B:** Phase contrast appearance of the same field as in a (2 days in vitro). **C:** Anti-fibronectin immunofluorescence: pleomorphic fibroblasts are classically positive in older cultures or have faint nontypical binding (10 days in vitro) for surface fibronectin, whereas Schwann cells *(arrows)* are negative (unfixed culture). **D:** Phase contrast appearance of the same field as in c. **E:** Fibroblasts that do not bind anti-NGFR have formed a monolayer (45 days in vitro), upon which lie surface anti-NGFR-positive spindle-shaped bipolar and multipolar Schwann cells. **F:** Phase contrast of the same field. ×162.

ated markers like galactocerebroside and P_0 myelin protein, which expression is lost after a few hours or days in culture; b) analysis of the effects of potential mitogenic agents; and c) induction of specific surface antigens. Although the availability of a method to isolate cultures highly enriched for human fetal Schwann cells has several potential uses, recent studies of developmental changes in peripheral nerves suggest that the expression of some markers by Schwann cells could be dependent on the age of the donor. Fields and McMenamin (72) observed that several monoclonal antibodies, isolated by Ciment and Weston (73), that react with nuclear and axonal structures also react with cytoskeletal elements in Schwann cells cultured from adult rats, but not with neonatal rat Schwann cells (SCs), astrocytes, or fibroblasts. Ciment and Weston (73) were able to distinguish between quail SCs and precursors by the use of S-100 protein, which is expressed late in development. We observed that cultures from human fetal nerves of 15 weeks or less contain fewer S-100-positive putative Schwann cells than cultures from more mature fetuses (74). These data have been recently confirmed by Jessen et al. (2), as previously stated. These authors described glial cells present in hindlimb nerves of 14–15 day old rat embryos that cannot survive in vitro in murine serum-containing media, do not express S-100 protein, and are strongly immunoreactive with the antibodies against the NGF receptor (192-IgG or 217 c-Ran 1), which has previously been established as a marker for cultured SC and allows these cells to be distinguished in culture from fibroblastic cells. On the other hand, the expression of the receptors for the NGF is restricted to immature or regenerating Schwann cells and absent in fully developed Schwann cells (14,19,75). The ability to establish cultures of SC opens the possibility of studying cultured Schwann cells isolated from animals subjected to experimental diseases such as experimental allergic neuritis (EAN), streptozotocin or alloxan-induced diabetes, and lead neuropathy. Moreover, the responsiveness of Schwann cells dissociated from adult nerves may be different from that of neonatal cells with respect to the response to growth factors or cytokines. The availability of a method for dissociating adult nerves that circumvents difficulties related to the large amount of connective tissue and my-

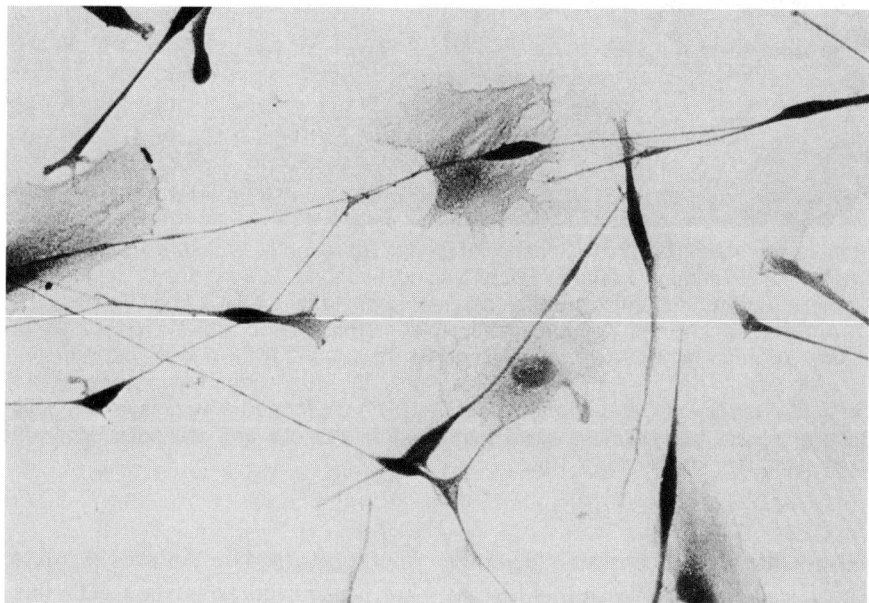

FIG. 4. Dissociated adult rat Schwann cells after staining with the anti S-100 protein antibody. There is strong cytoplasmatic and nuclear staining of Schwann cells. Fibroblasts are negative: the weak stain of the flat cells represents the counterstain with hematoxylin. Immunoperoxidase, $\times 250$.

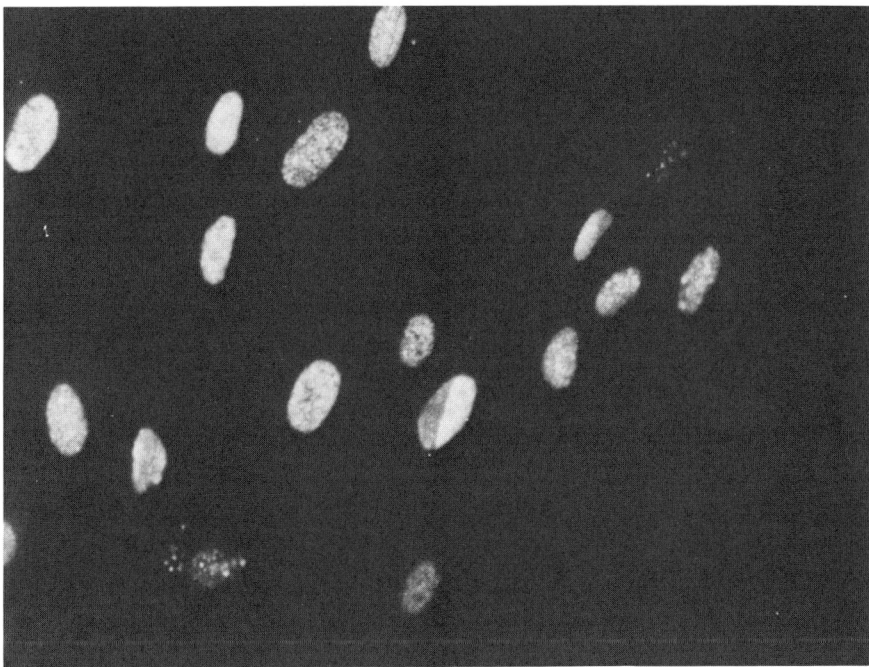

FIG. 5. Immunofluorescence with anti-BrdU antibody of adult rat Schwann cells after 7 days in vitro. Some cells incorporate BrdU into their nuclei. ×250.

elin could allow one to cultivate Schwann cells from human diagnostic nerve biopsies and autopsy material.

Moreover, in general, dissociated cell cultures are difficult to obtain from adult tissue because of its abundant connective tissue, and myelin and cell preparations from this tissue have a high percentage of fibroblasts that divide well in vitro and rapidly outnumber other cell types. A method to obtain Schwann cells from adult rat sciatic nerves by collagenase digestion has been described by Fields and McMenamin (72). The cell specific markers, anti-Ran-1, anti-Thy-1, anti-GFAP, and anti-intermediate filaments antibody, were used to identify cells isolated by this preparative method. Schwann cells were 10–30% of the isolated cells at 3 days in cultures. Another method for isolation, culture, and characterization of SC from adult rat sciatic nerve has been subsequently reported (68).

Enzymatic digestion with collagenase, dispase, and hyaluronidase yielded prepa-

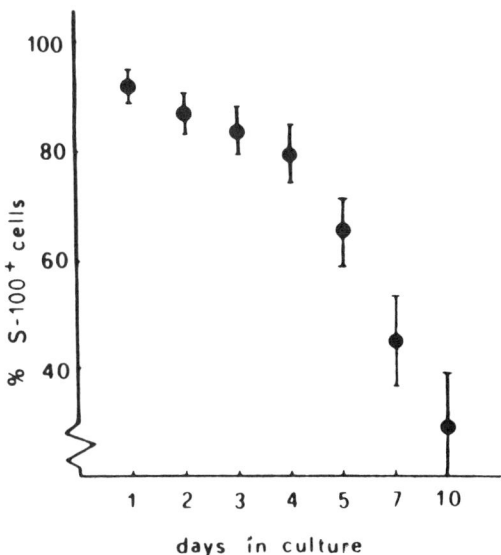

FIG. 6. Immunoperoxidase demonstration of anti-S-100 antibodies binding to adult rat Schwann cell cultures as a function of time in vitro. The means of five cultures are depicted.

rations from which cells attached readily to D-poly-L-lysine-coated glass coverslips. The cultures contained bipolar and round cells that were labeled specifically with anti-S-100 protein antibody, while the flat polymorphic cells were not labeled (Fig. 4). The percentage of Schwann cells identified by the S-100 protein was 92% at day 1. The proliferation rate of adult Schwann cells in culture using BrdU, an analog of thymidine, was also established (Fig. 5). The results show that these cells undergo proliferation in vitro even in the absence of mitogenic factors. However, because fibroblasts replicate faster than Schwann cells in culture, the proportion of fibroblasts increases, but at day 4, about 80% of the cells are still S-100 positive (Fig. 6).

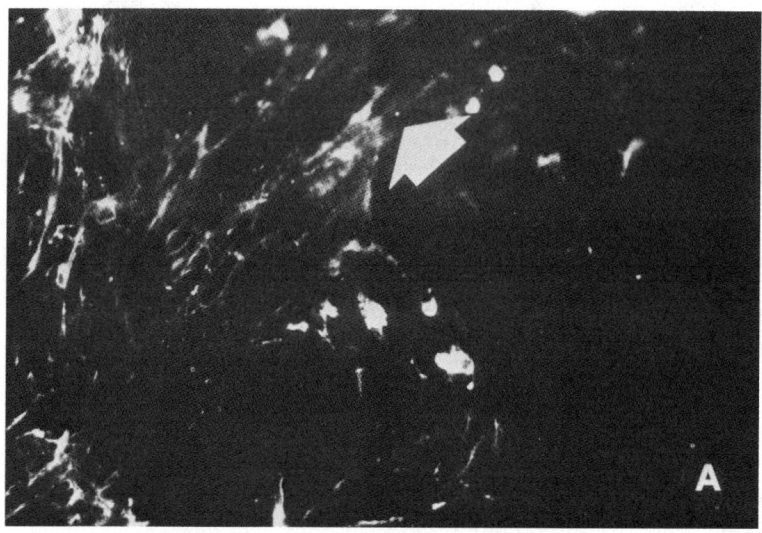

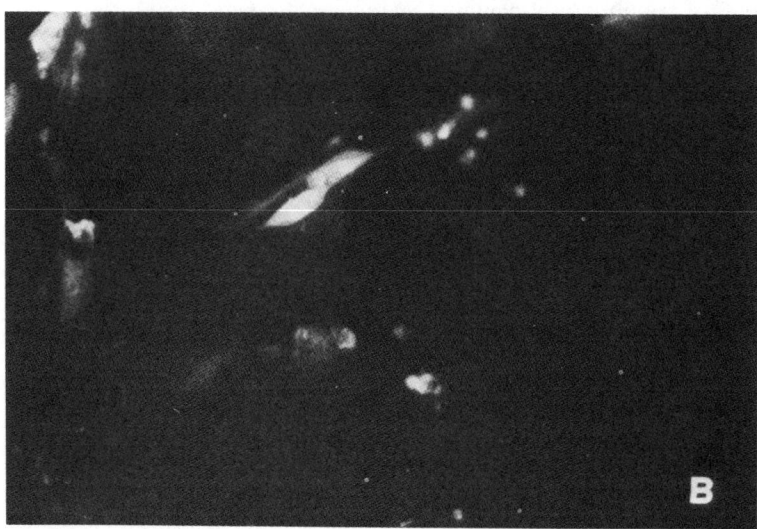

FIG. 7. FN immunofluorescence **(A)** and S-100 labeling **(B)** of adult Schwann cell culture. Most spindle-shaped S-100-positive cells are FN negative (*arrow*). ×250.

As previously reported for neonatal cultures, Schwann cells demonstrated the loss of myelin-associated phenotypic marker GalC by day 4. Laminin was used as cell-specific marker to confirm the light microscopic appearance of Schwann cells. Cultured Schwann cells did not express fibronectin during the first days in culture, but a few FN-positive Schwann cells were detectable after 4 days in culture, probably as a consequence of the increased production of extracellular matrix by the overgrowing fibroblasts (Fig. 7). Alternatively, some adult Schwann cells kept in culture for 7 days or more could conceivably produce small amounts of FN. The percentage of Schwann cells by immunocytologic or morphologic criteria is high (approximately 80%) at day 4, even without employing mitotic inhibitors or antibody-mediated cell lysis. This is believed to be a result of very accurate dissection and cleaning of connective tissue from the epineurium of the sciatic nerve under a dissecting microscope. Other measures that may have contributed to the results include a) the high yield due to extensive but gentle nerve digestion by the combination of three different enzymes employed for a very long time in the presence of FCS (the latter was necessary because cells were unable to stick on the coverslips in its absence, probably because the effects was too strong and toxic); b) the effect of poly-L-lysine-coated glass coverslips, which enhance a differential adhesion between Schwann cells and fibroblasts; and c) the reduction in FCS percentage after 48 h and use of RPMI 1640 medium in which Schwann cell mitosis is more frequent. This method seems to provide proliferating Schwann cells from normal adult rat nerves in quantity and time sufficient for a) morphological and immunocytological characterization, and b) analysis of the effects of mitogenic agents and induction of specific markers. It offers the advantages of speed, simplicity, higher yields, and the avoidance of exposure of cells to cytotoxic drugs, antisera, and complement in all cases in which the source from an adult nerve is more suitable.

MAJOR HISTOCOMPATIBILITY COMPLEX ANTIGENS

The major histocompatibility complex (MHC) is a tightly linked cluster of genes located on chromosome 17 in mouse and on chromosome 6 in humans. These genes encode for a series of highly polymorphic cell surface glycoproteins, which can be divided into two classes: Class I (H-2 in rodents and human lymphocyte antigen [HLA]-A,B,C in humans) and Class II (Ia in rodents and HLA-D system in humans). The MHC proteins are important in a phenomenon called MHC or T cell restriction. In the context of immune regulation, T lymphocytes cannot recognize an antigen on the cell surface if the appropriate MHC antigen is not simultaneously expressed by that cell. Class I proteins are the useful restriction elements for cytotoxic T cells, whereas Class II molecules are the restriction elements for helper T cells.

The appearance of the II Class histocompatibility molecules has been recently investigated in cultured human Schwann cells obtained from both fetal and adult normal nerves (76). Dissociated human Schwann cells were studied at different times in culture with anti-HLA-DR monoclonal antibodies (MAb). Some cultures were grown without fetal calf serum in the medium in order to avoid the possibility of antigenic induction due to agents like interferon which can be present in the serum. Cells were identified by two color immunofluorescence with anti S-100 protein antibody. Cultures obtained from both fetal and adult nerves contained HLA-DR-positive Schwann cells (Fig. 8). The percentage of positive cells markedly varied as a function of time, and no differences were found between cultures grown in the presence or absence of serum. This percentage was 35.5% at day 7 after dissociation, 70.6% at day 14,

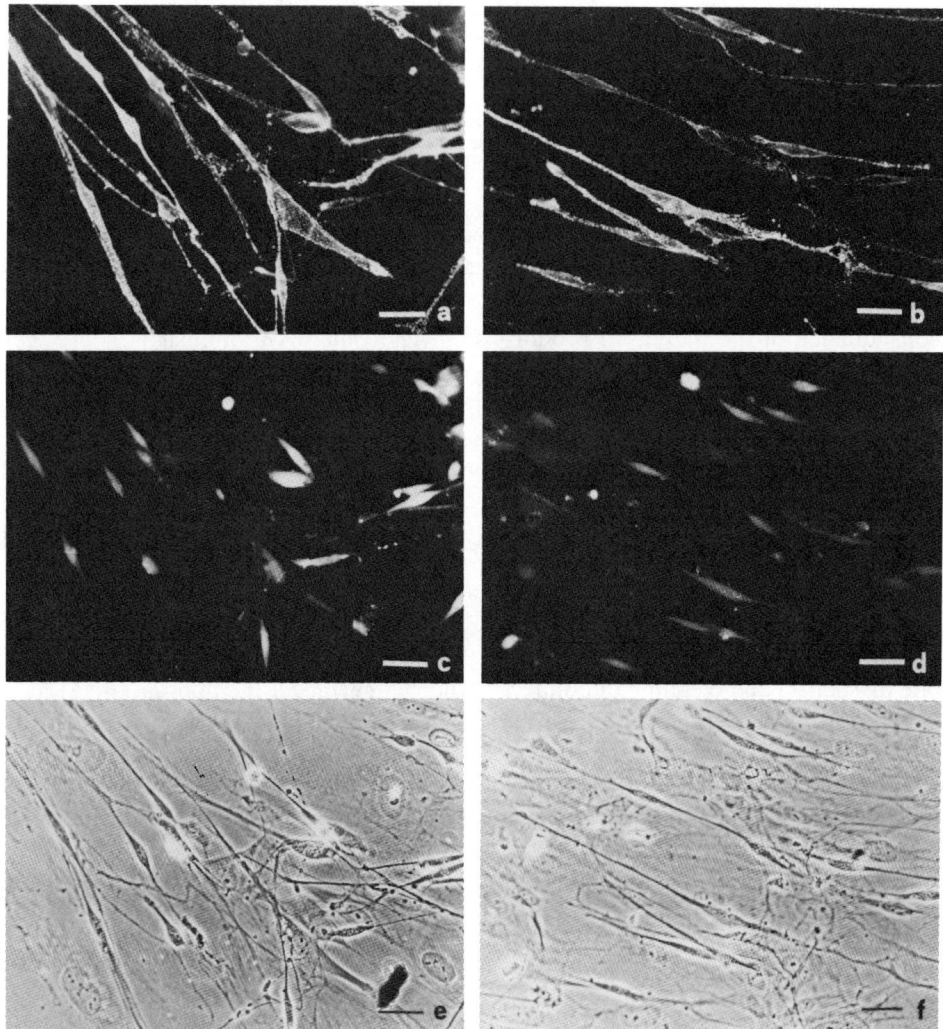

FIG. 8. a, c, e: Double labeling of cultured human Schwann immunostained with anti-S-100 and anti-HLA-DR antibodies. **b, d, f:** Parallel cultures grown in the absence of fetal calf serum. **a, b:** HLA-DR-rhodamine immunofluorescence; **c, d:** S-100-FITC immunofluorescence; **e, f:** phase-contrast microscopy. Bars = 50 μm.

and 81.8% at day 21 in cultures from four fetal nerves. At the same time in culture, percentages for Schwann cells from two normal adult and two pathologic nerves were, respectively, 66.7%, 69.95%, 76.6%, and 34.4%, 54.5%, 60.6%. No correlation was observed between the staining intensity in sections and the number of HLA-DR-positive Schwann cells in tissue culture.

These findings are contrary to previous studies which demonstrated the failure of detecting DR reaction on cultured human fetal Schwann cells (52,77) and on rat and mouse Schwann cells (78–80) without stimulation with gamma-interferon.

From these data, it is clear that human Schwann cells from both fetal and adult nerves are capable of expressing DR antigens also in absence of gamma interferon.

The detection of DR antigens on adult Schwann cells is in agreement with the results of Kim et al. (52), who demonstrated the presence of Ia antigens on the surface of certain populations of oligodendrocytes and astrocytes from normal adult human brains. A possible explanation for different results in fetal Schwann cells can be that the presence of DR molecules on the surface of the cell depends on the method employed. A strong chemical dissociation could imply a modification of the cell membrane and related structures. In any case, only with "in situ hybridization" with mRNA probes will it be possible to identify with certainty HLA-DR-producing cells and cells that take this material from the environment.

Whereas the meaning of DR presence on Schwann cells in some peripheral neuropathies can be easily explained, it is more difficult to understand why DR is strongly increased in neuropathies with no signs of inflammation such as CMT or is expressed in nerves during the fetal stage and on the Schwann cell membrane in tissue culture. These findings seem to confirm the hypothesis of Pollard et al. (81), who suggested that class II molecules can be expressed at a certain stage of differentiation or dedifferentiation in Schwann cells. In this case, DR antigen appearance on human SC may reflect not only an immunologically mediated phenomenon but also a dependence on axon-SC interaction.

NGF RECEPTOR

Human cultured SC were used to examine the expression of the receptors for NGF and of other molecules active during nerve development and repair. The relevance of that is related to the lack of experimental models in animals for some important human diseases in which SC are involved, such as neurofibromatosis. Staining of cultured human Schwann cells with anti-NGF receptor antibodies (Fig. 9) and binding of NGF to chick Schwann cells (75,82,83) demonstrate that this cell type is capable of NGF receptor expression. Recently NGF receptor expression was also detected on Schwann cells derived from traumatic neuromas and neurofibromas (19,84,85).

The role of the NGF receptor during neural development remains unclear. Schwann cells are capable of synthesizing NGF (86,87) so that a portion of the receptors may be occupied at any given time. NGF presented in this cell-bound concentrated form may be particularly effective for stimulation of developing sympathetic and sensory neurons (14). Once development is complete, the Schwann cell-associated NGF may be unnecessary since the innervated organ supplies NGF, and since the myelin sheath separates the neuron and the Schwann cell. It has been proposed that during nerve repair, Schwann cell-associated NGF also acts as a chemoattractant (14), and such a role in development is possible, since recent studies suggest that Schwann cells move ahead of developing axons and may guide the growth cones (88,89,36). A question raised by these studies is what developmental event induces the down-regulation of NGF receptor expression. It does not seem likely that cessation of Schwann cell division results in receptor down-regulation since human Schwann cells placed in culture without mitogens have an extremely low mitotic index but are positive for NGF receptor. Nor does it seem likely that myelination itself is the controlling element, since virtually all neural sheaths from adult sural nerve are negative, even though 80% of axons in the adult nerve are unmyelinated (90). Therefore, we suggested (68) that during this period there is a differentiation/maturation of both myelinating and nonmyelinating Schwann cells resulting from mature, functional Schwann cell-axon interactions (63). Disruption of these interations following nerve injury results in the dedifferentiation of the Schwann cells and a re-expression of

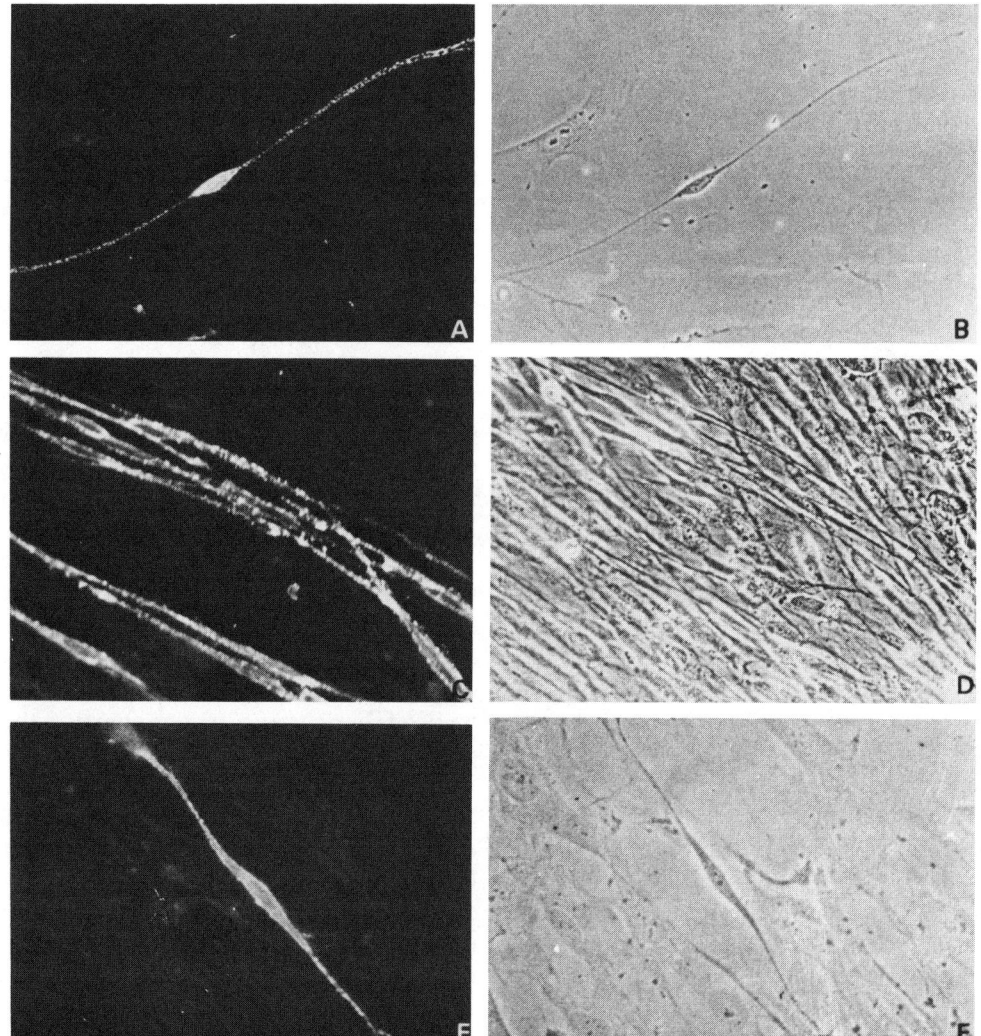

FIG. 9. Immunofluorescence staining with anti-NGF receptor MAb and phase contrast microscopy of cultured fetal Schwann cells. **A, B:** Cells from a 19 week nerve after 7 days in culture. **C, D:** Cells from the same nerve as in A and B after 35 days in culture. **E, F:** Cells from a 17 week nerve after 28 days in culture. The Schwann cells are positive, and the fibroblasts are negative. All at ×170.

the NGF receptor as observed by Taniuchi et al. (14). These results are supposed by the continued expression of NGF receptor by Schwann cells in culture in the absence of neurons, by the down-regulation of receptor in murine mixed cultures of neurons and Schwann cells (39), and during nerve development (Fig. 10). Daniloff et al. (91) have proposed a similar model for the expression of neural adhesion molecules during development and nerve repair. Expression of NGF receptor and neural adhesion molecules may be related since for PC12 pheochromocytoma cells NGF induces expression of the adhesion molecules (92) and for cultured murine Schwann cells NGF induces expression of L1, a molecule involved with fasciculation and initial Schwann cell-neuron interactions (18). L1 expression in developing nerves sharply

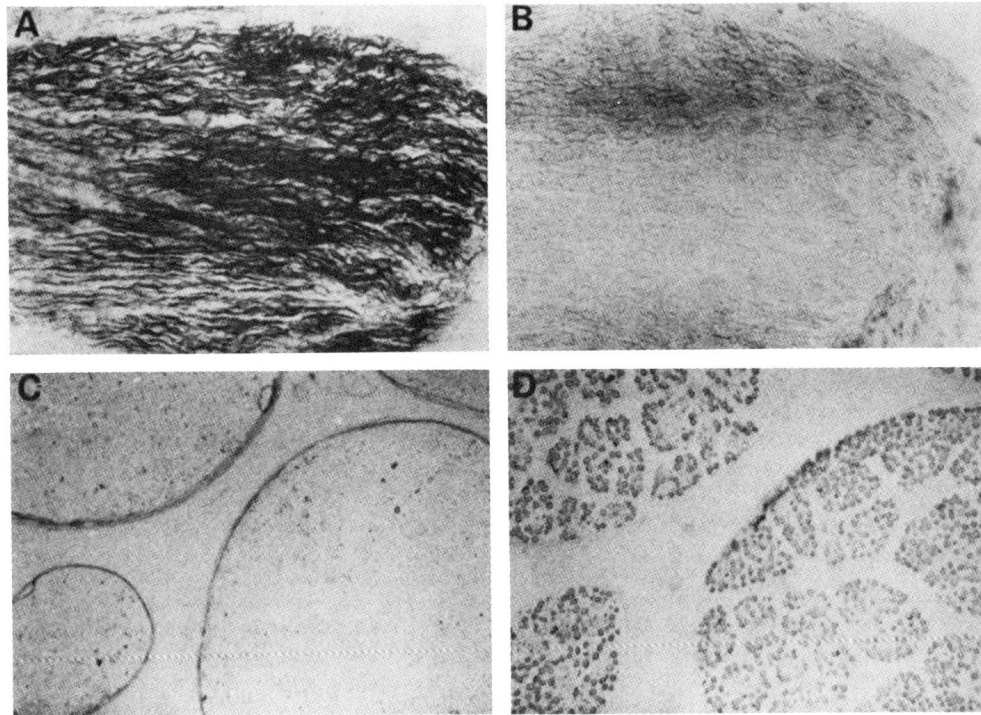

FIG. 10. Immunoperoxidase staining of frozen human peripheral nerves during development. **A:** Thirteen-week nerve stained with anti-NGF receptor MAb ME 20.4 shows intense immunoreactivity. **B:** Adjacent section of the same nerve as in A stained with MAb 4C5 (specific for myelin) shows no immunoreactivity. **C:** Adult nerve stained with anti-NGF receptor MAb shows immunoreactivity limited to the perineurium and a few endoneurial cells. **D:** Adjacent section of the same nerve as in C stained with MAb 4C5 shows strong staining of myelin sheaths. All at ×100.

decreases after Schwann cells wrap around the axons about 1.5 loops and just prior to the expression of myelin-related markers (13). This mechanism may also be relevant to development-dependent regulation of NGF receptor in other parts of the peripheral nervous system and the central nervous system (93,94).

TISSUE CULTURE STUDIES OF NEUROFIBROMATOSIS

Neurofibromatosis type 1 (NF-1, von Recklinghausen's disease) is characterized by the focal accumulation of Schwann-like cells to form subcutaneous and plexiform neurofibromas and schwannomas (95). In previous work, Pleasure et al. (96) have developed methods for the isolation and purification of neurofibroma Schwann-like cells and examined by tritiated thymidine autoradiography the baseline and mitogen-stimulated rates of proliferation of these cells during their maintenance in minimum essential medium (MEM)-serum. In these conditions, mitosis of neurofibroma Schwann-like cells like that of normal adult human Schwann cells is slow, but is stimulated by addition of partially purified GGF or rat CNS axolemmal fragments to the medium. Unlike neonatal rat Schwann cells, both neurofibroma Schwann-like cells and adult human Schwann cells respond to treatment with cAMP analogues or forskolin by a diminution in rate of mitosis (Table 3).

In order to determine the capacity of neurofibroma Schwann-like cells for axon-driven differentiation, we have shown that these cells co-cultured with fetal rat DRG neurons are induced to express immunoreactive galC and MAG, whereas Schwann-like cells (SLC) NGFR are down-regulated (97). The logistics of such co-culture experiments were the absence of species barrier problem since previous studies indicated that rat axolemma could drive the proliferation of human Schwann cells and neurofibroma Schwann-like cells (51,98,99) and that human Schwann cells were capable of myelinating rodent axons when transplanted in vivo (100).

These observations taken together indicate that neurofibroma Schwann-like cells do not differ markedly from normal human Schwann cells in baseline and mitogen-stimulated rates of proliferation during maintenance in this simple culture system. Moreover, Schwann neurofibroma, like normal Schwann cells, can be driven to differentiate by neuronal contact. These data, however, do not allow full assessment of whether the proliferation and differentiation of SLC is entirely normal. Further studies with human SC from normal adult nerves would be necessary to determine whether or not NF-SLC are entirely competent to differentiate in the presence of axons and to form myelin.

CONCLUSIONS

The importance of Schwann cells in the formation and maintenance of myelin in the PNS and in the understanding of the clinical problems of peripheral neuropathies is self-evident. One challenge of the future should be the possibility of isolating a large number of human Schwann cell from nerve biopsies and maintaining them in culture for long periods. Using these cultures, basic biological, physiological, and immunological properties and traits of Schwann cells could be investigated in the absence of other cell types, which may interfere with phenotypic expression of the cells in question. Using these cultured cells it will be also possible to study the effect of putative growth factors for Schwann cells, which are reported to be mitogenic for rodent Schwann cells.

Prior to the onset of myelination, a set of myelin specific genes is expressed in each myelinating Schwann cell. The timing of the expression of each of these genes is co-ordinately regulated and closely coupled to the onset of myelination. The major control of expression of this gene set is at the level of transcription. Since these genes are expressed in only Schwann cells, they are subject both to tissue specific as well as temporal control. Using molecular biology techniques currently available, study of myelin gene expression offers an excellent opportunity for analysis of these important aspects of gene regulation. Current theories of the regulation of eukaryotic gene expression suggest that transcription is controlled by the interaction of *trans* active factors (regulatory proteins), with specific DNA sequences proximal to the gene, (promoters and/or enhancers). Regulation of the myelin specific gene set will likely follow this model. Although transcriptional control is the major level of myelin gene regulation, other factors may also modulate gene expression. Alternative splicing has been demonstrated for many of the myelin genes, most notably MBP, and this process can modulate gene expression by producing a family of related mRNAs (and proteins) from a single primary transcript (62,101).

The majority of data currently available about the expression of PNS myelin proteins derives from morphological and biochemical studies. With the development of new molecular biological techniques it will now be possible to examine expression of myelin elements at the gene level and to probe the specific regulatory factors for each. Identification of *cis* and *trans* active regulatory factors, and delineation of promoter and or enhancer sequences will be important steps in understanding the biology of myelination. Finally, knowledge of the elements involved in myelin gene regulation will permit the search for the primary genetic defects that form the basis of inherited dismyelinating disorders of the PNS.

ACKNOWLEDGMENTS

The authors wish to thank Laura Geremia, Paola Doneda, and Anna Maria Conti for assistance in the preparation of this manuscript. These studies were supported by Associazione Amici del Centro Dino Ferrari, Associazione Italiana Sclerosi Multipla, and Istituto Superiore di Sanità-Progetto AIDS.

REFERENCES

1. Ritchie JM, Rang HP. Extraneuronal saxitoxin binding sites in rabbit myelinated nerve. *Proc Natl Acad Sci USA* 1983; 80: 2803–2807.
2. Jessen KR, Morgan L, Stewart HJ, Mirsky R. Three markers of adult non-myelin-forming Schwann cells, 217c (Ran-1), A5E3 and GFAP: development and regulation by neuron-Schwann cell interactions. *Development* 1990; 109: 91–103.
3. Wood P, Moya F, Eldridge C, et al. Studies of the initiation of myelination by Schwann cells. In: Duncan ID, Skoff RP, Colman D, eds. *Myelination and dysmyelination*, vol. 605. New York: Annals of the New York Academy of Sciences, 1990; 1–14.
4. Wood PM, Williams AK. Oligodendrocyte proliferation and CNS myelination in cultures containing dissociated embryonic neurologic and dorsal root ganglion neurons. *Dev Brain Res* 1984; 12: 225–241.
5. Wood PM, Bunge RP. Evidence that axons are mitogenic for oligodendrocytes isolated from adult animals. *Nature* 1986; 320: 756–758.
6. Eldridge CF, Bunge MB, Bunge RP, Wood PM. Differentiation of axon-related Schwann cells in vitro I, absorbic acid regulates basal lamina assembly and myilin formation. *J Cell Biol* 1987; 105: 1023–1034.
7. Bunge MB, Bunge RP, Carey DJ, Cornbrooks CJ, Eldridge CF, Williams AK, Wood PM. Axonal and nonaxonal influences on Schwann cell development. In: Coages PW, Markwold RR, Kenny AD, eds. *Developing and regenerating vertebrate nervous systems*. New York: Alan R. Liss, Inc.; 1983; 71–105.
8. Wood PM, Bunge RP. Evidence that sensory axons are mitogenic for Schwann cells. *Nature* 1975; 256: 662–664.
9. Manthorpe M, Skaper S, Varon S. Purification of mouse Schwann cells using neurite-induced proliferation in serum-free monolayer culture. *Brain Res* 1980; 196: 467–482.
10. Armati-Gulson P. Schwann cells, basement lamina and collagen in developing rat dorsal root ganglia in vitro. *Dev Biol* 1980; 77: 213–217.
11. Bunge MB, Williams AK, Wood PM. Neuron-Schwann cell interaction in basal lamina formation. *Dev Biol* 1982; 92: 449–450.
12. Ratner N, Elbein A, Bunge MB, Porter S, Bunge RP, Glaser L. Specific asparagine-linked oligosaccharides are not required for certain neuron-neuron and neuron-Schwann cell interactions. *J Cell Biol* 1986; 103: 159–170.
13. Martini R, Schachner M. Immunoelectron microscopic localization of neural cell adhesion molecules (LI, N-CAM, and MAG) and their shared carbohydrate epitope and myelin basic protein in developing sciatic nerve. *J Cell Biol* 1986; 103: 2439–2448.
14. Taniuchi M, Clark HB, Johnson EM. Induction of Nerve Growth Factor receptor in Schwann cells after axotomy. *Proc Natl Acad Sci USA* 1986; 83: 4094–4098.
15. Taniuchi M, Clark HB, Schweitzer JB, Johnson EM Jr. Expression of nerve growth factor receptors by Schwann cells of axotomized peripheral nerves: ultrastructural location, suppression by axonal contact, and binding properties. *J Neurosci* 1988; 8: 664–681.
16. Politis MJ, Sternberger N, Ederle K, Spencer PS. Studies on the control of myelinogenesis. IV. Neuronal induction of Schwann cell myelin-specific protein synthesis during nerve fiber regeneration. *J Neurosci* 1982; 2: 1252–1266.
17. Windebank AJ, Wood P, Bunge RP, Dyck PJ. Myelination determines the caliber of dorsal root ganglion neurons in culture. *J Neurosci* 1985; 5: 1563–1569.
18. Seilheimer B, Schachner M. Regulation of neural cell adhesion molecule expression on cultured mouse Schwann cells by nerve growth factor. *EMBO J* 1987; 6: 1611–1616.
19. Ross AH, Pleasure D, Sonnenfeld K, et al. Expression of melanoma-associated antigens by normal and neurofibroma Schwann cells. *Cancer Res* 1986; 46: 5887–5892.
20. Fryxell KJ. Synthesis of sulfatide by cultured rat Schwann cells. *J Neurochem* 1980; 35: 1461–1464.
21. Mirsky R, Winter J, Abney ER, Pruss RM, Gavrilovic J, Raff MC. Myelin-specific proteins and glycolipids in rat Schwann cells and oligodendrocytes in culture. *J Cell Biol* 1980; 84: 483–494.
22. Isaque A, Roomi MW, Szymanska I, Kowalski S, Eylar EH. The P_0 glycoprotein of peripheral nerve myelin. *Can J Biochem* 1980; 58: 913–919.
23. Sterberger NH, Quarles RH, Itoyama Y, Webster HdeF. Myelin-associated glycoprotein demonstrated immunocytochemically in myelin and myelin-forming cells of developing rats. *Proc Natl Acad Sci USA* 1979; 76: 1510–1514.
24. Shuman S, Hardy M, Pleasure D. Peripheral

nervous system myelin and Schwann cell glycoproteins: identification by lectin binding and partial purification of a peripheral nervous system myelin-specific 170,000 molecular weight glycoprotein. *J Neurochem* 1983; 41: 1277–1285.
25. Lees MB, Brostoff SW. Proteins of myelin. In: Morell P, ed. *Myelin,* second edition. New York: Plenum Press; 1984: 197–224.
26. Hahn AF, Kachar B, Webster H deF. Expression of myelin proteins in developing rat Schwann cells. *Soc Neurosci Abstr* 1985; 11: 331.5(A).
27. Zeller NK, Behar TN, Dubois-Dalcq M, Lazzarini RA. The timely expression of myelin basic protein gene in cultured rat brain oligodendrocytes is independent of continuous neuronal influences. *J Neurosci* 1985; 5: 2955–2962.
28. Puckett CL, Hudson L, Ono K, Friedrich V, Benecke J, Dubois-Dalcq M, Lazzarini RA. Myelin-specific proteolipid protein is expressed in myelinating Schwann cells but is not incorporated into myelin sheaths. *J Neurosci Res* 1987; 18: 511–518.
29. Ono K, Friedrich V Jr, Hudson L, Lazzarini R, Dubois-Dalcq M. The unexpected expression of the major CNS myelin protein, proteolipid protein, in Schwann cells in vivo and in vitro. In: *Proc. Second International Conference on Charcot Marie Tooth Disorders.* York York: Alan R. Liss, Inc.; 201–208.
30. Mokuno K, Baron P, Grinspan J, Sobue G, Kreider B, Pleasure D. Neurological lineages and neurological diseases. In: Kim S, ed. *Myelination and demyelination: implications for multiple sclerosis.* New York: Plenum Press; 1989: 17–28.
31. Kamholz J, Sessa M, Scherers T, et al. Structure and expression of proteolipid protein in the peripheral nervous system. *J Neurosci Res;* 1992: 31: 231–244.
32. Fields KL. Cell type-specific antigens of cells of the central and peripheral nervous system. *Curr Top Dev Biol* 1979; 13: 237–257.
33. Spencer PS. Neuronal regulation of myelinating cell function. In: Ferrendelli JA, ed. *Society for Neuroscience Symposia, Volume IV: Aspects of developmental neurobiology.* Bethesda, MD: Society for Neuroscience; 1979: 275–321.
34. Smith ME. Biosynthesis of peripheral nervous system myelin proteins in vitro. *J Neurochem* 1980; 35: 1183–1189.
35. Smith ME, Kocsis JD, Waxman SG. Myelin protein metabolism in demyelination and remyelination in the sciatic nerve. *Brain Res* 1983; 270: 37–44.
36. DiStefano PS, Johnson EM Jr. Nerve growth factor receptors on cultured Schwann cells. *J Neurosci* 1988; 8: 231–241.
37. Sobue G, Pleasure D. Schwann cell galactocerebroside induced by derivatives of adenosine 3',5' monophosphate. *Science* 1984; 224: 72–74.
38. Lemke G, Chao M. Axons regulate Schwann cell expression of the major myelin and NGF receptor genes. *Development* 1988; 102: 499–504.
39. Mokuno K, Sobue G, Reddy UR, Wurzer J, Kreider B, Hotta H, Baron P, Ross AH, Pleasure D. Regulation of Schwann cell nerve growth factor receptor by cyclic adenosine 3',5'-monophosphate. *J Neurosci Res* 1988; 21: 465–472.
40. Riopelle RJ, Haliotis T, Roder JC: Nerve growth factor receptors of human tumors of neural crest origin: characterization of binding site heterogeneity and alteration by theophylline. *Cancer Res* 1983; 43: 5184–5189.
41. Greene LA, Drexler SA, Connolly JL, Rukenstein A, Green SH. Selective inhibition of responses to nerve growth factor and of microtubule-associated protein phosphorylation by activators of adenylate cyclase. *J Cell Biol* 1986; 103: 1967–1978.
42. Kreider BQ, Corey-Bloom J, Lisak RP, Doan H, Pleasure D. Stimulation of mitosis of cultured rat Schwann cells isolated by differential adhesion. *Brain Res* 1982; 237: 238–243.
43. Sobue G, Kreider B, Asbury A, Pleasure D. Specific and potent mitogenic effect of axolemmal fraction on Schwann cells from rat sciatic nerves in serum-containing and defined media. *Brain Res* 1983; 280: 263–275.
44. Baron-van Evercooren A, Kleinman HK, Seppa EJ, Rentier B, Dubois-Dalcq M. Fibronectin promotes rat Schwann cell growth and motility. *J Cell Biol* 1982; 93: 211–216.
45. McGarvey ML, Baron-van Evercooren A, Kleinman HK, Dubois-Dalcq M. Synthesis and effects of basement membrane components in cultured rat Schwann cells. *Dev Biol* 1984; 105: 18–28.
46. Raff MC, Abney ER, Brockes JP, Hornby-Smith A. Schwann cell growth factors. *Cell* 1978; 15: 813–822.
47. Brockes JP, Lemke GE, Balzer DR. Purification and preliminary characterization of a glial growth factor from the bovine pituitary. *J Biol Chem* 1980; 225: 8374–8377.
48. Lemke GE, Brockes JP. Identification and purification of glial growth factor. *J Neurosci* 1984; 4: 75–83.
49. Lisak RP, Sobue G, Kuchmy D, Burns JB, Pleasure DE. Products of activated lymphocytes stimulate Schwann cell mitosis in vitro. *Neurosci Lett* 1985; 57: 105–111.
50. Sobue G, Brown MJ, Kim SU, Pleasure DE. Axolemma is a mitogen for human Schwann cells. *Ann Neurol* 1984a; 15: 449–452.
51. Sobue G, Pleasure D. Astroglial proliferation and phenotype are modulated by neuronal plasma membrane. *Brain Res* 1984b; 324: 175–179.
52. Kim SU, Moretto G, Shin DH. Expression of Ia antigens on the surface of human oligodendrocytes and astrocytes in culture. *J Neuroimmunol* 1985; 10: 141–149.
53. McGowan JA, Strain AJ, Bucher NLR. Synergistic effects of epidermal growth factor and

cyclic AMP on cell proliferation. *J Cell Physiol* 1981; 108: 353–363.
54. Roger PP, Dumont JE. Factors controlling proliferation and differentiation of canine thyroid cells cultured in reduced serum conditions: effects of thyrotropin, cyclic AMP and growth factors. *Mol Cell Endocrinol* 1984; 36: 79–93.
55. Westermark K, Westermark B, Karlsson FA, Ericson LE. Location of epidermal growth factor receptors on porcine thyroid follicle cells and receptor: regulation by thyrotropin. *Endocrinology* 1986; 118: 1040–1046.
56. Roger PP, Servais P, Dumont JE. Induction of DNA synthesis in dog thyrocytes in primary culture: synergistic effects of thyrotropin and cyclic AMP with epidermal growth factor and insulin. *J Cell Physiol* 1987; 130: 58–67.
57. Weinmaster G, Lemke G. Cell-specific cyclic AMP-mediated induction of the PDGF receptor. *EMBRO S* 1990; 9: 915–919.
58. Lai C, Brow MA, Nave KA, et al. Two forms of 1B236/myelin-associated glycoprotein, a cell adhesion molecule for postnatal neural development, are produced by alternative splicing. *Proc Natl Acad Sci USA* 1987; 84: 4337–4341.
59. Milner RJ, Lai C, Nave KA, Lenoir D, Ogata J, Sutcliffe JG. Nucleotide sequences of two mRNAs for rat brain proteolipid protein. *Cell* 1985; 42: 931–939.
60. Lemke G, Axel R. Isolation and sequence of a cDNA encoding the major structural protein of peripheral myelin. *Cell* 1985; 40: 501–508.
61. Roach A, Boylan K, Horvath S, Prusiner SB, Hood L. Characterization of a cloned cDNA representing rat myelin basic protein: absence of expression in shiverer mutant mice. *Cell* 1983; 34: 799–806.
62. Kamholz J, de Ferra F, Puckett C, Lazzarini RA. Identification of three forms of human myelin basic protein by cDNA cloning. *Proc Natl Acad Sci USA* 1986; 83: 4962–4966.
63. Bray GM, Rasminski M, Aguayo AJ. Interaction between axons and their sheats cells. *Annu Rev Neurosci* 1981; 4: 127–162.
64. Lemke G, Kuhn R, Monuki ES, Weinmaster G. Transcriptional controls underlying Schwann cell differentiation and myelination. In: Duncan ID, Skoff RP, Colman D, eds. *Myelination and demyelination*, vol. 605. New York: Annals of the New York Academy of Sciences; 1990: 248–253.
65. Lemke G, Chao M. Axons regulate Schwann cell expression of the major myelin and NGF receptor genes. *Development* 1988; 102: 499–504.
66. Campagnoni AT, Verdi JM, Verity AN, Amur-Umarjee S. Posttranscriptional events in the expression of myelin protein genes. In: Duncan ID, Skoff RP, Colman D, eds. *Myelination and dysmyelination*, vol. 605. New York: Annals of the New York Academy of Science; 1990: 270–279.
67. Peden KWC, Rutkowski JL, Gilbert M, Tennekoon GI. Production of Schwann cell lines using a regulated oncogene. In: Duncan ID, Skoff RP, Colman D, eds. *Myelination and dysmyelination*, vol. 605. New York: Annals of the New York Academy of Science; 1990: 286–293.
68. Scarpini E, Kreider BQ, Lisak RP, et al. Cultures of human Schwann cells isolated from fetal nerves. *Brain Res* 1988; 440: 261–266ò.
69. Kreider BQ, Messing A, Doan H, Kim SU, Lisak RP, Pleasure DE. Enrichment of Schwann cell cultures from neonatal rat sciatic nerve by differential adhesion. *Brain Res* 1981; 207: 433–444.
70. Askanas V, Engel WK, Dalakas M, Lawrence JV, Carter LS. Human Schwann cells in tissue culture. Histochemical and ultrastructural studies. *Arch Neurol* 1980; 37: 329–337.
71. Moretto G, Kim SU, Shin DH, Pleasure DE, Rizzuto N. Long-term cultures of human adult Schwann cells isolated from autopsy materials. *Acta Neuropathol* 1984; 64: 15–21.
72. Fields KL, McMenamin P. Schwann cells cultured from adult rats contain a cytoskeletal protein related to astrocyte filaments. *Dev Brain Res* 1985; 20: 259–269.
73. Ciment G, Weston JA. Early appearance in neural crest and crest-derived cells of an antigenic determinant present in avian neurons. *Dev Biol* 1982; 93: 355–367.
74. Scarpini E, Meola G, Baron P, et al. Cytochemical, ultrastructural and immunological studies of cultured human Schwann cells. *Basic Appl Histochem* 1987; 31: 33–42.
75. Raivich G, Zimmermann A, Sutter A. The spatial and temporal pattern of NGF receptor expression in the developing chick embryo. *EMBO J* 1985; 4: 637–644.
76. Scarpini E, Lisak RP, Beretta S, et al. Quantitative assessment of class II molecules in normal and pathological nerves. *Brain* 1990; 113: 659–675.
77. Samuel NM, Mirsky R, Grange JM, Jessen KR. Expression of major histocompatibility complex class I and class II antigens in human Schwann cell cultures and effects of infection with Mycobacterium leprae. *Clin Exp Immunol* 1987; 68: 500–509.
78. Lisak RP, Hirayama M, Kuchmy D, Rosenzweig A, Kim SU, Pleasure DE, Silberberg DH. Cultured human and rat oligodendrocytes and rat Schwann cells do not have immune response gene associated antigen (Ia) on their surface. *Brain Res* 1983; 289: 285–292.
79. Wekerle H, Schwab M, Linington C, Meyermann R. Antigen presentation in the peripheral nervous system: Schwann cells present endogenous myelin autoantigens to lymphocytes. *Eur J Immunol* 1986; 16: 1551–1557.
80. Bartlett PF, Wycherly K, Wong GH. Induction of histocompatibility antigens on neural cells by interferon-γ: lack of expression on sensory neurons. *Neurosci Lett* 1984; Supplement 15: S46.
81. Pollard JD, McCombe PA, Baverstock J, Gaterby PA, McLeod JG. Class II antigen expression and T lymphocyte subsets in chronic in-

flammatory demyelinating polyneuropathy. *J Neuroimmunol* 1986; 13: 123–134.
82. Rohrer H. Nonneuronal cells from chick sympathetic and dorsal root sensory ganglia express catecholamine uptake and receptors for nerve growth factor during development. *Dev Biol* 1985; 111: 95–107.
83. Hosang M, Shooter EM. Molecular characteristics of nerve growth factor receptors on PC12 cells. *J Biol Chem* 1985; 260: 655–662.
84. Pleasure D, Kreider BQ, Sobue G, Ross AH, Koprowski H, Sonnenfeld KH, Rubenstein AE. Schwann-like cells cultured from human dermal neurofibromas: immunohistological identification and response to Schwann cell mitogens. *Ann NY Acad Sci* 1986; 486: 227–240.
85. Sonnenfeld KH, Bernd P, Sobue G, Lebwhol M, Rubenstein AE. Nerve growth factor receptors on dissociated neurofibroma Schwann-like cells. *Cancer Res* 1986; 46: 1446–1452.
86. Rush RA. Immunohistochemical localization of endogenous nerve growth factor. *Nature* 1984; 312: 364–367.
87. Heumann R, Korsching S, Bandtlow C, Thoenen H. Changes of nerve growth factor synthesis in nonneuronal cells in response to sciatic nerve transection. *J Cell Biol* 1987; 104: 1623–1631.
88. Keynes RJ. Schwann cells during neural development and regeneration: leaders or followers? *Trends Neurosci* 1987; 10: 137–139.
89. Noakes PG, Bennett MR. Growth of axons into developing muscles of the chick forelimb is preceded by cells that stain with Schwann cell antibodies. *J Comp Neurol* 1987; 259: 330–347.
90. Ochoa J, Mair WGP. The normal sural nerve in man: I. Ultrastructure and numbers of fibers and cells. *Acta Neuropathol* 1969; 13: 197–206.
91. Daniloff JK, Levi G, Grumet M, Rieger F, Edelman GM. Altered expression of neuronal cell adhesion molecules induced by nerve injury and repair. *J Cell Biol* 1986; 103: 929–945.
92. Friedlander DR, Grumet M, Edelman GM. Nerve growth factor enhances expression of neuron-glia cell adhesion molecule in PC12 cells. *J Cell Biol* 1986; 102: 413–419.
93. Yan Q, Johnson EM. A quantitative study of the developmental expression of nerve growth factor (NGF) receptor in rats. *Dev Biol* 1987; 121: 139–148.
94. Buck CR, Martinez HJ, Black IB, Chao MV. Developmentally regulated expression of the nerve growth factor receptor gene in the periphery and brain. *Proc Natl Acad Sci USA* 1987; 84: 3060–3063.
95. Riccardi VM. von Recklinghausen neurofibromatosis. *N Engl J Med* 1981; 305: 1617–1627.
96. Pleasure D, Kreider B, Sobue G, Ross AH, Koprowski H, Sonnenfeld K, Rubinstein A. Schwann-like cells cultured from human dermal neurofibromas: immunohistological identification and response to Schwann cell mitogens. *Ann NY Acad Sci* 1986; 486: 227–240.
97. Baron P, Kreider BQ. Axons induce differentiation of neurofibroma Schwann-like cells. *Acta Neuropathol* 1991; 81: 491–495.
98. Sobue G, Sonnefeld K, Rubenstein A, Pleasure D. Tissue culture studies of neurofibromatosis: effect of axolemma fragments and cyclic adenosine 3′,5′ monophosphate analogues on proliferation of Schwann like and fibroblast like neurofibroma cells. *Ann Neurol* 1985; 18: 68–73.
99. Pleasure D, Kreider B, Shuman S, Sobue G. Tissue culture studies of Schwann cell proliferation and differentiation. *Dev Neurosci* 1985; 7: 364–373.
100. Aguayo A, Kasarjian J, Skamene E, Kongshavn P, Bray G. Myelination of mouse axons by Schwann cells transplanted from normal and abnormal human nerves. *Nature* 1977; 268: 753–755.
101. Kamholz J. Molecular genetics of myelin basic protein in mouse and humans. In: Kim S, ed. *Myelination and demyelination: implications for multiple sclerosis.* New York: Plenum Press, 1989: 49–59.

8

Nerve–Muscle Trophic Interaction

Alberto Cangiano, Mario Buffelli, and Efrem Pasino

Institute of Human Physiology, Medical School, University of Verona, 37134 Verona, Italy

The development of the nervous system as well as the repair of lesions by neuroregeneration are the result of complex processes among which an important role is played by medium- and long-term influences that neurons exert on each other (and with nonneuronal target cells) at the level of synapses. These influences are distinct from the short-term synaptic interactions through which the excitability of the innervated cells and thus their action potential discharge is regulated: They are often referred to as trophic.

To give just a brief account of the most important functions mediated by trophic interactions one may list 1) the regulation of neuronal number during development (matching the size of neuronal pools to that of their target territories), 2) the regulation of the process of synaptogenesis (controlling the development of the necessary pre- and postsynaptic specializations), 3) the induction in the follower cells of properties appropriate for the tasks imposed by the innervating neurons (for example, contraction speed of muscles innervated by tonic or phasic motoneurons), 4) the reestablishment of synaptic connections after damage.

Trophic interactions can be distinguished as anterograde and retrograde. In the latter the target cells regulate the properties, the degree of axonal arborization, and even the survival of the presynaptic neurons. The anterograde interactions work instead in the opposite direction; the neurons controlling a vast array of properties of the innervated cells, which can be other neurons, muscular elements, and still other cell types. The two kinds of interactions are far from being separate: A close link exists in fact at the level of target cells between anterograde and retrograde signaling. One important difference between the two orders of trophic effects is that while the retrograde ones are only mediated by chemical factors, such as nerve growth factor (NGF), the anterograde effects can in addition depend on synaptic activation of follower cells and therefore on the impulse activity thus evoked. Indeed a central question in the studies on forward interactions is that of the relative role of electrical activity and chemical factors in their mediation.

An extensively utilized experimental model of anterograde interactions, because of its relative simplicity, is the control operated by motoneurones on skeletal muscle fibers. Probably the longer known and most obvious evidence for this control is the profound muscle atrophy that follows denervation, with a reduction of overall mass, fiber diameter, and contractile proteins actin and myosin (1,2). In addition to the contractile apparatus, many surface membrane properties of the muscle fibers change after denervation, and the same is true following the establishment of innervation during development. In the course of this review the very general features of these anterograde nerve-muscle interactions will be described, but the focus of the attention will be on the nature of the neural signals by which they are mediated. Also, the main emphasis will be on the surface membrane properties of the muscle fibers, rather than on the properties of the contractile apparatus to which only brief references will be made.

It is important at the outset to distinguish the effects of the nerve on the sarcolemma in junctional and extrajunctional ones, since some striking differences (to be described later) exist in their neural control. The extrajunctional ones are generalized to the entire membrane outside the neuromuscular synapses, whereas the junctional effects are much more restricted (only about 0.1% of the entire fiber's membrane) but are of course of great importance for the process of synaptogenesis.

The single most important integral membrane protein of muscle fibers is the acetylcholine receptor (AChR). As a general overview of the importance of the anterograde neurotrophic control on this membrane property, we shall recall that AChRs are present and diffusely distributed at moderate density in the membrane of embryonic myotubes and fibers of newborn animals (3,4) but they rapidly accumulate at sites of contact of incoming motor nerve terminals, that is the initial neuromuscular synapses (4–6) (for a review, see refs. 7,8). After a few weeks these initial clusters of *junctional* receptors have become a permanent feature of the muscle fibers (some, however, disappear; see refs. 9,10 for a review), whereas the *extrajunctional* receptors have proceeded through a dramatic decrease in density (about four orders of magnitude) to substantial disappearance (11,7,8, for reviews). After denervation, in the adult life, acetylcholine receptors once again appear in the entire extrajunctional membrane (12,13), a phenomenon which has long been known by neurobiologists under the name of *denervation supersensitivity*. This has been for many years a classical field of studies on forward slow interactions, one in which the idea of a chemical anterograde trophic factor has been actively debated. It is for this reason that we begin the review of nerve-muscle interactions with the neural control of the extrajunctional membrane properties.

EXTRAJUNCTIONAL MEMBRANE PROPERTIES

The idea that the development of AChRs in the extrajunctional membrane after denervation is due to cessation of supply of a physiological neural factor normally exerting an inhibitory action on that membrane, is based on many striking experimental observations reviewed in (10). We will mention here the so-called effect of the nerve stump, consisting in a progressively delayed appearance of the extrajunctional AChRs when the nerve is cut at increasing distances from the muscle (see 10,14 for review). Longer stumps would act as a larger reservoir of the hypothetical inhibitory trophic substance and thus maintain the extrajunctional membrane free from AChRs for a longer time. This and other evidence described in references 10 and 14 might seem to negate a role for muscle evoked impulse activity (and its cessation after denervation) in the control of the extrajunctional membrane.

A turning point in the unraveling of this story is represented by the demonstration given by Lømo and Rosenthal (15; see also ref. 16) and Lømo and Westgaard (17) that in vivo direct electrical stimulation of denervated muscles prevents the development of ACh supersensitivity or suppresses it if already present. This inhibitory control exerted on the extrajunctional membrane by electrical stimulation also applies (18,17) to other changes developing after denervation, such as the appearance of tetrodotoxin (TTX)-insensitive action potentials (described by Redfern and Thesleff, ref. 19, and owing to the insertion in the membrane of voltage-dependent Na^+ channels resistant to TTX; ref 20).

Another important property acquired by the extrajunctional membrane after denervation and repressed by activity (that is by electrical stimulation) is the ability to accept foreign innervation (see section later in chapter on long-term effects): By paralyzing the muscle fibers without suppressing the original innervation, it is actually possible to hyperinnervate the fibers with the foreign axons (21). The innervability of the extrajunctional membrane is thus inhibited by activity, like extrajunctional AChRs: however, it must be a separate membrane property since not all denervated muscles accept foreign innervation, in spite of becoming supersensitive to ACh (see also ref. 9 for a discussion).

Denervation vs. Pure Paralysis: Short Term

A puzzling situation at this point is represented by the observation made in various laboratories that muscle paralysis induced by chronic nerve conduction block is, surprisingly enough, much less effective than denervation in inducing the extrajunctional membrane AChRs, TTX-resistant Na^+ channels, and other changes (22–25). Similar results have been shown for paralysis by botulinum toxin (26,27). This has revived the idea of a neurotrophic inhibitory factor, which would still function in the paralyzed muscle and maintain it in a condition intermediate between normal and denervated; in the normal muscle both the trophic factor and nerve impulses would combine their effects in keeping the extrajunctional membrane completely free of AChRs as well as normal in any other respects.

However, another interpretation is possible, namely that there is an additional factor that might induce effects in the extrajunctional membrane similar to those caused by inactivity. This factor is represented by the breakdown products of the degenerating intramuscular portion of the nerve, which would combine, in the denervated muscle, their effects with those of muscle paralysis to yield the full-blown effect: absence of Wallerian degeneration in the purely paralyzed muscle would thus explain why it becomes much less supersensitive to ACh and its action potentials become less resistant to TTX (28–32,14,17).

Our own approach to testing the hypothesis of nerve breakdown products has been based on two different experimental situations: partial denervation (29,30) and section of a transplanted foreign nerve (31). Important features are shared by the two preparations: 1) products of degeneration are from nerves that maintain their normal central connections; 2) the effects are observed on the extrajunctional regions of muscle fibers not innervated by the degenerating axons; and 3) since muscle denervation produces both nerve breakdown and inactivity, the study of the interaction between the two events has received special attention (this has been obtained by comparing the effects of products of nerve degeneration on muscle fibers either normally active or paralyzed).

In the partial denervation paradigm only one lumbar radicular nerve was cut in the rat, thus obtaining innervated and denervated fibers intermingled with one another in hindlimb muscles. Products of nerve degeneration transiently accumulate in the interstitium between the muscle fibers and their ability to induce extrajunctional AChRs can be tested by applying acetylcholine microiontophoretically while recording its effect on the transmembrane potential from individual *innervated* fibers (electrophysiological testing of development of TTX-resistant channels can be done in the same fibers). Extrajunctional AChRs and TTX-resistant channels do appear in such fibers (29) and their density becomes striking (*as large as in the denervated fibers*) when partial denervation is combined with inactivity of the fibers left innervated, by chronically blocking nerve conduction (30,31) (Fig. 1B,C). To appreciate this result fully it must be emphasized that the experiments are done relatively early after partial denervation, that is, when in control muscles inactivity alone has not yet caused ACh supersensitivity (or TTX resistance) to appear (Fig. 1A, solid columns), whereas total denervation has already attained nearly maximal effects (Fig. 1A, open columns).

Effects essentially similar to those observed after partial denervation are seen using a preparation in which nerve breakdown products are obtained through the process of degeneration of a foreign nerve (31). The superficial fibular nerve is transplanted early in life on the rat soleus muscle and allowed to grow over its surface for several weeks. No synapses are made, however, as the original soleus nerve is left intact. In the

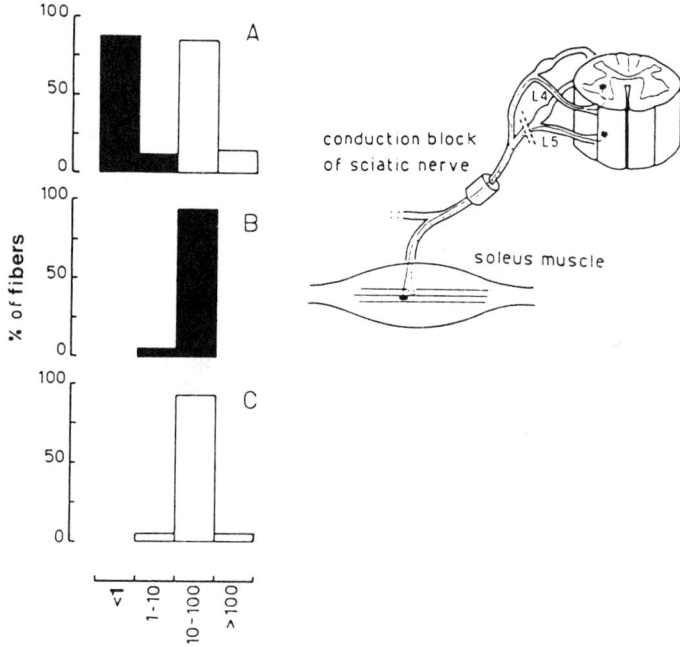

FIG. 1. Effect of partial denervation, by section of the radicular nerve L_5, on the extrajunctional ACh sensitivity of the innervated-paralyzed fibers of the rat soleus muscle, at about 3 days. **A** shows control muscles, purely paralyzed *(solid columns)* and totally denervated *(open columns)*. **B** and **C** illustrate the partially denervated muscles with innervated-inactive fibers *(solid columns in B)* and denervated fibers *(open columns in C)*. Each population is composed of 25–40 fibers from four to five muscles. Sensitivity to ACh is measured through the depolarization produced by its microiontophoretic application to the extrajunctional region (about 2 mm from the end-plates). Conduction block was obtained through tetrodotoxin-impregnated silastic cuffs. Note that in the partially denervated muscles the extrajunctional ACh sensitivity of the innervated paralyzed fibers (*B*) is equal in magnitude to that of denervated fibers, whereas in purely paralyzed muscles it is just appearing (*A, solid columns*). Accordingly, the time of onset of the extrajunctional sensitivity is identical in the two classes of fibers (not shown). This eliminates the possibility that the changes in the innervated fibers are mediated through the spinal cord or that they are a mere consequence, by contact, of those in the denervated fibers, because in both cases the ACh supersensitivity should be delayed in the innervated fibers. Results entirely similar to those shown for ACh sensitivity have been obtained for action potential resistance to tetrodotoxin in both soleus and extensor digitorum longus muscles (30,31). (From Cangiano, ref. 14, with permission.)

adult animal, when any effect of trauma has long disappeared, the transplanted nerve is sectioned, and about 3 days later the extrajunctional membrane, including the region of the foreign nerve outgrowth, is examined for the development of supersensitivity to ACh and TTX-resistant action potentials (the last parameter is that illustrated in Fig. 2). A crucial variable is represented by the presence or absence of activity in the soleus muscle fibers. When the muscle is normally active, denervation-like changes fail to develop under the degenerating nerve (Fig. 2, solid triangles). However, when section of the foreign nerve is combined with inactivity of the soleus muscle, a high level of TTX resistance (and of sensitivity to ACh, not shown) appears under the degenerating nerve and surrounding regions (Fig. 2, solid circles). The amount of the change is comparable to that produced after the same time (3 days) by plain denervation, obtained by section of the original soleus nerve (Fig. 2, open triangles); inactivity alone, on the other hand, has not yet produced any effects in most of the extrajunctional membrane (Fig. 2, open circles).

The above experiments indicate that

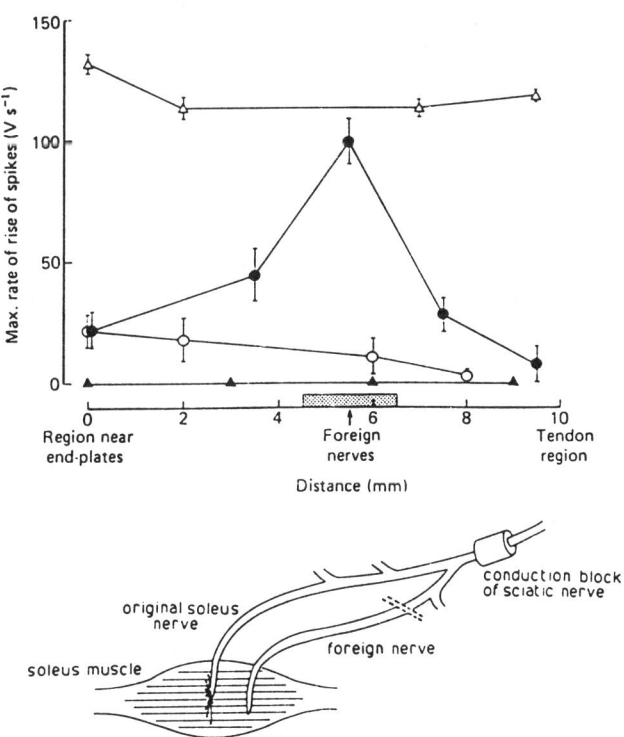

FIG. 2. Effect of sectioning a foreign nerve (superficial fibular), transplanted 2 months earlier, on resistance to TTX of directly elicited action potentials in rat soleus muscle fibers, at about 3 days. Effect of sectioning the foreign nerve on a paralyzed muscle *(solid circles)* and on a normally active one *(solid triangles)*. Control muscles: one denervated by section of its own nerve *(open triangles)*, the other purely paralyzed *(open circles)*; the latter also has an intact transplanted foreign nerve, for control purposes. Chronic paralysis obtained by conduction block of sciatic nerve with a tetrodotoxin-impregnated silicone cuff. Comparable results were obtained when the extrajunctional membrane change tested was sensitivity to ACh. This was true for the muscles illustrated above as well as for four other paralyzed soleus muscles with a degenerating foreign nerve. (Reproduced in modified form from Cangiano et al., ref. 31, with permission.)

nerve breakdown products are indeed very effective in inducing the appearance of AChRs and TTX-resistant channels provided inactivity of muscle fibers is also present. We are dealing here with a potentiation and not a mere summation of effects because at early times, such as those selected for the present experiments, either factor alone has weak effects, but their interaction induces changes as dramatic as those following denervation. In other words, at such early stages (a few days) a large gap exists between the negligible effects of pure inactivity and the already maximal effects of denervation. This gap is completely bridged by the effect of nerve destruction on inactive membranes, as seen locally with the foreign nerve paradigm and over the entire endplates-tendon region with the partial denervation paradigm (for details, see ref. 31). Thus the greater efficacy of denervation vs. pure inactivity can well be explained, at least at early times, by nerve breakdown products acting diffusely throughout the muscle on membranes highly reactive because of the concomitant muscle inactivity.

Denervation vs. Pure Paralysis: Long Term

While the interpretation based on nerve breakdown products can satisfactorily explain the greater efficacy of denervation with respect to paralysis alone over the initial time period, it could not easily do so on a long-lasting or permanent basis. This is because nerve breakdown products are only transiently present in the muscle interstitium. Therefore their effects should also be transient, with a progressive decline in the level of the extrajunctional membrane changes in the denervated muscles until they finally meet the slowly growing levels of the purely paralyzed muscles. This should be true unless 1) the levels in the denervated muscles remain high because once triggered they would survive their causal factor, and 2) a trophic factor continuously released from axons in the paralyzed muscles, exerting a normalizing action on their extrajunctional membrane, would keep the levels of AChRs and TTX-resistant channels permanently lower than in their denervated counterparts. Several studies do in fact support the possibility that the difference in efficacy between denervation and paralysis is maintained in time (33–35; see, however, 27,36).

We have recently reexamined the problem of the long-lasting effects of nerve conduction blocks with the working hypothesis that the reason for their lower efficacy with respect to denervation might reside in the difficulty to achieve a really complete blockade in large nerves such as the rat sciatic, for the duration of weeks (37). Rather than trying to record chronically from the paralyzed muscles, to evaluate any possible degree of residual spike activity (that is, other than fibrillation), we attempted instead to improve the block as much as possible. This was done in two ways: 1) performing a dose/response study, that is, exploring systematically the effects of increasing doses of TTX (the blocking agent commonly used), and 2) developing a cuff (a silicone structure for nerve application of the blocking agent) that can deliver the TTX solution all around the nerve instead of just on one point of its surface, for optimal distribution (Colorplate 1). Figure 3 illustrates the details of the cuff.

The comparison between denervation and paralysis alone was made on the rat extensor digitorum longus (EDL) and soleus muscles of the two sides (one side denervated, the other paralyzed) over times ranging from 2 to 5 weeks. In one group of rats, the paralyzed muscles were initially denervated by a close nerve crush but were quickly reinnervated by the electrically silent axons. This particular paradigm, already used by others (34), is probably superior to that of pure paralysis alone: In fact, the muscles of the two sides undergo initially the same denervation-like changes and one can later study whether and to what extent the reinnervating, electrically silent axons can shift toward normal the extrajunctional properties of the paralyzed muscle, as compared to the contralateral denervated control.

The properties studied are as usual AChRs and TTX-resistant channels, scanning the extrajunctional membrane over a distance of several millimeters from the end-plate to tendon region. The results obtained for EDL and soleus muscles can be summarized as follows:

1. In both muscle types at lower doses of TTX the reinnervated-paralyzed muscles exhibit an obvious picture of partial normalization, since they present denervation-like changes less pronounced than in the denervated partners (see example in Fig. 3A, for EDL): these baseline doses produce, on average, good behavioral hindlimb paralysis and have been utilized for this purpose in various studies (see, for example, 38,39).

2. In both EDL and soleus muscles increasing the TTX doses produces a clearcut increase in the level of extrajunctional membrane changes in the reinnervated-paralyzed muscles: for the EDL muscles the level of the denervated muscles is actually reached with the highest doses (Fig. 3B, C); for the soleus, the paralyzed muscles do not quite reach the denervated ones, even with the highest doses (not shown).

3. However, even with the soleus muscles equality of effects is obtained if one isolates the posterior tibial fascicle (containing the soleus axons) from the rest of the sciatic nerve and then blocks conduction only along this branch (Fig. 4), using a cuff with an appropriately smaller inner diameter.

All these results indicate that the long-term effects of muscle paralysis on the extrajunctional membrane properties become equal to those of denervation (in contrast with much previous evidence), provided that nerve conduction block is really complete (37,40). One might conceivably object, however, that impulse conduction block makes, in some way, the electrically

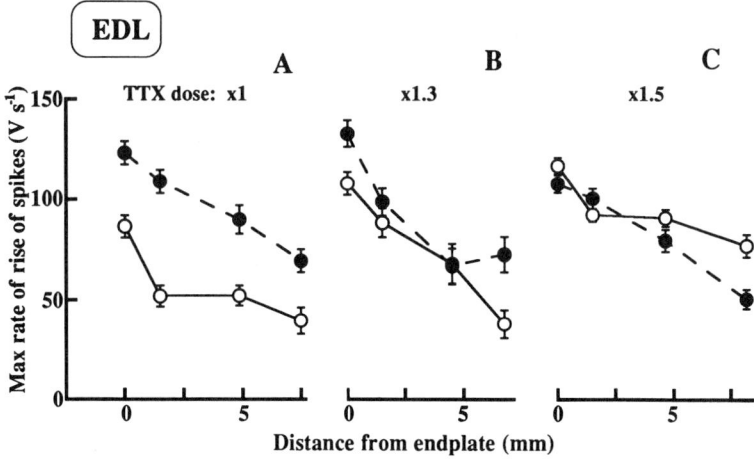

FIG. 3. Long-term effect (2–5 weeks, average 3) of reinnervating rat EDL muscles *(open circles)* with axons blocked with increasing doses of TTX. Comparison is made with contralateral, permanently denervated muscles *(solid circles)*. The TTX dose × 1 equals 6.6 μ/day. The membrane property measured is the resistance to TTX (10^{-6} M) of action potentials directly elicited in individual muscle fibers. Amount of resistance is measured as the maximal rate of rise of the action potential. Each data point is the mean ± S.E. of 6–12 fibers per muscle, in several muscles. **A, B,** and **C:** 7, 3, 7 muscle pairs, respectively.

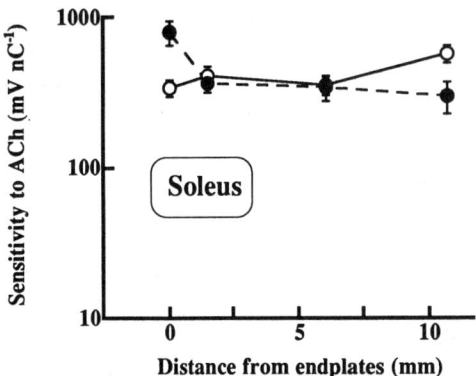

FIG. 4. Long-term effect (3–4 weeks) of reinnervating rat soleus muscles *(open circles)* with axons blocked with high doses of TTX (× 1.5: see Fig. 4). *Solid circles:* Contralateral permanently denervated muscles. The membrane property measured is sensitivity to microiontophoretically applied ACh in individual fibers. One unit of sensitivity equals 1 mV of depolarization obtained with 1 nC of charge passed through the microiontophoretic pipette. Each data point is the mean ± S.E. of 5–7 fibers per muscle, in three muscles. The silicone cuff is applied around the posterior tibial division of the sciatic nerve.

silent axons unable to deliver trophic chemical factors to the muscle: one possibility, not unreasonable, is, for example, that the silent axons no longer release the trophic factors. This idea does not quite fit with the behavior of the blocked nerves, which in our experiments are able to regenerate at normal speeds and, in addition, to *fully* reinnervate the EDL and soleus muscles with no delay (not shown). However, we wanted to look into this matter more closely and decided to utilize as an index of the *trophic competence* (in the sense of chemical factors) of the blocked nerve, its ability to induce in muscle clusters of acetylcholine receptors. This is a function that motor axons, through their terminals, exhibit typically during early synaptogenesis and probably also throughout adult life as a maintainance action. This *junctional* action is in fact the only generally undisputed *chemical* trophic action of motor nerves,

together with their ability to determine the site of deposit of the enzyme acetylcholinesterase (see section later in chapter on junctional properties). The specific point to test in connection with our experiments on chronically blocked nerves, is to see whether the same nerves are able to induce AChR clusters during novel synapse formation in muscles of adult rats, when sciatic nerve blockade is induced with our high TTX doses and our special cuff. For this purpose we examined ectopic synapse formation between the transplanted fibular nerve and the extrajunctional membrane of the soleus muscle, activated by cutting the original soleus nerve, a preparation well established in the literature (41–47) (see Fig. 9 and its legend, for more details). These procedures are performed bilaterally, but on one side, in addition, the sciatic nerve is chronically blocked with the maximal doses of TTX (× 1.5 the baseline dose) (Color Figure 2). Thus on the blocked side the innervating foreign fibular axons are electrically silent and the soleus muscle remains permanently paralyzed, unlike the control side where the fibular axons are normally active and reestablish muscle activity upon innervation. The results are evaluated with acute experiments performed 1 to 5 weeks after the initial bilateral section of the original soleus innervation. Small but clearcut contractions can be evoked *bilaterally* following foreign nerve stimulation, indicating that some muscle fibers have been reinnervated. Since synaptic transmission from the electrically blocked axons might occur before AChR clustering (48), we have applied the AChRs ligand α-bungarotoxin (conjugated to the red fluorescent probe rhodamine) to both soleus muscles to reveal the formation of new receptor clusters. Such clusters were easily found on both sides, if anything, more abundantly on the impulse-blocked one (Colorplate 2, upper left) (49). That these fluorescent dye accumulations are really sites of synaptic contact was indicated by the finding that they are in precise register with motor nerve terminals visualized with the new green fluorescent probe FM 1-43 (Molecular Probes) after uptake by endocytosis during a short period of transmitter release enhancement (Color Figure 2, upper right) (50).

Other interesting results that we have obtained with the comparison of denervated and long-term paralyzed muscles relate to overall mass and contractile properties: Consistently with the extrajunctional membrane properties, muscle weight and strength of contraction have shown a remarkably parallel behavior. In fact, equal decrease in the values of both parameters has occurred in fast EDL and slow soleus, when comparing the denervated with the purely paralyzed companions (51). This is at variance with a previous report (52). Detailed publications of all the results described so far with long-lasting conduction blocks will soon appear.

Summing up the experimental evidence presented so far on the neural factors controlling the extrajunctional membrane (as well as muscle weight and strength), the effects of denervation and paralysis coincide in the long term, thus indicating that muscle-evoked impulse activity is the main physiological factor controlling generalized properties of muscle. In the short term (approximately the first 10–15 days in rats), a transient difference appears between the effects of denervation and those of pure conduction block on the extrajunctional membrane, which can be explained as a combination, in the denervated muscle, of the actions of paralysis and of nerve breakdown products. Thus the long-suggested participation of neural substances in keeping the extrajunctional membrane in the normal state does not appear to be supported by experiments of muscle inactivation through block of nerve conduction.

What then about other evidence that instead supports a role for neural chemical factors in the physiological regulation of the nonsynaptic membrane?

Nerve Stump Effects; Nicotinic Influences

We have described earlier the clearcut action of the length of the distal nerve stump in delaying the extrajunctional denervation-induced changes.

Again, nerve breakdown products can offer an alternative interpretation to that based on neural physiological substances, as pointed out by Jones and Vrbová (28). In fact, nerve terminal degeneration is also delayed by a longer nerve stump (53) and the values of time increment are the same as those observed for the extrajunctional membrane changes (54). In the same study, the stump phenomenon is also shown to exist, with identical temporal characteristics, for foreign nerves that have never established synaptic connections (54). Finally, the possibility that the neural factor underlying the stump effect is the neurotransmitter acetylcholine is contradicted by the demonstration that neuromuscular preparations blocked with α-bungarotoxin in organ culture still exhibit the stump length effect on extrajunctional properties (55).

The participation of a nicotinic influence in the physiological control of the extrajunctional membrane has been implicated, on the other hand, by a number of studies that, by using muscle inactivation with α-bungarotoxin, alone (56) or in combination with botulinum toxin (26), have shown *even in the short term* development of levels of ACh supersensitivity and TTX resistance as large as after denervation. These results imply an additional mechanism, with respect to nerve breakdown products, explaining the greater efficacy of denervation versus inactivity alone observed at early times. Namely, this would be the removal of acetylcholine from the denervated muscle. Thus acetylcholine could act as a genuine trophic transmitter, that is, through a mechanism that is separate from that related to transmission of action potentials and production of muscle activity. (For a detailed discussion of this and other mechanisms related also to trophic substances, see refs. 14,10,9.) More recently, experiments using these poisons that interfere with ACh transmission have been done with the aim of measuring their effects on mRNAs involved in the expression of AChRs (57) and TTX-insensitive Na^+ channels (58). These interesting developments also introduce, however, a higher degree of complexity. As an example, while in most studies extrajunctional ACh sensitivity and TTX resistance are at 5–7 days definitely lower after botulinum toxin than after denervation (24,26,27), mRNA SkM2 (encoding the TTX-resistant channel) is much higher (about fourfold) and γAChR mRNA (encoding the homonimous subunit characteristic of extra-junctional receptors) is equal or moderately higher in botulinum-treated than in denervated muscles.

In any event, since *in the long term* reinnervating but electrically silent axons cannot repress to any extent the extrajunctional AChRs and TTX-insensitive channels of previously denervated muscles (37,40), while the same axons have 1) a maintained axonal transport (to be published), 2) spontaneous quantal (59) and nonquantal acetylcholine release (to be published), 3) a normal ability to fully reinnervate muscles, and 4) an intact trophic competence of establishing new ectopic synapses (46) and of inducing completely new clusters of AChRs (49), it appears unlikely that the transmitter acetylcholine or other neural influences different from nerve impulses have any major role in the physiology of regulation of the extrasynaptic AChRs and related properties.

JUNCTIONAL MEMBRANE PROPERTIES

The experiments already described and illustrated in Color Figure 2 are a good starting point for reviewing the evidence indicating that chemical factors of neural origin have a major, albeit not exclusive, role in the regulation of junctional properties. In fact, the normal ability of motor axon terminals to induce the accumulation of AChRs at their site of contact with the muscle fibers is maintained if the axons are electrically silent because of impulse conduction block along their course to the muscle. These experiments indicate that neither pre- nor postsynaptic evoked spike activity is required for cluster formation. That also acetylcholine transmission, end-plate potential, or ionic currents are not required is shown by the demonstration in culture that clusters form during AChRs blockade with α-bungarotoxin (5). The ability to cluster AChRs in muscle is specific to motor nerve endings since this is not exhibited in vitro by sympathetic or primary sensory neurons (60). Since impulse transmission begins soon after contact is established, and in the embryo even before clustering of receptors (48), and since activity has an inhibitory influence on extrajunctional AChRs (see previous section), it follows that clustered AChRs very quickly become resistant to the effects of activity (43,42).

The above evidence indicates that in all likelihood a chemical substance, specific to motor nerve endings, has the ability to accumulate AChRs in precise register with the site of contact, overcoming the inhibitory effect that the activity thus evoked in the muscle fiber would otherwise exert on the same receptors. The effect leaves a persistent trace even after denervation, since high density accumulations of AChRs can be observed for a long time at the vacated endplate *in spite of continuous and actually accelerated turnover* of the receptors (reviewed in ref. 7) (a slow rundown anyway clearly occurs; see ref. 61). This relative persistence is also true if the denervated muscle is subjected to chronic direct electrical stimulation (42). We shall see ahead that the persistent trace probably resides in the extracellular matrix facing the subsynaptic membrane (synaptic basal lamina).

There are now various good candidates for a neurotrophic substance(s) having the

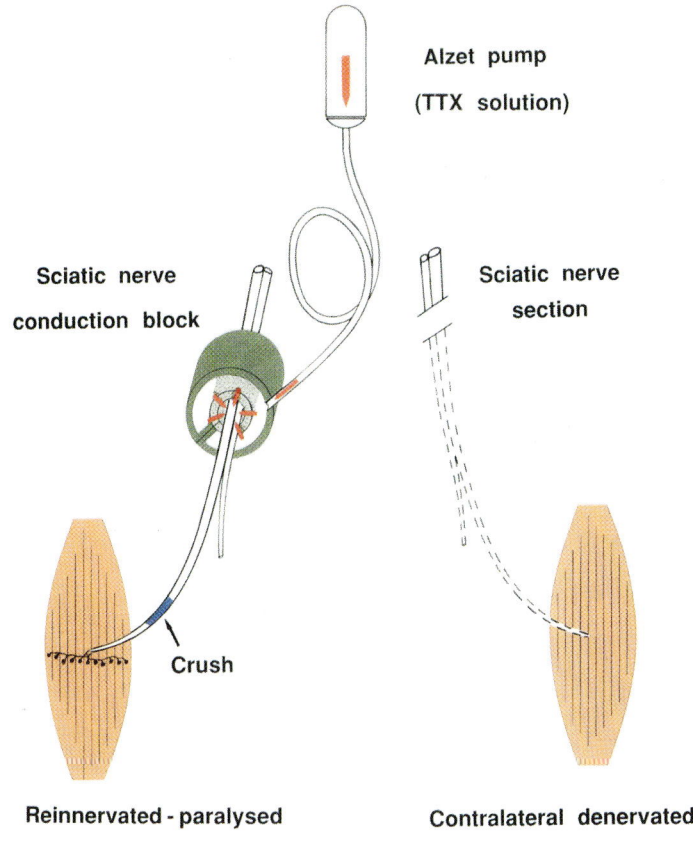

Colorplate 1. Chronic conduction block of sciatic nerve. A TTX solution in saline of appropriate concentration is delivered to a silicone cuff placed around the nerve from an Alzet pump 2 ML4 (flow rate 2.5 µl/hr). The cuff is double walled, the inner wall being permeable to the solution. Although only one muscle is shown on each side, both EDL and soleus are experimented on.

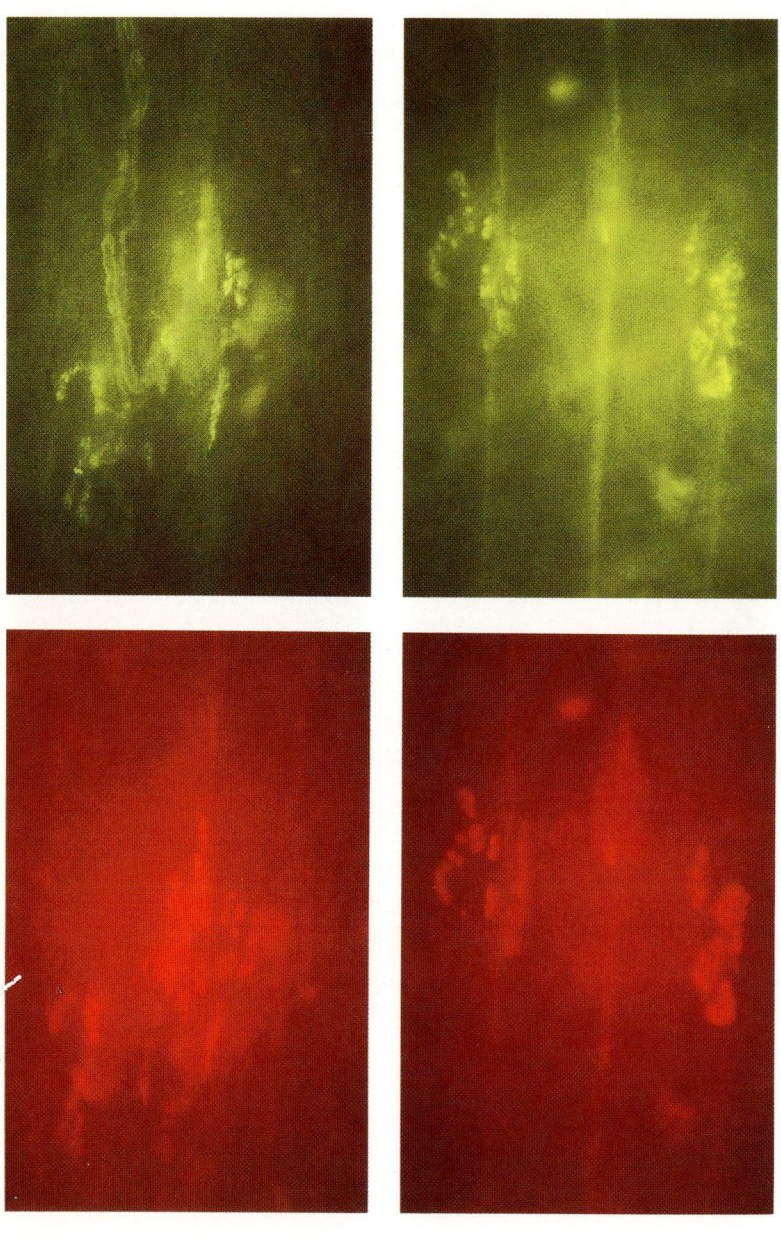

Colorplate 2. Ectopic neuromuscular junctions formed by the foreign fibular nerve and the soleus muscle in rats. Synapse formation is activated by section of the original soleus innervation. After about 5 weeks, pre- and postsynaptic components of the same synapses are visualized with fluorescent probes, in a soleus muscle innervated by impulse blocked fibular axons (*upper row*) and in the contralateral control soleus where the foreign axons and thus the myofibers are normally active (*lower row*). *Right*: pictures with green fluorescence show motor axon terminals visualized with FM 1–43, a fluorescent probe (Molecular Probes) taken up by endocytosis during 10 min of depolarization by bath application of high potassium; also axons are visible in the upper picture because in the same plane of focus of the terminals (see ref. 50 for more information). *Left*: pictures with red fluorescence show AChR clusters visualized with rhodamine-α-bungarotoxin. Bar = 50 μm.

function of establishing and maintaining the AChRs aggregate at the neuromuscular junction. We shall limit our review to three candidates that in recent years have received most of the attention: *agrin* and related basal lamina factors, so-called *ARIA* (acetylcholine receptor-inducing activity), and *CGRP* (calcitonin gene-related peptide). Before proceeding, however, we must introduce two other important points. First, AChRs accumulate under the motor terminal with two mechanisms: One is aggregation by lateral migration of receptors already present in the membrane, and the other is de novo synthesis and insertion in the membrane (the relative importance varies with species and interpretations) (5,62,63). Second, two are the synaptic specializations on which the function of the neuromuscular junction is critically dependent: AChRs and acetylcholinesterase (AChE), both of which will thus be considered.

Basal Lamina

The role in synaptogenesis of that part of the extracellular matrix (an acellular network of glycoproteins ensheathing like a scaffolding the muscle fibers and other cells) (for a review, see ref. 64) that is closest to the muscle fiber's membrane, the *basal lamina,* was first discovered by McMahan and coworkers with experiments on regeneration of muscle fibers in the adult animal. Only the basal lamina runs through pre- and postsynaptic components of the neuromuscular junction, the *synaptic* basal lamina. The basic structure of the experiments is actually to destroy both muscle and nerve, and then let one regenerate but not the other or vice versa. All that remains is a "ghost" of the muscle, the extracellular scaffolding including the synaptic basal laminae [the Schwann cells remain (65) or not (66) depending on how the muscle is damaged]. If one prevents reinnervation, only the muscle fibers regenerate, which they readily do inside the basal lamina sheaths. What is striking is that they form again AChR aggregates in precise register with the very discrete areas of the old synaptic basal laminae, in spite of the absence of motor nerve terminals. This is true whether Schwann cells are present (65) or absent (66) (Fig. 5). That the AChR cluster is in register with previous synaptic basal lamina is demonstrated by the fact that these lamina sites clearly stain for AChE: in fact the major synaptic location of AChE is just the basal lamina (67) where it also remains (at least in part) for long times after damage. The indication of these experiments is that some basal lamina molecule(s) directs the clustering of AChRs during muscle regeneration. A variation of the above experimental plan allows one to show that synaptic basal lamina also directs the accumulation of AChE on regenerating muscle fibers: this requires that the original AChE is eliminated so that any AChE observed after regeneration must have been formed de novo (68). This is done by transferring in vitro a frog muscle at the time of the planned lesion, incubating it with the irreversible AChE inhibitor DFP, and then replacing the muscle in the frog until myofiber regeneration has occurred (while reinnervation is prevented, as usual). A few weeks later AChE can be stained at high concentration on the basal lamina sheaths in register with the regenerated AChR clusters, that is, at the original synaptic sites.

The basal lamina also directs the formation of *presynaptic* specializations, during synapse regeneration. In a reverse experiment of those described above, after damage, only the nerve was let to regenerate, but not the muscle. After a few weeks the regenerating axons reinnervated the original synaptic sites on the vacated basal lamina sheaths. In spite of the absence of the myofibers, normal terminals formed not only containing synaptic vesicles but exhibiting active zones in precise register with the places where the synaptic cleft and junctional fold basal laminae meet (69).

In order to identify the active molecule(s)

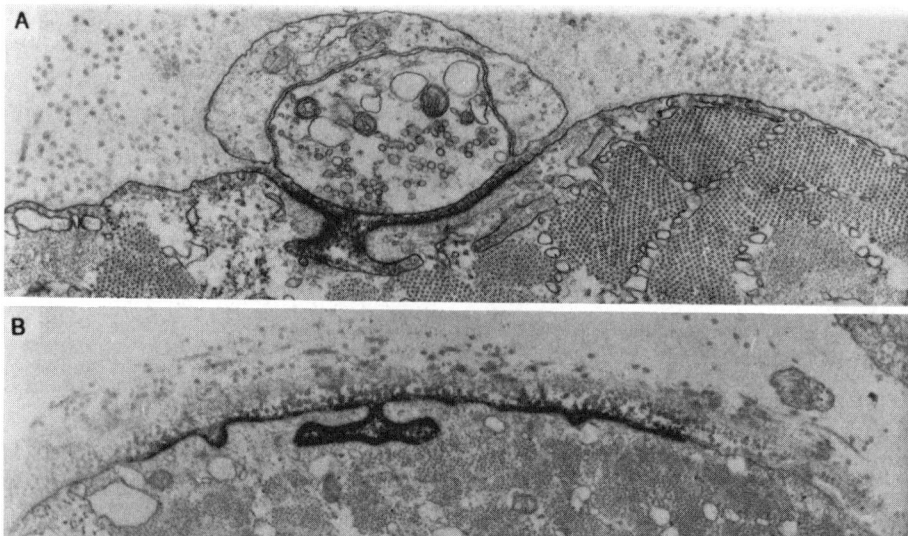

FIG. 5. AChRs in frog muscle that has regenerated after freeze damage, while nerve regeneration has been prevented. Electron microscope view of cross section through the junctional region of normal myofiber **(A)** and 30 days regenerated myofiber **(B)**. AChRs are concentrated on the surface of the myofiber and along the edges of a junctional fold, corresponding in B to old synaptic basal lamina (see text). AChRs labeled with HRP-α-bungarotoxin. (From McMahan and Slater, ref. 66, with permission.)

of the basal lamina, McMahan and coworkers prepared basal lamina extracts of the synapse-rich Torpedo electric organ, a collection of modified cholinergic neuromuscular synapses, and isolated two polypeptide fractions (150 and 95 kD) that aggregate AChRs in chick myotubes in culture. It is important to note that the extracts induce the clusters by aggregating AChRs preexisting in the membrane, without increasing their overall number: Consistently, their efficacy is not affected by inhibition of protein synthesis (reviewed in 70). Each of the two fractions also induces AChE accumulations at the same sites. This and other experiments reviewed (70) demonstrated that the two protein fractions that aggregate AChRs and AChE (and possess other activities as well), represent the basal lamina aggregating factor, which was given the name of *agrin*. Furthermore anti-agrin monoclonal antibodies (mABs) were prepared that stain fish, frog and chicken neuromuscular junctions (not rat, however) (71). The stain fills the synaptic cleft (Fig. 6A). That the molecules recognized by the mABs are indeed part of the basal lamina was demonstrated in experiments on damaged muscles where all cells were absent but the extracellular matrix present (71). The mABs stained the synaptic basal lamina (Fig. 6B). The persistence of agrin in the synaptic basal lamina after denervation is not absolute since the stain undergoes a progressive diminution over time (72). Finally, lack of staining in the rat is likely to reflect variations in agrin structure (73).

An important development with the anti-agrin mABs is that they stain also motoneurons cell bodies (and not other neurons): this can be shown early in the embryo, at the time when motoneurons begin to innervate the muscles (Fig. 7) (74). This permits the establishment of a link between the role of agrin during regeneration with a suggested role during development. It thus seems likely that during initial neuromuscular synapse formation in the embryonic

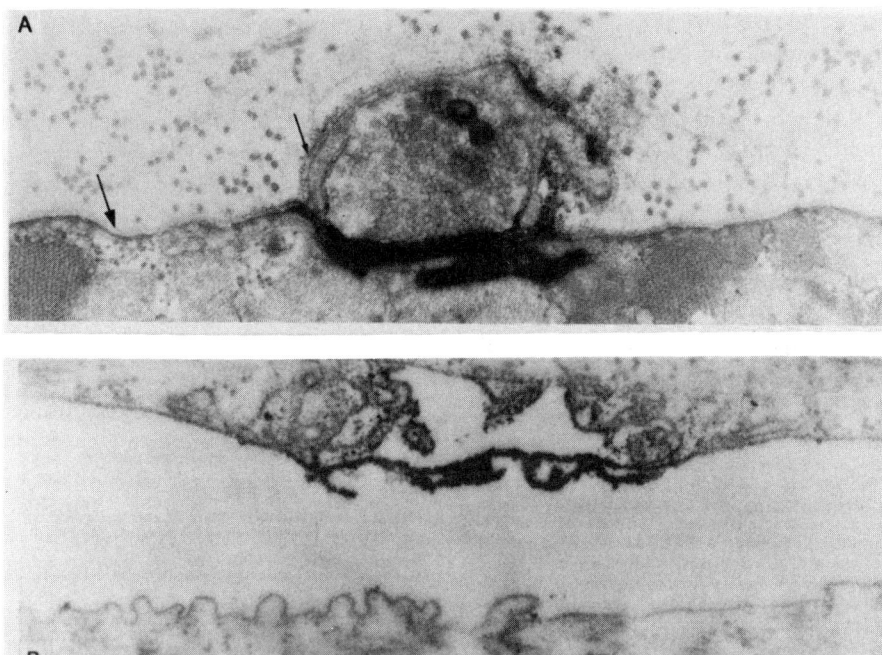

FIG. 6. Anti-agrin mABs recognize molecules concentrated in and stably bound to the synaptic basal lamina at frog neuromuscular junctions. **A:** Normal junction. **B:** Site of a neuromuscular junction 3 weeks after crush-damage of the muscle. Myofiber, axon terminal, and Schwann cell degenerated and were phagocytized in response to the trauma but the basal laminae of the myofiber and of the Schwann cell persisted. Antibody binding in the damaged muscle is localized to the synaptic portion of the myofiber basal lamina, presenting a staining pattern identical with that at the normal neuromuscular junction. Bar = 1 μm. (From Reist et al., ref. 71, with permission.)

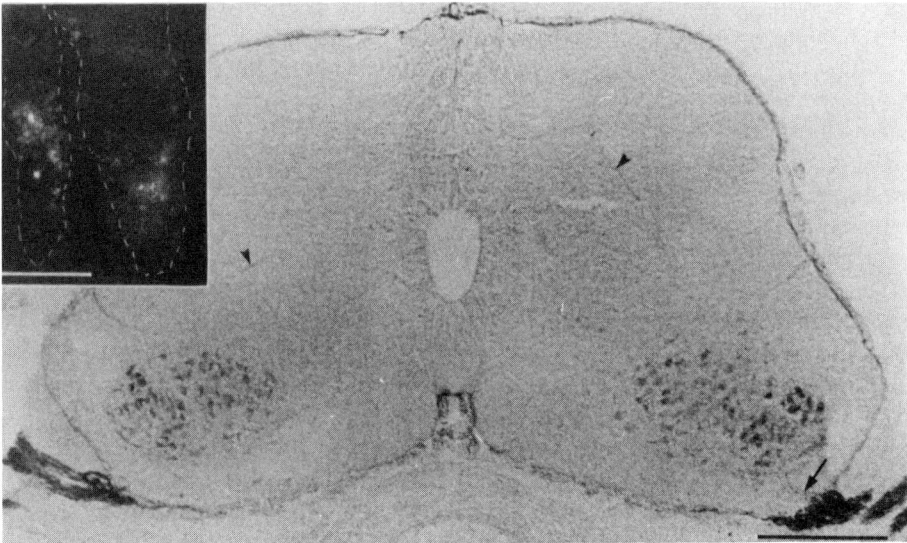

FIG. 7. Cross-section of the lumbosacral region of a spinal cord from a day 10 chick embryo incubated with an anti-agrin mAB. Motor neurons and the pial surface of the spinal cord are intensely stained. Capillaries *(arrowheads)* are lightly stained. The intensely stained structures outside the spinal cord are ventral roots; much of the stain is probably in the Schwann cells basal lamina, which is known to stain intensely in the adult. Bar = 200 μm. (From Magill-Solc and McMahan, ref. 74, with permission.)

life, agrin is released at motor nerve terminals and, by acting on agrin receptors, induces AChR clustering in the myofibers and formation of essential constituents of the synaptic basal lamina to which AChE (with a participation of muscle activity, see ahead) and other molecules can bind. Agrin itself then becomes stably anchored to this developing synaptic basal lamina, replenished with continued release from motor nerve endings, thus maintaining the postsynaptic specializations or directing their regeneration (70).

Acetylcholine Receptor-Inducing Activity (ARIA)

A 42,000-D glycoprotein has been purified by Usdin and Fischbach from chick brain that induces the accumulation in chick myotube membrane of AChRs and that produces a larger number and size of their clusters, working at extremely low concentrations (picomolar), by increasing severalfold the rate of membrane insertion of the receptors (75). The increase was accompanied by an increased synthesis of the receptors and an increase in the level of mRNA encoding for their α-subunit, without a change in γ- and δ-subunit (76). The action appears to be very selective in that ARIA does not affect total protein synthesis. ARIA only acts on ACh receptors since it does not induce any increase in AChE. From this and other results, the main mechanism of action is therefore envisaged as ARIA being released from motor nerve endings during neuromuscular synapse formation, stimulating transcription in the subsynaptic nuclei of the α-subunit gene, this subunit being perhaps present in limiting amounts in the chick myotubes. Thus ARIA is like agrin—a putative mediator of the anterograde trophic influence of the nerve on *junctional* properties—but it is quite distinct from agrin in every respect, except the common final result of receptor membrane accumulation. It is difficult at this time to see the relationship between Agrin and ARIA, apart from noting that they may not be alternative since one aggregates by lateral migration ACh receptors preexisting in the membrane, whereas the other increases receptor synthesis and membrane insertion. Certainly they are present in the same species, chicken, for example.

Calcitonin Gene-Related Peptide (CGRP)

CGRP is a 37 amino acid peptide that is present in various neurons, including motoneurons and their terminals (see later for qualifications) and that has been shown to increase the number of AChRs in chick myotubes (77,78). There are some similarities in mechanism with ARIA: For example CGRP increases receptor synthesis by increasing levels of α-subunit AChR mRNA, both the processed and the unspliced form, and it is thought to increase α-subunit gene transcription (79–81). There is no evidence so far that CGRP, in addition to increasing AChRs membrane incorporation, also induces receptor clustering. Another difference with ARIA is that the CGRP mechanism is probably cAMP dependent (82) whereas ARIA does not increase cAMP levels. Finally, the effect of CGRP is not as pronounced as that of ARIA, both on the message and on the receptor.

We have recently reexamined the action of CGRP to see if its accumulating action of AChRs in the muscle fiber's membrane, is not only present in cultured myotubes, but can also be demonstrated in vivo in an adult rat muscle. We have therefore applied CGRP through a very thin polyethylene tubing on the surface of the soleus muscle and observed a striking development of extrajunctional AChRs while the solvent alone is without effect (Fig. 8) (83).

CGRP has been shown to be localized in the dense-core vesicles of the motor nerve terminals (84). However the peptide is not always equally expressed: In fact, it is present in the motor nerve endings of the new-

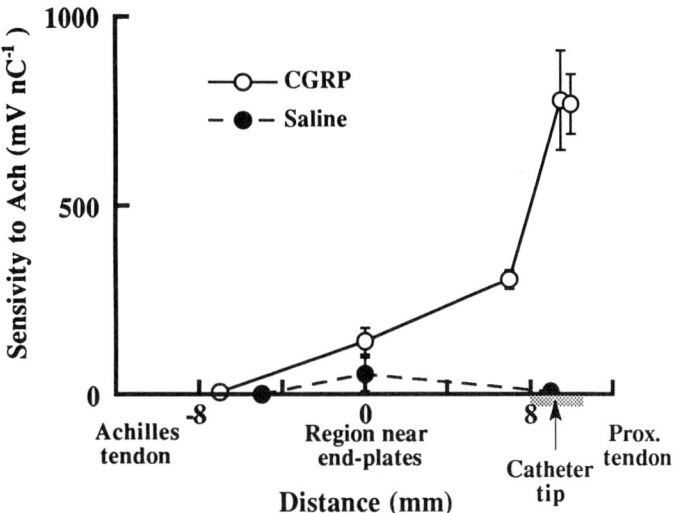

FIG. 8. Accumulation of AChRs in soleus muscle fibers of an adult rat *(open circles)* at the site of continuous in vivo application of CGRP. Iontophoretic electrophysiological mapping of individual fibers. The saline solution containing the peptide was delivered to the soleus surface through a 200 μm diameter polyethylene tubing from a Alzet osmotic pump placed under the skin of the back (flow rate 0.5 μl/hr). The CGRP dose was 4.6 μg/day. Good AChRs accumulations were obtained already at 0.2 μg/day. The soleus muscle was chronically paralyzed with a TTX-impregnated cuff (described in 31) placed around the sciatic nerve. *Solid circles:* Three control muscles, also chronically paralyzed, in which only saline was applied. Durations of in vivo treatments were 62–66 hr, for experimental and control muscles. In each muscle, 6–8 fibers were assayed for ACh sensitivity at each position. Bars represent standard errors.

born rat but slowly decreases thereafter to completely disappear in the adult from the endings (85), to be reexpressed transiently during reinnervation.

Summing up, it is possible that CGRP plays a role in synaptogenesis as a trophic transmitter, but the precise function and the relation with AChRs clustering remains to be elucidated.

Acetylcholinesterase

AChE is, like the acetylcholine receptor, an essential postsynaptic specialization, whose main function is to quickly terminate the action of acetylcholine (by hydrolyzing it), thus permitting the transmission of action potentials at high frequency. Another important function is to protect the myofibers from calcium accumulation and dependent protease activation, that would otherwise result owing to excessive calcium entry through active AChRs channels (reviewed in refs. 86,87). There are many molecular forms of AChE (reviewed in refs. 87,88) and we have already described the association of the asymmetric form (with collagen tail) with the synaptic basal lamina, this being the functional form of the enzyme in synaptic transmission.

From the point of view of the neural regulation of synaptic AChE, there is good evidence that both an anterograde neural chemical signal and muscle-evoked activity play a role. In the section on basal lamina we have already seen that synaptic agrin can induce AChE accumulation colocalized with AChRs clusters. In addition, as we have seen in the myofiber regeneration experiments, basal lamina agrin is sufficient in inducing regeneration of at least some

AChE (at least in frogs), in the absence of impulse activity. Moreover, nerve extracts have a maintenance effect on AChE of rat diaphragm in organ culture (89). On the other hand, experiments of cholinergic blockade (90), muscle direct stimulation (45), and nerve conduction block (46) shed light on the role of activity and on the interplay between the anterograde chemical factor and activity.

In chick spinal cord explant-myotube cultures curare blocks the appearance of AChE at neuromuscular junctions, which otherwise form normally (90). The importance of activity, and its relationship with an *imprinting* action of the motor nerve endings, is clearly demonstrated in experiments of Lømo and Slater on synapse formation between a foreign nerve and the adult rat soleus muscle in vivo, a preparation already described in an earlier section. A few weeks after transplantation of the foreign fibular nerve on an extrajunctional region of the soleus muscle, the soleus is denervated by cutting its original innervation. This activates formation of synapses by the foreign nerve, a number of them forming rather synchronously around the third day in the extrajunctional region occupied by the nerve. At this time synaptic potentials become detectable and AChR clusters demonstrable. Histochemical appearance of AChE instead is delayed, occurring only after a further 3–4 days (Fig. 9A). If at the time of initial synapse formation (approximately 3 days), the foreign nerve is also cut, its motor nerve endings are made to degenerate shortly after they have made contact with the myofibers. A search during the following days for hystochemically demonstrable AChE accumulations, not surprisingly gives negative results in the foreign nerve region but shows plenty of mature AChE plaques in the original synaptic region (Fig. 9C,E). The striking result is that if, in other similar preparations, one starts in vivo chronic direct stimulation of the soleus muscle beginning at the time of foreign nerve section, after a few days many AChE plaques can be demonstrated in the region of the degenerating foreign nerve (Fig. 9B,D). They have an appearance entirely similar to those forming in the control preparation, that is when the reinnervating fibular nerve is left intact (Fig. 9A). Thus there are two distinct neural signals that induce the development of AChE at ectopic neuromuscular junctions. With the first signal (probably a chemical one), the nerve endings set the sites where AChE should accumulate. With the second signal, which is the activity evoked in the myofibers through the freshly formed sites of cholinergic transmission, the nerve makes AChE appear at those sites. Consistent with this interpretation is the finding that a foreign fibular nerve does not induce (or only to a very minor extent in some of the muscle fibers) AChE plaques, if its conduction is blocked and nerve-evoked muscle activity does not resume (46). Muscle fibrillatory activity however develops in this preparation and it could lead to the formation of some AChE. This might be particularly true if one carried on the experiment for a time longer than the 2 weeks explored.

There are species in which a neurotrophic factor certainly plays a more extensive role in AChE formation than just dictating the site of its accumulation. This is true for the *Xenopus laevis* where it has been shown that block of activity of the entire embryo with a local anesthetic does not prevent the formation of functionally active AChE at the neuromuscular junctions (91).

AChR Properties: Channel Kinetics and Metabolic Stability

During development AChRs undergo marked changes in some of their properties. Changes that, at least in many species, depend on nerve influences, rather than on an inherent developmental plan, are the gating

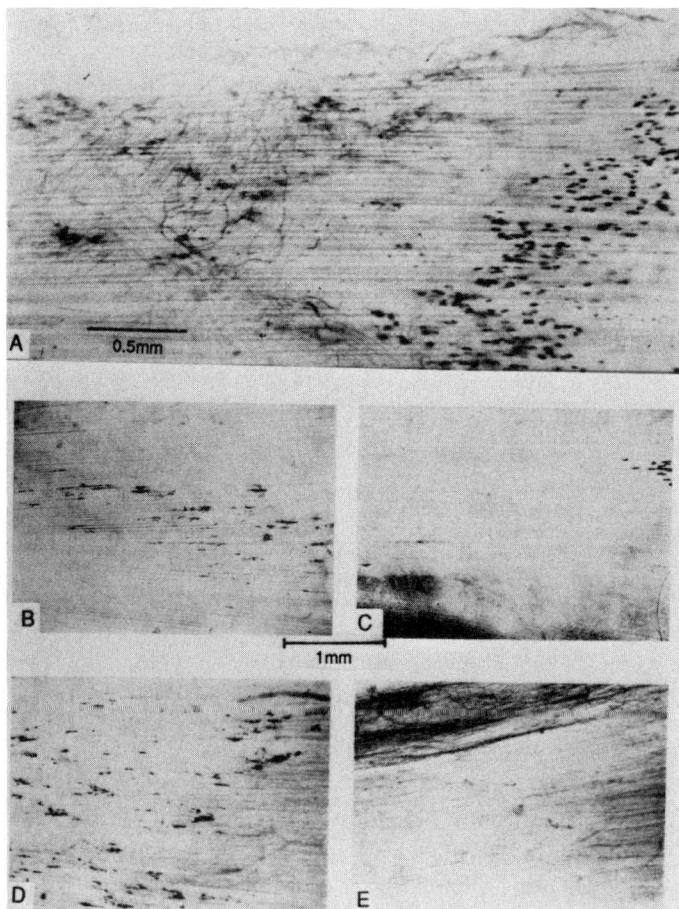

FIG. 9. Development of ACh esterase plaque in soleus myofibers after degeneration of foreign fibular nerve sprouts, induced by direct electrical stimulation of the muscle. **A** illustrates the basic preparation in which a transplanted foreign fibular nerve forms ectopic synapses when the soleus nerve is cut (14 days earlier in this case): fibular axons stained with methylene blue and the underlying end-plates, visualized through an AChE stain, are visible to the left. To the right AChE plaques of the original denervated end-plates devoid of nerve fibers, with the exception of a narrow strand which may or may not contact original end-plates. **B** and **D**: AChE plaques in the region of the degenerated fibular nerve after cutting first the soleus nerve and 3(B) or 7(D) days later the fibular nerve in chronically stimulated muscles. **C** and **E**: Lack of AChE plaques in nonstimulated but otherwise similarly treated contralateral muscles. Fibular nerve cut 3 (B and C) and 7 (D and E) days after cutting soleus nerve. Muscles stimulated for the last 7 days in B and 12 days in D. Acute experiment 11 (B and C) and 19 (D and E) days after cutting soleus nerve. (From Lømo and Slater, ref. 45, with permission.)

characteristics of the ion channel and the metabolic stability of the receptor.

Channel Kinetics

Embryonic AChR channels when they open conduct somewhat smaller current and remain open for a longer time (3–5 times) than adult end-plate channels. After denervation in the adult life the AChRs that develop in the extrajunctional membrane are again similar to the embryonic receptors. The developmental change in synaptic AChR channel conductance (γ) and mean open time (τ) occurs in various species, with the exception of chick muscle. In rat muscles it takes place approximately during the first 3 weeks of postnatal life (reviewed in 8). Approximate τ values for slow channels are 4–6 msec and for fast channels are ~1 msec. The physiological significance of the change in kinetics is not obvious. While a long open time appears useful at immature synapses to increase the safety of synaptic transmission, after maturation the decrease in open time might be necessary to limit calcium influx through the open AChR channels and thus damage (8). This would then be similar to one of the functions of AChE, as mentioned above.

An important development in this field has been the demonstration that mammalian (calf) fast and slow AChR channels are different proteins with different subunit composition of their pentameric structure. Five subunits, $\alpha,\beta,\gamma,\delta$ and a more recently discovered ϵ in calf, are assembled to form two different pentameric combinations: $\alpha_2\beta\gamma\delta$ and $\alpha_2\beta\delta\epsilon$, representing the slow and the fast channel, respectively. This was done by first transcribing bovine cDNAs for the five subunits and then co-expressing in *Xenopus* oocytes the four mRNAs of the two mixtures. After translation, full functional AChRs were inserted in the oocyte membrane, slow when the injected mRNAs mixture contained γ and fast when the mixture contained ϵ (92).

It has been shown in rats that the developmental switch from slow to fast channels is dependent on innervation, since it is prevented by muscle denervation soon after birth (93). The information that activity evoked in muscle (and perhaps also a trophic factor) is important in mediating the neurally determined switch, has come from in vivo experiments on ectopic innervation of the adult soleus muscle, entirely similar to those already described for AChE. In fact, if the innervating foreign fibular axons are cut and made to degenerate after they have briefly contacted the denervated myofibers, the switch to fast gating occurs anyway, provided the muscle is kept active by chronic direct stimulation (94). In *Xenopus* the shift of channels from slow to fast does occur, but is independent from innervation and thus appears to be part of an intrinsic developmental program of the myofibers (reviewed in 8).

Metabolic Stability

Turnover of AChRs in the membrane is neurally controlled. In noninnervated myotubes turnover is fast, with half-life of about 1 day and the same is true for receptors that develop in the extrajunctional membrane of the denervated adult muscle fibers (reviewed in 7). When innervation occurs during development, the receptors that cluster under the motor nerve terminals initially are of the unstable extrajunctional type but in a few days they become stable (half-life of about 10 days) (7). After denervation the junctional receptors are replaced in about 2–3 weeks by AChRs with a short half-life (95). Recent experiments have indicated that the nerve controls metabolic stabilization through the evoked muscle activity. First, it has been shown that chronic TTX block of nerve conduction in rats is as effective as denervation in making short-life AChRs to replace the stable receptors at the neuromuscular junctions (96). Second, chronic direct muscle stimulation prevents junctional receptor destabilization at denervated mouse endplates (97). Third, direct muscle stimulation in rats induces metabolic stability at long-term denervated junctions (61).

How muscle activity stabilizes the AChRs is unknown. Direct muscle stimulation also induces the switch from slow γ-subunit to fast ε-subunit channels. However metabolic stabilization does not depend on this change in structure of the AChRs, because 1) it occurs during synapse development before change to fast channel kinetics (rats) (98,99) or without any such change (chick), and 2) junctional AChRs after denervation are destabilized before fast kinetics disappears (100,47).

CONCLUSIONS

We have reviewed a number of mechanisms through which the anterograde long-term control of motoneurons on the membrane of muscle fibres is expressed both during development and adult life. We did not aim to be exhaustive and to give a complete account of all the most recent findings, especially of those related to the quickly expanding field of molecular biology. Rather, we concentrated on the control of the principal membrane properties both junctional and extrajunctional and selected those aspects on which the agreement is more general. Also we have presented our own recent data on the effects of long-term muscle disuse, a more controversial topic. The other main emphasis was on the nature of the neural signals that mediate the anterograde control of muscle.

In spite of the extreme diversity of the variables controlled, the neural signals so far identified are rather few: nerve impulses, which appear to work essentially through the evoked muscle activity and chemical physiological signals of which only agrin and ARIA are relatively well characterized both in nature and biological activity. Another class that we have been concerned with is what we called nerve breakdown products: In spite of the rather vague impression that this term may communicate, they have clearcut effects on myofiber's membrane and explain satisfactorily a prominent difference in muscle changes, observed approximately during the first 2 weeks, between denervation and paralysis free from nerve degeneration. Whether they may be of relevance for other fields, for example, that of pathology of diseases involving nerve degeneration, remains to be determined.

The mechanism of the response of the muscle membrane to products of nerve degeneration, is unknown. That an inflammatory reaction, with any of its cellular or biochemical components, is the only explanation of this response, seems unlikely. In fact even very high doses of an anti-inflammatory agent such as cortisone are completely ineffective in antagonizing the induction of AChRs and TTX-insensitive Na^+ channels by a degenerating foreign nerve (31). This and other data presented (31) may instead suggest the hypothesis that nerve breakdown products induce their membrane effects through direct action of some factor normally contained in axons and/or their terminals. This becomes particularly attractive, because of greater simplicity, if one assumes that this factor coincides with one of the neurotrophic factors that has the action of inducing, during development, the junctional accumulation of AChRs. When an adult muscle is denervated, the AChR-inducing factor could be released in the interstitium, because of nerve breakdown. It thus would become able to act at a distance and be highly effective because the concomitant inactivity has made the membrane much more responsive, thus explaining the greater efficacy of denervation vs. inactivity alone.

Going back to the physiological factors that control the muscle in general, it should be pointed out that the evidence accumulated so far on the control of the most diverse properties reviewed here indicates that generalized properties of muscle, both of the membrane and of the contractile apparatus, are controlled by nerve-evoked muscle activity. Discrete, localized properties are instead controlled by neurotrophic chemical factors released by motor nerve terminals: these are the synaptic cluster of acetylcholine receptors and the instruction on where to accumulate the enzyme acetylcholinesterase. These are in fact the two properties that one would predict to necessitate a highly concentrated local action. Properties of the junctional AChRs (metabolic stability and fast kinetics) are instead controlled, perhaps entirely, by muscle activity. The same appears to be true, at least in some species, for AChE accumulation. In other words it seems possible that a control has been developed during evolution, through which, with minor exceptions, only the necessary local instructions have been assigned to chemical, nerve-released factors whereas any other property, local or general, has been left to control by the nonlocalized signal represented by the muscle action potential.

ACKNOWLEDGMENT

The financial support of Telethon-Italy for part of the experiments is gratefully acknowledged.

REFERENCES

1. Tower SS. The reaction of muscle to denervation. *Physiol Rev* 1939; 19: 1–48.
2. Close R. Dynamic properties of mammalian skeletal muscle. *Physiol Rev* 1972; 52: 129–197.
3. Diamond J, Miledi R. A study of fetal and newborn rat muscle fibres. *J Physiol (Lond)* 1962; 162: 393–408.
4. Bevan S, Steinbach JH. The distribution of α-bungarotoxin binding sites on mammalian skeletal muscle developing in vivo. *J Physiol (Lond)* 1977; 267: 195–213.
5. Anderson MJ, Cohen MW. Nerve-induced and spontaneous redistribution of acetylcholine receptors on cultured muscle cells. *J Physiol (Lond)* 1977; 268: 757–773.
6. Frank E, Fischbach GD. Early events in neuromuscular junction formation in vitro. *J Cell Biol* 1979; 83: 143–158.
7. Salpeter MM, Loring RH. Nicotinic acetylcholine receptor in vertebrate muscle: properties, distribution and neural control. *Prog Neurobiol* 1985; 25: 297–325.
8. Schuetze SM, Role LW. Developmental regulation of nicotinic acetylcholine receptors. *Annu Rev Neurosci* 1987; 10: 403–457.
9. Grinnell AD. Trophic interaction between nerve and muscle. In: Engel AG, Banker BQ, eds. *Myology*. New York: McGraw Hill, 1986: 359–391.
10. Purves D, Lichtman JW. *Principles of neural development*. Sunderland, MA: Sinauer Assoc.; 1985.
11. Fambrough DM. Control of acetylcholine receptors in skeletal muscle. *Physiol Rev* 1979; 59: 165–227.
12. Axelsson J, Thesleff S. A study of supersensitivity in denervated mammalian muscle. *J Physiol (Lond)* 1959; 147: 178–193.
13. Miledi R. The acetylcholine sensitivity of frog muscle fibres after complete or partial denervation. *J Physiol (Lond)* 1960; 151: 1–23.
14. Cangiano A. Denervation supersensitivity as a model for the neural control of muscle. *Neuroscience* 1985; 14: 963–971.
15. Lømo T, Rosenthal J. Control of ACh-sensitivity by muscle activity in the rat. *J Physiol (Lond)* 1972; 221: 493–513.
16. Jones R, Vrbová G. Effect of muscle activity on denervation hypersensitivity. *J Physiol (Lond)* 1970; 210: 144–145.
17. Lømo T, Westgaard RH. Control of ACh sensitivity in rat muscle fibres. *Cold Spring Harbor Symp Quant Biol* 1976; 40: 263–274.
18. Lømo T, Westgaard RH. Further studies on the control of ACh sensitivity by muscle activity in the rat. *J Physiol (Lond)* 1975; 252: 603–626.
19. Redfern P, Thesleff S. Action potential generation in denervated rat skeletal muscle. II. The action of tetrodotoxin. *Acta Physiol Scand* 1971; 82: 70–78.
20. Weiss RE, Horn R. Functional difference between two classes of sodium channels in developing rat skeletal muscle. *Science* 1986; 233: 361–364.
21. Jansen JKS, Lømo T, Nicolaysen K, Westgaard RH. Hyperinnervation of skeletal muscle fibers. Dependence on muscle activity. *Science* 1973; 181: 559–561.
22. Cangiano A, Lutzemberger L, Zorub DS. Effects of inactivity on muscle membrane properties in rats. *Neurosci Abstracts* 1975; 1: 766 (1178).
23. Lavoie PA, Collier B, Tenenhouse A. Comparison of α-bungarotoxin binding to skeletal muscle after inactivity or denervation. *Nature* 1976; 260: 349–350.
24. Pestronk A, Drachman DB, Griffin JW. Effect of muscle disuse on acetylcholine receptors. *Nature* 1976; 260: 352–353.
25. Cangiano A, Lutzemberger L, Nicotra L. Non-

25. equivalence of impulse blockade and denervation in the production of membrane changes in rat skeletal muscle. *J Physiol (Lond)* 1977; 273: 691–706.
26. Mathers DA, Thesleff S. Studies on neurotrophic regulation of murine skeletal muscle. *J Physiol (Lond)* 1978; 282: 105–114.
27. Brown MC, Hopkins WG, Keynes RJ. Comparison of effects of denervation and botulinum toxin paralysis on muscle properties in mice. *J Physiol (Lond)* 1982; 327: 29–37.
28. Jones R, Vrbová G. Two factors responsible for the development of denervation hypersensitivity. *J Physiol (Lond)* 1974; 236: 517–538.
29. Cangiano A, Lutzemberger L. Partial denervation affects both denervated and innervated fibres in mammalian skeletal muscle. *Science* 1977; 196: 542–545.
30. Cangiano A, Lutzemberger L. Partial denervation in inactive muscle affects innervated and denervated fibres equally. *Nature* 1980; 285: 233–235.
31. Cangiano A, Magherini PC, Pasino E, Pellegrino M, Risaliti R. Interaction of inactivity and nerve breakdown products in the origin of acute denervation changes in rat skeletal muscle. *J Physiol (Lond)* 1984; 355: 345–365.
32. Brown MC, Holland RL, Ironton R. Degenerating nerve products affect innervated muscle fibers. *Nature* 1978; 275: 652–654.
33. Gilliatt RW, Westgaard RH, Williams JI. Acetylcholine sensitivity of denervated and inactivated baboon muscles. *J Physiol (Lond)* 1978; 280: 499–514.
34. Bray JJ, Hubbard JI, Mills RG. The trophic influence of tetrodotoxin-inactive nerves on normal and reinnervated rat skeletal muscles. *J Physiol (Lond)* 1979; 297: 479–491.
35. Eldridge L, Liebhold M, Steinbach JH. Alterations in cat skeletal neuromuscular junctions following prolonged inactivity. *J Physiol (Lond)* 1981; 313: 529–545.
36. Stanley EF, Drachman DB. Effects of disuse on the resting membrane potential of skeletal muscle. *Exp Neurol* 1979; 64: 231–234.
37. Cangiano A, Buffelli M, Pasino E. Does reinnervation with electrically silent axons affect the extrajunctional membrane properties of denervated skeletal muscles? *Soc Neurosci Abstr* 1989; 15 (Part 2): 1259.
38. Betz WJ, Caldwell JH, Ribchester RR. Sprouting of active nerve terminals in partially inactive muscles of the rat. *J Physiol (Lond)* 1980; 303: 281–297.
39. Spector SA. Effects of elimination of activity on contractile and histochemical properties of rat soleus muscle. *J Neurosci* 1985; 5: 2177–2188.
40. Pasino E, Arancio O, Buffelli M, Cangiano A. Essential role of impulse activity in the recovery of muscle extrajunctional properties upon reinnervation. *Neurosci Lett* 1990; Suppl 39: S165.
41. Fex S, Thesleff S. The time required for innervation of denervated muscles by nerve implants. *Life Sci* 1967; 6: 635–639.
42. Frank E, Jansen JKS, Lømo T, Westgaard RH. The interaction between foreign and original motor nerves innervating the soleus muscle of rats. *J Physiol (Lond)* 1975; 247: 725–743.
43. Lømo T, Slater CR. Control of acetylcholine sensitivity and synapse formation by muscle activity. *J Physiol (Lond)* 1978; 275: 391–402.
44. Lømo T, Slater CR. Acetylcholine sensitivity of developing ectopic nerve-muscle junctions in adult rat soleus muscles. *J Physiol (Lond)* 1980; 303: 173–189.
45. Lømo T, Slater CR. Control of junctional acetylcholinesterase by neural and muscular influences in the rat. *J Physiol (Lond)* 1980; 303: 191–202.
46. Cangiano A, Lømo T, Lutzemberger L, Sveen O. Effects of chronic nerve conduction block on formation of neuromuscular junctions and junctional AChE in the rat. *Acta Physiol Scand* 1980; 109: 283–296.
47. Reiness CG, Weinberg CB. Metabolic stabilization of acetylcholine receptor at newly formed neuromuscular junction in the rat. *Dev Biol* 1981; 84: 247–254.
48. Dennis MJ. Development of the neuromuscular junction: inductive interactions between cells. *Annu Rev Neurosci* 1981; 4: 43–68.
49. Pasino E, Buffelli M, Busetto G, Cangiano A. Chronic conduction block differentially affects extrajunctional and junctional membrane properties in skeletal muscle. In: *XV Annual Meeting of the European Neuroscience Association.* Munich, 1992; in press.
50. Betz WJ, Mao F, Bewick GS. Activity-dependent fluorescent staining and destaining of living vertebrate motor nerve terminals. *J Neurosci* 1992; 12: 363–375.
51. Buffelli M, Pasino E, Cangiano A. Effects of reinnervation with normal and tetrodotoxin-inactive nerves on contractile properties of mammalian skeletal muscle. *Neurosci Lett* 1990; Suppl 39: S36.
52. Spector SA. Trophic effects on the contractile and histochemical properties of rat soleus muscle. *J Neurosci* 1985; 5: 2189–2196.
53. Miledi R, Slater CR. On the degeneration of rat neuromuscular junctions after nerve section. *J Physiol* 1970; 207: 507–528.
54. Arancio O, Buffelli M, Cangiano A, Pasino E. Nerve stump effects in muscle are independent of synaptic connections and are temporally correlated with nerve degeneration phenomena. *Neurosci Lett* (in press).
55. Rochel S, Robbins N. Is a nicotinic influence involved in denervation-induced depolarization of muscle? *J Neurosci* 1985; 5: 2331–2335.
56. Drachman DB, Stanley EF, Pestronk EF, Griffin JW, Price DL. Neurotrophic regulation of two properties of skeletal muscle by impulse dependent and spontaneous acetylcholine transmission. *J Neurosci* 1982; 2: 232–243.
57. Witzemann V, Brenner HR, Sakmann B.

Neural factors regulate AChR subunit mRNAs at rat neuromuscular junctions. *J Cell Biol* 1991; 114: 125–141.
58. Yang JS-J, Sladky JT, Kallen RG, Barchi RL. TTX-sensitive and TTX-insensitive sodium channel mRNA transcripts are independently regulated in adult skeletal muscle after denervation. *Neuron* 1991; 7: 421–427.
59. Gundersen K. Spontaneous activity at long-term silenced synapses in rat muscle. *J Physiol (Lond)* 1990; 430: 399–418.
60. Cohen MW, Weldon PR. Localization of acetylcholine receptors and synaptic ultrastructure at nerve muscle contacts in culture: dependence on nerve type. *J Cell Biol* 1980; 86: 388–401.
61. Furnagalli G, Balbi S, Cangiano A, Lømo T. Regulation of turnover and number of acetylcholine receptors at neuromuscular junctions. *Neuron* 1990; 4: 563–569.
62. Ziskind-Conhaim L, Geffen I, Hall ZW. Redistribution of acetylcholine receptors on developing rat myotubes. *J Neurosci* 1984; 4: 2346–2349.
63. Role LW, Matossian VR, O'Brien RJ, Fischbach GD. On the mechanism of acetylcholine receptor accumulation at newly formed synapses on chick myotubes. *J Neurosci* 1985; 5: 2197–2204.
64. Sanes JR. The extracellular matrix. In: Engel AG, Banker BQ, eds. *Myology*. New York: McGraw Hill; 1986: 155–175.
65. Burden SJ, Sargent PB, McMahan UJ. Acetylcholine receptors in regenerating muscle accumulate at original synaptic sites in the absence of the nerve. *J Cell Biol* 1979; 82: 412–425.
66. McMahan UJ, Slater CR. The influence of basal lamina on the accumulation of acetylcholine receptors at synaptic sites in regenerating muscle. *J Cell Biol* 1984; 98: 1453–1473.
67. McMahan UJ, Sanes JR, Marshall LM. Cholinesterase is associated with the basal lamina at neuromuscular junction. *Nature* 1978; 271: 172–174.
68. Anglister L, McMahan UJ. Basal lamina directs acetylcholinesterase accumulation at synaptic sites in regenerating muscle. *J Cell Biol* 1985; 101: 735–743.
69. Sanes JR, Marshall LM, McMahan UJ. Reinnervation of muscle fiber basal lamina after removal of myofibers. *J Cell Biol* 1978; 78: 176–198.
70. McMahan UJ, Wallace BG. Molecules in basal lamina that direct the formation of synaptic specializations at neuromuscular junctions. *Dev Neurosci* 1989; 11: 227–247.
71. Reist NE, Magill C, McMahan UJ. Agrin-like molecules at synaptic sites in normal, denervated, and damaged skeletal muscle. *J Cell Biol* 1987; 105: 2457–2469.
72. Nitkin RM, Smith MA, Magill C, Fallon JR, Yao Y-M M, Wallace BG, McMahan UJ. Identification of agrin, a synaptic organizing protein from Torpedo electric organ. *J Cell Biol* 1987; 105: 2471–2478.
73. Ruff F, Payan DG, Magill-Solc C, Cowan DM, Scheller H. Structure and expression of rat agrin. *Neuron* 1991; 6: 811–823.
74. Magill-Solc C, McMahan UJ. Motor neurons contain agrin-like molecules. *J Cell Biol* 1988; 107: 1825–1833.
75. Usdin TB, Fischbach GD. Purification and characterization of a polypeptide from chick brain that promotes the accumulation of acetylcholine receptors in chick myotubes. *J Cell Biol* 1986; 103: 493–507.
76. Harris DA, Falls DL, Dill Devor RM, Fischbach GD. Acetylcholine receptor-inducing factor from chicken brain increases the level of mRNA encoding the receptor α-subunit. *Proc Natl Acad Sci USA* 1988; 85: 1983–1987.
77. Fontaine B, Klarsfeld A, Hökfelt T, Changeux JP. Calcitonin gene-related peptide, a peptide present in spinal cord motoneurons, increases the number of acetylcholine receptors in primary cultures of chick embryo myotubes. *Neurosci Lett* 1986; 71: 59–65.
78. New HV, Mudge AW. Calcitonin gene-related peptide regulates muscle acetylcholine receptor synthesis. *Nature* 1986; 323: 809–811.
79. Fontaine B, Klarsfeld A, Changeux JP. Calcitonin gene-related peptide and muscle activity regulate acetylcholine receptors α-subunit mRNA levels by distinct intracellular pathways. *J Cell Biol* 1987; 105: 1337–1342.
80. Österlund M, Fontaine B, Devillers-Thiery A, Geoffroy B, Changeux JP. Acetylcholine receptor expression in primary cultures of embryonic chick myotubes-I. discoordinate regulation of α-, γ- and δ-subunit gene expression by calcitonin gene related peptide and by muscle electrical activity. *Neuroscience* 1990; 32: 279–287.
81. Moss SJ, Harkness PC, Mason IJ, Barnard EA, Mudge AW. Evidence that calcitonin gene-related peptide and cAMP increase transcription of AChR α subunit gene, but not of other subunit genes. *J Mol Neurosci* 1991; 3: 101–108.
82. Laufer R, Changeux JP. Calcitonin gene-related peptide elevates cyclic AMP levels in chick skeletal muscle: possible neurotrophic role for a coexisting neuronal messenger. *EMBO J* 1987; 6: 901–906.
83. Buffelli M, Arancio O, Pasino E, Cangiano A. Acetylcholine receptors and TTX-resistant action potentials development in mammalian skeletal muscle following chronic *in vivo* application of calcitonin gene-related peptide. *Neurosci Lett* 1990; Suppl 39: S36.
84. Matteoli M, Haimann C, Torri-Tarelli F, Polak JM, Ceccarelli B, De Camilli P. Differential effect of α-latrotoxin on exocytosis from small synaptic vesicles and from large dense core vesicles containing calcitonin gene-related peptide at the frog neuromuscular junction. *Proc Natl Acad Sci USA* 1988; 85: 7366–7370.
85. Matteoli M, Balbi S, Sala C, Chini B, Cimino M, Vitadello M, Fumagalli G. Developmentally regulated expression of calcitonin gene-related

86. Salpeter MM, Kasprzak H, Feng H, Fertuk H. End-plates after esterase inactivation in vivo: correlation between esterase concentration, functional response and fine structure. *J Neurocytol* 1978; 8: 95.
87. Rotundo RL, Fambrough. Function and molecular structure of acetylcholinesterase. In: Engel AG, Banker BQ, eds. *Myology*. New York: McGraw Hill; 1986: 791–808.
88. Massoulie J, Bon S. The molecular forms of cholinesterase and acetylcholinesterase in vertebrate. *Annu Rev Neurosci* 1982; 5: 57–106.
89. Younkin SG, Brett RS, Davey B, Younkin LH. Substances moved by axonal transport and released by nerve stimulation have an innervation-like effect on muscle. *Science* 1978; 200: 1292–1295.
90. Rubin L, Schuetze C, Weill C, Fischbach GD. Regulation of acetylcholinesterase appearance at the neuromuscular junction in vitro. *Nature* 1980; 287: 264–267.
91. Cohen MW, Greschner M, Tucci M. In vivo development of cholinesterase at neuromuscular junction in the absence of motor activity in Xenopus laevis. *J Physiol (Lond)* 1984; 348: 57–66.
92. Mishina M, Takai T, Imoto K, Noda M, Takahashi T, Numa S, Methfessel C, Sakmann B. Molecular distinction between fetal and adult forms of muscle acetylcholine receptor. *Nature* 1986; 321: 406–411.
93. Schuetze SM, Vicini S. Neonatal denervation inhibits the normal postnatal decrease in end-plate channel open time. *J Neurosci* 1984; 4: 2297–2302.
94. Brenner HR, Lømo T, Williamson R. Control of end-plate channel properties by neurotrophic effects and by muscle activity in rat. *J Physiol (Lond)* 1987; 388: 367–381.
95. Shyng SL, Salpeter MM. Degradation rates of acetylcholine receptors inserted into denervated vertebrate neuromuscular junctions. *J Cell Biol* 1989; 108: 647–651.
96. Cangiano A, Fumagalli G, Lømo T. Acetylcholine receptors at rat neuromuscular junctions turn over rapidly after nerve block by TTX. *J Physiol (Lond)* 1987; 390: P 174.
97. Brenner HR, Rudin W. On the effect of muscle activity on the end-plate membrane in denervated mouse muscle. *J Physiol (Lond)* 1989; 410: 501–512.
98. Brenner HR, Sakmann B. Neurotrophic control of channel properties at neuromuscular synapses of rat muscle. *J Physiol (Lond)* 1983; 337: 159–171.
99. Levitt TA, Salpeter MM. Denervated endplates have a dual population of junctional acetylcholine receptors. *Nature* 1981; 291: 239–241.
100. Michler A, Sakmann B. Receptor stability and channel conversion in the subsynaptic membrane of the developing mammalian neuromuscular junction. *Dev Biol* 1980; 80: 1–17.

9

Nonregenerative Approaches to Spinal Cord Injury

Wise Young

Department of Neurosurgery, New York University Medical Center, New York, New York 10016

Regeneration has long been regarded to be the only hope for recovery from spinal cord injury (1). However, the spinal cord possesses remarkable capabilities for spontaneous recovery. Quantitative analyses of injured cat spinal cords indicate that very few (5–10%) spinal axons will support recovery (2,3). Most surviving axons are demyelinated (4,5) and dysfunctional (4,6,7), suggesting that even fewer functioning axons are necessary for recovery. The spinal cord possesses much motor circuitry that can operate independently of descending influences (8–10). Spinal pathways can substitute for each other to mediate complex motor behaviors (11–16).

Many treatments have been reported to be beneficial in spinal cord injury. These include cooling (17,18), glucocorticosteroids (19–23), opiate receptor blockers (24–26), high dose steroids (27–29) and other inhibitors of lipid peroxidation (30–34), glutamate receptor blockers (35–39), serotonin receptor blockers (40–42), calcium channel blockers (43–45), inhibitors of cyclo-oxygenase (46–49), proteinase inhibitors (50,51), and others (52,53). Drugs such as 4-aminopyridine (54,55) and GABA receptor blockers (56,57) can improve conduction in injured spinal axons.

Humans also recover from severe spinal cord injury. "Incomplete" spinal-injured patients admitted with residual motor or sensory function generally will recover (58). Patients may show remarkable functional preservation despite major spinal cord lesions (59–62). While "complete" patients with no motor or sensory function below the lesion tend not to improve much (63), the recent National Acute Spinal Cord Injury Study (NASCIS 2) showed that methylprednisolone given shortly after injury significantly improved neurologic recovery in such patients (64,65). Monosialic ganglioside (GM1) also improved motor recovery in spinal-injured patients at 1 year after injury (66). These findings provide a basis for optimism in spinal cord injury.

WHAT IS NECESSARY AND SUFFICIENT FOR FUNCTIONAL RECOVERY?

More than three decades ago, Windle et al. (67) reported that cats can recover from near-complete sections of the spinal cord. Cats with as little as 10% of their spinal cord tracts often recover locomotory behavior. Guth et al. (68), in studies examining the effects of enzyme therapy on transected spinal cords, found that rats sometimes recovered locomotory function and evoked potentials after apparently total transection of the spinal cord. Histological assessments revealed that these rats often had a thin strand of ventral white matter. Unfortunately, they viewed this as a problem rather than a reason for hope. They subsequently formulated strict criteria verifying completeness of spinal transections before regeneration can be claimed (69).

Blight et al. (70,2,3) carried out the first detailed morphometric studies of cats after severe spinal cord injury. The spinal cords invariably showed a centripetal pattern of tissue destruction with greater loss of deeper axons. A majority of surviving axons concentrated in a thin rim located within 0.5 mm of the pial surface. Larger axons were selectively lost. Most of the surviving axons were demyelinated. Cats that recovered locomotion generally had axon counts in the range of 25,000–50,000 axons or 5–10% of normal counts of approximately 500,000 myelinated axons. Many of these cats were able to walk, run, and jump. Some cats with as few as 10,000–20,000 axons or 2–4% of normal showed recovery of somatosensory evoked potentials (70) and return of locomotory ability.

Humans appear to be able to recover motor and sensory function even after lesions involving 90% of the spinal cord. Several reports suggest that people can have some motor function despite documented lesions that leave only a thin strand of white matter crossing the injury site (60,61,71,72,62). Likewise, neurosurgeons have long known that patients with spinal tumors can show relatively few neurological deficits until the tumor occupies 90% or more of the width of the spinal cord. The time course of compression appears to be important in determining the degree of deficit manifested by such patients. If spinal axons are lost slowly over a prolonged period, patients may show little motor deficits.

The observation that 5–10% of spinal axons can support substantive functional recovery has important implications for spinal cord injury research. Since spinal cord transections are very rare, even very severely injured patients are likely to have some surviving axons. Many of these axons are probably demyelinated. These patients are likely to be perched close to the threshold of recovery. The addition of relatively few axons to or improving conduction in some of the surviving axons in the existing population of surviving axons may well push the patients over that threshold. Thus, treatments do not need to rescue, repair, or regenerate a large number of axons to affect functional recovery.

REDUNDANCY OF SPINAL PATHWAYS

The ability of the spinal cord to recover from extensive lesions raises important questions. How can so few axons support complex motor behavior? Is 90% of the spinal cord redundant? What spinal pathways are necessary and sufficient for recovery? The observation that 5–10% of the spinal pathways can support functional recovery suggests strongly that many spinal tracts can substitute for each other. Alstermark et al. (73–76,11,77,12–14) studied the ability of cats to use their forepaw to retrieve food morsels after lesions of the corticospinal, rubrospinal, vestibulospinal, reticulospinal, propiospinal, and other descending tracts. Cats often recovered from combined lesions of two or more tracts. However, propriospinal pathways, which modulate spinal interneuronal activity (78), appear to be important for such substitution to occur. Lesions that include the cervical propiospinal tract often compromised recovery of motor recovery in the forelimbs. The propriospinal tracts and short intraspinal tracts are situated close to the gray matter (79) and are particularly sensitive to mechanical (80) and ischemic insults (81) that cause centrally located lesions.

Some spinal pathways appear to play a critical role in locomotory recovery. Eidelberg et al. (15,82,16,83–87) systematically examined the effects of selective spinal cord lesions on locomotory recovery animals ranging from ferrets to primates. They confirmed that a small percentage of spinal axons can support locomotory recovery but that preservation of some ventral pathways was critical for recovery. These tracts contain the descending systems that initiate and maintain locomotory and postural mechanisms.

The spinal cords can operate relatively independently of the brain. For example, the scratching behavior of dogs is largely programmed in the spinal cord (88). Chronically spinalized frogs retain a similar wiping reflex (89). Cats (8,90,91,10) and rats (92) with severed spinal cord can be trained to walk. Isolated spinal cords are capable of complex neuronal output (93–96) resembling locomotory activity. Such "fictive" locomotion can be initiated and modulated with drugs that manipulate spinal excitability (97,98,9,99–101). Such behavior, however, differs from normal locomotion. It is not under descending control, hindlimbs are not coordinated with upper limb movements (102), and rhythmic sensory feedback is required (103).

ROLE OF AXONAL DYSFUNCTION IN SPINAL CORD INJURY

Axonal dysfunction is seldom considered in spinal cord injury. The neurological deficits are often assumed to be due to axonal loss. A majority of axons crossing the spinal lesion site in chronically injured cats are demyelinated and dysfunctional (6,5,3). These axons are sensitive to temperature changes and cannot conduct high frequency trains of action potentials. Such abnormalities are consistent with demyelination and partial remyelination (104–106). Inability of axons to carry high frequency spike trains severely limits information transmission. Spinal-injured patients may have sufficient axons but still do not recover because the axons are dysfunctional.

Many investigators have reported demyelination in animals after spinal cord injury (107–113). Oligodendroglial cells are exquisitely sensitive to trauma and ischemia. Conditions at the lesion site contribute to demyelination. The profound and prolonged decreases in extracellular calcium ionic activity observed at the injury site (114–116) probably contribute to demyelination (117,118). Excessive Ca entry into cells activates neutral proteases and myelinases (119,109,110,120), which break down myelin (121,122). Macrophages (5) may play a role in demyelination (123,124). Finally, injured spinal cords generate inflammatory and immunological products (125–127) that cause demyelination, i.e., activated complement (128–132) and tumor necrosis factor (133).

Conduction of demyelinated axons can be improved by treatment. For example, 4-aminopyridine (4-AP), a blocker of fast voltage-sensitive potassium channels located underneath myelin (134–136), can improve conduction of axons crossing lesions (7,54,55,137). Blockade of K channels reduces the K release associated with white matter activation in unmyelinated (138) or premyelinated (139,140) preparations. 4-AP improves function of patients with multiple sclerosis (141,142) and in animals after demyelination (143–147). However, 4-AP also affects neuronal activity (148) and synaptic activity (101). The in vivo effects of 4-AP may be partly due to these effects (100,149). Axons also possess receptors to gamma amino butyric acid, which influences axonal conduction (56,57)

REMYELINATION OF SPINAL AXONS

Oligodendroglial cells can remyelinate axons (150–156). Such remyelination, however, is constrained by several factors. Although adult oligodendroglial cells can be stimulated to proliferate after injury (157), their ability to divide is strictly limited (158,159). Oligodendroglial remyelination is restricted to the distance that these cells can migrate. More often than not, the remyelinated spinal axons tend to have thin myelin sheaths and abnormal internodal distances (4,70,2,5).

Schwann cells also will remyelinate central axons (160–166,151–156,4) and improve the safety factor of axonal conduction

(163). Schwann cells will invade the lesion sites of injured spinal cords to remyelinate (164) axons and improve somatosensory evoked potentials in cats (4). Since few axons are required for functional recovery, remyelination should contribute to functional recovery.

Remyelination therapy of injured spinal cords is feasible. Unlike multiple sclerosis (167,168), spinal cord injury results in a stable demyelinated region. Schwann cell remyelination is of interest because Schwann cells lack factors that inhibit axonal elongation (169–176) and therefore may provide an appropriate environment for axonal regeneration. Peripheral nerves also provide a ready source of Schwann cells homografts, which pose less risk for immunologic rejection (177). Adult Schwann cells can be cultured (178,179) and are sensitive to (180–184) growth factors. Note that regenerated axons are unmyelinated and may need to be myelinated to contribute to functional recovery.

Finally, although drugs that improve conduction in demyelinated spinal cords, such as 4-AP and GABA receptor blockers, may have too many side-effects for chronic administration, they may serve a useful purpose in identifying patients for biological remyelination therapy. Because such therapy will probably require the introduction of cells to the lesion site and procedures to transplant cells to the lesion site may require surgery, it would be helpful if patients who would benefit from remyelination can be identified. Drugs that improve conduction in demyelinated axons may provide an important diagnostic tool.

RECOVERY IN HUMAN SPINAL CORD INJURY

Spinal cord injury assessment is often oriented toward identification of deficits on the assumptions that deficits reflect axonal loss. Recovery, however, is determined not by what has been lost but by what survives the injury. Clinical experience suggests that spinal-injured patients admitted to the hospital with any residual motor or pinprick sensation (58) below the injury level have an excellent prognosis for recovery. The propensity for recovery in "incomplete" spinal cord injury is shown clearly by data from NASCIS 1 (185) and NASCIS 2 (64,65). Figure 1 summarizes the 1 year motor change scores of patients treated with low, high, and megadose methylprednisolone. The patients were grouped into "plegic," "plegic+," and "paretic," which, respectively, mean patients with no motor or sensory, no motor and some sensory, and some motor and sensory function below the lesion on admission.

"Plegic" patients with no motor or sensory function below the lesion site generally have a poor prognosis for recovery (63,186). As shown in Fig. 1, placebo-treated "plegic" patients recovered less than 5 points compared to 12 and 31 points in paretic and plegic+ patients at 1 year after injury. However, very high dose methylprednisolone given within 8 hours after injury improved recovery of "plegic" to a level comparable to those of "paretic" patients. The finding that a treatment given to "plegic" patients significantly improves sensory and motor recovery implies that "plegic" patients have some residual spinal pathways.

The concept that "complete" spinal cord injury patients have some residual spinal pathways is supported by other data. A majority of patients with chronic "complete" spinal cord injury can continue to exert some motor control (187,188), especially suprasegmental motor control over reflexes elicited by vibration stimuli (189). Many so-called complete patients can learn to voluntarily suppress or enhance their spasticity or spasms that occur. The term "discomplete" has been coined to distinguish these patients with subclinical motor and sensory function (190). Thus "complete" typically does not necessarily mean complete loss of all connections between the brain and the spinal cord.

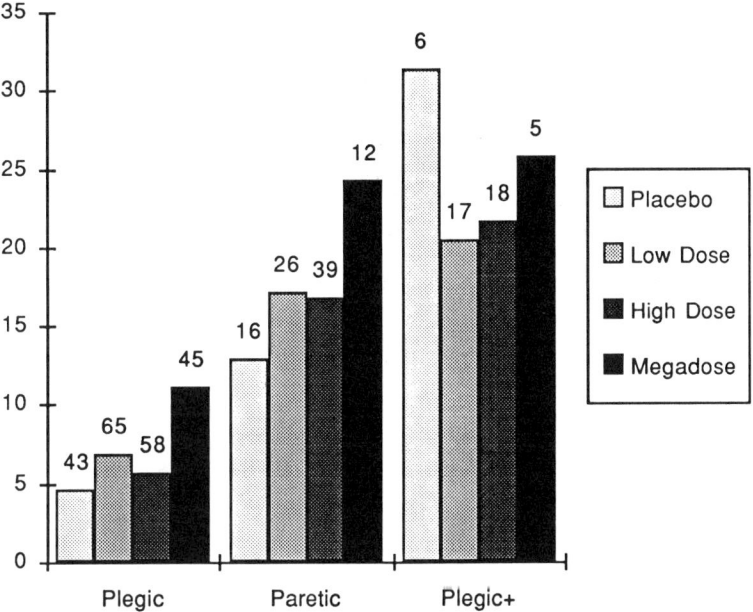

FIG. 1. Effect of methylprednisolone on motor change scores in NASCIS 1 and 2. Motor scores were obtained by summing motor strength scores from 14 muscle groups, graded on the clinical scale of 0–5, for a total of 70 points. Data from NASCIS 1 (185) and 2 (64,65) are shown, comparing three doses of methylprednisolone: low dose (100 mg/day for 10 days), high dose (1,000 mg/day for 10 days), and megadose (30 mg/kg bolus given within 8 hours followed by 5.4 mg/kg/hr for 23 hours). *Plegic* refers to patients admitted with no motor or sensory function below the lesion level. *Paretic* indicates patients admitted with some motor function below the lesion level. *Plegic* + refers to plegic patients admitted with some sensory preservation. Numbers of patients are given on the top of each column.

Combined, these findings strongly suggest that many patients with severe spinal cord injury may be perched on the threshold of recovery. The addition of a small percentage of axons on top of the existing population of surviving axons will push them over the threshold. Treatments do not have to rescue, restore, or regenerate many axons to improve functional recovery. This provides a basis for hope that effective treatments will be available not only for acute but chronic spinal cord injury.

TIME COURSE OF NEUROLOGIC RECOVERY

Traumatic injury transiently abolishes all conduction across the lesion site. Ion-selective microelectrodes studies (191) have shown a very large rise in extracellular potassium ionic activity, which should depolarize all axons crossing the lesion site. Other ionic shifts and blood flow changes (116) take place. Recovery of surviving spinal pathways should occur when the environment at the injury site returns to normal within a few hours. Indeed, animals recover within minutes from selective lesions made in the spinal cord with surgical instruments (192,193).

Recovery from severe spinal cord injury is very slow, requiring months or even years to manifest. Figures 2 and 3 illustrate the motor and sensory recover in placebo-treated plegic and paretic patients in NASCIS 2 (64,65,194). At 6 weeks, plegic patients show only 25% and 50% of the motor and sensory recovery observed at 1 year after injury. At 6 months, motor recovery was

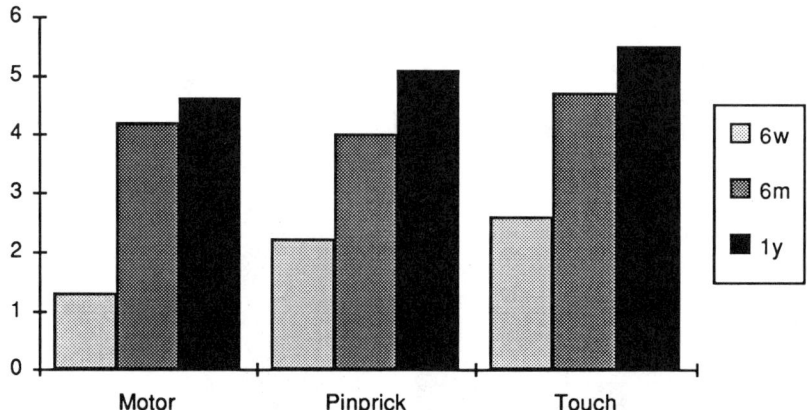

FIG. 2. Motor and sensory change scores in placebo-treated plegic patients (n = 43). Time course of motor and sensory recovery in placebo-treated plegic patients in NASCIS 2 (64,65,194). *Motor* change scores were obtained as described in Fig. 1. *Pinprick* and *touch* scores were graded on a scale of 0–2 in 29 dermatomes, summed, and subtracted from admission scores at 6 weeks *(6w)*, 6 months *(6m)*, and 1 year *(1y)* after injury.

close to 1 year but some improvement could still be observed between 6 months and 1 year. Patients who were examined 13–15 months after injury continued to show significant improvements compared to 12 months (185). Recovery due to methylprednisolone treatment, however, required 6 months to manifest fully (65). In contrast, recovery from less severe injuries occur quickly, as shown in Fig. 3.

The slow pace of recovery in severe spinal cord injury suggests the presence of recovery processes that occur over months after injury. Reorganization of the central nervous system distal and proximal to the lesion site may play a role in recovery of function. In addition to trans-synaptic degeneration of cells in the lumbosacral spinal cord (195,196) and brain (197–200), local dorsal root afferents sprout to occupy (201)

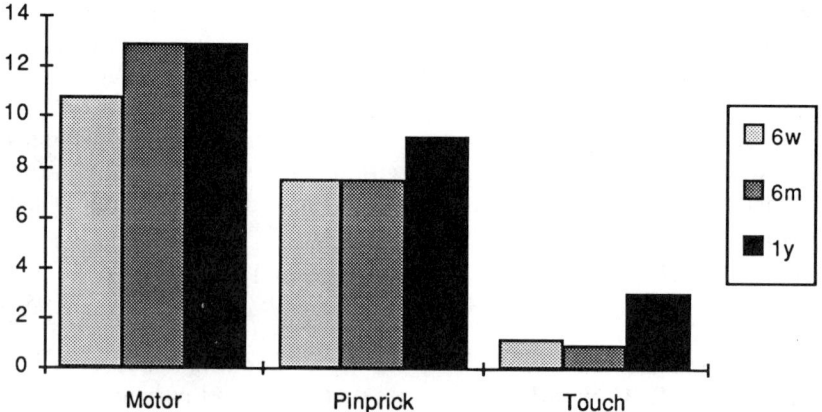

FIG. 3. Motor and sensory change scores in placebo-treated paretic patients (n = 16). Time course of motor and sensory recovery in placebo-treated paretic patients in NASCIS 2 (64,65,194). *Motor, pinprick,* and *touch* scores were obtained as described in Fig. 2.

vacated synapses (202–207). Studies of neonatal spinal cord injury suggest that plasticity plays a major role in recovery of function (208). Glucocorticosteroids have been reported to inhibit (209–211) while gonadal steroids enhance (212) sprouting. While sprouting is commonly viewed as potentially contributory to recovery, it may be deleterious by increasing spasticity (213).

Demyelination and remyelination of surviving axons may be another reason for the slow pace of recovery in severe spinal cord injuries. Demyelination peaks at several days after spinal cord injury (5,3). Remyelination is a relatively slow process. Oligodendroglia may have to migrate several centimeters and Schwann cell invasion is likely to take months (4). Treatments that speed the remyelination process, for example, may improve the rate of recovery.

MECHANISMS OF RECOVERY

The finding that functional recovery is common in animals and humans despite massive losses of axons suggests that efficient and effective recovery mechanisms exist in the spinal cord. The recovery observed in spinal-injured animals and humans probably involve at least three nonregenerative mechanisms: redundancy of spinal pathways, reorganization of the nervous system proximal and distal to the lesion site, and remyelination. Redundancy of spinal pathways subserving motor and sensory function is an efficient means of ensuring rapid recovery from incomplete spinal cord injuries. During evolution of the vertebrate central nervous system, spinal pathways and connections were superimposed upon existing structures. Because newer and specialized tracts were added to the spinal cord without replacing or eliminating the older tracts, many functions may be masked under normal conditions. Multiple routes are available for motor and sensory communication. These overlapping systems can substitute for each other in situations of injury.

Since Ramón y Cajal (214) described the abortive attempts of central axons to grow after injury, the inability of the spinal cord to regenerate has been widely acknowledged. Much evidence, however, suggests that central axons are capable of regeneration. For example, many primitive vertebrates regenerate spinal axons (215–221). Spontaneous regeneration has been reported in spinal dorsal columns (222–224,216) and brain (225–227). Central axons grow well in peripheral nerves (228–234) and reconnect with target neurons (235–240). The problem is not inability of central axons to regenerate. Rather mammals have evolved specific mechanisms to inhibit axonal regeneration in the central nervous tissues (173–175).

Regeneration offers little adaptive advantage for mammals because it is simply too slow and inefficient to contribute to recovery. In larger mammals, the distance that axons have to grow may exceed a meter. At the rate of 1 mm per day (the rate of hair growth, for example), an axon may require several years to reach its target site. A spinal-injured animal does not have the luxury of waiting months or even years for the function to return. Redundant pathways represent a surer and faster means of recovery. Furthermore, incorrect connections by regenerating axons may increase spasticity or pain. Given this situation, it is not surprising that regeneration did not evolve as a mechanism for recovery and, in fact, its occurrence may be strongly inhibited to avoid interference with existing effective recovery mechanisms.

SUMMARY

Much evidence suggests that recovery from spinal cord injury can occur by means other than regeneration. Spinal cord injury victims admitted to the hospital with even the slightest preservation of sensory or motor function below the injury level generally have a much better prognosis for substantial recovery than those admitted with no function below the lesion level. Animals often recover from severe lesions which interrupt >90% of spinal cord pathways. Morphometric and physiological studies in spinal-injured cats have shown that as little as 10% of spinal axons can support locomotory recovery. Since most of the surviving axons are demyelinated and dysfunctional, this indicates that remarkably few conducting axons, probably <5% of normal, are sufficient for recovery. The ability of the spinal cord to function with minimal descending control explains why drugs can improve neurologic recovery when given to animals and people shortly after severe spinal cord injury. Treatments need not rescue large numbers of axons to have a beneficial effect. In addition, improving conduction in demyelinated axons may restore function. For example, 4-aminopyridine, a blocker of fast potassium channels that has been shown to improve conduction in patients with multiple sclerosis, was recently found to improve conduction in injured spinal cords. Although these drugs do not have lasting effects on conduction and may be unsuitable for chronic use, they may be useful for identifying patients who would benefit from remyelination. Longer-term solutions to the problem will require a combination of biological and pharmacological approaches. For example, remyelination of surviving axons by injecting or facilitating Schwann and oligodendroglial cells from adult or fetal sources thus is a therapeutic option that is being intensely explored. Because regenerated axons require remyelination, these solutions may be helpful to maximize the contributions of regenerated axons to function. Finally, much of the dysfunction after spinal cord injury stems from imbalance of excitatory and inhibitory inputs. Selective neuropharmacology and even surgical lesions may help restore balance and thereby improve function. Nonregenerative approaches to chronic spinal cord injury hold much promise.

ACKNOWLEDGMENT

This work was supported in part by grants NS10164, NS15590, and NS27226 from the National Institutes of Health.

REFERENCES

1. Windle WF. *Regeneration in the central nervous system*. Springfield, IL: Charles C Thomas; 1955.
2. Blight AR. Cellular morphology of chronic spinal cord injury in the cat: analysis of myelinated axons by line sampling. *Neuroscience*. 1983; 10: 521–543.
3. Blight AR, DeCrescito V. Morphometric analysis of experimental spinal cord injury in the cat: the relation of injury intensity to survival of myelinated axons. *Neuroscience* 1986; 19: 321–341.
4. Blight A, Young W. Central axons in injured cat spinal cord recover electrophysiological function following remyelination by Schwann cells. *J Neurol Sci* 1989; 91: 15–34.
5. Blight AR. Delayed demyelination and macrophage invasion: a candidate for secondary cell damage in spinal cord injury. *Cent Nerv Syst Trauma* 1985; 2: 299–315.
6. Blight AR. Axonal physiology of chronic spinal cord injury in the cat: intracellular recording in vitro. *Neuroscience* 1983; 10: 1471–1486.
7. Blight AR. Effect of 4-aminopyridine on axonal conduction-block in chronic spinal cord injury. *Brain Res Bull* 1989; 22: 47–52.
8. Barbeau H, Rossignol S. Recovery of locomotion after chronic spinalization in the adult cat. *Brain Res* 1987; 412: 84–95.
9. Barbeau H, Rossignol S. Initiation and modulation of the locomotor pattern in the adult chronic spinal cat by noradrenergic, serotonergic and dopaminergic drugs. *Brain Res* 1991; 546: 250–260.
10. Lovely RG, Gregor RJ, Roy RR, and Edgerton VR. Weight-bearing hindlimb stepping in treadmill-exercised adult spinal cats. *Brain Res* 1990; 514: 206–218.
11. Alstermark B, Lundberg A, Pinter M, Sasaki S. Subpopulations and functions of long C3-C5 propriospinal neurones. *Brain Res* 1987; 404: 395–400.
12. Alstermark B, Lundberg A, Sasaki S. Integration in descending motor pathways controlling the forelimb in the cat. 10. Inhibitory pathways to forelimb motoneurones via C3-C4 propriospinal neurones. *Exp Brain Res* 1984; 56: 279–292.
13. Alstermark B, Lundberg A, Sasaki S. Integration in descending motor pathways controlling the forelimb in the cat. 11. Inhibitory pathways from higher motor centres and forelimb afferents to C3-C4 propriospinal neurones. *Exp Brain Res* 1984; 56: 293–307.
14. Alstermark B, Lundberg A, Sasaki S. Integra-

tion in descending motor pathways controlling the forelimb in the cat. 12. Interneurones which may mediate descending feed-forward inhibition and feed-back inhibition from the forelimb to C3-C4 propriospinal neurones. *Exp Brain Res* 1984; 56: 308–322.
15. Eidelberg E, Nguyen L, Deza L. Recovery of locomotor function after hemisection of the spinal cord in cats. *Brain Res Bull* 1986; 16: 507–515.
16. Eidelberg E, Story JL, Walden JG, Meyer BL. Anatomical correlates of return of locomotor function after partial spinal cord lesions in cats. *Exp Brain Res* 1981; 42: 81–88.
17. Albin MS, White RJ, Acosta RG, Yashon D. Study of functional recovery produced by delayed localized cooling after spinal cord injury in primates. *J Neurosurg* 1968; 29: 113–120.
18. Albin MS, White RJ, Yashon D, Harris LS. Effects of localized cooling on spinal cord trauma. *J Trauma* 1969; 9: 1000–1008.
19. Campbell JB, DeCrescito V, Tomasula JJ, Demopoulos HB, Flamm ES, Ransohoff J. Experimental treatment of spinal cord contusion in the cat. *Surg Neurol* 1973; 1: 102–106.
20. Ducker TB, Hamit HF. Experimental treatments of acute spinal cord injury. *J Neurosurg* 1969; 30: 693–697.
21. Kuchner EF, Hansebout RR. Combined steroid and hypothermia treatment of experimental spinal cord injury. *Surg Neurol* 1976; 6: 371–376.
22. Lewin MG, Pappius HM, Hansebout RR. Effects of steroids on edema associated with injury of the spinal cord. In: Reulen HJ, Schurmann K, eds. *Steroids and brain edema.* Berlin: Springer-Verlag; 1972.
23. Parker AJ, Smith CW. Functional recovery from spinal cord trauma following dexamethasone and chlorpromazine therapy in dogs. *Res Vet Sci* 1976; 21: 246–247.
24. Faden AI, Jacobs TP. Opiate antagonist WIN 44,441-3 stereospecifically improves neurologic recovery after ischemic spinal injury. *Neurology* 1985; 35: 1311–1315.
25. Faden AI, Jacobs TP, Holaday JW. Opiate antagonist improves neurologic recovery after spinal injury. *Science* 1980; 211: 493–494.
26. Faden AI, Takemori AE, Portghese PS. K-selective opiate antagonist norbinaltorphimine improves outcome after traumatic spinal cord injury in rats. *Cent Nerv Syst Trauma* 1987; 4: 227–234.
27. Hall ED. Effects of the 21-aminosteroid U74006F on posttraumatic spinal cord ischemia in cats. *J Neurosurg* 1988; 68: 462–465.
28. Hall ED, Braughler JM. Effects of methylprednisolone on spinal cord lipid peroxidation and (Na^+-K^+)-ATPase activity: dose response analysis during the first hour after contusion injury in the cat. *J Neurosurg* 1982; 57: 247–253.
29. Hall ED, Braughler JM. Role of lipid peroxidation in post-traumatic spinal cord degeneration: a review. *Cent Nerv Syst Trauma* 1986; 3: 281–294.
30. Anderson DK, Braughler JM, Hall ED, Waters TR, McCall JM, Means ED. Effects of treatment with U74006F on neurological outcome following experimental spinal cord injury. *J Neurosurg* 1988; 69: 562–567.
31. Anderson DK, Hall ED, Braughler JM, McCall JM, Means ED. Effect of delayed administration of U74006F (Tirilazad Mesylate) on recovery of locomotor function after experimental spinal cord injury. *J Neurotrauma* 1991; 8: 187–192.
32. Anderson DK, Means ED. Lipid peroxidation in spinal cord. $FeCl_2$ induction and protection with antioxidants. *Neurochem Pathol* 1983; 1: 249–264.
33. Anderson DK, Means ED. δ-Tocopherol, mannitol, and methylprednisolone prevention of $FeCl_2$ initiated free radical induced lipid peroxidation in spinal cord. In: Novelli U, eds. *Oxygen free radicals in shock.* Basel: Karger; 1986.
34. Saunders RD, Dugan LL, Demediuk P, Means ED, Horrocks LA, Anderson DK. Effects of methylprednisolone and the combination of alpha-tocopherol and selenium on arachidonic acid metabolism and lipid peroxidation in traumatized spinal cord tissue. *J Neurochem* 1987; 49: 24–31.
35. Bakshi R, Faden AI. Competitive and non-competitive NMDA antagonists limit dynorphin A-induced rat hindlimb paralysis. *Brain Res* 1990; 507: 1–5.
36. Faden AI, Ellison JA, Noble LJ. Effects of competitive and non-competitive NMDA receptor antagonists in spinal cord injury. *Eur J Pharmacol* 1990; 175: 165–174.
37. Faden AI, Lemke M, Simon RP, Noble LJ. N-methyl-D-aspartate antagonist MK801 improves outcome following traumatic spinal cord injury in rats: Behavioral, anatomic, and neurochemical studies. *J Neurotrauma* 1988; 5: 33–45.
38. Faden AI, Simon RP. A potential role for excitotoxins in the pathophysiology of spinal cord injury. *Ann Neurol* 1988; 23: 623–626.
39. Yum SW, Faden AI. Comparison of the neuroprotective effects of the N-methyl-D-aspartate antagonist MK-801 and the opiate-receptor antagonist nalmefene in experimental spinal cord ischemia. *Arch Neurol* 1990; 47: 277–281.
40. Puniak MA, Freeman GM, Agresta CA, Van Newkirk L, Barone CA, Salzman SK. Comparison of a serotonin antagonist, opioid antagonist, and TRH analog for the acute treatment of experimental spinal trauma. *J Neurotrauma* 1991; 8: 193–203.
41. Salzman SK, Hirofuji E, Llados EC, MacEwen GD, Beckman AL. Monoaminergic responses to spinal trauma. Participation of serotonin in posttraumatic progression of neural damage. *J Neurosurg* 1987; 66: 431–439.
42. Salzman SK, Puniak MA, Liu Z-j, Maitland-Heriot RP, Freeman GM, Agresta CA. The serotonin antagonist mianserin improves functional recovery following experimental spinal trauma. *Ann Neurol* 1991; 30: 533–541.
43. Guha A, Tator CH, Piper I. Increase in rat spi-

nal cord blood flow with the calcium channel blocker, nimodipine. *J Neurosurg* 1985; 63: 250–259.
44. Guha A, Tator CH, Piper I. Effect of a calcium channel blocker on posttraumatic spinal cord blood flow. *J Neurosurg* 1987; 66: 423–430.
45. Madden KP, Clark WM, Marcoux FW, et al. Treatment with conotoxin, an 'N-type' calcium channel blocker, in neuronal hypoxic-ischemic injury. *Brain Res* 1990; 537: 256–262.
46. Faden AI, Lemke M, Demediuk P. Effects of BW755C, a mixed cyclo-oxygenase-lipoxygenase inhibitor, following traumatic spinal cord injury in rats. *Brain Res* 1988; 463: 63–68.
47. Fujita Y, Shingu T, Kurihara M, et al. Evaluation of a low dose administration of aspirin, dipyridamol and steroid. Therapeutic effects on motor function and protective effects on Na^+-K^+-activated ATPase activity against lipid peroxidation in an experimental model of spinal cord injury. *Paraplegia* 1985; 23: 56–57.
48. Siegal T, Lossos F. Experimental neoplastic spinal cord compression: effect of anti-inflammatory agents and glutamate receptor antagonists on vascular permeability. *Neurosurgery* 1990; 26: 967–970.
49. Siegal T, Shohami E, Shapira Y. Comparison of soluble dexamethasone sodium phosphate with free dexamethasone and indomethacin in treatment of experimental neoplastic spinal cord compression. *Spine* 1988; 13: 1171–1176.
50. Iizuka H, Iwasaki Y, Yamamoto T, Kadoya S. Morphometric assessment of drug effects in experimental spinal cord injury. *J Neurosurg* 1986; 65: 92–98.
51. Iwasaki Y, Yamamoto H, Iizuka H, Yamamoto T, Konno H. Suppression of neurofilament degradation by protease inhibitors in experimental spinal cord injury. *Brain Res* 1987; 406: 99–104.
52. Janssen L, Hansebout RR. Pathogenesis of spinal cord injury and newer treatments. A review. *Spine* 1989; 14: 23–32.
53. Young W. Pharmacological therapy of acute spinal cord injury. In: Errico T, Waugh T, Bauer RD, eds. *Spinal cord injury*. Philadelphia: J. B. Lippincott; 1991, pp. 415–433.
54. Blight AR, Gruner JA. Augmentation by 4-aminopyridine of vestibulospinal free fall responses in chronic spinal-injured cats. *J Neurol Sci* 1987; 82: 155–159.
55. Blight AR, Toombs JP, Bauer MS, Widmer WR. The effects of 4-aminopyridine on neurological deficits in chronic cases of traumatic spinal cord injury in dogs: a phase I clinical trial. *J Neurotrauma* 1991; 8: 103–119.
56. Sakatani K, Chesler M, Hassan AZ. $GABA_A$ receptors modulate axonal conduction in dorsal columns of neonatal rat spinal cord. *Brain Res* 1991; 542: 273–279.
57. Sakatani K, Chesler M, Hassan AZ. GABA-sensitivity of dorsal column axons: an in vitro comparison between adult and neonatal rat spinal cords. *Neurosci Lett* (in press).
58. Crozier KS, Graziani V, Ditunno JFJ, Herbison GJ. Spinal cord injury: prognosis for ambulation based on sensory examination in patients who are initially motor complete. *Arch Phys Med Rehabil* 1991; 72: 119–121.
59. Kakulas BA. Pathology of spinal injuries. *Cent Nerv Syst Trauma* 1984; 1: 117–129.
60. Kakulas BA. Pathomorphological evidence for residual spinal cord functions. In: Eccles JC, Dimitrijevic MR, eds. *Upper motor neuron function and dysfunction*. Basel: Karger; 1985, pp. 163–169.
61. Kakulas BA. The clinical neuropathology of spinal cord injury. A guide to the future. *Paraplegia* 1987; 25: 212–216.
62. Puchala E, Windle WF. The possibility of structural and functional restitution after spinal cord injury: a review. *Exp Neurol* 1977; 55: 1–42.
63. Brown PJ, Marino RJ, Herbison GJ, Ditunno JFJ. The 72-hour examination as a predictor of recovery in motor complete quadriplegia. *Arch Phys Med Rehabil* 1991; 72: 546–548.
64. Bracken MB, Shepard MJ, Collins WF, et al. Methylprednisolone or naloxone in the treatment of acute spinal cord injury: one year follow-up results of the second National Acute Spinal Cord Injury Study. *J Neurosurgery* 1992; 76: 23–31.
65. Bracken MB, Shepard MJ, Collins WF, et al. A randomized controlled trial of methylprednisolone or naloxone in the treatment of acute spinal-cord injury: results of the Second National Acute Spinal Cord Injury Study. *N Engl J Med* 1990; 322: 1405–1411.
66. Geisler FH, Dorsey FC, Coleman WP. Recovery of motor function after spinal-cord injury—a randomized, placebo-controlled trial with GM-1 ganglioside. *N Engl J Med* 1991; 324: 1829–1838.
67. Windle WF, Smart JO, Beers JJ. Residual function after subtotal spinal cord transection in adult cats. *Neurology* 1958; 8: 518–521.
68. Guth L, Albuquerque EX, Deshpande SS, Barrett CP, Donati EJ, Warnick JE. Ineffectiveness of enzyme therapy on regeneration in the transected spinal cord of the rat. *J Neurosurg* 1980; 52: 73–86.
69. Guth L, Brewer CR, Collins WF, Goldberger ME, Perl ER. Criteria for evaluating spinal cord regeneration experiments. *Exp Neurol* 1980; 69: 1–3.
70. Blight A, Young W. Axonal morphometric correlates of evoked potentials in experimental spinal cord injury. In: Salzman S, eds. *Neural monitoring*. New York: Humana Press; 1990, pp. 87–113.
71. Kakulas BA, Bedbrook GM. A correlative clinicopathological study of spinal cord injury. *Proc Aust Assoc Neurol* 1969; 6: 123–132.
72. Kakulas BA, Bedbrook GM. Pathology of injuries of the vertebral spinal cord—with emphasis on the microscopic aspects. In: Vincken PJ, eds. *In: Handbook of clinical neurology*. Amsterdam: Elsevier, 1976, pp. 27–42.
73. Alstermark B, Gorska T, Johannisson T, Lund-

berg A. Effects of dorsal column transection in the upper cervical segments on visually guided forelimb movements. *Neurosci Res* 1986; 3: 462–466.
74. Alstermark B, Gorska T, Johannisson T, Lundberg A. Hypermetria in forelimb target-reaching after interruption of the inhibitory pathway from forelimb afferents to C3-C4 propriospinal neurones. *Neurosci Res* 1986; 3: 457–461.
75. Alstermark B, Johannisson T, Lundberg A. The inhibitory feedback pathway from the forelimb to C3-C4 propriospinal neurones investigated with natural stimulation. *Neurosci Res* 1986; 3: 451–456.
76. Alstermark B, Lundberg A, Pinter M, and Sasaki S. Long C3-C5 propriospinal neurones in the cat. *Brain Res*. 1987; 404: 382–388.
77. Alstermark B, Lundberg A, Pinter M, Sasaki S. Vestibular effects in long C3-C5 propriospinal neurones. *Brain Res* 1987; 404: 389–394.
78. Jankowska E, Lundberg A, Stuart D. Propriospinal control of interneurons in spinal reflex pathways from tendon organs in the cat. *Brain Res* 1983; 261: 317–320.
79. Benoist G, Kausz M, Rethelyi M, Pasztor E. Sensitivity of the short range spinal interneurones of the cat to experimental spinal cord trauma. *J Neurosurg* 1979; 51: 834–840.
80. Blight AR. Mechanical factors in experimental spinal cord injury. *J Am Paraplegia Soc* 1988; 11: 26–34.
81. Blumbergs PC, Byrne E. Hypotensive central infection of the spinal cord. *J Neurol Neurosurg Psychiatry* 1980; 43: 751–753.
82. Eidelberg E, Story JL, Meyer BL, Nystel J. Stepping by chronic spinal cats. *Exp Brain Res* 1980; 40: 241–246.
83. Eidelberg E, Straehley D, Erspamer R. Relationship between residual hindlimb assisted locomotion and surviving axons after incomplete spinal cord injuries. *Exp Neurol* 1977; 56: 312–322.
84. Eidelberg E, Walden J, Nguyen L. Locomotor control in macaque monkeys. *Brain* 1981; 104: 647–663.
85. Eidelberg E, Woolf B, Kreinick CJ, Davis F. Role of dorsal funiculi in movement control. *Brain Res* 1976; 114: 427–438.
86. Eidelberg E, Yu J. Effects of corticospinal lesions upon treadmill locomotion in cats. *Exp Brain Res* 1981; 43: 101–103.
87. Eidelberg E, Yu J. Effects of vestibulospinal lesions upon locomotor function in cats. *Brain Res* 1981; 22: 179–183.
88. Sherrington CS. *The integrative action of the nervous system*. (Paperbound edition, 1963). Cambridge, England: Cambridge University Press; 1947.
89. Fukson OI, Berkinblit MB, Feldman AG. The spinal frog takes into account the scheme of its body during the wiping reflex. *Science* 1980; 209: 1261–1263.
90. Belanger M, Drew T, Rossignol S. Spinal locomotion: a comparison of the kinematics and the electromyographic activity in the same animal before and after spinalization. *Acta Biol Hung* 1988; 39: 151–154.
91. Lovely RG, Gregor RJ, Roy RR, Edgerton VR. Effects of training on the recovery of full-weight-bearing stepping in the adult spinal cat. *Exp Neurol* 1986; 92: 421–435.
92. Meisel RL, Rakerd B. Induction of hindlimb stepping movements in rats spinally transected as adults or as neonates. *Brain Res* 1982; 240: 353–356.
93. Dubuc R, Cabelguen JM, Rossignol S. Rhythmic fluctuations of dorsal root potentials and antidromic discharges of primary afferents during fictive locomotion in the cat. *J Neurophysiol* 1988; 60: 2014–36.
94. Gossard JP, Cabelguen JM, Rossignol S. Intra-axonal recordings of cutaneous primary afferents during fictive locomotion in the cat. *J Neurophysiol* 1989; 62: 1177–1188.
95. Gossard JP, Cabelguen JM, Rossignol S. Phase-dependent modulation of primary afferent depolarization in single cutaneous primary afferents evoked by peripheral stimulation during fictive locomotion in the cat. *Brain Res* 1990; 537: 14–23.
96. Gossard JP, Cabelguen JM, Rossignol S. An intracellular study of muscle primary afferents during fictive locomotion in the cat. *J Neurophysiol* 1991; 65: 914–926.
97. Barbeau H, Julien C, Rossignol S. The effects of clonidine and yohimbine on locomotion and cutaneous reflexes in the adult chronic spinal cat. *Brain Res* 1987; 437: 83–96.
98. Barbeau H, Rossignol S. The effects of serotonergic drugs on the locomotor pattern and on cutaneous reflexes of the adult chronic spinal cat. *Brain Res* 1990; 514: 55–67.
99. Christenson J, Bongianni F, Grillner S, Hökfelt T. Putative GABAergic input to axons of spinal interneurons and primary sensory neurons in the lamprey spinal cord as shown by intracellular Lucifer yellow and GABA immunohistochemistry. *Brain Res* 1991; 538: 313–318.
100. Dubuc R, Rossignol S. The effects of 4-aminopyridine on the cat spinal cord: rhythmic antidromic discharges recorded from the dorsal roots. *Brain Res* 1989; 491: 335–348.
101. Jankowska E, Lundberg A, Rudomin P, Sykova E. Effects of 4-aminopyridine on synaptic transmission in the cat spinal cord. *Brain Res* 1982; 240: 117–129.
102. Kato M, Murakami S, Yasuda K, Hirayama H. Disruption of fore- and hindlimb coordination during overground locomotion in cats with bilateral serial hemisection of the spinal cord. *Neurosci Res* 1984; 2: 27–47.
103. Andersson O, Grillner S. Peripheral control of the cat's step cycle. II. Entrainment of the central pattern generators for locomotion by sinusoidal hip movements during "fictive locomotion". *Acta Physiol Scand* 1983; 118: 229–239.
104. Waxman SG. Conduction in myelinated, unmyelinated, and demyelinated fibers. *Arch Neurol* 1977; 34: 585–589.
105. Waxman SG. Prerequisites for conduction in

demyelinated fibers. *Neurology* 1978; 28: 27–33.
106. Waxman SG. Biophysical mechanisms of impulse conduction in demyelinated axons. In: Waxman SG, eds. *Functional recovery in neurological disease.* New York: Raven Press; 1988, pp. 185–213.
107. Balentine JD. Pathology of experimental spinal cord trauma. II. Ultrastructure of axons and myelin. *Lab Invest* 1978; 39: 254–255.
108. Balentine JD, Hilton CW. Ultrastructural pathology of axons and myelin in calcium induced myelopathy. *J Neuropathol Exp Neurol* 1980; 39: 339–345.
109. Banik NL, Hogan EL, Whetstine LJ, Balentine JD. Changes in myelin and axonal proteins in $CaCl_2$-induced myelopathy in rat spinal cord. *Cent Nerv Syst Trauma* 1984; 1: 131–138.
110. Banik NL, Powers JM, Hogan EL. Effects of spinal cord trauma on myelin. *J Neuropathol Exp Neurol* 1980; 39: 232–244.
111. Gledhill RF, Harrison BM, McDonald WI. Demyelination after acute spinal cord compression. *Exp Neurol* 1973; 28: 472–487.
112. McDonald WI. Mechanisms of functional loss and recovery in spinal cord damage. In: eds. *Symposium on the outcome of severe damage to the central nervous system.* Amsterdam: Elsevier; 1974, pp. 24–35.
113. Wakefield CL, Eidelberg E. Electron microscopic observations of the delayed effects of spinal cord compression. *Exp Neurol* 1975; 48: 637–646.
114. Stokes BT, Fox P, Hallinden G. Extracellular calcium activity in the injured spinal cord. *Exp Neurol* 1983; 80: 561–572.
115. Young W, Flamm ES. Effect of high dose corticosteroid therapy on blood flow, evoked potentials, and extracellular calcium in experimental spinal injury. *J Neurosurg* 1982; 57: 667–673.
116. Young W, Yen V, Blight A. Extracellular calcium activity in experimental spinal cord contusion. *Brain Res* 1982; 253: 115–123.
117. Blank WDJ, Bunge MB, Bunge RP. The sensitivity of the myelin sheath, particularly the Schwann cell axolemmal junction, to lowered calcium levels in cultured sensory ganglia. *Brain Res* 1974; 67: 503–518.
118. Frankenhaeuser B. The effect of calcium on the myelinated nerve fibre. *J Physiol (Lond)* 1957; 137: 245–260.
119. Banik NL, Hogan EL, Powers JM, Whetstine LJ. Degradation of cytoskeletal proteins in experimental spinal injury. *Neurochem Res* 1982; 7: 1465–1475.
120. Banik NL, Powers JM, Smith KP. Ca^{2+} activated neutral proteinase in normal and traumatized spinal cord. *Soc Neurosci Abstr* 1979; 5: 396.
121. Trotter JL, Clark HB, Collins KG, Wegeschiede CL, Scarpellini JD. Myelin proteolipid protein induces demyelinating disease in mice. *J Neurol Sci* 1987; 79: 173–188.
122. Waxman SG, Kocsis JD, Nitta KC. Lysophosphatidyl choline-induced focal demyelination in the rabbit corpus callosum. *J Neurol Sci* 1979; 44: 45–53.
123. Tipperman R, Kasckow J, Herndon RM. The fine structure of macrophages in lysolecithin-induced demyelination: a freeze-fracture study. *J Neuropathol Exp Neurol* 1984; 43: 522–530.
124. Triarhou LC, Herndon RM. Effect of macrophage inactivation on the neuropathology of lysolecithin-induced demyelination. *Br J Exp Pathol* 1985; 66: 293–301.
125. Hsu CY, Halushka PV, Hogan EL, Banik NL, Lee WA, Perot PL. Alterations of thromboxane and prostacyclin levels in experimental spinal cord injury. *Neurology* 1985; 35: 1003–1009.
126. Palladini G, Grossi M, Maleci A, Lauro GM, Guidetti B. Immunocomplexes in rat and rabbit spinal cord after injury. *Exp Neurol* 1987; 95: 639–651.
127. Rebhun J, Madorsky JG, Glovsky MM. Proteins of the complement system and acute phase reactants in sera of patients with spinal cord injury. *Ann Allergy* 1991; 66: 335–338.
128. Lassmann H, Stemberger H, Kitz K, Wisniewski HM. In vivo demyelinating activity of sera from animals with chronic experimental allergic encephalomyelitis. Antibody nature of the demyelinating factor and the role of complement. *J Neurol Sci* 1983; 59: 123–137.
129. Liu WT, Vanguri P, Shin ML. Studies on demyelination in vitro: the requirement of membrane attack components of the complement system. *J Immunol* 1983; 131: 778–782.
130. Rodriguez M, Lucchinetti CF, Clark RJ, Yakash TL, Markowitz H, Lennon VA. Immunoglobulins and complement in demyelination induced in mice by Theiler's virus. *J Immunol* 1988; 140: 800–806.
131. Triarhou LC, Herndon RM. The effect of dexamethasone on L-alpha-lysophosphatidyl choline (lysolecithin)-induced demyelination of the rat spinal cord. *Arch Neurol* 1986; 43: 121–125.
132. Vanguri P, Shin ML. Hydrolysis of myelin basic protein in human myelin by terminal complement complexes. *J Biol Chem* 1988; 263: 7228–7234.
133. Selmaj KW, Raine CS. Tumor necrosis factor mediates myelin and oligodendrocyte damage in vitro. *Ann Neurol* 1988; 23: 339–346.
134. Baker M, Bostock H, Grafe P, Martius P. Function and distribution of three types of rectifying channel in rat spinal root myelinated axons. *J Physiol (Lond)* 1987; 383: 45–67.
135. Blight AR, Someya S. Depolarizing afterpotentials in myelinated axons of mammalian spinal cord. *Neuroscience* 1985; 15: 1–12.
136. Kaars C, Faber DS. Myelinated central vertebrate axon lacks voltage sensitive potassium conductance. *Science* 1981; 212: 1063–1065.
137. Gruner JA. Comparison of vestibular and auditory startle responses in the rat and cat. *J Neurosci Methods* 1989; 27: 13–23.
138. Young W, Rosenbluth J, Wojak JC, Sakatani K, Kim H. Extracellular potassium activity

and axonal conduction in spinal cord of the myelin-deficient mutant rat. *Exp Neurol* 1989; 106: 41–51.
139. Kocsis JD, Eng DL, Gordon TR, Waxman SG. Functional differences between 4-aminopyridine and tetraethylammonium-sensitive potassium channels in myelinated axons. *Neurosci Lett* 1987; 75: 193–198.
140. Kocsis JD, Ruiz JA, Waxman SG. Maturation of mammalian myelinated fibers: changes in action-potential characteristics following 4-aminopyridine application. *J Neurophysiol* 1983; 50: 449–63.
141. Jones RE, Heron JR, Foster DH, Snelgar RS, Mason RJ. Effects of 4-aminopyridine in patients with multiple sclerosis. *J Neurol Sci* 1983; 60: 353–362.
142. Stefoski D, Davis FA, Faut M, Schauf CL. 4-Aminopyridine improves clinical signs in multiple sclerosis. *Ann Neurol* 1987; 21: 71–77.
143. Bowe CM, Kocsis JD, Targ EF, Waxman SG. Physiological effects of 4-aminopyridine on demyelinated mammalian motor and sensory fibers. *Ann Neurol* 1987; 22: 264–268.
144. Eng LF, Gordon TR, Kocsis JD, Waxman SG. Development of 4-AP and TEA sensitivities in mammalian myelinated nerve fibers. *J Neurophysiol* 1988; 60: 2168–2179.
145. Kaji R, Sumner AJ. Effects of 4-aminopyridine in experimental CNS demyelination. *Neurology* 1988; 38: 1884–1887.
146. Sherratt RM, Bostock H, Sears TA. Effects of 4-aminopyridine on normal and demyelinated mammalian nerve fibers. *Nature* 1980; 283: 570–572.
147. Targ EF, Kocsis JD. 4-Aminopyridine leads to restoration of conduction in demyelinated rat sciatic nerve. *Brain Res* 1985; 328: 358–361.
148. Crain SM, Crain B, Peterson ER, Hiller JM, Simon EJ. Exposure to 4-aminopyridine prevents depressant effects of opiates on sensory-evoked dorsal-horn network responses in spinal cord cultures. *Life Sci* 1982; 31: 235–240.
149. Dubuc R, Rossignol S, Lamarre Y. The effects of 4-aminopyridine on the spinal cord: rhythmic discharges recorded from the peripheral nerves. *Brain Res* 1986; 369: 243–259.
150. Blakemore WF. Observations on remyelination in the rabbit spinal cord following demyelination induced by lysolecithin. *Neuropathol Appl Neurobiol* 1978; 4: 47–59.
151. Blakemore WF. Limited remyelination of CNS axons by Schwann cells transplanted into the sub-arachnoid space. *J Neurol Sci* 1984; 64: 265–276.
152. Blakemore WF, Crang AJ. The use of cultured autologous Schwann cells to remyelinate areas of persistent demyelination in the central nervous system. *J Neurol Sci* 1985; 70: 207–223.
153. Blakemore WF, Crang AJ, Evans RJ, Patterson RC. Rat Schwann cell remyelination of demyelinated cat CNS axons: evidence that injection of cell suspensions of CNS tissue results in Schwann cell remyelination. *Neurosci Lett* 1987; 77: 15–19.
154. Blakemore WF, Crang AJ, Patterson RC. Schwann cell remyelination of CNS axons following injection of cultures of CNS cells into areas of persistent demyelination. *Neurosci Lett* 1987; 77: 20–24.
155. Dal Canto MC, Lipton HL. Schwann cell remyelination and recurrent demyelination in central nervous system of mice infected with attenuated Theiler's virus. *Am J Pathol* 1980; 98: 101–122.
156. Harrison B. Schwann cell and oligodendrocyte remyelination in lysolecithin-induced lesions in irradiated rat spinal cord. *J Neurol Sci* 1985; 67: 143–159.
157. Raine CS, Moore GR, Hintzen R, Traugott U. Induction of oligodendrocyte proliferation and remyelination after chronic demyelination. Relevance to multiple sclerosis. *Lab Invest* 1988; 59: 467–476.
158. Arenella LS, Herndon RM. Mature oligodendrocytes. Division following experimental demyelination in adult animals. *Arch Neurol* 1984; 41: 1162–1165.
159. Dutly F, Schwab ME. How is oligodendrocyte differentiation and myelin formation regulated? *Schweiz Arch Neurol Psychiatr* 1989; 140: 19–21.
160. Blakemore WF. Remyelination by Schwann cells of axons demyelinated by intraspinal injection of 6-aminonicotinamide in the rat. *J Neurocytol* 1975; 4: 745–757.
161. Blakemore WF. Remyelination of CNS axons by Schwann cells transplanted from the sciatic nerve. *Nature (Lond)* 1981; 266: 68–69.
162. Feigin I, Ogata J. Schwann cells and peripheral myelin within human central nervous tissues: the mesenchymal character of Schwann cells. *J Neuropathol Exp Neurol* 1971; 30: 603–612.
163. Felts PA, Smith KJ. Schwann cell remyelination restores secure conduction to central demyelinated fibers. *Soc Neurosci Abstr* 1987; 13: 499.
164. Harrison BM, Pollard JD. Pattern of Schwann cell remyelination in a spinal cord lesion. *Neurosci Lett* 1984; 52: 275–280.
165. Itoyama Y, Webster HD, Richardson EPJ, Trapp BD. Schwann cell remyelination of demyelinated axons in spinal cord multiple sclerosis lesions. *Ann Neurol* 1983; 14: 339–346.
166. Raine CS. On the occurrence of Schwann cells in normal central nervous system. *J Neurocytol* 1976; 5: 371–380.
167. Prineas JW, Connell F. Remyelination in multiple sclerosis. *Ann Neurol* 1979; 5: 22–31.
168. Prineas JW, Kwon EE, Cho ES, Sharer LR. Continual breakdown and regeneration of myelin in progressive multiple sclerosis plaques. *Ann NY Acad Sci* 1984; 436: 11–32.
169. Caroni P, Savio T, Schwab ME. Central nervous system regeneration: oligodendrocytes and myelin as non-permissive substrates for neurite growth. *Prog Brain Res* 1988; 78: 363–370.
170. Caroni P, Schwab ME. Two membrane protein

fractions from rat central myelin with inhibitory properties for neurite growth and fibroblast spreading. *J Cell Biol* 1988; 106: 1281–1288.
171. Caronni P, Schwab ME. Codistribution of neurite growth inhibitors and oligodendrocytes in rat CNS: appearance follows nerve fiber growth and precedes myelination. *Dev Biol* 1989; 136: 287–295.
172. Savio T, Schwab ME. Rat CNS white matter, but not gray matter, is nonpermissive for neuronal cell adhesion and fiber outgrowth. *J Neurosci* 1989; 9: 1126–1133.
173. Savio T, Schwab ME. Lesioned corticospinal tract axons regenerate in myelin-free rat spinal cord. *Proc Natl Acad Sci USA* 1990; 87: 4130–4133.
174. Schnell L, Schwab ME. Axonal regeneration in the rat spinal cord produced by an antibody against myelin-associated neurite growth inhibitors. *Nature* 1990; 343: 269–272.
175. Schwab ME. Myelin-associated inhibitors of neurite growth. *Exp Neurol* 1990; 109: 2–5.
176. Schwab ME, Caroni P. Oligodendrocytes and CNS myelin are nonpermissive substrates for neurite growth and fibroblast spreading in vitro. *J Neurosci* 1988; 8: 2381–2393.
177. Wekerle H, Schwab M, Linington C, Meyermann R. Antigen presentation in the peripheral nervous system: Schwann cells present endogenous myelin autoantigens to lymphocytes. *Eur J Immunol* 1986; 16: 1551–1557.
178. Brockes JP, Fields KL, Raff MC. Studies on cultured rat Schwann cells. I. Establishment of purified populations from cultures of peripheral nerve. *Brain Res* 1979; 165: 105–118.
179. Seil FJ, Blank NK. Myelination of central nervous system axons in tissue culture by transplanted oligodendrocytes. *Science* 1981; 212: 1407–1408.
180. DiStefano PS, Johnson EMJ. Nerve growth factor receptors on cultured rat Schwann cells. *J Neurosci* 1988; 8: 231–241.
181. Johnson EMJ. Regulation of nerve growth factor receptor expression on Schwann cells. *Prog Brain Res* 1988; 78: 327–331.
182. Johnson EMJ, Taniuchi M, DiStefano PS. Expression and possible function of nerve growth factor receptors on Schwann cells. *Trends Neurosci* 1988; 11: 299–304.
183. Taniuchi M, Clark HB, Johnson EMJ. Induction of nerve growth factor receptor in Schwann cells after axotomy. *Proc Natl Acad Sci USA* 1986; 83: 4094–4098.
184. Taniuchi M, Clark HB, Schweitzer JB, Johnson EMJ. Expression of nerve growth factor receptors by Schwann cells of axotomized peripheral nerves: ultrastructural location, suppression by axonal contact, and binding properties. *J Neurosci* 1988; 8: 664–681.
185. Bracken MB, Shepard MJ, Hellenbrand KG, et al. Methyprednisolone and neurological function 1 year after spinal cord injury. *J Neurosurg* 1985; 63: 704–713.
186. Frankel HL, Hancock DO, Hyslop G, et al. The value of postural reduction in the initial management of closed injuries of the spine with paraplegia and tetraplegia. I. *Paraplegia* 1969; 7: 179–192.
187. Dimitrijevic MR, Dimitrijevic MM, Sherwood AM, Faganel J, et al. Neurophysiological evaluation of chronic spinal cord stimulation in patients with upper motor neuron disorders. *Int Rehab Med* 1980; 2: 82–85.
188. Dimitrijevic MR, Faganel J, Lehmkuhl D, Sherwood AM. *Motor control in man after partial or complete spinal cord injury*. New York: Raven Press; 1983.
189. Dimitrijevic MR, Dimitrijevic MM, Faganel J, Sherwood AM. Suprasegmentally induced motor unit activity in paralyzed muscles of patients with established spinal cord injury. *Ann Neurol* 1984; 16: 216–221.
190. Dimitrijevic MR. *Residual motor functions in spinal cord injury*. New York: Raven Press; 1988.
191. Young W, Koreh I, Yen V, Lindsay A. Effects of sympathectomy on extracellular potassium activity and blood flow in experimental spinal cord contusion. *Brain Res* 1982; 253: 105–113.
192. Cohen AR, Young W, Ransohoff J. Intraspinal localization of somatosensory evoked potentials. *Neurosurgery* 1981; 9: 157–162.
193. Young W, Cohen AR, Hunt CD, Ransohoff J. Acute physiological effects of ultrasonic vibrations on nervous tissue. *Neurosurgery* 1981; 8: 689–694.
194. Young W, Bracken MB. The Second National Acute Spinal Cord Injury Study. In: Jane J, Torner J, Anderson D, and WY eds. *NIH Central Nervous System Status Report 1991*. New York: Mary Ann Liebert; 1991.
195. Eidelberg E, Nguyen LH, Polich R, Walden JG. Transsynaptic degeneration of motoneurones caudal to spinal cord lesions. *Brain Res Bull* 1989; 22: 39–45.
196. Kaelan C, Jacobsen PF, Kakulas BA. An investigation of possible transynaptic neuronal degeneration in human spinal cord injury. *J Neurol Sci* 1988; 86: 231–237.
197. Feringa ER, Gilbertie WJ, Vahlsing HL. Histologic evidence for death of cortical neurons after spinal cord transection. *Neurology* 1984; 34: 1002–1006.
198. Feringa ER, Lee GW, and Vahlsing HL. Cell death in Clarke's column after spinal cord transection. *J Neuropathol Exp Neurol* 1985; 44: 156–164.
199. Feringa ER, Lee GW, Vahlsing HL, Gilbertie WJ. Cell death in the adult rat dorsal root ganglion after hindlimb amputation, spinal cord transection, or both operations. *Exp Neurol* 1985; 87: 349–357.
200. Feringa ER, Vahlsing HL. Labelled corticospinal neurons one year after spinal cord transection. *Neurosci Lett* 1985; 58: 283–286.
201. Liu CN, Chambers WW. Intraspinal sprouting of dorsal root axons. *Arch Neurol Psychiatr* 1958; 79: 46–61.

202. Goldberger EM, Murray M. Recovery of movement and axonal sprouting may obey some of the same laws. In: Cotman CW, eds. *Neuronal plasticity*. New York: Academic Press; 1978, pp. 174–182.
203. Goldberger ME, Murray M. Restitution of function and collateral sprouting in the cat spinal cord: the deafferented animal. *J Comp Neurol* 1974; 158: 37–54.
204. Hulsebosch CE, Coggeshall RE. Quantitation of sprouting of dorsal root axons. *Science* 1981; 213: 1020–1021.
205. Hulsebosch CE, Perez-Polo JR, Coggeshall RE. In vivo ANTI-NGF induces sprouting of sensory axons in dorsal roots. *J Comp Neurol* 1987; 259: 445–451.
206. Murray M, Goldberger ME. Restitution of function and collateral sprouting in the cat spinal cord: the partially hemisected animal. *J Comp Neurol* 1974; 158: 19–36.
207. Prendergast J, Murray M, Goldberger ME. Sprouting and reflex recovery after spinal nerve lesions in cats. *Exp Neurol* 1981; 73: 732–749.
208. Bregman BS, Goldberger ME. Anatomical plasticity and sparing of function after spinal cord damage in neonatal cats. *Science* 1982; 217: 553–555.
209. Scheff SW, Benardo LS, Cotman CW. Hydrocortisone administration retards axon sprouting in the rat dentate gyrus. *Exp Neurol* 1980; 68: 195–201.
210. Scheff SW, Cotman CW. Chronic glucocorticoid therapy alters axon sprouting in the hippocampal dentate gyrus. *Exp Neurol* 1982; 76: 644–654.
211. Scheff SW, Dekosky ST. Steroid suppression of axon sprouting in the hippocampal dentate gyrus of the adult rat: dose-response relationship. *Exp Neurol* 1983; 82: 183–191.
212. Morse JK, Scheff SW, Dekosky ST. Gonadal steroids influence axon sprouting in the hippocampal dentate gyrus: a sexually dimorphic response. *Exp Neurol* 1986; 94: 649–658.
213. McCouch GP, Austin GM, Liu CN, Liu CY. Sprouting as a cause of spasticity. *J Neurophysiol* 1958; 21: 205–216.
214. Ramón y Cajal S. *Degeneration and regeneration of the nervous system*. London: Oxford University Press; 1928.
215. Anderson MJ, Swanson KA, Waxman SG, Engl LF. Glial fibrillary acidic protein in regenerating teleost spinal cord. *J Histochem Cytochem* 1984; 32: 1099–1106.
216. Borgens RB, Roederer E, Cohen MJ. Enhanced spinal cord regeneration in lamprey by applied electrical fields. *Science* 1981; 213: 611–617.
217. Mackler SA, Selzer ME. Regeneration of functional synapses between individual recognizable neurons in the lamprey spinal cord. *Science* 1985; 229: 774–776.
218. Mackler SA, Selzer ME. Specificity of synaptic regeneration in the spinal cord of the larval sea lamprey. *J Physiol (Lond)* 1987; 388: 183–198.
219. MacVicar BA, Llinas RR. Barium action potentials in regenerating axons of the lamprey spinal cord. *J Neurosci Res* 1985; 13: 323–335.
220. Masuda NLM, Nicholls JG. Extracellular matrix molecules in development and regeneration of the leech CNS. *Philos Trans R Soc Lond [Biol]*. 1991; 331: 323–35.
221. Wood MR, Cohen MJ. Synaptic regeneration in identified neurons of the lamprey spinal cord. *Science* 1979; 206: 344–347.
222. Borgens RB, Blight AR, Murphy DJ. Axonal regeneration in spinal cord injury: a perspective and new technique. *J Comp Neurol* 1986; 250: 157–167.
223. Borgens RB, Blight AR, Murphy DJ, Stewart L. Transected dorsal column axons within the guinea pig spinal cord regenerate in the presence of an applied electric field. *J Comp Neurol* 1986; 250: 168–180.
224. Lampert P, Cressman M. Axonal regeneration in the dorsal columns of the spinal cord of adult rats. An electron mircoscopic study. *Lab Invest* 1964; 13: 825–839.
225. Foerster AP. Spontaneous regeneration of cut axons in adult rat brain. *J Comp Neurol* 1982; 210: 335–356.
226. Khan T, Dauzvardis M, Sayers S, Carbon filament implants promote axonal growth across the transected rat spinal cord. *Brain Res* 1991; 541: 139–145.
227. Richardson PM, Verge VMK. Axonal regeneration in dorsal spinal roots is accelerated by peripheral axonal transection. *Brain Res* 1987; 411: 406–408.
228. Aguayo AJ, Benfey M, David S. A potential for axonal regeneration in neurons of the adult mammalian nervous system. *Birth Defects* 1983; 19: 327–340.
229. Benfey M, Aguayo AJ. Extensive elongation of axons from rat brain into peripheral nerve grafts. *Nature* 1982; 296: 150–152.
230. Bray GM, Vidal SM, Aguayo AJ. Regeneration of axons from the central nervous system of adult rats. *Prog Brain Res* 1987; 71: 373–379.
231. Bray GM, Villegas-Perez MP, Vidal-Sanz M, Aguayo AJ. The use of peripheral nerve grafts to enhance neuronal survival, promote growth and permit terminal reconnections in the central nervous system of adult rats. *J Exp Biol* 1987; 132: 5–19.
232. David S, Aguayo AJ. Axonal elongation into peripheral nervous system "bridges" after central nervous system injury in adult rats. *Science* 1981; 214: 931–933.
233. David S, Aguayo AJ. Axonal regeneration after crush injury of rat central nervous system fibres innervating peripheral nerve grafts. *J Neurocytol* 1985; 14: 1–12.
234. Richardson PM, Issa VM, Aguayo AJ. Regeneration of long spinal axons in the rat. *J Neurocytol* 1984; 13: 165–182.
235. Aguayo AJ, Vidal SM, Villegas-Perez MP, Bray GM. Growth and connectivity of axotomized retinal neurons in adult rats with optic nerves

substituted by PNS grafts linking the eye and the midbrain. *Ann NY Acad Sci* 1987; 495: 1–9.
236. Benfey M, Bunger UR, Vidal SM, Bray GM, Aguayo AJ. Axonal regeneration from GABAergic neurons in the adult rat thalamus. *J Neurocytol* 1985; 14: 279–296.
237. Carter DA, Bray GM, Aguayo AJ. Regenerated retinal ganglion cell axons can form well-differentiated synapses in the superior colliculus of adult hamsters. *J Neurosci* 1989; 9: 4042–4050.
238. Keirstead SA, Rasminsky M, Fukuda Y, Carter DA, Aguayo AJ, Vidal SM. Electrophysiologic responses in hamster superior colliculus evoked by regenerating retinal axons. *Science* 1989; 246: 255–257.
239. Munz M, Rasminsky M, Aguayo AJ, Vidal-Sanz M, Devor MG. Functional activity of rat brainstem neurons regenerating axons along peripheral nerve grafts. *Brain Res* 1985; 340: 115–125.
240. Vidal-Sanz M, Bray GM, Villegas-Perez MP, Thanos S, Aguayo AJ. Axonal regeneration and synapse formation in the superior colliculus by retinal ganglion cells in the adult rat. *J Neurosci* 1987; 7: 2894–2909.

10

Traumatic Brain Injury

The Pathobiology of Injury and Repair

John T. Povlishock

Department of Anatomy, Medical College of Virginia/Virginia Commonwealth University, Richmond, Virginia 23298-0709

When basic scientists experimentally evaluate those issues relevant to central nervous system injury and repair, it is often stated that the purpose of such investigations is to provide new and useful information that may ultimately lead to the better management and treatment of brain-injured man. Despite the fact that numerous papers commonly reflect this theme, it is remarkable how few actually consider the pathobiological phenomena directly relevant to traumatically brain-injured man. This shortcoming stems, in part, from the fact that the majority of the literature dealing with traumatic brain injury resides in the clinical realm, which frequently provides the basic scientist with a sometimes incomplete appreciation of those events operant with traumatic brain injury. In view of these factors, the goal of the present communication is to provide an overview of those basic science issues of immediate relevance to traumatic brain injury. In this context, this chapter not only will focus on mechanisms of traumatic brain injury but also will consider mechanisms of posttraumatic reorganization and repair. Obviously, no chapter can consider all aspects of traumatic brain injury; thus, in the present overview, we have chosen to focus only on those aspects of traumatic brain injury that constitute the major substrates of the morbidity and recovery associated with the traumatic condition.

THE BRAIN PARENCHYMAL RESPONSE TO TRAUMA

When considering the brain's response to trauma, it is important to recall that all traumatic events do not influence the brain in precisely the same fashion. Thus, the pathobiology associated with assaults, falls from limited heights, or missile injuries is different from that associated with a high-speed automobile accident. With assaults, falls, or missile injuries focal changes predominate, whereas with motor vehicle accidents involving considerable acceleration/deceleration of the brain, diffuse change generally occurs throughout the brain parenchyma. The purpose of this chapter is not to review all the pathobiology of focal versus diffuse injury. Rather, the purpose of this text is to alert the reader that such differences exist and, as such, must be taken into consideration when evaluating specific mechanisms of brain injury and repair.

Most information suggests that when the brain is traumatically injured, several types of change occur, and as such, these changes impact upon both the morbidity and recovery associated with the injury. Typically, both brain parenchymal and cerebral vascular changes are triggered by the traumatic event, and depending upon the severity of the injury as well as the nature of the primary insult (fall versus motor vehicle accident) various forms of brain parenchymal and vascular abnormalities have been described. These include focal and diffuse brain parenchymal changes ranging from a net phase of neural excitation to traumatically induced axotomy in addition to vascular changes ranging from subtle perturbation of the blood-brain barrier to overt hematoma formation. In the following passages, we will review those changes suggested to occur with traumatic brain injury.

Traumatically Induced Changes in the Brain Parenchyma

Neuroexcitation/Abnormal Agonist Receptor Interaction

Perhaps, one of the newest and most rapidly developing areas in traumatic brain injury research centers on the question as to whether or not a net phase of excitation, triggered by the traumatic episode, directly contributes to some of the morbidity associated with injury. In this scenario, it is envisioned that, in the case of mild, moderate, and severe traumatic brain injury, the tensile forces of the traumatic episode cause mass depolarization with the release of multiple transmitter systems. In this process, it is believed that these transmitters act at their receptor sites to trigger agonist-receptor interactions that have enduring adverse affects upon their postsynaptic targets. (For a detailed review, see Hayes et al., ref. 1.) In the process of traumatically induced neuroexcitation, considerable attention has been focused on the potential role of the cholinergic and glutaminergic systems (1–14). It is believed that the cholinergic muscarinic receptor and the glutamate N-methyl-D-aspartate (NMDA) receptor play pivotal roles in the damaging sequelae of injury and, thus, are direct contributors to the morbidity associated with injury (1–14). Support for the role of abnormal agonist-receptor interactions in the pathobiology of traumatic injury has emerged from several lines of evidence. Specifically, in the case of moderate and severe traumatic brain injury, it been shown that the traumatic episode is associated with a net tissue increase in excitatory amino acids such as glutamate (4,5). This has been confirmed by in vivo microdialysis with the suggestion that the excitatory amino acids have been derived through traumatically induced neurotransmitter release (4,5). In these studies, considerable interest has focused on the potentially damaging consequences of such glutamate release; however, at present, new information is beginning to suggest that multiple transmitter systems may be implicated in the pathobiology of trauma. Although work in this area is just evolving, various receptor antagonists have been shown to be beneficial in blunting some of the damaging consequences of injury. Pretreatment with phencyclidine, a glutamate-NMDA receptor antagonist, has improved the behavioral deficits seen following experimental traumatic brain injury in rats (9). Similarly, the use of MK-801, a noncompetitive NMDA antagonist, has also been associated with considerable protection in brain-injured rats (12,13). Further, pretreatment or early posttreatment with pharmacological antagonists of the muscarinic cholinergic receptor can afford protection from the pathophysiology associated with TBI. For example, pretreatment or immediate posttreatment with scopolamine (1.0 mg/kg intraperitoneally) significantly reduces the functional motor deficits associated with fluid percussion TBI in the rat (6,14). Of further interest is the observation that combinations of multiple receptor antagonists also translate into significant cerebral protection. It has been recognized that the combination of mild traumatic brain injury with mild ischemic insult results in hippocampal cell loss in the selectively vulnerable areas of the brain despite the fact that independently these insults are incapable of evoking any brain parenchymal change (15). However, when animals subjected to such dual insults were pretreated with both glutamate-NMDA and cholinergic muscarinic receptor antagonists (phencyclidine and scopolamine), complete protection was afforded, with sparing of the hippocampus (16). Collectively, then, all the above information points to the involvement of multiple agonist-receptor interactions in the pathobiology of injury. Parenthetically, it should be pointed out that the above-described sequence of events described in brain-injured animals may also be operant in humans who have sustained severe traumatic brain injuries. Preliminary in vivo microdialysis conducted in such patients has identified elevated glutamate levels with the suggestion that this was contributing to the morbidity seen in this patient population (17).

Although in animals and humans there is now compelling evidence that traumatic brain injury elicits the release of multiple neurotransmitter systems, it is unclear precisely how this transmitter surge translates into the morbidity associated with the traumatic condition. As can be gleaned from those studies demonstrating protection afforded through the use of receptor antagonists, some event involving the agonist receptor interface must be pivotal in the pathobiology of trauma. Some have speculated that the agonist-receptor surge contributes to postsynaptic change, which then translates into morbidity (1,2). In this scenario, it is envisioned that the excitatory activity translates into possible nonlethal intracellular calcium nonregulation, which, in turn, affects cell function (1). Such a postulated pathway constitutes a significant departure from previous thought, which held that all neuroexcitotoxic events result in the lethal activation of calcium-sensitive neuronal effector-systems leading to cell death (18–20). Therefore, in the context of traumatic brain injury, the suggestion of sublethal neuroexcitotoxicity is novel and implies that this nonlethal event may be potentially amenable to therapeutic intervention.

Axonal Damage

Despite the fact that data are beginning to emerge regarding the pathobiological implications of traumatically induced agonist-receptor interactions, many questions still remain unresolved. In contrast to this situation, however, there is now considerable evidence that the tensile forces of the traumatic event also alter axons in animals and man and thereby directly contribute to morbidity (21–45). In animals and humans surviving the traumatic event for periods ranging from days to several weeks, evidence of traumatically induced axonal injury is found in the occurrence of reactive axonal swellings or retraction balls seen scattered throughout the brain parenchyma (21,22,24, 26–28,30,31). Such reactive axonal swellings or retraction balls are seen as enlarged spheroid masses of axoplasm capping an axonal shaft, which appears disconnected from its downstream/distal partner (Figs. 1 and 2). This appearance has led to the often-stated belief that these axonal profiles were formed, at the moment of injury, by traumatic forces that tear the axon, causing it to retract and expel a ball of axoplasm (21,22,28,30). It was envisioned that these traumatically torn axons would then disconnect from their target sites and, thereby, result in the morbidity associated with the injury (30).

With continued survival (several weeks to months), these axonal events were associated with microglia clustering, followed, in time, by the occurrence of Wallerian degeneration involving the distal, disconnected axonal segment (23,27). Collectively, the pathological recognition of reactive axonal

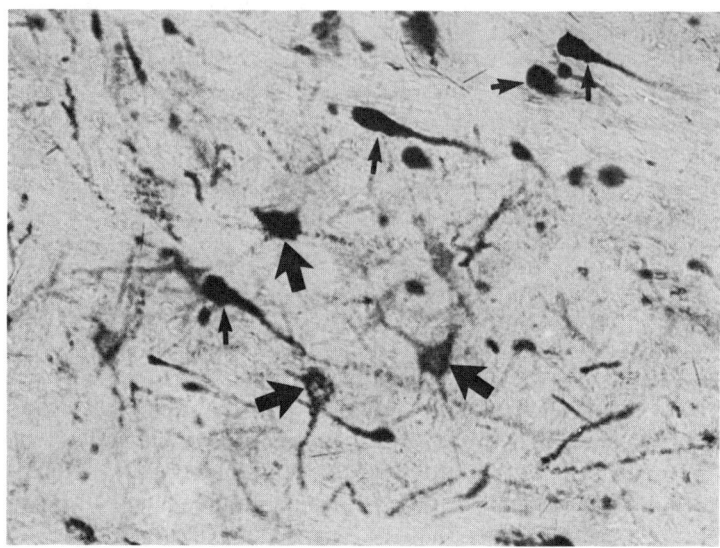

FIG. 1. This light micrograph reveals traumatically induced axonal damage in an experimental animal. Through the use of anterogradely transported HRP, damaged axons can be recognized as enlarged tracer-containing swellings *(arrows)* that occur at the site of axonal disconnection. Note that despite the presence of these reactive axonal swellings, other intact axons can also be seen in the field. *Block arrows* demarcate the appendages of neurons in the field that have been retrogradely labeled with HRP. × 500.

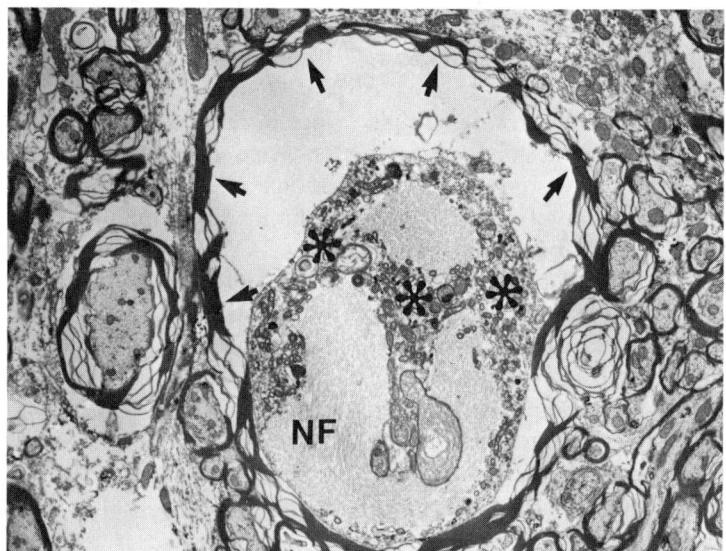

FIG. 2A and B. In this electron micrograph, a reactive axonal swelling can be seen 24 hr postinjury. Note that the swelling contains organelles *(asterisks)* that cap a neurofilamentous core *(NF)*. Also note that this swelling, which is detached from the distal axonal segment, is completely encompassed by a thinned distended myeline sheath *(arrows)*. ×2,500.

swellings, microglia clustering, and/or Wallerian change have been taken as evidence for the occurrence of traumatically induced axonal change. Based upon the identification of these features, axonal injury has now been identified following mild, moderate, and severe traumatic brain throughout the brain, in multiple foci wherein other intact and undamaged fiber systems were also seen (21–29,31). The widespread or diffuse occurrence of such axonal damage has led to its characterization as diffuse axonal injury (DAI), and at present, this term has gained widespread use in both the clinical and laboratory setting (28,30). Considerable significance has been attached to the occurrence of diffusely damaged axons, as it has been suggested that diffuse axonal injury, independent of any other brain change, can result in serious neurological impairment. In subhuman primates sustaining severe traumatic brain injury, Gennarelli et al. (30) have reported that the coma occurring in these animals was directly related to the occurrence of diffuse axonal injury. Originally, in the study of human traumatic brain injury, the identification of macroscopic changes within the corpus callosum and brainstem were considered a prerequisite for the occurrence of diffuse axonal injury (26,28). However, since the original description of this phenomenon, it has been recognized that DAI can occur without concomitant lesions in these structures (25). Thus, at present, most are refraining from such overly restrictive classifications of diffuse axonal injury. In humans, as well as some animal studies, damaged axons have been described throughout the subcortical white matter, the basal ganglia, and thalamus as well as multiple brainstem sites (28,31,32,34,35,42,45). In both animals and man, the damaged axons were once exclusively associated with large caliber fibers; however, currently, more rigorous studies are beginning to suggest that fibers of all caliber are subject to failure (37). Typically, axonal damage is visualized in axons just as they begin to change their anatomical course. In both man and animals, axonal change is found in foci where axons change course to turn around blood vessels, cross in decussating bundles, or turn to enter target (synaptic) sites (26, 29,37,42).

Historically, most have assumed that the tensile forces of injury mechanically tear or sever the axon at the moment of injury (21,22,28,30). Thus, there was little hope that any therapeutic and/or management strategy could reverse this immediate traumatically induced event. Recently, laboratory investigations have reexamined the issue of the pathogenesis of these traumatically injured axons in order to ascertain the correctness of the above-stated premise. To evaluate this issue fully, anterogradely transported tracers were employed in experimentally injured animals in the belief that if the axons were indeed torn at the moment of injury, then this would elicit the immediate formation of tracer-containing reactive swelling. Contrary to expectations, however, no tracer-laden swellings were identified early in the posttraumatic course. In fact, it was observed that the traumatic event did not immediately tear axons and cause an expulsion of axoplasm. Rather, it was observed that the traumatic event elicited a focal impairment of anterograde axoplasmic transport that, over time, resulted in continued local axonal swelling due to the continued delivery of anterogradely transported materials (32). With continued survival, this progressive swelling resulted in local lobulation that preceded the separation of the axon cylinder into a proximal segment in continuity with the sustaining somata and a distal segment now detached from the sustaining soma (32). With disconnection, the proximal swelling showed continued expansion owing to the delivery of anterogradely transported substances, ultimately (over a 12–24 hr period) forming the mature retraction ball of classical description (32) (Figs. 1 and 2). The distal segment, on the other hand, underwent rapid degenerative Wallerian change. The above-described studies were first conducted in animals subjected to minor traumatic brain injury, in order to obviate any concern regarding the generation of concomitant ischemic/hypoxic change (32). However, since this initial description these results have also been confirmed in animals sustaining moderate and severe injuries (34,35,38,40). Although in the case of severe traumatic injury the time to disconnection was accelerated in comparison to mildly injured state, no evidence was found to suggest immediate traumatically induced tearing/disconnection (40). Clearly, the traumatic event somehow altered axonal function to elicit a local swelling followed by disconnection. Since our initial description of this process in 1983, other laboratories have both directly or indirectly confirmed our observations. Gennarelli et al. (39) and Maxwell et al. (41,46), in various animal models of injury, have also suggested that the axonal damage seen with traumatic injury does not result from immediate tearing. Rather, they, too, advocate a traumatic induction of a focal axonal change that progresses over time to form a reactive swelling or retraction ball. Precisely what initial subcellular intraaxonal event leads to this local failure with subsequent swelling and disconnection remains an area of intense debate. Obviously, if one could identify the initiating factor in this reactive cascade, then perhaps one could rationally design appropriate therapeutic approaches. Moving on the observations of Maxwell et al. (46), who described early posttraumatic blebbing of the nodal axolemma, Adams et al. (47) have assumed that this axonal event reflected focal axolemmal change involving altered axolemmal permeability that allowed for the increased influx of extracellular calcium. In this scenario, it was envisioned that the resulting increase in intracellular calcium triggered the activation of neutral proteases and/or related agents, which then caused neurofilamentous degradation (47). This, in turn, was envisioned to impair axoplasmic transport ultimately leading to axonal disconnection (47). Although, from the general neurobiological perspective, this argument appeared credible, published descriptions of the progression of reactive axonal change did not appear consistent with this concept (32,34,38,40,42). In fact, in our published studies, we found no evidence of the neurofilament degradation, and/or granular disorganization typically associated with damaging calcium influx (48–51). Thus, the evidence to support the premise of Adams et al. (41) seems limited. Perhaps, increased intraaxonal calcium has a role in this process, but its role is most likely not associated with the activation of neutral proteases with subsequent neurofilament degradation and/or granular degeneration. Based upon our own detailed descriptive studies, our laboratories questioned whether the traumatic event could perhaps elicit direct cytoskeletal/neurofilament change resulting in impaired axoplasmic transport leading to axonal detachment. To this end, we utilized antibodies targeting all the neurofilament subunits and found that within 15 min of the traumatic event, the 68 kD core neurofilament subunit demonstrated increased immunoreactivity that correlated with local distention and dramatic infolding of the axolemma (37). Over time (1–2 hr postinjury) (Fig. 3a–d), the 68 kD immunoreactivity increased, and as such, this increase paralleled continued expansion of the axon cylinder (42). At this stage, the related axolemma displayed little of the infolding seen in the initial postinjury period. Despite this fact, however, the 68 kD immunoreactive neurofilaments now began to show changes in their alignment (42) (Fig. 4). Unlike the control situation, in which these neurofilament subunits move in a linear fashion paralleling the axon's long axis, however, by 2 hr postinjury, these immunoreactive neurofilament subunits lost their linear alignment (Fig. 4). Some now moved in a course oblique to the axon's axis, while others formed spiraling profiles. With continued survival this process continued, and

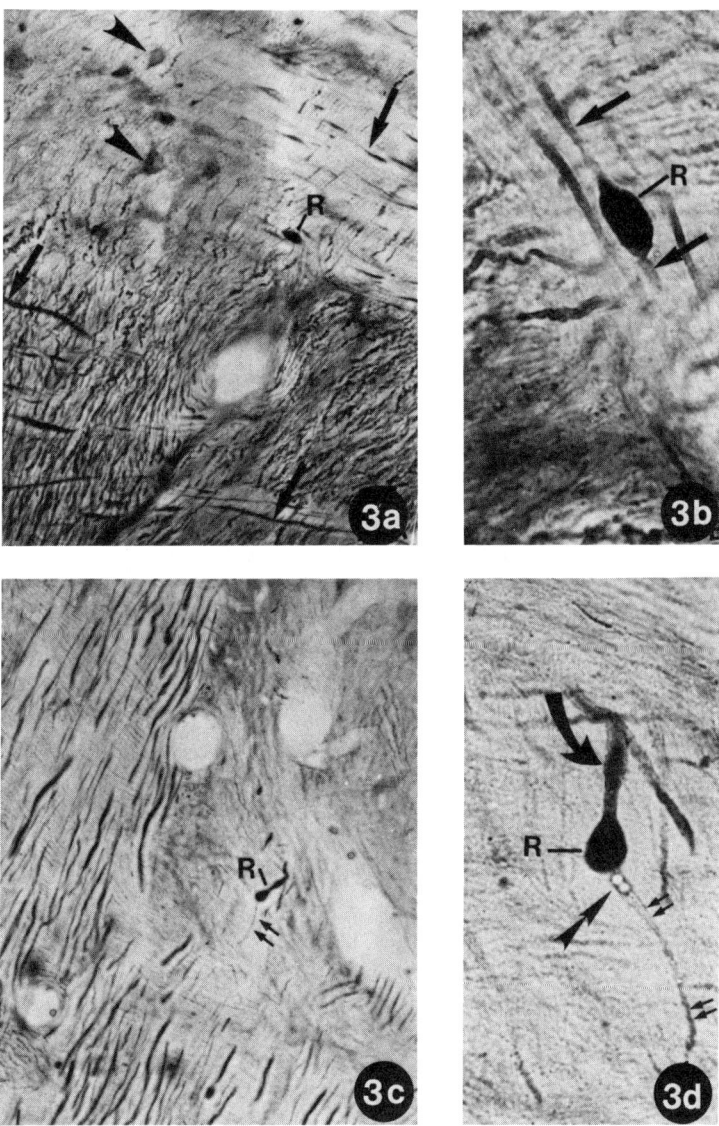

FIG. 3. In these photomicrographs at 2 hr postinjury, reactive axonal change (R) is easily distinguished from surrounding altered axons (arrows) through the use of monoclonal antibodies targeting the 68 kD subunit. In **A**, a low power view of the vestibular nucleus reveals an intensely immunoreactive axon (R) which can be seen in relation to normal immunoreactive axons (arrows) and somata (arrowheads). In **B**, the same reactive segment (R) shows at high magnification focal distention in relation to its attached proximal and distal segments (arrows). At the site of injury, increased immunoreactivity, associated with the 68 kD subunit has occurred, and as such, this closely follows a contour change seen within the axon cylinder. **C** again shows another reactive axonal segment (R), seen using antibodies targeted to the 68 kD subunit. Note that the reactive segment is seen to consist of a proximal axonal segment in continuity with the reactive axonal swelling (R) and a distal collapsed axonal segment (double arrows). **D** shows at high magnification this immunoreactive change. Note that the vacuolated distal axonal segment (double arrowheads) is most likely in the process of detaching from the proximal axonal segment (curved arrow) and its reactive swelling (R). a and c, ×125; b and d, ×500. (Reproduced with permission from Yaghmai and Povlishock, ref. 42.)

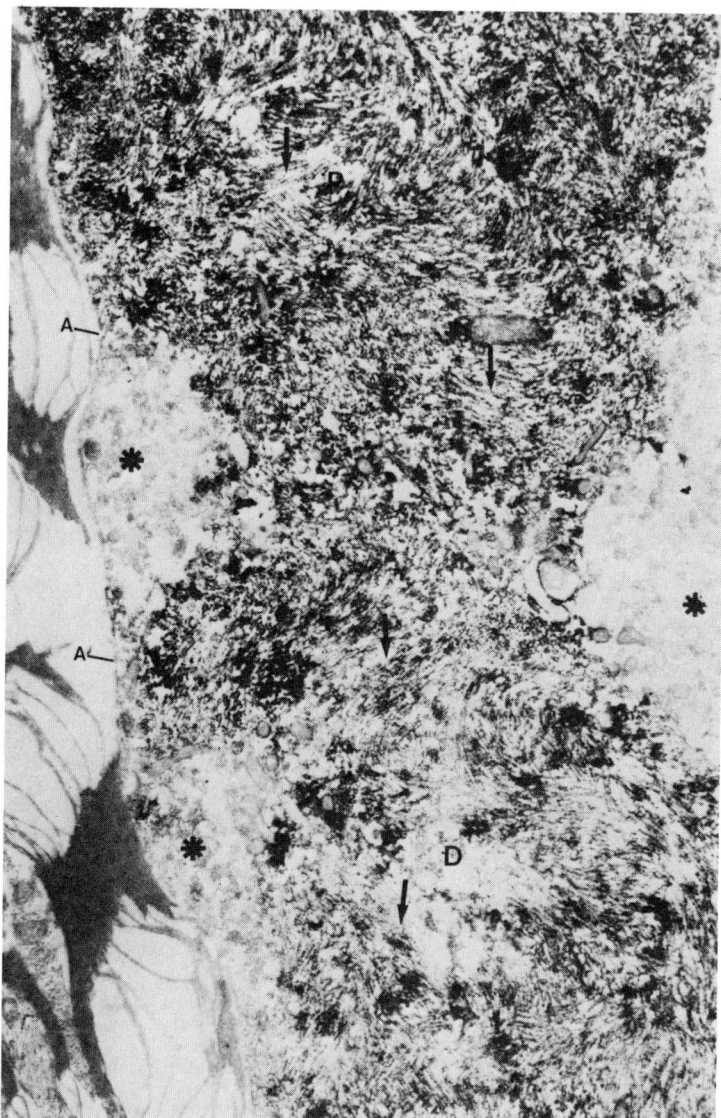

FIG. 4. In this electron micrograph, a reactive swelling is seen in the process of constriction within 2 hr of the traumatic episode. Note that the reactive axonal segment consists of a neurofilament-laden immunoreactive core that is sequestered into proximal *(P)* and distal segments *(D)*. Note at the point of constriction that the immunoreactive 68 kD neurofilament subunits appear to have withdrawn *(*)* from the overlying intact axolemma *(A)* to aggregate more centrally within the swelling. Last, note that the immunoreactivity is localized in individual neurofilaments *(arrows)*, some of which appear to be deviating from their normal linear intraaxonal course. ×12,000. (Reproduced with permission from Yaghmai and Povlishock, ref. 42.)

in some cases, the neurofilament subunits detached from an isolated segment of the axolemma withdrawing deeper into the axon cylinder (42) (Fig. 4). This traumatically induced process of neurofilament misalignment and regional detachment from the axolemma paralleled the subsequent impairment of axoplasmic transport. In fact, as the 68 kD neurofilaments continued to show disordered alignment, organelles began to accumulate at these sites, obviously due to the impaired anterograde transport elicited by the collapse of neurofilament/cytoskeletal architecture (42). As was noted with the use of anterograde tracers (32), the continued delivery of organelles and their accumulation at the site of impaired transport resulted in a continued focal expansion of the axon cylinder that preceded disconnection. These findings regarding traumatically induced change in the 68 kD neurofilament subunit confirmed our initial description that the tensile forces of injury did not tear axons. Further, they confirmed that some subtle intraaxonal event impaired anterograde transport, and apparently, this intraaxonal event involved neurofilament/cytoskeletal change early in the posttraumatic course. Precisely what triggered this neurofilament change is unclear; yet, several lines of indirect evidence suggest that the traumatic episode may exacerbate normally occurring intraaxonal events (37,42). Although the literature on this issue is just evolving, there is a growing consensus that the axonal neurofilament structure can no longer be viewed as a stable entity. Rather, most now consider the neurofilament to undergo constant modification (52). In this regard, it is of interest that, in studies of uninjured axons, the 68 kD subunit undergoes disassembly and exchange between a stable filamentous pool and a soluble yet kinetically active pool in the axoplasm (52). It has been posited that this subunit disassembly and exchange are controlled by the action of protein kinase C on the amino acid heads of the 68 kD subunit and that this kinase is regulated by changing phosphorylation states (52). In view of these findings, we have recently posited that the traumatic episode may trigger altered phosphorylation states that elicit excessive 68 kD subunit exchange resulting in disordered neurofilament structure (42). We are currently exploring this issue and considering various therapeutic approaches to blunt this damaging event. Our long-term goal would be to block neurofilament disassembly and prevent axonal disconnection.

The obvious issue in relation to all of the above experimental studies is whether these fascinating events described in experimental animals are operant in traumatically brain-injured humans. Perhaps the findings are species specific. Alternatively, perhaps, the models of injury generate a repertoire of change not found in humans. To obviate these valid concerns, we recently used the above-described immunocytochemical strategies in a postmortem study of brain-injured humans (53). In this study of traumatically brain-injured humans, the same neurofilament changes described in experimental animals were seen and, as such, these contributed to local axonal change, focal axonal swelling, and ultimate disconnection (Figs. 5 and 6). Interestingly, although our findings in man did replicate the pattern of change seen in experimental animals, there was one significant difference. Specifically, in man, the time of disconnection was significantly longer than that seen in animals, suggesting that the window for potential therapeutic intervention may be longer in brain-injured humans (53).

As noted above, considerable interest exists in the concept of diffuse axonal injury and the factors involved in its pathogenesis; yet, it is also important to recall that the actual morbidity triggered by such axonal damage is caused by the Wallerian degeneration of the distal axon and its synaptic terminal projections. With the development of reactive axonal swelling, the axonal segment distal to the site of disconnection is

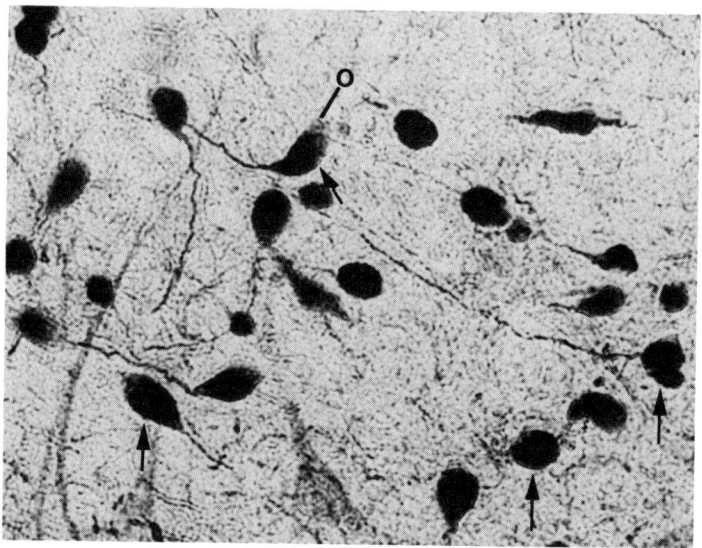

FIG. 5. In this light micrograph, antibodies to the 68 kD subunits reveal in traumatically brain-injured humans numerous reactive axonal swellings. Note that the immunoreactive neurofilaments appear confined to the core of the swelling (*arrows*) with some evidence of a nonimmunoreactive cap, most likely containing organelles (*O*). ×500. These immunoreactive swellings seen the hippocampus 80 hr postinjury confirm the presence of DAI. ×500.

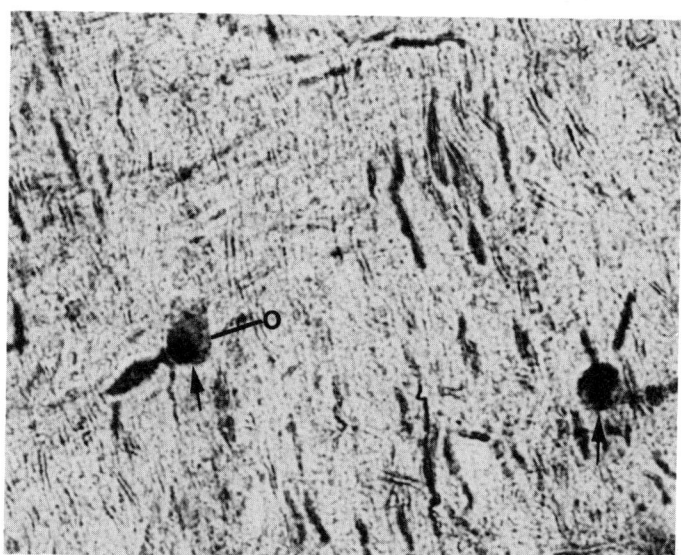

FIG. 6. Again, with antibodies targeting the 68 kD subunit, this sample harvested from the basal ganglia of a traumatically brain-injured human shows reactive axonal swellings. Note that these swellings again demonstrate a immunoreactive neurofilament core *(arrow)* as well as a nonimmunoreactive organelle (*o*) cap. ×400.

removed from the sustaining somata. This results in the rapid degeneration of its synaptic terminals, which then functionally disconnect their target neuronal populations (36,37,54) (Figs. 7 and 8). Thus, the diffuse axonal injury actually translates into diffuse synaptic terminal degeneration, which results in rapid diffuse deafferentation. Typically, within 24 hr of the axonal injury, the various target sites of these axonal projections demonstrate scattered synaptic profiles that reveal either increased electron density or neurofilamentous hyperplasia (36,37,54) (Figs. 7 and 8). Over the next several days, these degenerating terminals detach from their synaptic sites and are engulfed by reactive glia, which ultimately cover the now deafferented site. In reality, it is this process of degeneration and deafferentation that most likely results in much of the morbidity associated with the traumatic condition. Importantly, as will be developed in another section of this chapter, these same diffuse degenerative/deafferentation-mediated changes may also set the stage for the recovery seen following mild and moderate traumatic brain injury.

Neuronal Somatic Change

In addition to the above-described phase of neural excitation and axonal injury, traumatic injury to the brain has also been associated with other forms of perturbation to the brain parenchyma including structural and metabolic abnormalities in the neuronal somata. With the most severe injuries, contusion and/or other destructive processes can directly destroy neurons. Also, owing to a traumatically induced reduction in blood flow leading to ischemia, neuronal ischemic cell change and cell death can occur. Additionally, when axotomy occurs close to the sustaining soma, neuronal chromatolysis has been described, with the suggestion that some chromatolytic neurons go on to die (55). In the case of more moderate to mild traumatic brain injuries, the above-described somatic responses are

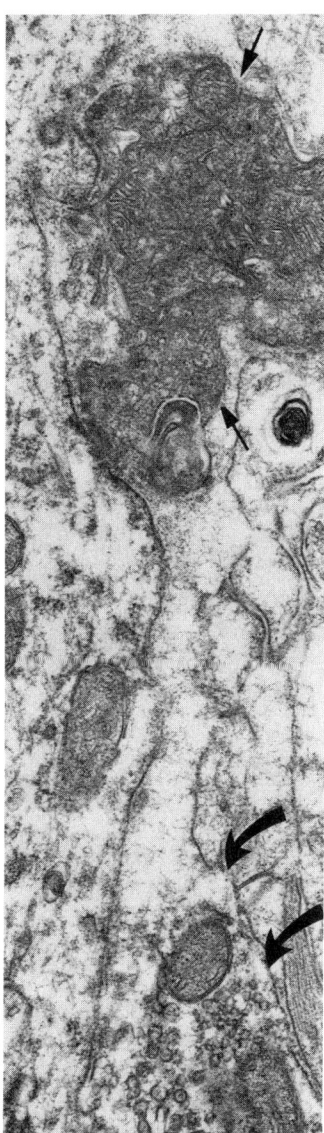

FIG. 7. This electron micrograph shows an example of the diffuse deafferentation occurring after diffuse axonal injury. Note that following DAI, target areas reveal damaged electron-dense boutons (arrows) which sit adjacent to intact undamaged synaptic terminals (curved arrows). ×25,000.

not commonly observed; however, in these situations, there is evidence to suggest that the traumatic event evokes metabolic changes that are independent of widespread axotomy and/or primary ischemia. Primarily, through the use of 2-deoxyglucose, var-

the traumatic event evokes foci of glucose hypermetabolism that correlate with the previously described phase of neuroexcitation. In general, such hypermetabolism is maximal in the first hour following injury (56), followed, over time, by a more sustained period of reduced metabolism (57,58). Although, in most cases, this reduced glucose metabolism is global in nature, there are reports of isolated hypermetabolic foci interspersed in regions showing reduced metabolism (57,58). At present, the overall neurobiological implications of such altered glucose metabolism are unclear. Surely, these somatic metabolic changes reflect a neuronal response to injury, yet, it is unknown whether these changes contribute to the morbidity associated with the condition.

Traumatically Induced Vascular Change

As noted above, traumatic injury to the brain typically involves both focal and diffuse changes. In falls, assaults, or motor vehicle accidents, contusions are a common manifestation of focal injury to the brain. Again, generally related to the nature and site of impact, contusions can be found in multiple cortical sites. Most commonly they are seen in the frontal and temporal lobes, where these cortical regions normally cross the relatively rough surfaces of the anterior and middle cranial fossae, respectively. Contusion manifests itself in varied forms, sometimes involving hemorrhagic change in the crest of the gyri, while in other cases eliciting hemorrhage at the grey/white interface. It frequently originates as a hemorrhage resulting from vascular damage sustained at the moment of impact, and can evolve and enlarge over a several-day posttraumatic course. Such hemorrhage may lead to infarction within the related cortical gray, and thus, in some cases, a contusion resembles a hemorrhagic infarction confined to the cortical surface.

In addition to contusion seen within the

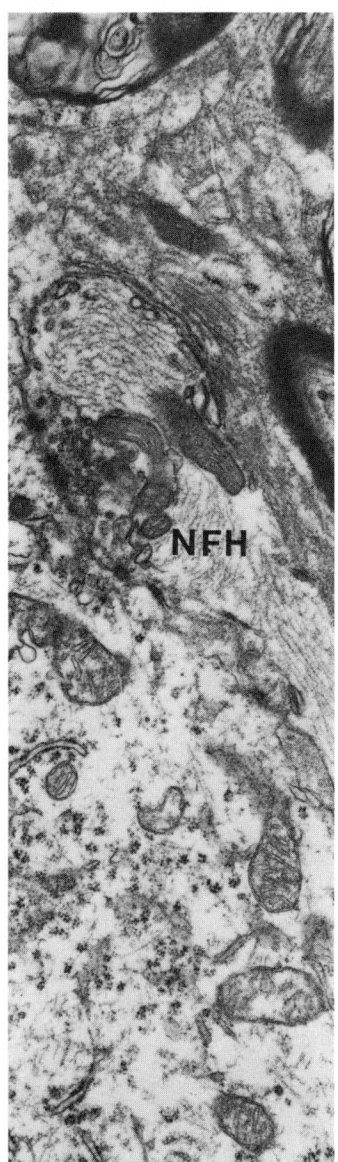

FIG. 8. This figure demonstrates that following diffuse axonal injury, other forms of diffuse synaptic terminal change can be seen. Note the presence of neurofilamentous hyperplasia (NFH) within a synaptic terminal. ×20,000.

ious patterns of altered glucose metabolism have been described following trauma. Although it is difficult to detail a precise pattern of altered glucose metabolism following injury due to differences in animal modeling and injury levels, it appears that

superficial cortices, traumatic brain injury can also be associated with other forms of vascular change. As is well recognized, assaults, falls, and motor vehicle accidents can be associated with tearing of the epidural vessels. This results in bleeding into the epidural compartment, creating a mass effect that can displace the brain, elevate intracranial pressure, and generate life-threatening physiologic changes. Similarly, the shear and tensile forces of traumatic injury can also disrupt the bridging veins, causing the development of a subdural hematoma, which over a more prolonged posttraumatic course can result in a mass lesion with its damaging consequences. In addition to these intra- or extradural vascular abnormalities, traumatic brain injury is almost invariably associated with some degree of subarachnoid hemorrhage, caused by the rupture of pial vessels within the subarachnoid space. While little is known about the long-range consequences of such subarachnoid blood, recent evidence suggests that such blood can contribute to the onset of vasospasm, which, in turn, could result in reduced regional cerebral blood flow, with devastating consequences to the injured brain (59). Traumatic brain injury can also give rise to intraparenchymal vascular injury. Foci of hematoma can be identified within subcortical white matter, basal ganglia, and brainstem sites, which, dependent upon their localization, may also contribute to significant morbidity. Diffuse petechial hemorrhage can also be associated with head injury; however, when recognized, it is almost invariably associated with severe morbidity or mortality (60).

In concert to the above-described structural vascular changes, it is also well known that various forms of functional vascular change also occur following traumatic brain injury. Depending upon the severity of the initial traumatic brain insult, such functional vascular change can include the impairment or loss of autoregulation (62,63), impaired physiologic cerebral vascular responsiveness to changes in arterial blood gases (64,65), altered cerebral blood flow (65–70), and/or altered blood-brain barrier status (71). With the most severe traumatic brain injuries in both animals and man, autoregulation may be significantly impaired or lost (61,62,63), allowing flow to the brain to become dependent upon the systemic arterial pressure. In this regard, elevated blood pressure would result in hyperemia, whereas decreased blood pressure would result in hypoperfusion. Traumatically induced shifts in the autoregulatory curve or range could be of particular significance in those patients sustaining secondary insults (vida supra). As noted, these autoregulatory abnormalities appear most pronounced in severe injury; however, less dramatic autoregulatory changes have also been described with more moderate injuries.

Impaired vascular responsiveness to blood gas change has also been described in both animals and man sustaining severe traumatic brain injury. In animals, impaired vascular responsiveness to hypocapnia has been described (64), and in man, CO_2 vasomotor responsiveness can also be impaired following severe injury. Normally, hyperventilation will reduce pCO_2, causing arteriolar vasoconstriction. With injury, this pCO_2-related vasoconstriction can be impaired, with the degree of impairment reflecting, to some extent, the type of injury (65). In addition to these abnormalities in autoregulation and in CO_2 responsiveness, laboratory studies have also shown other forms of impaired cerebral vascular function following traumatic brain injury. Perhaps one of the most intriguing findings concerns endothelial-dependent relaxation in traumatically brain-injured animals. Normally, agents such as acetylcholine induce dilation through the release of endothelium-derived relaxing factor (EDRF), which, in turn, acts on the vascular smooth muscle. In the traumatic condition, however, the normal vasodilatory endothelial-dependent response is converted to vasoconstriction (72). In fact, in the early posttraumatic period, the topical application of acetylcholine to traumatically brain-injured animals results in sustained vasoconstriction, which appears to lessen over a prolonged posttraumatic course (72). Although the overall relevance of these endothelial-dependent phenomena to brain-injured man is at the moment unclear, it is our impression that the impaired endothelial-dependent relaxation, coupled with changes in autoregulation and in CO_2 vasoresponsiveness, suggest that the cerebral blood vessels may not be well equipped to maintain homeostasis in the face of declining blood pressure and/or changed blood gas composition. Conceivably, all these factors can explain the brain's vulnerability to secondary posttraumatic insult, and this will be discussed in a later section of this chapter.

Paralleling the above-described vascular changes that occur with traumatic brain injury, other functional changes, particularly those involving cerebral blood flow, can also occur. Primary traumatically induced ischemia has been suggested on the basis of the postmortem analyses of severely brain-injured humans (73); however, the recognition of posttraumatic ischemia in patients has not been a common event. In fact, most blood flow studies have provided a rather confusing picture of the cerebral blood flow (CBF) changes occurring after severe injury. Some investigators, such as Barclay et al. (74) have noted global CBF reductions in head-injured patients in comparison to age-matched controls. Further, they found an association between low regional cerebral blood flow and focal brain injury, while observing that increased regional CBF correlated with improved cognition. In contrast, however, other investigators have reported that increased blood flow is a finding common to traumatically brain-injured patients (69,70,75). Recently, however, new information has emerged that suggests that these discrepant findings may relate to the timing of the posttraumatic blood-flow studies. Specifically, in patients without surgical mass lesions, Marion et al. (65) reported that, in the first hours of injury, global CBF is low, followed over time by a hyperemic phase that peaks at 24 hr. Further, these same investigators demonstrated that global CBF values varied to some extent with the type of traumatic brain injury. These important studies have been extended recently in our own institution, where new evidence has emerged that the above-described, reduced CBF values can reach ischemic levels early in the posttraumatic course of some severely injured patients (66). Importantly, these new cerebral blood flow studies demonstrate that only when the blood flow studies are performed within the first hours after injury can reduced or ischemic blood flows be recognized. Typically, reduced flows seen in the early posttraumatic phase tend to normalize or reach increased levels over time. Thus, based upon these recent studies, one may conclude that the blood flow abnormalities seen after injury most likely reflect the timing of the flow studies.

Concomitant with the above-described overt structural, functional, and flow changes, traumatic brain injury also elicits perturbations of the blood-brain barrier. As has long been recognized, the blood-brain barrier resides in the cerebral vascular endothelium, which serves as an interface to regulate the movement of various solutes from the blood to brain front, thereby allowing for the maintenance of a stable brain microenvironment. With traumatic brain injury, however, both overt as well as subtle endothelial changes allow for the passage of normally excluded substances into the brain parenchyma (71). In some cases, normally excluded serum proteins can enter the brain together with a host of other substances normally confined to the blood front. In this regard, it has long been assumed that, with disruption of the barrier, the passage of serum proteins contributes to an osmotic gradient, which, in turn, translates into a temporally delayed increase in brain water, termed edema. In this scenario, it has been assumed that the edema, in turn, contributes to elevation in intracranial pressure (ICP) with the damaging consequences associated with this. Within the scope of this review, it is impossible to consider all issues relevant to traumatically related induced edema and attendant ICP change, and in this matter, the reader is referred to one of several reviews in this area (76). Suffice to say that contemporary thought on the role of the barrier perturbation in the generation of edema has become much more complex. Blood-brain barrier perturbation in itself is an acute event, whereas the genesis of edema with attendant ICP rise is a more delayed phenomenon in both animals and man. Further, although the passage of serum proteins may be important for the concept of brain edema, there is now compelling evidence that the passage of other blood-borne factors may be equally or perhaps more significant in the pathobiology of traumatic brain injury. In this regard, the passage of blood-borne neurotransmitters as well as other related solutes may directly contribute to some of the cellular dysfunction seen with injury.

In regard to the myriad of vascular abnormalities described above in relation to traumatic brain injury, many factors have been postulated to contribute to their genesis. Clearly, the shear and tensile strains of trauma may act directly upon the cerebral vessels and elicit both structural and functional change. Similarly, the pressor responses associated with traumatic injury may also be contributing factors. Recent studies have also begun to appreciate that both the traumatic event and its accompanying hypertensive episode result in the accelerated metabolism of arachidonate with the increased production of prostaglandins (64,77–79). With the increased production of prostaglandins, there is a concomitant production of oxygen radicals in which the superoxide anion figures prominently (80–82). To date, the superoxide anion has been clearly linked to many of the vascular abnormalities described in the previous section. The superoxide anion has been shown to have direct effects upon both the cerebral vascular endothelium and the arteriolar smooth muscle wall. In the context of the endothelium, the associated radical production has been linked to altered endothelial-dependent responses (72), alterations in blood-brain barrier status (83), overt endothelial change (84), and the potential for enhanced platelet aggregation. Similarly, this same superoxide anion surge has been associated with change in vascular diameter as well as abnormal vasoreactivity. Collectively, then, it appears that the superoxide anion, in particular, may be responsible for many of the vascular abnormalities associated with traumatic injury, which, as such, may contribute to morbidity and mortality. In the experimental setting, the use of superoxide anion scavengers, such as superoxide dismutase, has blunted virtually all of the above-described abnormalities, and this compelling evidence has led to the use of superoxide dismutase in clinical trials. Although the trials to assess this in the clinical population are currently underway, the long-range hope is that the early use of such drugs after injury will lead to a significant improvement in the morbidity and mortality associated with this devastating condition.

SPECTRUM OF TRAUMATIC BRAIN INJURY

In the previous passages, considerable effort has been expended to fully develop the possible neural and vascular changes that occur with traumatic brain injury. As noted in the opening paragraph, it is erroneous to assume that all of the described neuronal and vascular events occur across the spectrum of mild through severe traumatic brain injury. Further, as noted in the opening paragraph, different types of injury will also translate to differential focal and diffuse responses within the context of mild, moderate, and severe injuries. Although it is beyond the scope of the present communication to closely detail the pathobiology of mild, moderate, and severe traumatic brain injury, the following passages are presented to provide the reader with a brief overview of some of the assumed brain parenchymal and vascular changes associated with mild through severe injury.

Historically, information on mild to moderate brain injury has been relatively limited owing to the fact that such injuries are not associated with mortality, and thus, these patients do not come to routine postmortem examination. However, with the advent of detailed imaging studies, coupled with limited postmortem analyses in addition to information gleaned from the experimental animal setting, a better impression of mild to moderate injury is now evolving. Specifically, in the case of mild traumatic brain injury, there is little evidence to support the concept direct vascular involvement. Other than isolated instances of transient perturbation of the blood-brain barrier, there is no direct evidence of traumatically induced reduction of cerebral blood flow and/or ischemia (85). Similarly, there is no evidence to suggest impaired autoregulation and/or vascular reactivity. Despite the absence of enduring vascular changes of minor head injury, there is evidence from both the laboratory and the human setting that minor injury may be associated with sublethal neuroexcitotoxic events as well as with limited diffuse axonal injury (1,24,31,32,44,85). As mild traumatic brain injury is associated with some morbidity, one could speculate that these primary brain parenchymal events are the major contributors to the posttraumatic behavioral/neurological dysfunction. With more moderate injury, many of the above-described brain parenchymal changes are exacerbated, and as such, neuroexcitation as well as more widespread axon injury appear to correlate with moderate insult to the brain (1,35,37,42). In addition to these more diffuse changes, moderate injuries are also associated with localized contusional changes in the cortex. Thus, in the case of moderate injury, focal contusional change can superimpose its damaging effects upon the already diffusely injured brain. On the vascular front moderate injury is associated with alterations in the blood-brain barrier and perhaps with modest impairments in vascular reactivity (35). However, once again, there is little evidence to support the premise that primary ischemia constitutes a primary event in the pathobiology of moderate injury. With the most severe injuries, a myriad of changes occur through the neuraxis. Not only is the number and distribution of damaged axons significantly increased, but also now their damaging consequences may be further complicated by the possibility of primary ischemia, mass lesion formation, and multifocal contusion. Collectively, then, these events in severe traumatic brain injury so adversely damage the brain as to result in enduring morbidity.

SECONDARY INSULTS

In the previous passages, much detail has focused on those brain parenchymal and vascular changes occurring with traumatic brain injury. Although these changes are the most likely determinants of both morbidity and recovery, it is important to bear in mind that the damaging consequences of mild, moderate, and severe injury can be significantly exacerbated by the superimposition of a secondary posttraumatic insult. As alluded to in a previous section, the injured brain is quite susceptible to moderate secondary insults that the normal brain would tolerate well. Typically, because trauma involves damage to multiple organ systems, traumatic brain injury may be complicated by hypotension due to blood loss or by hypoxia secondary to pulmonary obstruction/dysfunction or hypoventilation. In cases in which the traumatic event is complicated by a concomitant hypoxic or hypotensive insult, there is evidence emerging from the clinical setting that the outcome of these patients is significantly worse than anticipated on the basis of the traumatic brain injury alone (J.D. Miller, personal communication). This clinical impression has been more than confirmed in the laboratory setting, where various investigators have subjected head-injured animals to secondary insults, such as hypoxia (86,87). In this setting, hypoxic challenges that are normally well tolerated become devastating and contribute to severe morbidity and mortality (86,87). Although the actual pathobiological factors involved in this increased sensitivity to secondary insults are not entirely known, it has been widely speculated that the impaired vascular function occurring with traumatic brain injury provides inadequate vasomotor responsiveness to the injured brain in the face of a secondary challenge. Although this argument appears quite credible, other laboratory evidence suggests that the damaging consequences of secondary insult may be much more complex. In fact, as previously noted in animals subjected to traumatic brain injury followed by a sublethal ischemic challenge, there is compelling evidence that blood flow may not be the major factor in determining morbidity and mortality (15,16). In these studies, it appears that the secondary ischemic insult is capable of triggering additional abnormal agonist/receptor interactions that impact upon the previously injured brain parenchyma (15,16). In this setting, if secondary insults are imposed, pretreatment with antagonists targeted to specific receptor systems have not only afforded significant protection of the brain parenchyma but also significant functional recovery (16). Thus, in man, the damaging consequences of secondary insult most likely reflect a summation of events mediated by the brain vasculature as well as by the brain parenchyma.

REPAIR AND RECOVERY FOLLOWING CENTRAL NERVOUS SYSTEM INJURY

In the preceding passages, considerable detail has been provided to carefully describe those brain parenchymal and vascular changes that occur with traumatic brain injury so that the reader may appreciate the complexity of those issues at work with injury and any potential repair process. As can be gleaned from the previous passages, mild and moderate injury would appear to offer some potential for recovery, while severe traumatic injury would entail the most daunting obstacles to any successful recovery. The rationale for such statement stems from the fact that mild and moderate injuries are typically associated with diffuse changes that occur in an otherwise normal brain parenchyma, not significantly influenced by concomitant vascular compromise. Thus, it is not unreasonable to suggest that, in this situation, the unaltered brain parenchyma may be capable of restoring some degree of function to the injured patient. In the case of mild traumatic injury, it is known that morbidity seen in the early posttraumatic period successfully resolves over a 3–6 month period (61). Similarly, in the case of moderate injury, significant, yet incomplete, recovery can also occur. Unfortunately, in both patient populations, however, there is no evidence to indicate how this recovery is accomplished. In the following passages, I will attempt to detail some of those neuronal responses thought to participate in the recovery seen following injury. Although, in most cases, the literature supporting each of the purported responses is limited, this narrative should provide some insight into those processes potentially operant in the brain's attempt to repair itself following injury.

In the study of those reparative processes potentially at work following injury, three particular lines of thought have developed. First, there are those that adhere to the premise that undamaged brain tissue may be capable of taking over the function of the damaged foci. Second, there are others who contend that the diffusely damaged axons mount a sustained and perhaps targeted regenerative response, and last, there are those who suggest that adaptive neuroplasticity is the major factor in all reparative processes. In the following passages, I will address each of these aspects.

Evidence for Brain Reorganization Following Traumatic Injury

One of the most enduring concepts in the field of neural injury is the premise that once brain injury occurs, unaltered/undamaged areas of the brain can reorganize and therefore, over time, restore the brain function previously lost. Additionally, there has also been some support for the concept that the injurious event itself elicits generalized neural shock (diaschisis), the dissipation of which ultimately leads to recovery (88). Historically, most studies dealing with either brain reorganization and/or dissipation of neural shock have not been conducted in animal models of experimental traumatic brain injury. Rather, most have relied on cortical contusion, ablation, or undercutting purportedly employed to replicate the important features of traumatic brain injury. In such studies conducted in various species, a rather confusing set of data has emerged neither convincingly supporting nor rejecting the potential for brain rearrangement and/or the dissipation of diaschisis. For example, in rhesus monkeys, the undercutting of the cortical thumb area was suggested to elicit the reorganization of the adjacent cortex to assume the ability to generate thumb movement (89). This intriguing finding, however, was not confirmed in a similar study using cats wherein the adjacent uninjured cortex was never capable of eliciting an appropriate response (90). The controversy surrounding cortical reorganization also carries over into the question of diaschisis, as the numerous studies neither support nor reject the possibility of such a biological occurrence (91,92). To date, the issue of cortical reorganization and/or diaschisis following traumatic brain injury has remained highly controversial; however, a recent well-designed and -conducted experimental study has shed considerable doubt on the premise that local brain reorganization postinjury contributes to the recovery process. Boyeson et al. (93), through the generation of ablation, laceration, and contusional cortical injuries, followed by microstimulation of adjacent cortical areas to evoke movement, could find no evidence to support the premise of postinjury reorganization and/or transient shock within the adjacent uninjured cortices. Despite this fact, however, these same authors have, in parallel investigations, proposed that remote brain sites may participate in recovery. Thus, although denying the potential for adjacent cortical reorganization, these authors also suggest the possibility that reorganization in remote sites may have some adaptive influence on the recovery process (93).

Evidence for Axonal Regeneration

Targeted axonal regeneration of a damaged axon has long been a goal of those involved in the study of CNS injury. Unfortunately, in the eyes of most critical investigators, this goal seemed totally unrealistic, as numerous reports suggested that all CNS regenerative efforts proved rapidly abortive as glial scarring and/or the lack of a growth-sustaining environment led to the demise of any regenerative attempt (94–96). For some, the work of Aguayo et al. (97,98) demonstrating sustained CNS axonal growth in a peripheral nerve environment rekindled interest in CNS regeneration; yet, here, it was unclear as to how this approach would prove efficacious in traumatic brain injury. Thus, it would not be inaccurate to state that contemporary thought holds little enthusiasm for the concept of sustained, targeted growth of damaged axons. Although, in general, one can appreciate why such an impression exists, one would urge caution in assuming that these premises must necessarily apply to the axonal injury seen with trauma. In this regard, one must recall that virtually all information on potential CNS axonal regeneration has been gleaned from lesioning paradigms that do not replicate those axonal changes seen with TBI. For example, virtually all lesioning paradigms create large focal lesions that cause localized and complete axonal damage generally associated with reactive gliosis, hemorrhage, and collagen ingrowth. Although such lesioning paradigms may replicate some of the important features of a traumatically induced contusion, they certainly do not replicate those pathological findings associated with diffuse axonal injury, wherein damaged axons are typically found in a brain environment lacking other forms reactive to neuronal and/or glial change (32). Thus, this suggests that the fate of these diffusely damaged axons may be quite different from those found in focal lesions. The fate of diffusely damaged axons was recently evaluated in our laboratories, and much to our surprise, the diffusely damaged axons were observed to mount a sustained regenerative response (34,43). In the early period postinjury, reactive axonal swellings were seen giving rise to numerous sprouts (43) (Fig. 9). By the end of the first week postinjury, these sprouts continued to elongate, and on occasion, they filled the cavity found between the reactive swelling and the overlying encompassing myelin (43). With continued survival, growth cones were also observed originating from the reactive swellings whose overall size now decreased as their axoplasmic volume was redirected into the elongated growth cone and sproutlike processes (34,43) (Figs. 10 and 11). Similar to the situation in the peripheral nervous system, it appeared that successfully regenerating fibers lost their swollen reactive segment as their axoplasm was redistributed onto the growing neurites (99). With the decrease in reactive swelling volume, difficulty was encountered following continued axonal growth, as with continued axonal swelling shrinkage, no point of orientation could be found for detecting regenerating neurites. Despite this serious obstacle, detailed studies did reveal that occasional growth cones could penetrate the myelin sheath of the reactive axon and course distally through the brain parenchyma, sometimes traveling in the distal myelin sheath undergoing Wallerian change (97,34) (Fig. 10). Although the ultimate fate of these regenerating neurites was impossible to ascertain, the sustained growth, demonstrated by these diffusely injured axons, constituted a clear departure from the traditional literature wherein only brief and abortive regenerative efforts were described (94–96). What was puzzling in our original description of these regenerative events was the observation that some reactive swellings mounted a sustained regenerative effort while others rapidly degenerated and died (Fig. 11). Upon re-review of our original data, it appeared that those neurites damaged as they coursed through nuclear groups showed the most sustained regenerative efforts, while those in the white matter revealed the least regenerative effort. In light of Martin Schwab's pioneering studies (100–104), these findings seem to support his observations that inhibitory factors released from the white matter oligodendroglia suppress the neurite outgrowth that was sustained in the noninhibitory nuclear environment. At present, we are further exploring this possibility. However, irrespective of our ultimate findings, we believe that the initial description of sustained regeneration occurring with diffuse axonal injury demonstrates that the diffusely injured brain may not be responding in fashion comparable to that seen with focal injury. This is not to say that the diffusely injured brain is capable of functional regenerative efforts; yet, the sustained regeneration seen gives hope that future therapies

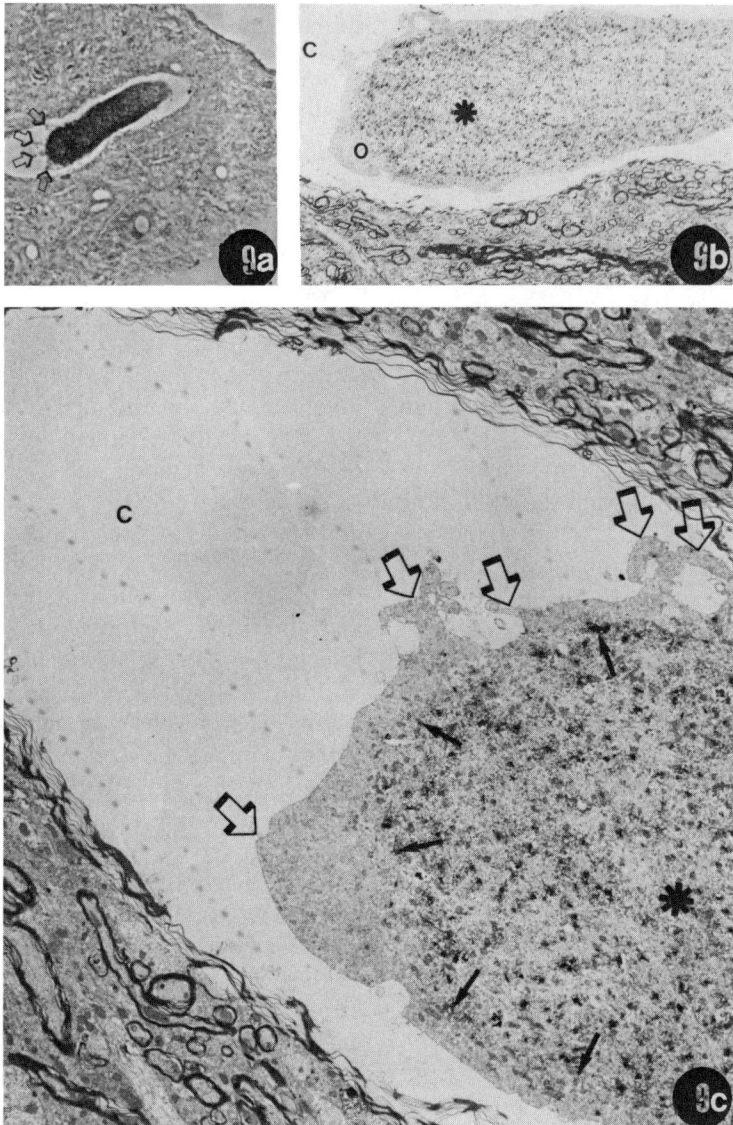

FIG. 9. These figures reveal evidence of axonal sprouting following traumatically induced axonal injury and disconnection. **a** reveals, 24 hr postinjury, the presence of numerous growth cones and sprouts *(arrows),* which appear to arise from the reactive swelling. **b** shows the same reactive swelling and contains a 68 kD immunoreactive neurofilamentous core *(*)* which is encompassed by an organelle mass *(o)* from which the sprouts arise. These details are better seen in **c**, where the sprout-like or growth-cone like processes *(open block arrows)* can be seen originating from the reactive swelling *(*)* to course in the clear cavity *(c)* that separates the reactive swelling from the overlying distended myelin sheath. Note once again that the sprout or growth-cone-like processes arise from region devoid of 68 kD immunoreactivity *(arrows)*. a, ×300; b, ×1,200; and c, ×4,500. (Reproduced with permission from Yaghmai and Povlishock, ref. 42.)

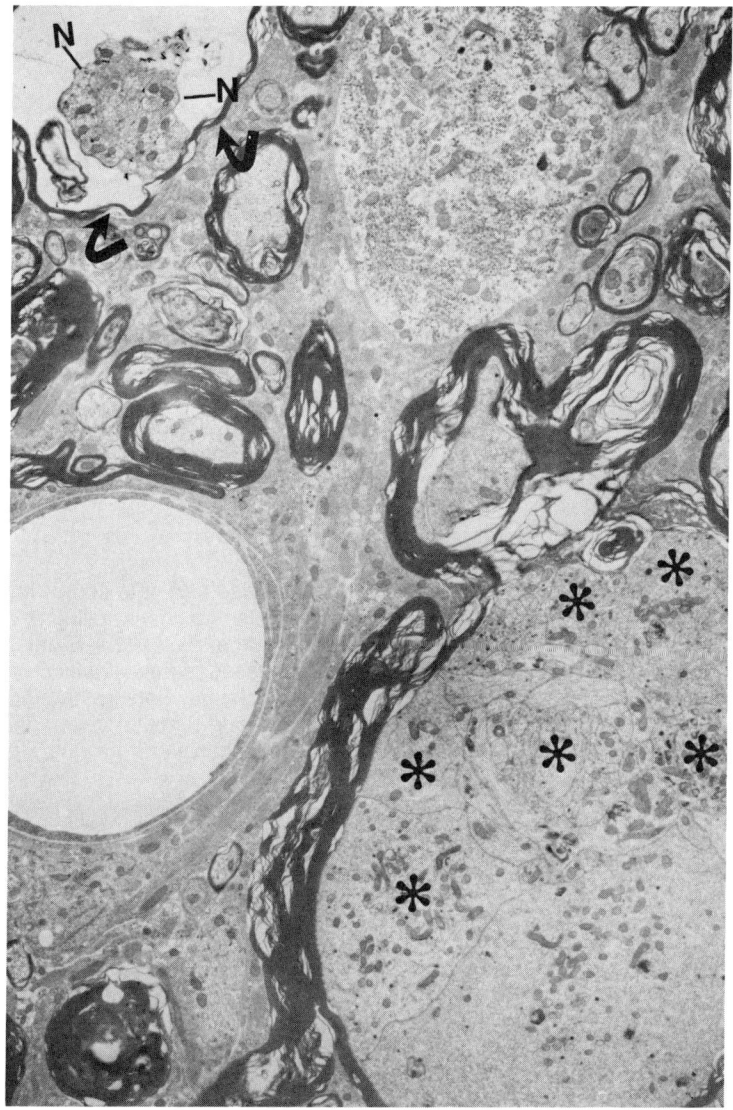

FIG. 10. This figure reveals, at a much later stage of postinjury, the presence of numerous growth cones and sprouts (*) packing the cavity once found surrounding the reactive axonal swelling. Note that in addition to these numerous reactive sprout and growth cone-like processes, found in relation to the reactive swelling, downstream sites showing Wallerian change *(curved arrows)* reveal the presence of neurites *(N)* which have obviously originated from the sprout and growth-cone-containing region to grow distally along the course of the degenerating axonal profile. ×5,000.

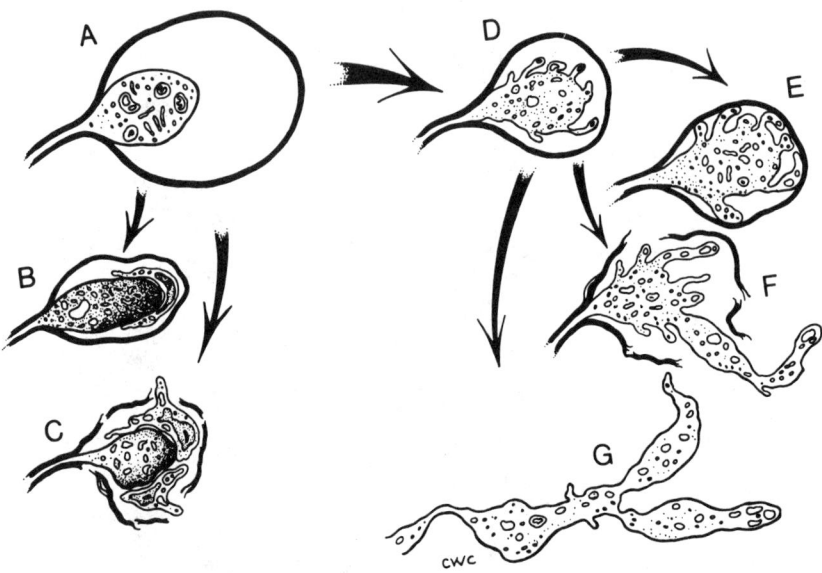

FIG. 11. The sequence of those degenerative or regenerative attempts seen with reactive axonal swelling formation following traumatic brain injury. The reactive axonal swelling **(A)** is seen in some cases to undergo degenerative change **(B** and **C)**, while in other cases **(D—G)** the reactive swelling gives rise to numerous sprout and growth cone-like processes, some of which break through the overlying myelin sheath **(F)** to elongate into the brain parenchyma. Note in the process of sprouting and growth cone formation, the overall size of reactive swelling tends to decrease as its volume is redirected into these growing neurites. (Reproduced with permission from Povlishock and Kontos, ref. 34.)

targeted at potentiating such outgrowth will favorably impact upon outcome.

Evidence for Neuroplasticity: Adaptive Versus Maladaptive Change

When considering traumatic brain injury, most concur that some degree of neuroplasticity must be operant following injury and thereby contributes to some of the partial recovery seen in head-injured patients, particularly those sustaining mild and moderate injury. Although this theme is common to most reviews regarding the recovery of brain function following injury, again it is remarkable how few studies have actually addressed this issue. Historically, considerations of neuroplasticity have derived their experimental foundation primarily through the use of isolated/discrete lesions of various areas of the neuraxis. In general, most paradigms exploring the potential for neuroplasticity used discrete or focal lesions to allow for relatively complete deafferentation of a target field, at least in terms of those projections derived from the area lesioned. Through such experimental approaches, various degrees of neuroplasticity have been demonstrated, and these findings have carried over into the clinical literature dealing with the recovery associated with traumatic brain injury. Unfortunately, in this scenario, there has been little consideration of the fact that the diffuse axonal injury, triggered by traumatic brain injury, may set the stage for a series of neuroplastic responses quite dissimilar from those occurring with large focal lesions. Thus, the question arises as to whether much of the information generated in the field of experimental plasticity can be immediately translated to the field of traumatic brain injury and repair. Recently, in a comprehensive review of those neuroplastic responses occurring with CNS injury, Oswald Steward recognized that the neuroplastic responses seen following focal versus diffuse injury may be dissimilar (105). In fact, Steward postulated that with diffuse axonal injury, the neuroplastic response may be more complete and adaptive than that seen following focal lesioning (102). He based this theory upon the premise that diffusely damaged axons would be found interspersed with the intact fibers, perhaps of the same functional type. Moving on the premise that the proximity of an intact fiber to a deafferentated site was predictive of the potential for reactive synaptic replacement, i.e., neuroplastic return, Steward hypothesized that the retention of intact fibers interspersed in foci of diffuse deafferentation could allow for a relatively complete neuroplastic (synaptic) recovery (102) (Figs. 12 and 13). Thus, in the case of mild traumatic brain injury, not only would the diffuse deafferentation cause the morbidity associated with the condition, but also it would set the stage for the ensuing adaptive neuroplasticity, which would explain the recovery ultimately seen following this injury. Having raised this provocative possibility, Steward acknowledged, however, that the experimental verification of this hypothesis would be difficult, as both complex animal modeling studies as well as extremely tedious experimental approaches would be needed to validate this assumption. Because of the importance of this issue, however, our laboratories initiated several studies of traumatic brain injury and the ensuing neuroplasticity. To this end, we chose to study the neuroplastic response in mild to moderate traumatic brain injury in that we wished to avoid the damaging consequences of ischemia and/or secondary insults. In the setting of mild to moderate injury, we focused on target nuclei known to be the sites of diffuse axonal injury with diffuse deafferentation. Additionally, we restricted our analysis to those target nuclei containing relatively homogeneous neurotransmitter populations (54). Our strategy, in this regard, was to utilize immunocytochemistry to follow terminal loss and neuroplastic recovery, and in this context, a homogeneous projection simplified the interpretation and analysis of our data. Initially, we confined our research efforts to the dorsolateral vestibular nucleus of the cat where we have previously identified traumatically induced reactive axonal change (54). The presence of reactive axonal change within this nucleus suggested the possibility of terminal loss within the same anatomical region. Further, since the majority of damaged axons within the dorsolateral vestibular nucleus are GABAergic, and since the somata in this region receive only GABAergic input, it appeared reasonable to assume that the diffuse axonal injury would correlate with GABAergic terminal loss. Also, since undamaged GABAergic fibers course through this nucleus, it appeared reasonable that these could provide for the ingrowth of GABAergic fibers to the traumatically deafferentated sites. Using both light microscopic and ultrastructural immunocytochemical analyses, with antibodies targeted against the neurotransmitter GABA, we confirmed the basic premise first articulated by Steward. Following traumatic brain injury, the presence of reactive axonal swellings within the dorsolateral vestibular nucleus correlated with the loss of perisomatic immunoreactive puncta/terminals. As posited, the loss of immunoreactive puncta/terminals did not occur at a highly focal fashion but occurred in a diffuse fashion throughout the nucleus (54). Some neuronal somata showed a control-like continuous perisomatic band of GABAergic immunoreactivity (Fig. 14a), whereas other somata demonstrated loss of perisomatic immunoreactive terminals in a scattered fashion (Fig. 14b,c). Parallel ultrastructural analyses confirmed that a direct correlation existed between a loss of immunoreactive and

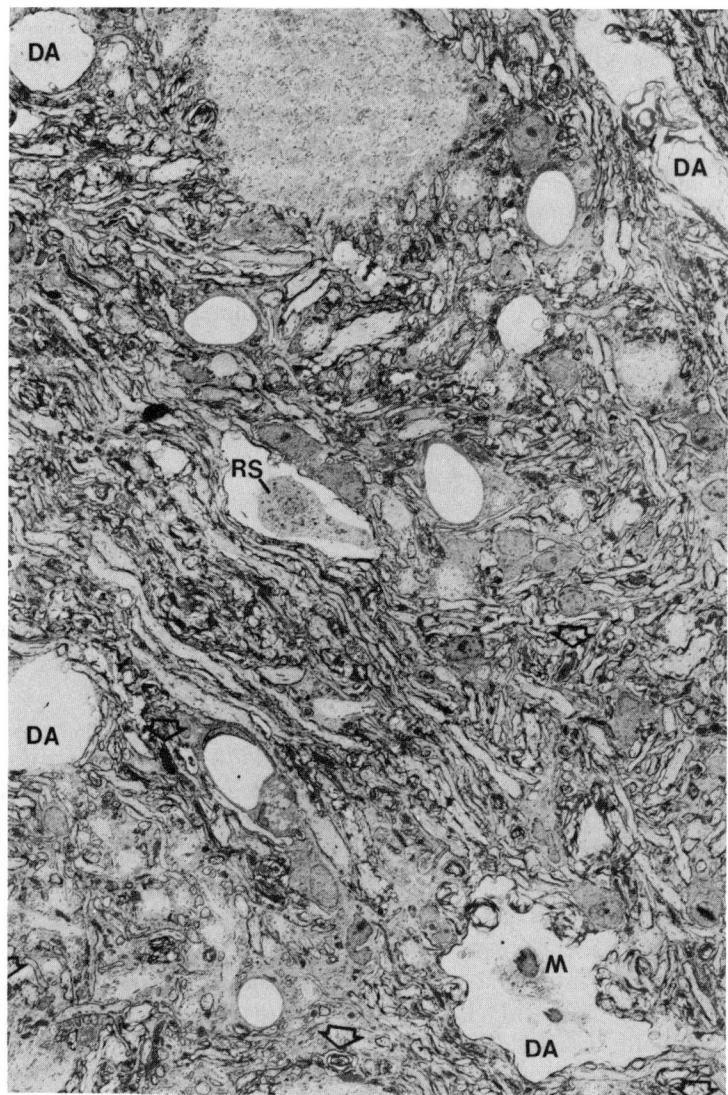

FIG. 12. This micrograph, harvested from the vestibular nucleus 7 days posttrauma, graphically illustrates some of the key features of diffuse axonal injury that underpin many of the concepts articulated by Steward. Note the presence of one reactive swelling *(RS)* as well as numerous damaged distal axonal segments *(DA)* undergoing collapse with macrophage *(m)* invasion and the formation of Wallerian debris *(open block arrows)*. Note that despite the presence of these diffusely reactive axonal changes, the balance of the brain parenchyma reveals intact and unaltered fibers and vascular elements. Thus, it is reasonable to suggest that this environment would promote repair following DAI and its attendant diffuse deafferentation. ×800. (Reproduced with permission from Erb and Povlishock, ref. 54.)

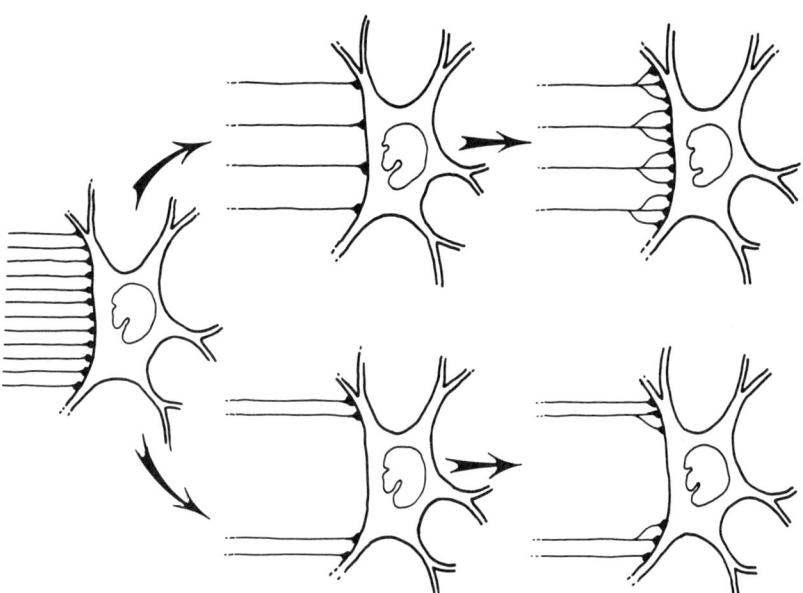

FIG. 13. Changes purported to occur following diffuse axonal injury with diffuse deafferentation. The *upper panel* of this cartoon illustrates that following diffuse axonal injury, diffuse deafferentation occurs. Note that the deafferentated neuron still shows the retention of related undamaged fiber systems. Over time *(arrows)*, these fiber systems are illustrated to sprout and functionally reoccupy the previously deafferentated domains, translating it to 100% reinnervation. In the *lower panel*, the results of large focal deafferentation are shown illustrating that a large area of deafferentation ensues and that this area lacks other intact fiber systems. This large focal deafferentation results in less-than-optimal synaptic return with an illustrated reinnervation of only 25% of control values. This cartoon emphasizes the fact that diffuse deafferentation may allow for more significant recovery than seen with focal deafferentation insults. (Reproduced with permission from Povlishock et al. ref. 85.)

terminal degeneration (54) (Fig. 15a,b). Of particular interest was the finding that over time postinjury, a progressive return of GABAergic terminals occurred (Fig. 14d). Contrary to expectations, however, this recovery was not rapid (54). The adapative recovery of GABAergic synaptic terminals required a prolonged period of posttraumatic survival to attain preinjury levels (54). Even by 6 months postinjury, the number of immunoreactive terminals encompassing the previously deafferentated somata had reached only 75% of control values. In fact, almost a year was required before the traumatically deafferentated soma had achieved a terminal density comparable to the controls. Although this prolonged adaptive terminal recovery seems to contradict existing laboratory studies of lesion induced neuroplasticity, this may relate to some features unique to diffuse axonal injury with diffuse deafferentation. The obvious criticism that can be directed against our studies, conducted in the cat dorsolateral vestibular nucleus, is that the sequence of deafferentation, followed by adaptive plasticity, may be unique to the respective nucleus with this relatively homogeneous synaptic input. Could similar events occur in target sites receiving much more complex and diffuse synaptic input? In such sites, diffuse deafferentation would occur, but it is not known if a complete return of homologous neurotransmitter systems could be achieved. We have begun to explore this issue in nuclei known both to receive diverse synaptic input and to demonstrate deafferentation. We have

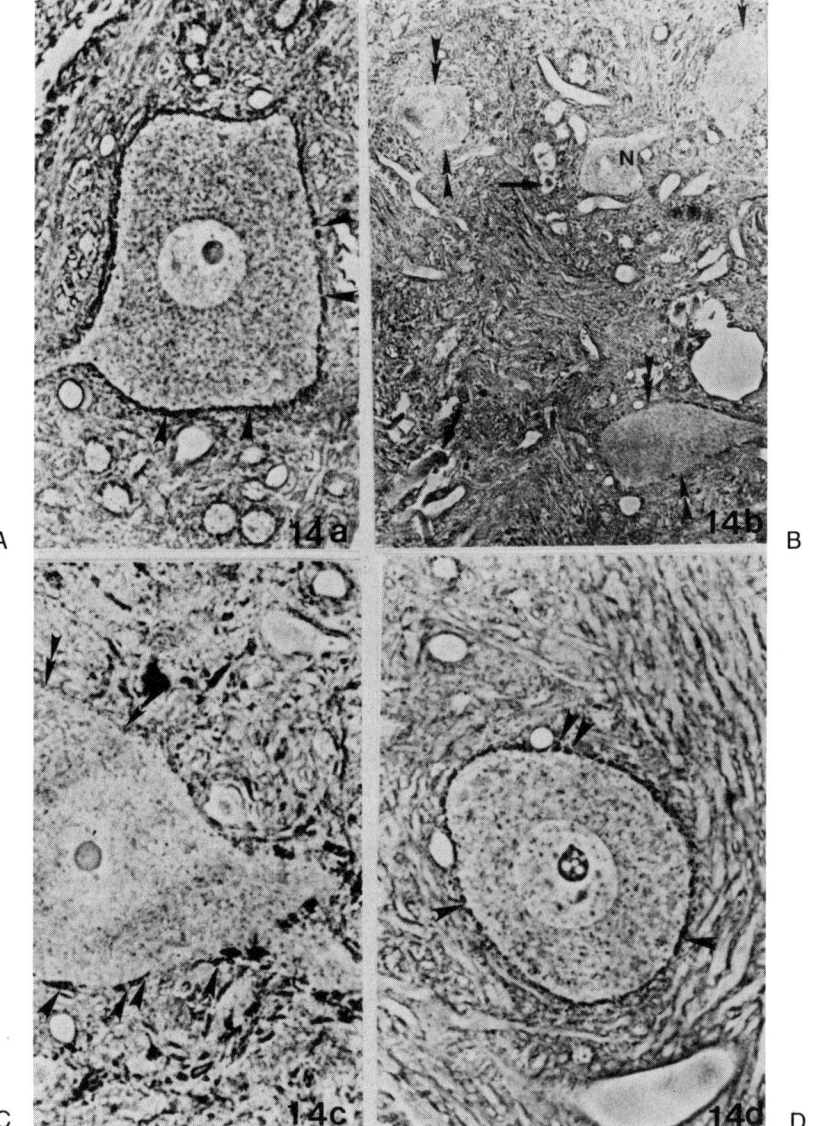

FIG. 14. These figures illustrate light micrographs taken through the vestibular nucleus processed for the immuncytochemical visualization of GABAergic terminal distribution. **A** reveals a control vestibular soma revealing numerous GABAergic-immunoreactive puncta *(arrowheads)* in relation to the somatic surface. **B** illustrates the loss of some immunoreactive puncta 7 days after traumatic brain injury. Note that the continuous band of perisomatic immunoreactivity seen in **A** is now disrupted with large areas of the somal surface revealing terminal/puncta loss *(double arrowheads)*. Note that this diffuse deafferentation occurs in the presence of diffusely damaged axons *(arrows)* seen scattered in the field. **C** reveals a neuronal soma from the vestibular nucleus 30 days after diffuse axonal injury. Note that despite the presence of some immunoreactive profiles *(arrowheads)*, large regions of the somal surface lack immunoreactive puncta (between double arrowheads). **D** is a light micrograph showing a neuronal soma harvested from the vestibular nucleus 1 year after injury. Note that the neuronal soma now displays a continuous band of immunoreactive puncta terminals *(arrowheads)* reminiscent of the control situation. a, ×750; b, ×250; c, ×800; d, ×750. (Reproduced with permission from Erb and Povlishock, ref. 54.)

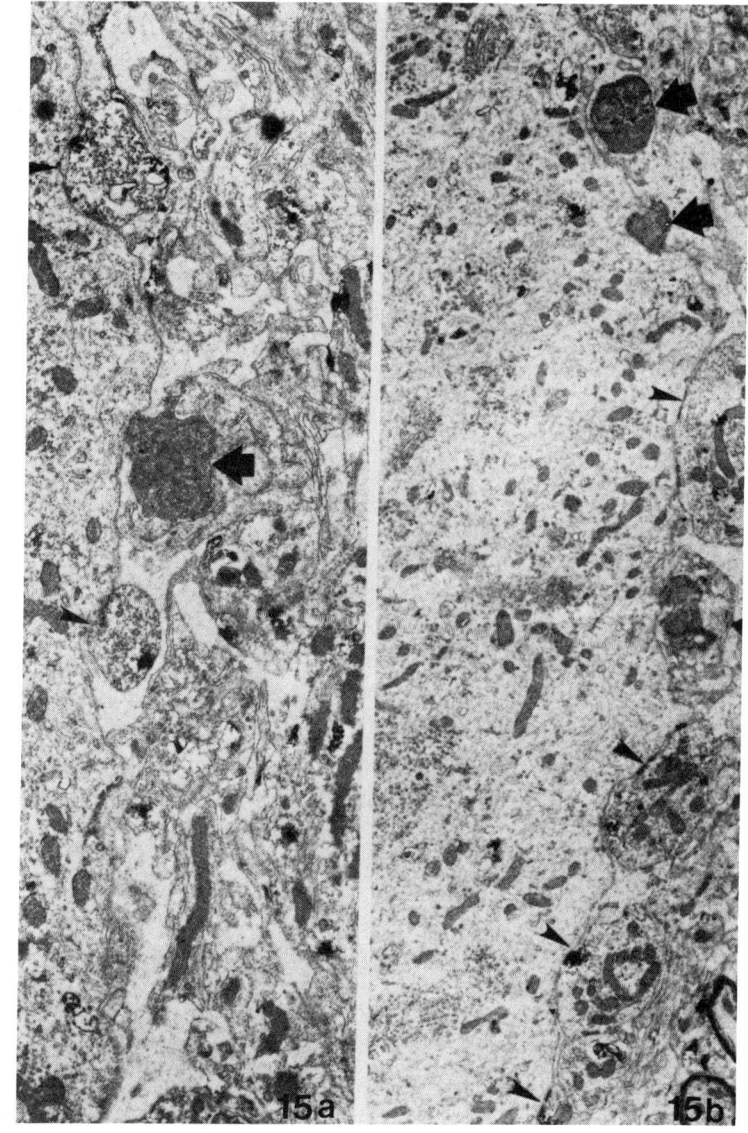

FIG. 15. These electron micrographs reveal the somal surface 7 days following the induction of diffuse axonal injury. Note that the number of immunoreactive terminals *(arrowheads)*, seen in both **A** and **B**, is reduced. As numerous terminals lose immunoreactivity and become electron dense *(block arrows)* they detach from the somal surface to be invested by reactive glial cells. These electron microscopic observations confirm the impression obtained in the previous light micrographs that a direct correlation exits between the loss of terminal immunoreactivity and neuronal degeneration. Thus, the following of neurotransmitter loss and return adequately reflects the actual loss and recovery of GABAergic immunoreactive puncta. a, ×10,000; b, ×10,000. (Reproduced with permission from Erb and Povlishock, ref. 54.)

initiated an investigation of deafferentation following traumatic brain injury in the cat red nucleus. Although our studies are by no means complete, the basic repertoire of change and repair described above appears operant, again supporting the assumption that the neuroplasticity, triggered by diffuse axonal injury and its subsequent deafferentation, may be more complete than that seen in other injurious/damaging conditions.

What is unknown in relation to the concept of diffuse deafferentation, followed by adaptive neuroplastic recovery, is the overall functional correlates of these events. Functional/behavioral studies have not been conducted in the experimental animals studied to date for various technical as well as animal welfare considerations. These issues are of obvious critical importance as it is imperative to understand if these neuroplastic changes translate into functional recovery. Indirect evidence, however, would suggest that these mechanisms are most likely operant in head-injured man, particularly those patients sustaining mild traumatic brain injury. In this patient population, Levin et al. (61) have described a distinct pattern of morbidity that is most likely correlated with modest diffuse deafferentation. Importantly, in this same population, Levin et al. (61) have also described over time a relatively complete recovery within this same patient population. Interestingly, the time to recovery typically entails 6 months to a year postinjury which, as such, is consistent with the prolonged adaptive recovery described in the cat model of traumatic brain injury. Whether such events are fully operant in the situation of human moderate traumatic brain injury remains to be determined. Again, based upon our animal studies, I predict that adaptive neuroplastic change is occurring following moderate human traumatic brain injury. In the human condition, however, the concomitant concurrence of focal lesions, such as contusion in hematoma formation, as well as the generation of secondary insults, may allow these damaging consequences to mask any potential adaptive recovery and, thereby, blunt its effectiveness. Last, in the case of severe human traumatic brain injury, the likelihood of adaptive recovery seems remote. Typically, with severe injury, mass lesion formation, focal lesions, and secondary insult clearly superimpose their damaging consequences upon any attempt of the brain to reorganize itself. Additionally, in this scenario, it is quite possible that the diffuseness of diffuse axonal injury, coupled with the large number of fibers involved, may allow for the ingrowth of nonadaptive systems and, thereby, contribute to maladaptive recovery. Clearly, many of these issues are purely speculative; yet, again, they would appear entirely consistent with a clinical impression of the morbidity and limited recovery seen in the case of severe traumatic brain injury.

REFERENCES

1. Hayes RL, Jenkins LW, Lyeth BC. Neurotransmitter-mediated mechanisms of traumatic brain injury: acetylcholine and excitatory amino acids. *J Neurotrauma* 1992; 9: S173–S183.
2. Bullock R, Fujisawa H. The role of glutamate antagonists for the treatment of CNS injury. *J Neurotrauma* 1992; 9: S443–S462.
3. Lyeth BG, Dixon CE, Hamm RJ, Jenkins LW, Young HF, Stonnington HH, Hayes RL. Effects of anticholinergic treatment on transient behavioral suppression and physiological responses following concussive rain injury to the rat. *Brain Res* 1988a; 448: 88–97.
4. Katayama Y, Becker DP, Tamura T, Hovda DA. Massive increases in extracellular potassium and the indiscriminate release of glutamate following concussive brain injury. *J Neurosurg* 1990; 73: 889–900.
5. Faden AI, Demediuk P, Panter SS, Vink R. The role of excitatory amino acids and NMDA receptors in traumatic brain injury. *Science* 1989; 244: 798–800.
6. Lyeth BG, Dixon CD, Jenkins LW, et al. Effects of scopolamine treatment on long-term behavioral deficits following concussive brain injury to the rat. *Brain Res* 1988b; 452: 39–48.
7. Lyeth BG, Jenkins LW, Hamm RJ, et al. Pretreatment with MK-801 reduces behavioral def-

icits following traumatic brain injury (TBI) in rats. *Soc Neurosci Abstr* 1989; 15: 1113.
8. Hayes RL, Stonnington HH, Lyeth BG, Dixon CE, Yamamoto T. Metabolic and neurophysiological sequelae of brain injury: a cholinergic hypothesis. *J CNS Trauma* 1986; 3(2): 163–173.
9. Hayes RL, Jenkins LW, Lyeth BG, et al. Pretreatment with phencyclidine, an N-methyl-D-aspartate receptor antagonist, attenuates long-term behavioral deficits in the rat produced by traumatic brain injury. *J Neurotrauma* 1988; 5(4): 287–302.
10. Hayes RL, Lyeth BG, Jenkins LW. Neurochemical mechanisms of mild and moderate head injury: Implications for treatment. In: Levin HS, Eisenberg HM, and Benton AL, eds. *Mild head injury*. New York: Oxford University Press; 1989: 54–79.
11. Hayes RL, Lyeth BG, Jenkins LW, Dixon CE, Hamm RJ. NMDA receptor antagonist reduce long-term behavioral deficits in rats produced by traumatic brain injury: role of hypothermia and time of administration. *J Neurotrauma* (in review).
12. McIntosh TK, Vink R, Soares H, Hayes RL and Simon R. Effects of N-methyl-D-aspartate receptor blocker MK-801 on neurologic function after experimental brain injury. *J Neurotrauma* 1989; 6: 247–259.
13. McIntosh TK, Vink R, Soares H, Hayes RL and Simon R. Effects of noncompetitive blockade of N-methyl-D-aspartate receptors on neurochemical sequelae of experimental brain injury. *J Neurochem* 1990; 55: 1170–1179.
14. Robinson SE, Fox SD, Posner MG, et al. The effect of M_1 muscarinic blockade on behavior following traumatic brain injury in the rat. *Brain Res* 1990; 511: 141–148.
15. Jenkins LW, Moszynski K, Lyeth G, et al. Increased vulnerability of the mildly traumatized brain to cerebral ischemia: the use of controlled secondary ischemia as a research tool to identify common or different mechanisms contributing to mechanical and ischemic brain injury. *Brain Res* 1989; 477: 211–224.
16. Jenkins LW, Lyeth BG, Lewelt W, et al. Combined pre-trauma scopolamine and phencyclidine attenuates post-traumatic increased sensitivity to delayed secondary ischemia. *J Neurotrauma* 1988a; 5(4): 303–315.
17. Persson L, Hillered L. Chemical monitoring of neurosurgical intensive care patients using intracerebral microdialysis. *J Neurosurg* 1992; 76(1): 72–80.
18. Siesjo BK, Wieloch T. Molecular mechanisms of ischemic brain damage: Ca^2 related events. In: *Cerebrovascular*
19. Meldrum B, Garthwaite J. Excitatory amino acid neurotoxicity and neurodegenerative disease. *TIPS* 1990; 11: 379–387.
20. Choi DW, Koh JY, Peters S. Pharmacology of glutamate neurotoxicity in cortical cell culture: attenuation by NMDA antagonists. *J Neurosci* 1988; 8: 185–196.
21. Strich SJ. Diffuse degeneration of the cerebral white matter in severe dementia following head injury. *J Neurol Neurosurg Psychiatry* 1956; 19: 163–185.
22. Strich SJ. Shearing of nerve fibers as a cause of brain damage due to head injury. *Lancet* 1961; 2: 443–448.
23. Oppenheimer DR. Microscopic lesions of the brain following head injury. *J Neurol Neurosurg Psychiatry* 1968; 31: 299–306.
24. Peerless SJ, Rewcastle NB. Shear injuries of the brain. *Can Med Assoc J* 1967; 96: 577–582.
25. Adams JH, Doyle D, Ford I, Gennarelli TA, Graham DI, McLellan D. Diffuse axonal injury in head injury: definition, diagnosis and grading. *Histopathology* 1989; 15: 49–59.
26. Adams JH, Mitchell DE, Graham DI, Doyle D. Diffuse brain damage of immediate impact type: Its relationship to 'primary brainstem damage' in head injury. *Brain* 1977; 100: 487–502.
27. Adams JH, Graham DI, Gennarelli TA. Head injury in man animals. *Acta Neurochir* 1983; 32: 15–30.
28. Adams JH, Graham DI, Murray LS, Scott G. Diffuse axonal injury due to nonmissile head injury in humans: An analysis of 45 cases. *Ann Neurol* 1982; 12: 557–563.
29. Adams JH, Graham DI, Scott G, Parker L, Doyle D. Brain damage in fatal non-missile head injury. *J Clin Pathol* 1980; 33: 1132–1145.
30. Gennarelli TA, Thibault LE, Adams JH, Graham DI, Thompson CJ, Marcincin RP. Diffuse axonal injury and traumatic coma in the primate. *Ann Neurol* 1982; 12: 564–574.
31. Pilz P. Axonal injury in head injury. *Acta Neurochir* 1983; 32: 119–126.
32. Povlishock JT, Becker DP, Cheng DLY, Vaughan GW. Axonal change in minor head injury. *J Neuropathol Exp Neurol* 1983; 42: 225–242.
33. Povlishock JT. Traumatically induced axonal damage without concomitant change in focally related neuronal somata and dendrites. *Acta Neuropathol* 1986; 70: 53–79.
34. Povlishock JT, Kontos HA. Continuing axonal and vascular change following experimental brain trauma. *Cent Nerv Syst* 1985; 2: 285–297.
35. Povlishock JT. The morphopathologic responses to experimental head injuries of varying severity. In: Becker D, Povlishock J, eds. *Central nervous system status report 1985*. Richmond: William Byrd Press; 1985: 443–452.
36. Povlishock JT. Diffuse deafferentation as the major determinant of morbidity and recovery following traumatic brain injury. *Adv Neurotrauma Res* 1990; 2: 1–11.
37. Povlishock JT. Traumatically induced axonal injury: pathogenesis and pathobiological implications. *Brain Pathology* 1991; 2: 1–12.
38. Cheng CLY, Povlishock JT. The effect of traumatic brain injury on the visual system: a morphologic characterization of reactive axonal change. *J Neurotrauma* 1988; 5: 47–60.

39. Gennarelli TA, Thibault LE, Tipperman R, et al. Axonal injury in the optic nerve: a model stimulating diffuse axonal injury in the brain. *J Neurosurg* 1989; 71: 244–253.
40. Erb DE, Povlishock JT. Axonal damage in severe traumatic brain injury: an experimental study in the cat. *Acta Neuropathol* 1988; 76: 347–358.
41. Maxwell WL, Kansagra AM, Graham DI, Adams JH, Gennarelli TA. Freeze-fracture studies of reactive myelinated nerve fibers after diffuse axonal injury. *Acta Neuropathol* 1988; 76: 395–406.
42. Yaghmai A, Povlishock JT. Traumatically induced reactive change as visualized through the use of monoclonal antibodies targeted to the neurofilament subunits. *J Neuropathol Exp Neurol* 1991; 51(2): 158–176.
43. Povlishock JT, Becker DP. Fate of reactive axonal swellings induced by head injury. *Lab Invest* 1985; 52: 540–552.
44. Jane AJ, Steward O, Gennarelli T. Axonal degeneration induced by experimental noninvasive minor head injury. *J Neurosurg* 1985; 62: 96–100.
45. Vanezis P, Chan KK, Scholtz CL. White matter damage following acute head injury. *Forensic Sci Int* 1987; 35: 1–10.
46. Maxwell WL, Graham AI, Adams JH, Gennarelli TA. Tipperman R, Sturatis M. Focal axonal injury: the early axonal response to stretch. *J Neurocytol* 1991; 20: 157–164.
47. Adams JH, Graham DI, Gennarelli TA, Maxwell WI. Diffuse axonal injury in non-missile head injury. *J Neurol Neurosurg Psychiatry* 1991; 54: 481–483.
48. Balentine JD, Hilton CW. Ultrastructural pathology of axons and myelin in calcium induced myelopathy. *J Neuropathol Exp Neurol* 1980; 39: 339.
49. Balentine JD. Hypotheses in spinal cord trauma research. In: Becker D, Povlishock JT, eds. *Central nervous system status report*. Richmond: William Byrd Press; 1985: 455–461.
50. Schlaepfer WW. Calcium-induced degeneration of axoplasm in isolated segments of rat peripheral nerve. *Brain Res* 1974; 69: 203–215.
51. Schlaepfer WW. Neurofilaments: structure, metabolism and implications in disease. *J Neuropathol Exp Neurol* 1987; 46: 117–129.
52. Angelides KJ, Smith KE, Tameda M. Assembly and exchange of intermediate filament proteins of neurons; neurofilaments are dynamic structures. *J Cell Biol* 1989; 108: 1495–1506.
53. Grady MS, McLaughlin MR, Christman CW, Valadka AB, Fligner CL, Povlishock JT. The use of antibodies targeted against the neurofilament subunits for the detection of diffuse axonal injury in humans. *J Neuropathol Exp Neurol* (in press).
54. Erb DE, Povlishock JT. Neuroplasticity following traumatic brain injury: a study of GABAergic terminal loss and recovery in the cat dorsal lateral vestibular nucleus. *Exp Brain Res* 1991; 83: 253–267.
55. Friede RL. Experimental concussion acceleration. *Arch Neurol* 1961; 4: 109–120.
56. Yoshino A, Hovda DA, Kawamata T, Katayama Y, Becker DP. Dynamic changes in local cerebral glucose utilization following cerebral concussion in rats: Evidence of a hyper- and subsequent hypometabolic state. *Brain Res* (in press).
57. Hayes RL, Pechura CM, Katayama Y, Povlishock JT, Yeatts ML, Becker DP. Activation of midbrain cholinergic sites implicated in unconsciousness following cerebral concussion in the cat. *Science* 1984; 223: 301–303.
58. Hayes RL, Katayama Y, Jenkins LW, Lyeth BG, Clifton GL, Gunter J, Povlishock JT, Young HF. Regional rates in glucose utilization in the cat following concussive head injury. *J Neurotrauma* 1988; 5(2): 121–127.
59. Doberstin C, Martin NA, Caron MJ, Zane C, Johnson JP, Kathleen T, Becker DP. Detection of posttraumatic arterial spasm using transcranial doppler and Xenon-133 rCBF monitoring. *Proceedings for the Society for Neurotrauma Society,* St. Louis, 1990.
60. Adams J, Graham D, Gennarelli T. Contemporary neuropathological considerations regarding brain damage in head injury. In: Becker DP, Povlishock J, eds. *Central nervous system status report*. Richmond: William Byrd Press; 1985: 65–77.
61. Levin HS, Mattis S, Ruff RM. Neurobehavioral outcome following minor head injury: A three-center study. *J Neurosurg* 1987b; 66: 234–243.
62. Lewelt W, Jenkins LW, Miller JD. Autoregulation of cerebral blood flow after experimental fluid percussion injury. *J Neurosurg* 1980; 53: 500–511.
63. Enevoldsen EM, Jensen FT. Autoregulation and CO_2 responses of cerebral blood flow in patients with acute severe head injury. *J Neurosurg* 1978; 48: 689–703.
64. Wei EP, Dietrich WD, Povlishock JT, Kontos HA. Functional, morphologic, metabolic abnormalities of the cerebral microcirculation after concussive brain injury in cats. *Circ Res* 1980; 46(1): 37–47.
65. Marion DW, Darby J, Yonas H. Acute regional/cerebral blood flow changes caused by severe head injuries. *J Neurosurg* 1991; 74: 407–414.
66. Bouma GJ, Muizelaar JP, Choi SC, Newlon PG, Young HF. Cerebral circulation and metabolism after severe traumatic brain injury; the elusive role of ischemia. *J Neurosurg* 1991; 75: 685–693.
67. DeWitt DS, Jenkins LW, Wei EP, et al. Effects of fluid-percussion brain injury on regional cerebral blood flow and pial arteriolar diameter. *J Neurosurg* 1986; 64(5): 787–794.
68. Yamakami I, McIntosh TK. Effects of traumatic brain injury on regional cerebral blood

69. Muizelaar JP, Ward JD, Marmarou A, Newlon PG, Wachi A. Cerebral blood flow and metabolism in severely head-injured children. Pat 2: Autoregulation. *J Neurosurg* 1989; 71: 72–76.
70. Obrist WD, Gennarelli TA, Segawa H, et al. Relation of cerebral blood flow to neurological status and outcome in head-injured patients. *J Neurosurg* 1979; 51: 292–300.
71. Povlishock JT, Becker DP, Sullivan HG, Miller JD. Vascular permeability alterations to horseradish peroxidase in experimental brain injury. *Brain Res* 1978; 153: 223–239.
72. Ellison MD, Erb DE, Kontos HA, Povlishock JT. Recovery of impaired endothelium-dependent relaxation after fluid-percussion brain injury in cats. *Stroke* 1989; 20: 911–917.
73. Graham DI, Adams JH, Doyle D. Ischemic brain damage in fatal non-missile head injuries. 1978; 39: 213–234.
74. Barclay L, Zemcov A, Reichert W, et al. Cerebral blood flow decrements in chronic head injury syndrome. *Biol Psychiatry* 1985; 20: 146–157.
75. Obrist WD, Langfitt TW, Jaggi JL, et al. Cerebral blood flow and metabolism in comatose patients with acute head injury. Relationship to intracranial hypertension. *J Neurosurg* 1984; 61: 241–253.
76. Tornheim PA. Traumatic edema in head injury. In: Becker DP, Povlishock JT, eds. *Central nervous system trauma status report*. Richmond: William Byrd Press; 1985: 431–439.
77. Kontos HA, Wei EP, Povlishock JT, Dietrich WD, Ellis EF, and Magiera CJ. Cerebral arteriolar damage by arachidonic acid and prostaglandin G. *Science* 1980; 209: 1242–1245.
78. Kontos HA, Wei EP, Ellis EF, Dietrich WD, Povlishock JT. Prostaglandins in physiological and in certain pathological responses of the cerebral circulation. *Fed Proc* 1981; 40: 2326–2330.
79. Kontos HA, Wei EP, Povlishock JT. Pathophysiology of vascular consequences of experimental concussive brain injury. *Trans Am Clin Climatol Assoc* 1981; 30: 111–121.
80. Kontos HA, Wei EP, Christman CW, Povlishock JT, Ellis EF. Free oxygen radicals in cerebral vascular response. *Physiologist* 1983; 26: 265–269.
81. Kontos HA, Wei EP, Povlishock JT, Christman CW. Oxygen radicals mediate the cerebral arteriolar dilation from arachidonate and bradykinin in cats. *Circ Res* 1984; 55: 295–303.
82. Wei EP, Christman CW, Kontos HA, Povlishock JT. Effects of oxygen radicals on cerebral arterioles. *Am J Physiol* 1985; 248: 157–162.
83. Wei EP, Kontos HA, Ellison MD, Povlishock JT. Oxygen radicals in arachidonate-induced increased blood-brain barrier permeability to proteins. *Am J Physiol* 1986; 251: H693–H699.
84. Kontos HA, Povlishock JT. Oxygen radicals in brain injury. *Cent Nerv Syst Trauma* 1986; 3: 257–263.
85. Povlishock JT, Erb DE, Astruc J. Axonal response to traumatic brain injury: reactive axonal change, deafferentation, and neuroplasticity. *J Neurotrauma* 1992; 9(1): S189–200.
86. Ishige N, Pitts LH, Carlson S et al. Effects of hypoxia on rat brain with traumatic injury. *J Cereb Blood Flow Metabol* 1987; 7(1): s638.
87. Ishige N, Pitts LH, Pogliani L, Hashimoto T, Nishimjura BS, Bartkowski HM, James TL. Effect of hypoxia on traumatic brain injury in rats: Part 2: Changes in high energy phosphate metabolism. *Neurosurgery* 1987; 20: 854–858.
88. Von Monakow C. Diaschisis (Harris G, translator). In: Pribram, ed. *Brain and behavior, 1. Mood, states and mind*. Baltimore: Penguin Books: 1969.
89. Glees P, Cole, J. Recovery of skilled motor functions after small repeated lesions of motor cortex in macaque. *J Neurophysiol* 1950; 13: 137–148.
90. Glassman RB, Malamut BL. Recovery from electroencephalographic slowing and reduced evoked potentials after somatosensory cortical damage in cats. *Behav Biol* 1976; 17: 333–354.
91. Feeney DM, Sutton RL. Pharmacotherapy for recovery of function after brain injury. *CRC Crit Rev Neurobiol* 1987; 13: 135–197.
92. Feeney DM, Baron JC. Diaschisis. *Stroke* 1986; 17–817.
93. Boyeson MG, Feeney DM, Dail WG: Cortical microstimulation thresholds adjacent to sensorimotor cortex injury. *J Neurotrauma* 1991; 8: 205–217.
94. Gilson BC, Stensaas LJ. Early axonal changes following lesions of the dorsal columns in rats. *Cell Tissue Res* 1974; 149: 1.
95. Lampert PW. A comparative electron microscopic study of reactive, degenerating, regenerating and dystrophic axons. *J Neuropathol Exp Neurol* 1967; 26: 345.
96. Lampert PW, Cressman M. Axonal regeneration in the dorsal columns of the spinal cord of adult rats. *Lab Invest* 1964; 13: 825.
97. David S, Aguayo AJ. Axonal elongation into peripheral nervous system "bridges" after central nervous system injury in adult rats. *Science* 1981; 214: 931–933.
98. Richardson PM, Issa VMK, Aguayo AJ. Regeneration of long spinal axons in the rat. *J Neurocytol* 1984; 13: 165–182.
99. Friede RL, Bischhausen R. The fine structure of stumps of transected nerve fibers in subserial sections. *J Neurol Sci* 1980; 44: 181.
100. Caroni P, Schwab ME. Antibody against myelin-associated inhibitor of neurite growth neutralizes nonpermissive substrate properties of CNS white matter. *Neuron* 1988b; 1: 85–96.
101. Savio T, Schwab ME. Rat CNS white matter, but not gray matter, is nonpermissive for neuronal cell adhesion and fiber outgrowth. *J Neurosci* 1989; 9: 1126–1133.
102. Savio T, Schwab ME. Lesioned corticospinal

tract axons regenerate in myelin-free rat spinal cord. *Proc Natl Acad Sci USA* 1990; 87: 4930–4133.
103. Schnell L, Schwab ME. Axonal regeneration in the rat spinal cord produced by an antibody against myelin-associated neurite growth inhibitors. *Nature* 1990; 343: 269–272.
104. Schwab ME. Myelin-associated inhibitors of neurite growth and regeneration in the CNS. *Trends Neurosci* 1990; 13: 452–456.
105. Steward O. Reorganization of neural connections following CNS trauma. Principles and experimental paradigms. *J Neurotrauma* 1989; 6: 99–152.

11

Molecular Cascades in Adaptive Versus Pathological Plasticity

Carl W. Cotman, Brian J. Cummings, and Christian J. Pike

Department of Psychobiology, University of California, Irvine, California 92717

Plasticity processes are essential for properly maintaining normal brain function (e.g., learning and memory) but they are also critical in that they can contribute to the recovery of function after injury or disease. As the brain ages, it must depend more and more on its regulatory and plasticity capacities. The aged brain is subject to increased challenges (e.g., cell loss, toxic insults, metabolic losses, etc.), which often accumulate and increase the risk of dysfunction and age-related neurodegenerative conditions such as Alzheimer's disease. The goals of basic regenerative research include identifying key plasticity mechanisms, understanding what regulates them, and applying this information to better understand normal function and eventually treat disease in man.

The hippocampal formation provides an excellent system for studies of synaptic growth and plasticity in the mature or aged brain (see Fig. 1). The hippocampus has extensive involvement in the plastic processes of learning and memory, has a well-defined anatomy, and sprouts and/or forms new synapses (reactive synaptogenesis) in response to lesions of its extrinsic and intrinsic circuitry. Previous work has shown that following such circuitry lesions, hippocampal reactive growth begins within a few days and continues for several weeks (1,2). Changes in the morphology and number of glia during this response are known, as are the functional properties of the new synapses. In addition to the observed reactive growth, these lesions result in the retrograde degeneration of neurons that project to the hippocampus and have lost contact with their targets. These changes in the hippocampus allow for not only study of the processes of degeneration and regeneration, but also evaluation of possible interventions. Interestingly, some of the same neuronal populations examined in these animal studies undergo similar degeneration and regeneration in Alzheimer's disease (AD), making it possible to evaluate predictions from animal studies to this progressive neurodegenerative disease.

In this chapter we discuss the molecular components that appear to regulate reactive synaptogenesis and, conversely, the factors that contribute to neuronal degeneration. Regenerative growth, characterized by the enhanced viability and reactive sprouting of neurons surviving an insult, requires two components: growth factors and suitable substrates. The influence of these factors and their importance in hippocampal and cortical plasticity has been demonstrated in both tissue culture and animal models. Basic fibroblast growth factor (bFGF) and the glycosaminoglycan heparan sulfate (HS) exemplify the pivotal roles in growth regulation played by trophic factors and substrates, respectively. We will discuss the nature of in vitro data supporting a role of

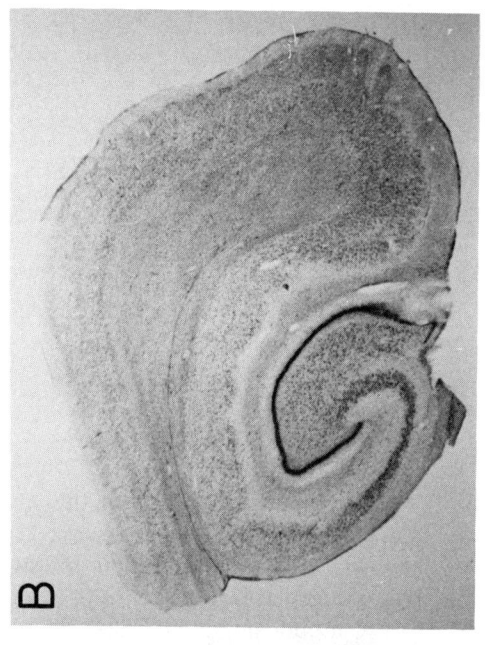
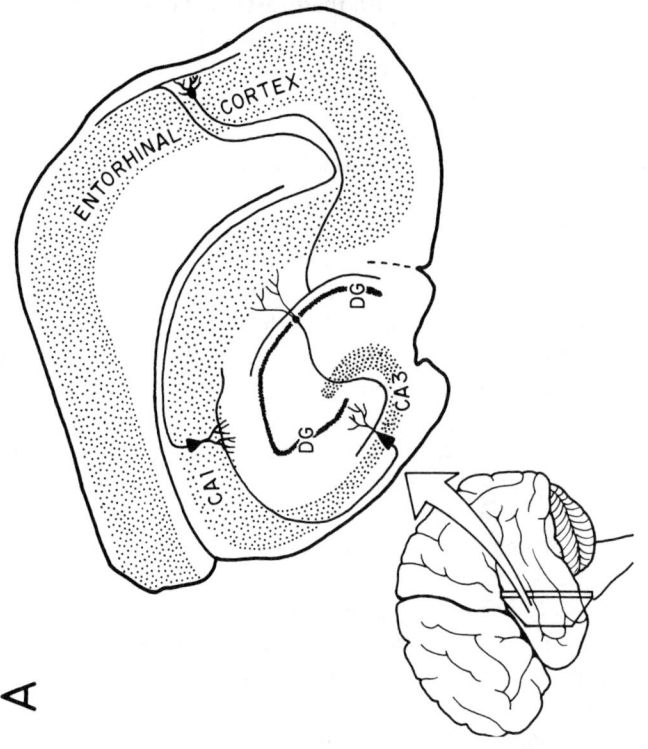

FIG. 1. The hippocampus is a highly plastic brain region. **A:** The hippocampal formation is located in the temporal lobe. Its circuitry includes projections from the entorhinal cortex to the dentate gyrus (DG) granule cells. These cells in turn form downstream connections with the hippocampal CA3 and CA1 subfields, which then return projections to the cortical mantle. **B:** A Nissl-stained section of human hippocampus illustrates the cellular distribution of hippocampal subfields CA1, CA3, and the dentate gyrus.

bFGF and HS in sprouting and regeneration, and then examine the extent to which such data apply to in vivo conditions. Next we describe the characteristics of bFGF induction in response to partial denervation. The data imply that injury, even in a degenerative disease, may be associated with molecular conditions that stimulate growth. Finally, we describe cellular and molecular tests of this hypothesis in AD brains, comparing predictions from animal models to AD. We suggest that though initially adaptive, over time plasticity processes in the AD brain ironically may accelerate dysfunction. For example, cellular events associated with regenerative growth in AD appear to interact positively with the β-amyloid protein. However, this interaction may ultimately contribute to neuronal degeneration.

GROWTH FACTORS AND SUBSTRATE MOLECULES INCREASE NEURONAL SURVIVAL AND NEURITE OUTGROWTH IN VITRO

Cultured central nervous system neurons are responsive to a variety of growth factors and substrates. Among the most effective growth factors for cultures of hippocampal and cortical neurons are fibroblast growth factors, in particular bFGF. Developing cortical (3–5) and hippocampal (6–8) cultures treated with bFGF at concentrations as low as 1 picomolar show greatly enhanced survival relative to nontreated control cultures. Also, bFGF enhances survival in in vitro regeneration paradigms using axotomized adult retinal cells (9) and wounded hippocampal neurons (10). In addition, in vitro bFGF treatment yields large increases in both the lengths and branching of hippocampal axons and dendrites (5,6,8). Thus, conditions that increase the availability of bFGF to hippocampal and cortical neurons will likely promote corresponding gains in neuronal sprouting and resiliency.

Substrate factors also provide important support for plastic and regenerative responses. The microenvironment in which cells exist is called the extracellular matrix and consists of many different substrate components, including laminin, fibronectin, and glycosaminoglycans. Substrate factors in the extracellular matrix are believed to interact with cells, affecting adhesion, neurite outgrowth, differentiation, and a variety of other biological activities (11–13). One substrate factor that has gained considerable research attention recently is the glycosaminoglycan HS.

We have observed that neurons grown on an HS substrate show dramatically increased axonal elongation in culture. As shown in Fig. 2, after 24 hours in vitro, hippocampal neurons grown on a HS-coated tissue culture dish extend significantly longer neurites than those grown on noncoated dishes (C.J.P. and C.W.C., unpublished observations). This effect is concentration dependent (data not shown) and appears quite specific since the related glycosaminoglycan (GAG) chondroitin sulfate is ineffective in neurite promotion (Fig. 2B).

We have also observed that both HS and CS substrates yield significant increases in the survival of hippocampal neurons; however only HS is effective at very low concentrations (data not shown). Increased survival by these substrates is transient, as the enhancement diminishes over time. Thus, the increases in neuritic outgrowth and neuronal survival are probably related to adhesive properties rather than true trophic activity. HS and CS substrates may facilitate both survival and neuritic outgrowth by promoting cellular attachment, but alone are insufficient for the maintenance of healthy neurons.

bFGF and HS Interact Synergistically In Vitro

Since growth factors and substrates often exist in the same environment, study of their interactions can yield a more complete

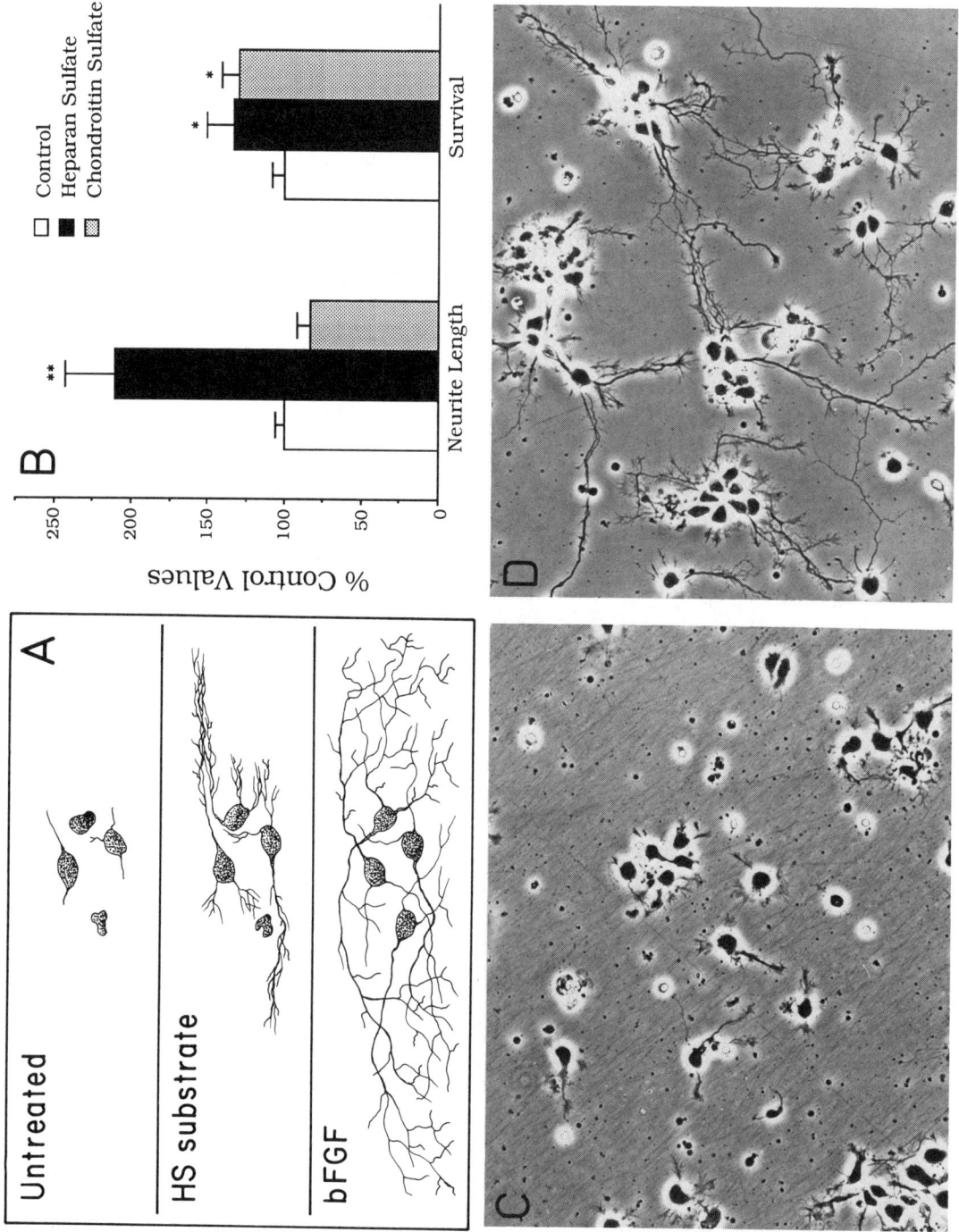

understanding of their functional properties. In the case of bFGF and HS, accumulating evidence suggests substantial interactions at many levels. First, bFGF has a strong binding affinity for HS and the closely related GAG heparin (14,15). When bound to HS or heparin, bFGF has a larger effective radius from its source due to increased diffusion (16) and is protected from proteolytic degradation (17,18). In addition, recent evidence suggests that bFGF is internalized into cells only when it is bound to heparin (19). Thus, the growth factor activity of bFGF would appear to require interaction with the substrate factors HS or heparin. In fact, the in vitro neurite-promoting activity of bFGF discussed above is potentiated on HS and heparin substrates (20,21).

In summary, evidence from in vitro studies suggests that both bFGF and HS stimulate neuritic outgrowth and enhance survival. Thus, effective regenerative responses should utilize both growth factors and substrate components. However, these substances also function in a variety of interactions, some of which may be relevant to disease states. It is essential to expand observations from in vitro models to in vivo paradigms.

GROWTH FACTORS ENHANCE REGENERATIVE SPROUTING AND CELL SURVIVAL IN ANIMAL MODELS

While there is an established body of literature about the effects of both trophic and substrate factors in vitro, less is known about the involvement of these substances in regenerative responses in vivo. One of the first examples was the finding that nerve growth factor (NGF), when administered intraventricularly after injury, can ameliorate cholinergic cell loss in rodents (22,23). It has also been demonstrated that infusion of bFGF can prevent the death of septal cholinergic neurons after transection of the fimbria-fornix (24). As mentioned above, bFGF is trophic in vitro to a wide variety of neuronal types, including noncholinergic neurons.

In order to determine if bFGF is also trophic in vivo to noncholinergic neurons, it is necessary to identify a suitable neuronal system. In considering the type of system to study, we sought to identify one naturally vulnerable to degenerative conditions. The entorhinal cortex is ideal in many ways since it degenerates in AD, and its layer II and III neurons project to the dentate gyrus and appear to utilize the neurotransmitter glutamate. Accordingly, we carried out experiments to determine if these neurons undergo atrophy or degeneration after axotomy and if these changes are affected by bFGF (see Fig. 3).

When the perforant pathway from the entorhinal cortex to the dentate gyrus is axotomized, approximately 30% of the neurons in layer II of entorhinal cortex die within 2 weeks as determined by cell counts. Remaining cells often demonstrate atrophy. Continuous intraventricular infusion of bFGF for 2 weeks following the knife cut is capable of reducing this cell loss to less than 5% (Table 1) (25). Thus, bFGF expresses in vivo trophic activity on a variety of cell types, making it the most general growth factor known.

FIG. 2. Growth factors and substrate components promote neuronal survival and process outgrowth in vitro. **A:** The diagram depicts the neurotrophic properties of HS and bFGF. **B:** Although both heparan sulfate (HS) and chondroitin sulfate (CS) enhance survival, only the more sulfated glycosaminoglycan HS increases neurite elongation. In comparison to cultured hippocampal neurons in the untreated control condition **(C)**, those in the **(D)** HS substrate condition rapidly extend longer, more branched neurites. Data were obtained from rat hippocampal cultures grown for 24 hours on dishes with either polylysine alone or polylysine treated with 100 µg/ml HS or CS.

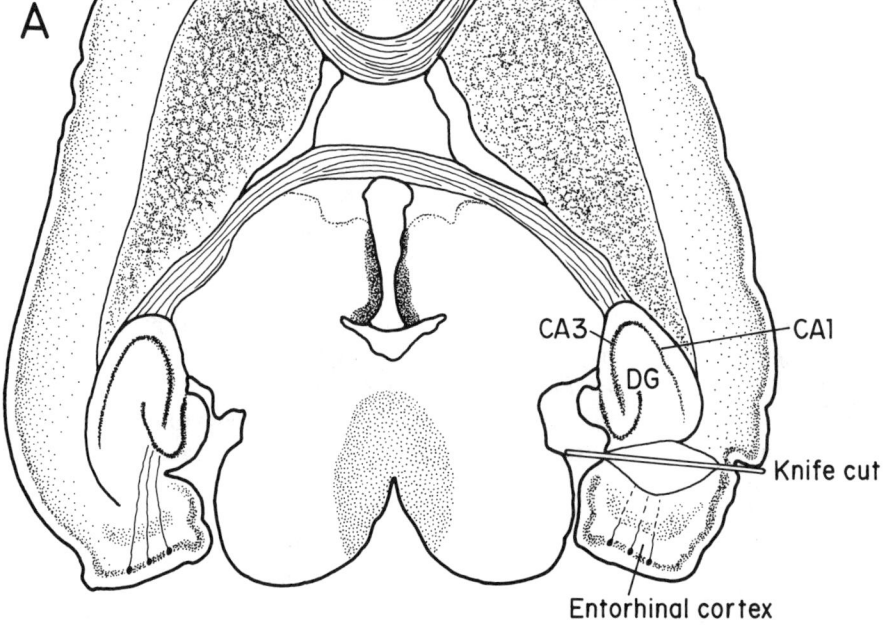
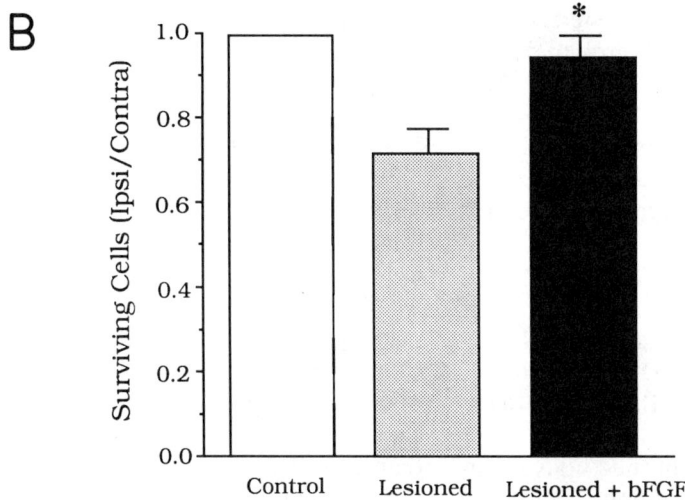

FIG. 3. bFGF rescues entorhinal cortical neurons in mature rats following axotomy. **A:** The diagram illustrates a lesion of the perforant pathway, which severs the axons of layer II stellate cells in the entorhinal cortex and results in approximately 30% loss of these cells. **B:** Continuous intraventricular infusion of 25 ng/hr bFGF over a period of 14 days reduces the cell loss to only 5% (25).

TABLE 1. *bFGF prevents neuronal loss after perforant path axotomy*[a]

Group	Ipsi/contra ratio	Standard error
Naive animals	1.00	.02
Lesioned	.72	.04
Lesioned + bFGF	.94	.04

[a]Neurons in layer II of entorhinal cortex from ipsilateral and contralateral sides relative to a unilateral knife cut of the perforant pathway were counted in nine 20 μm sections each, 14 days after the lesion. There was a 28% cell loss on the lesion side in control animals that received a knife cut. Intraventricular infusion of bFGF (25 ng/hr) for 14 days significantly reduced this loss to approximately 5%. (Student's T-test, $p \leq .005$.)

bFGF Levels Increase After CNS Injury

Previously, we have demonstrated that injury to the CNS evokes a time-dependent increase in neurotrophic factor activity (26), but the identity of these factors was not determined. Accordingly, we evaluated the possibility that bFGF might increase as a result of injury (see Fig. 4).

After a unilateral entorhinal cortex lesion, the hippocampus ipsilateral to the lesion showed an enhancement of bFGF immunoreactivity in the dentate gyrus (DG) outer molecular layer where the entorhinal fibers terminate. An increase in the number of bFGF immunopositive astrocytes was already evident at postlesion day 2, reached a maximum by day 7 and decreased to about normal levels by day 14. Computer densitometry showed an increase in bFGF immunoreactivity within individual astrocytes in the DG outer molecular layer reaching significance by postlesion day 7 and remaining through postlesion day 14, relative to the contralateral side and untreated controls. Astrocytes surrounding lesion areas showed increased bFGF immunoreactivity in their processes, and their cell bodies appeared to be enlarged and more darkly stained than bFGF-immunoreactive astrocytes in normal rats. The extracellular matrix surrounding bFGF-positive astrocytes also showed an increase in bFGF immunoreactivity with a similar time course. Parallel serial sections histochemically stained for acetylcholinesterase (AChE), a marker of axon sprouting by septal cells in the hippocampus (27), also showed enhanced staining of the DG outer molecular layer. The time course of AChE-staining intensification was similar to that observed with bFGF antibody staining (28).

The fact that an increase in bFGF immunoreactivity was detected in the extracellular matrix of the dentate gyrus ipsilateral to the lesion suggests that bFGF is released from astrocytes and becomes available to neural elements. Our observations that normal astrocytes show bFGF in the nucleus and perinuclear area and that hyperreactive astrocytes around the lesion show bFGF in the cytoplasm suggest a possible translocation of bFGF toward secretion pathways. The mechanism of release of bFGF is largely unknown but probably utilizes a series of post translational processing and compartmentalizations in the cytoplasm (29). In addition, evidence indicates that bFGF reaches the cell surface in a dynamic way, not exclusively as the result of cell death (30). Together, these data suggest that in response to degenerative events, bFGF is made more available to local neurons and may aid in cell survival and the reestablishment of synaptic connections. Thus, as predicted by both tissue culture and animal models, bFGF may function in compensatory regenerative processes.

HS Levels Increase After CNS Injury?

Although considerable in vitro data implicates HS as an important element in plastic responses, in vivo corroboration of such a role is only beginning to accumulate. At present, there is no data on whether or not HS levels are increased after injury in the central nervous system. However, there is growing evidence for a role in neurite outgrowth in vivo. HS and other GAG levels

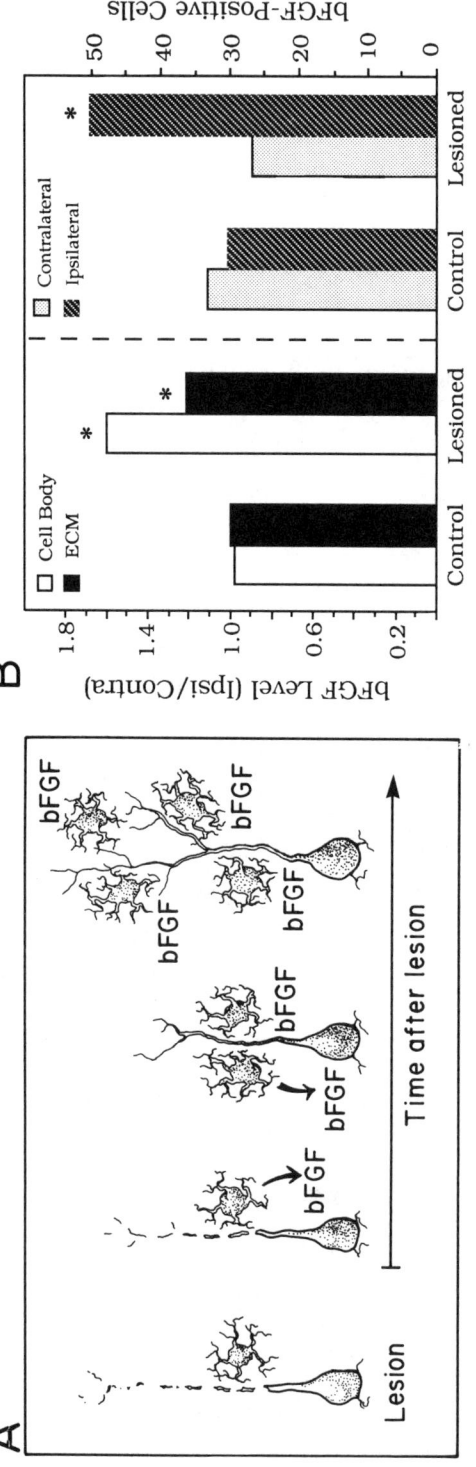

FIG. 4. bFGF levels increase after brain injury. **A:** Brain lesions result in a local increase in bFGF production and astrocyte number. These changes likely stimulate neuronal regeneration. **B:** The graph illustrates lesion-induced increases of bFGF-immunoreactivity within astrocytes and the surrounding neuropil (as measured by computerized densitometry). An increase in the number of bFGF-immunoreactive astrocytes ipsilateral to the lesion was also found. *$p < .05$.

are developmentally regulated (13,31) and some increase after injury (32). HS, for example, undergoes a fourfold increase in metabolic turnover during the phase of development associated with axonal growth and connectivity (33). Suggested developmental and regenerative roles of these extracellular matrix substrate components include the hydration and formation of guiding channels for axonal growth or regrowth (34), formation of extracellular binding sites for cell adhesion, and the binding and regulation of tropic factors (13, 35, 16).

REGENERATIVE SPROUTING IN NORMAL AGING AND IN ALZHEIMER'S DISEASE

There is evidence that, as in animal models, the adult and even the aged human brain are capable of regenerative and plastic responses. Although the normal human brain exhibits some regional decline in neuronal number with increasing age, it appears capable of compensatory dendritic sprouting and synaptic reestablishment. For example, pyramidal neurons in layer II of the parahippocampal gyrus show a significant increase in dendritic arborization during aging in the normal human brain (36,37). Similar age-related dendritic growth has also been reported in primate models (for a review, see 38). However, regional dendritic regression also occurs in human and primate aging, leading to speculation that normal aging may follow a course of neuronal loss, compensatory dendritic sprouting, and ultimately dendritic regression (38).

In addition to normal age-related sprouting, regenerative responses can also occur in response to brain injuries resulting from disease conditions. For example, hippocampal tissue excised from children and adult epileptics reveals sprouting and synaptic reestablishment in the mossy fibers (for a review, see 39). Individuals with AD also show evidence of compensatory regeneration. On the basis of animal studies, we would predict that regenerative sprouting in AD brains occurs primarily within those regions that experience cell loss. As such, AD may represent a model of the brain's ability to respond not only to age-related synaptic losses, but also to lesion-associated atrophy.

In AD, major neuronal loss occurs in the temporal lobe, particularly in layers II and III of the entorhinal cortex (38,40,41). The layer II stellate cells of the entorhinal cortex form the perforant pathway and comprise 86% of the synapses within the outer two-thirds of the molecular layer of the dentate gyrus (1). Thus, the degeneration of the entorhinal cortex may contribute to the functional disconnection of the hippocampus from the cerebral cortex (42).

Based on findings in rodents with entorhinal lesions, we would expect enhanced AChE staining in the dentate gyrus of AD if regenerative sprouting occurs. In fact, the dentate gyrus exhibits a faint pattern of AChE staining (from cholinergic input) in nondiseased brains, but an intensified pattern within the denervated zone in AD brains. We suggest that following initial cell loss during the early course of the disease, the remaining cells sprout new connections in a compensatory fashion in order to maintain some state of circuitry completion (43). This re-innervation may compensate for early synaptic losses and maintain cognitive functions longer.

THE MICROENVIRONMENT OF SENILE PLAQUES: LOCUS OF MISDIRECTED PLASTICITY

From a neuropathological perspective, AD is characterized not only by neuronal cell loss, but also by the presence of senile plaques and neurofibrillary tangles, predominantly within the cortex and hippocampal formation (see Fig. 5). Senile plaques are insoluble extracellular deposits comprising

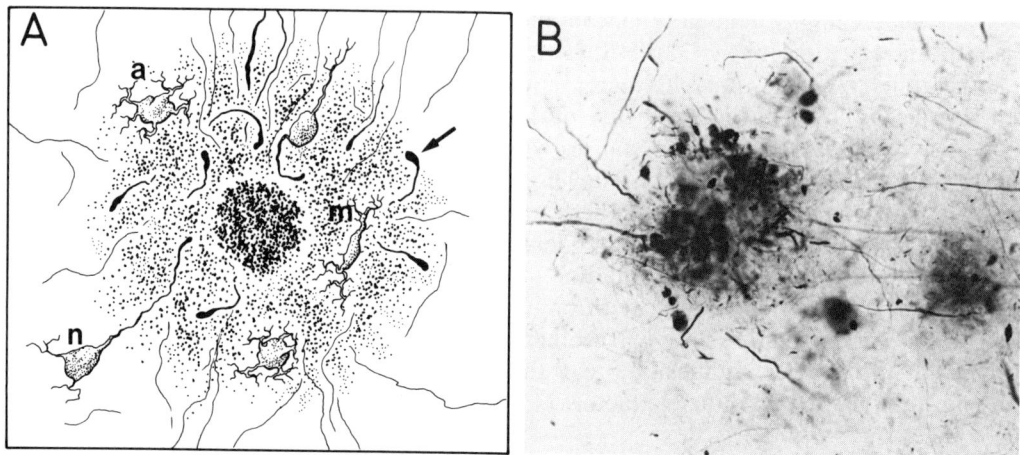

FIG. 5. Senile plaques of Alzheimer disease contain neurite-promoting factors. **A:** A classical senile plaque contains dystrophic neurites *(arrow)* and several cell types implicated in plaque formation: neurons *(n)*, astrocytes *(a)*, and microglia *(m)*. **B:** This photomicrograph shows a classical senile plaque from an Alzheimer brain, as stained by the Bielschowsky silver method. Numerous neurites appear to enter the plaque.

primarily β-amyloid protein (βA4). Senile plaques have a distribution that generally co-localizes with the regional selectivity of atrophied projections (44) and βA4 deposition has been suggested as the primary marker for AD pathology (45).

In addition to the intense AChE staining within the molecular layer of the dentate gyrus in AD brains, we noticed structures that were not predicted from animal models: small, round, cholinesterase-positive material usually surrounded by astrocytes. As revealed by thioflavin staining, a marker for amyloid plaques, these cholinesterase-rich deposits corresponded to senile plaques. They appeared to form along the areas of interface between degeneration and neuronal sprouting, and thus be the loci of these opposing processes. We suggested that the sprouting reactions might both be stimulated by and contribute to plaque formation (46,47). These findings support the hypothesis that the aged brain is capable of reactive synaptogenesis. However, this plasticity may be misdirected. As the sprouting reaction progresses, it appears to be directed at senile plaques rather than at functional targets. In fact, this observation is not new. In 1928 Cajal suggested the following:

> They [sprouts] appear to have been preceded by the deposit of a certain stimulating substance which is expelled from the expansional protoplasm, and which is destroyed later. . . . One may note that some of the new dendrites end in bulbs and tumefactions, which remind one of the buds of newly formed axons. Thus we may infer from what has been said that, in man as in laboratory animals, the regenerative act commences, and may even attain a certain strength, on condition that the traumatic commotion be sufficient to stir the axons out of their lethargy. . . . It appears as if the sprouts had been attracted toward the region of the plaque under the influence of some special neurotropic substance (48).

Other more recent observations similarly conclude the presence of regenerative growth in AD. For example, Ihara (49) described massive dendritic sprouting within the cortex in AD tissue using antibodies to the cytoskeletal protein tau. We have reported that tubulin alpha-1, a fetal isoform of the cytoskeletal protein tubulin, is upregulated in the deafferented hippocampus of both entorhinal-lesioned rodents and human AD patients (50). Several molecular markers of sprouting or synaptogenesis are elevated in rodent models of lesions and in the AD hippocampus: tau (51,52), synaptosomal-associated protein (SNAP-25) (53,54), and GAP-43 (55). This expression of proteins associated with either development and/or synapse formation confirms the occurrence of sprouting responses in AD.

Thus, growth and degeneration co-exist in AD. If sprouting is misdirected into plaques, the key issue becomes the identification of the specific molecules driving such growth. From the in vitro and in vivo studies described above, it would be predicted that trophic and substrate elements play a critical role. Significantly, higher levels of trophic activity have been observed in cortical cultures treated with AD brain extract in comparison to cultures treated with control brain extract (56). However, the molecules responsible were not isolated.

bFGF Is Associated With Senile Plaques in AD

Accordingly, we evaluated the possibility that bFGF is present in or around senile plaques. Using AD brain tissue, we found immunocytochemically that many plaques contain bFGF immunoreactivity. These bFGF-positive plaques are found both in the entorhinal cortex and along the middle of the DG molecular layer in a linear organization. bFGF-immunoreactivity was also localized in astrocytes, NFTs, and a few neuronal groups (57).

It appears as if bFGF-positive plaques are at a relatively early stage of development. The strongest bFGF-immunoreactivity was present in the plaques within the molecular layer of the dentate gyrus (Fig. 6). Most plaques in the DG showed weak staining with thioflavin fluorescence and Bielschowsky silver staining. In contrast, plaques across the hippocampus and entorhinal cortex that stained strongly for thioflavin or Bielschowsky silver staining, indicating they are at a more advanced stage, exhibited weaker bFGF-immunostaining. Rarely were burnt out or core plaques co-localized with bFGF-immunoreactivity, though these types of plaques were present in the AD brains examined. Burnt out plaques are believed to be a late stage in plaque formation.

As mentioned previously, entorhinal lesions in rodents cause an increase in bFGF-immunoreactivity. Frequently, plaques which immunostained positive for bFGF were found in areas with a high density of cells that also expressed bFGF-immunoreactivity. Most bFGF-positive cells around plaques were shown to be astrocytes with anti-GFAP immunohistochemistry, and some extended processes into the plaques. Within the molecular layer of the AD brain, we observed both an increase and an apparent reorganization of GFAP-positive astrocytes in a pattern also seen following entorhinal cortex ablation in rodents (57). Thus, astrocytes may contribute to the bFGF increase seen in plaques.

Other investigators have shown that whole brain levels of bFGF are elevated in AD compared to normal aged brains (58). Recently, Kato and colleagues demonstrated that exogenous bFGF can bind to plaques and neurofibrillary tangles in sectioned AD tissue, and this binding can be reduced by pretreatments which remove endogenous HS (59). Perry and colleagues have recently confirmed that bFGF binding to tangles is HS-mediated (60).

Thus, the data derived from AD brains parallel that from animal studies and support the hypothesis that in response to degenerative events, astrocytes produce and release bFGF, which then stimulates neuronal plasticity. However, in the case of AD, bFGF appears localized to senile plaques and may misdirect plastic responses

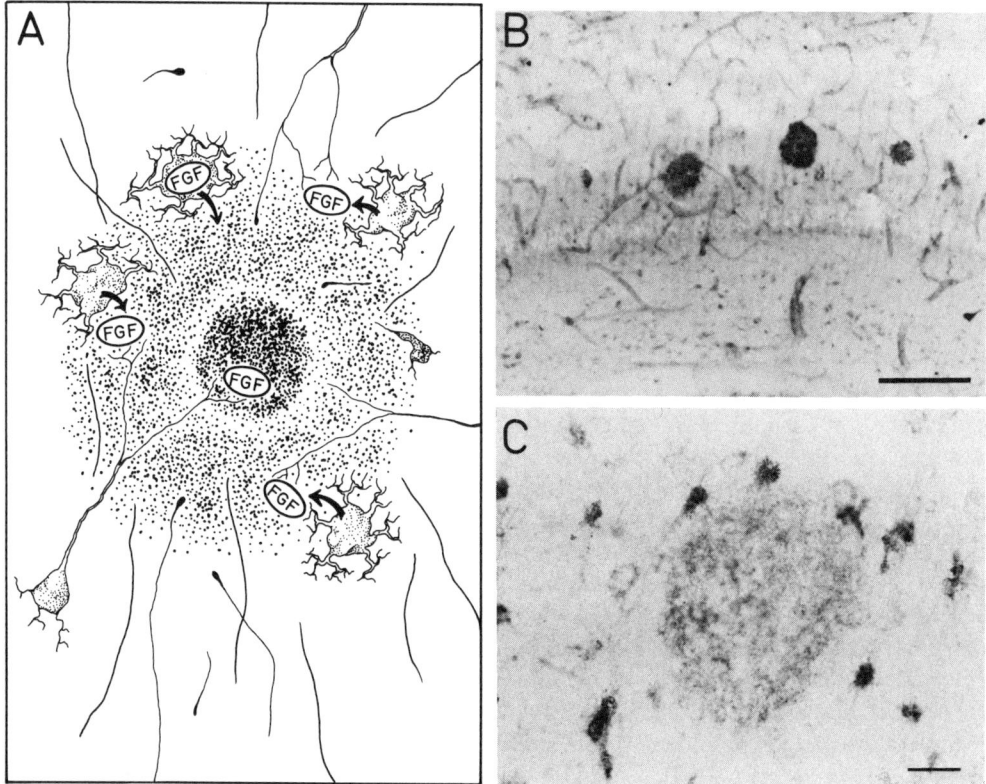

FIG. 6. bFGF is present in the senile plaque environment. **A:** The diagram illustrates the potential sites of bFGF involvement in plaque formation and misdirected plasticity. **B:** Basic FGF-immunoreactivity detects senile plaques located in the dentate gyrus molecular layer of Alzheimer brains (scale bar = 100 μm). **C:** The photomicrograph illustrates the presence of bFGF-immunoreactive astrocytes surrounding a bFGF-immunoreactive senile plaque (scale bar = 10 μm).

toward senile plaques rather than denervated targets, just as Cajal predicted.

HS Is Associated With Senile Plaques in AD

In addition to bFGF, substrate components might also contribute to the AD regenerative response. Previous work has shown that glycosaminoglycans are elevated in AD (61) and associated with plaques (62). More specifically, using monoclonal antibodies to HS and HS proteoglycan, Snow and colleagues have shown positive HS-immunoreactivity within plaques as well as in selected neurons and tangles. On the basis of these and other data, they hypothesized that HS is one of the earliest constituents of developing plaques (63,64). Recently, we have confirmed and extended these findings.

We observed that HS-immunoreactivity, in addition to being present in β-amyloid positive plaques, appears to accumulate within neurons. Select neurons show immunopositive deposits in the cytoplasm and/or heavy staining of the nuclei. We also identified HS-positive neurites entering plaques and microglia around plaques which were strongly HS-positive as well (Fig. 7) (65).

Thus, bFGF and HS may accumulate in concentrated areas associated with senile plaques, providing a microenvironment that could divert sprouting and plasticity processes away from potentially beneficial functions.

βA4 Peptide May Stimulate Aberrant Plasticity and Enhance Susceptibility to Cell Death

Although bFGF, HS, and numerous minor components are associated with senile plaques, the primary component of plaques in AD is a polypeptide called β-amyloid. Since senile plaques appear to be centers of both degeneration and regeneration, knowledge of β-amyloid's contribution to these processes is vital. In fact, deposition of β-amyloid peptides is generally believed to proceed neuritic involvement and plaque formation. Accordingly, we investigated the source, deposition, and biological activity of β-amyloid using two approaches: in vitro studies of amyloid peptides and in vivo immunocytochemistry for both the amyloid precursor protein (APP) and the β-amyloid peptide.

In order to investigate how the β-amyloid protein may affect the degenerative and/or regenerative responses seen in the AD brain, we treated neuronal cultures with synthetic homologs of β-amyloid. Using a low-density culture system optimized for measurement of trophic effects, we have reported that peptides corresponding to both the initial 28 residues (β1-28) and the full length β-amyloid protein (β1-42) increase the survival of developing hippocampal neurons (66,67). In addition, β1-42 causes significant axonal elongation and dendritic arborization in these cultures (67,68). Thus, like bFGF, soluble β-amyloid exhibits both survival- and neurite-enhancing properties in vitro.

However, β-amyloid peptide can express both neurotrophic and neurotoxic effects in vitro. Although it initially enhances the survival of immature neurons, we found that the β-amyloid peptide makes older cultures more vulnerable to insults, including excitotoxicity (69). Subsequently, Yanker and colleagues reported that β-amyloid directly causes neurotoxicity in older cultures, an effect potentiated by nerve growth factor (NGF) (70,71). In addition, a larger peptide that includes both β-amyloid and the C-terminus of APP is toxic to PC12 cultures

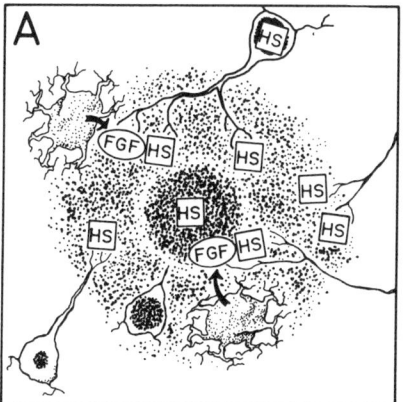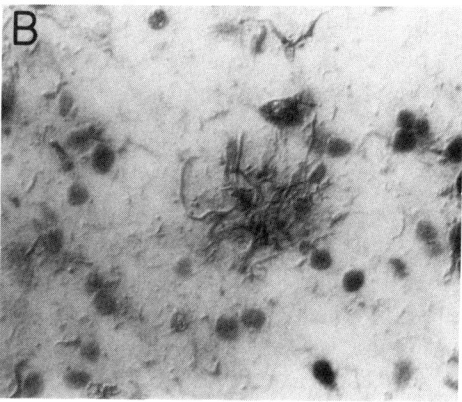

FIG. 7. Heparan sulfate is present in the senile plaque environment. **A:** The diagram illustrates the location of HS in the senile plaque environment. HS is found in neurons, their neurites, and glia and is hypothesized to co-localize with bFGF in select developing senile plaques. **B:** Heparan sulfate-immunoreactivity is observed within senile plaques, the neurites which enter them, and surrounding neurons and glial cells.

when these cells are differentiated by NGF (72). Recently, it was reported that in vivo injections of β-amyloid caused local toxicity (73). Thus, β-amyloid appears to have multiple biological actions and may be involved in a delicate balance between regenerative and degenerative processes. It is clearly important to determine the basis for this apparent opposing activity.

On the basis of recent experiments, we have suggested that the neurotoxic effects of β-amyloid may be primarily related to an aggregated form of the protein and perhaps to the age or the health of the neurons. We and other investigators have observed that β-amyloid has an inherent ability to spontaneously form insoluble aggregations in vitro, which parallels the self-assembly of β-amyloid hypothesized to occur in AD following its aberrant processing from APP (74–76). The aggregation of β1-42 is time, concentration, and pH dependent: Aggregation is maximized by incubation of solutions with high β-amyloid concentration and pH 5.5 (76). Stable forms of sheet-like aggregations, visible at the light microscope level, are maintained at physiological pH levels in incubated solutions of β1-42 but not β1-28(76). Similarly, after incubation only β-amyloid fragments that contain a hydrophobic domain, such as β1-42, show an altered electrophoresis profile, which includes a prominent, apparently insoluble band at the top of the stacking gel (68,76). Further, these aggregations show positive Congo Red and thioflavin-staining characteristics similar to senile plaques (76).

On the basis of these observations and our own data, we examined the possibility that the biological properties of β-amyloid may vary as a function of its aggregation state. In studies using cultured neurons, various conditions need to be met in order to distinguish trophic from toxic influences. To identify trophic influences, we have used low density cultures in defined media since their cells quickly degenerate unless a trophic factor is added. We detect toxic effects in a higher density culture system in which the cells survive longer, probably because they produce sufficient trophic factors themselves. In this higher density culture system, immature hippocampal neurons treated with newly solubilized, nonaggregated β1-42 showed greatly enhanced neurite outgrowth and no toxicity. However, sister cultures treated with the incubated, aggregated β1-42 exhibited a dose-dependent toxicity that approached 100% at a concentration of 100 µg/ml (see Fig. 8)(68). We also treated cultures with incubated β1-28, but this treatment lacked toxicity (77). In agreement with the findings of Burdick and colleagues, we also found that at physiological pH, incubated β1-28 solutions did not contain visible aggregates (77). Thus it appears that both the self-aggregation and toxic-promoting properties of β-amyloid require β-amyloid fragments longer than β1-28 (77). In addition, we have observed that aggregates of β-amyloid induce dystrophic changes in the necrites of cultured neurons which are similar to those observed in AD tissue (94). An amyloidogenic protein not associated with AD does not induce degenerative changes.

In summary, β-amyloid protein is capable of enhancing neuritic growth and survival but it can also promote and even cause toxicity. Within the AD brain, the senile plaque environment likely includes both soluble and aggregated β-amyloid protein, as well as bFGF, HS, and other lesser components. Although neuritic sprouting would be expected in this region, the resulting involvement with aggregated β-amyloid may prove detrimental to the regenerative response. Prediction of neuronal responses in AD is further complicated by the probability of interactions between the senile plaque components and various other bioactive substances.

Aberrant Growth Factor Cascades May Contribute to β-Amyloid Formation

There appear to be a number of interwoven molecular cascades contributing to the formation of plaques. The trophic fac-

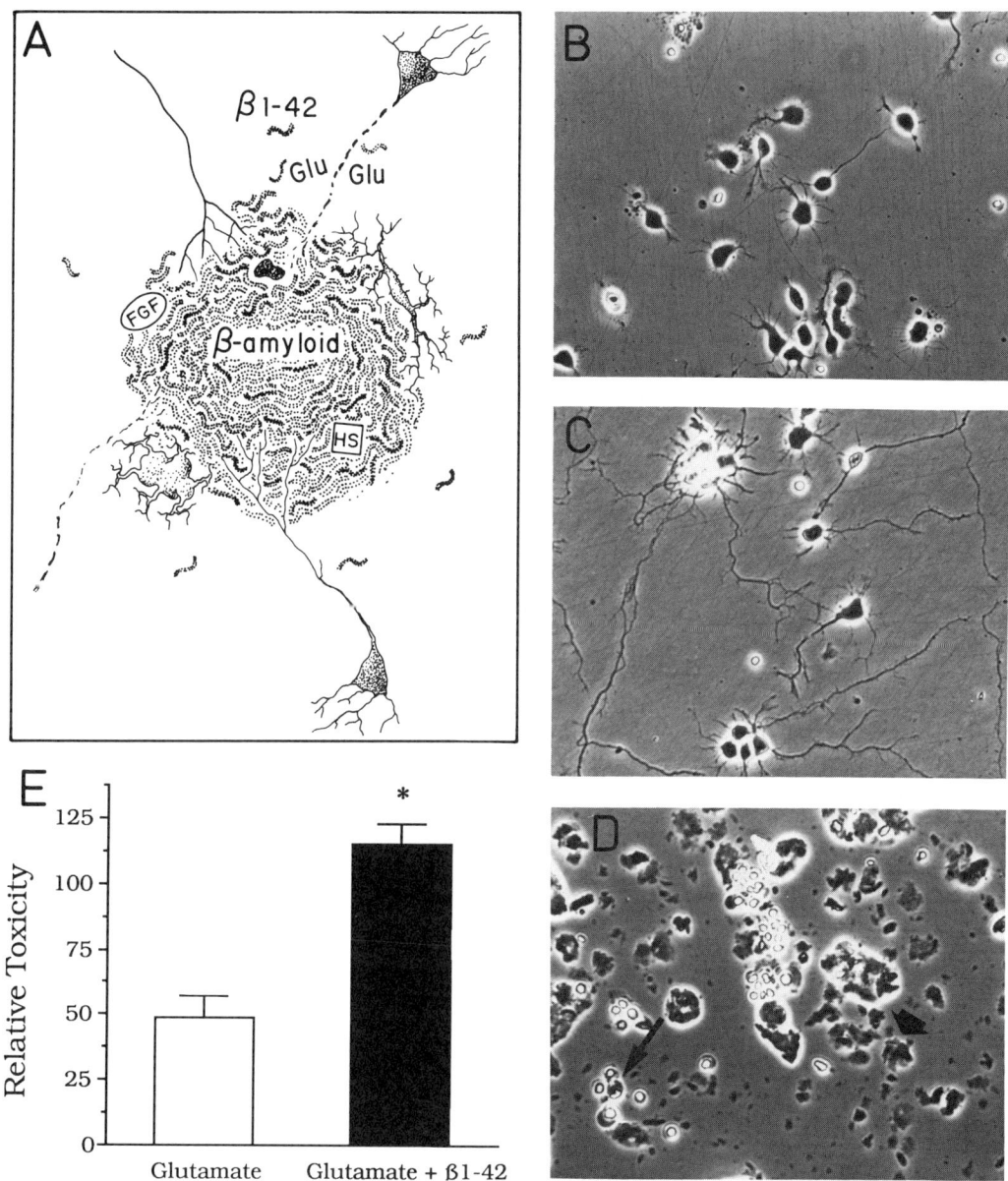

FIG. 8. β-amyloid can both stimulate neurite outgrowth and increase neuronal susceptibility to toxicity. **A:** Senile plaques are composed of a core of β-amyloid surrounded by diffuse amyloid fragments such as β1-42. These components are believed to not only stimulate neuritic growth, but also contribute to and/or cause neurotoxicity. **B:** Control hippocampal neurons show normal growth and survival in the absence of β-amyloid. **C:** After 24 hour exposure to soluble β1-42, these neurons exhibit dramatic neuritic growth and no significant cell loss. **D:** However, after exposure to "aged," aggregated β1-42 *(arrowhead)*, these cells degenerate *(arrow)* within 24 hours. **E:** Sublethal doses of glutamate become toxic to mature cortical cultures when preceded by a 2–4 day exposure to soluble β1-42.

tors involved in supporting plasticity are frequently involved in a number of regulatory pathways. Basic FGF is implicated in several regulatory pathways that are relevant to AD. For example, bFGF stimulates the production of APP mRNA in cultured glial cells (78). Thus, increases in bFGF may stimulate production of β-amyloid.

A positive feedback cycle would greatly exacerbate the process of β-amyloid accumulation and is consistent with the extensive β-amyloid deposition characteristic of AD. In support of this hypothesized cycle, not only does bFGF increase APP, but our laboratory recently demonstrated that the addition of β-amyloid to purified astrocyte cultures increases their release of bFGF (79). The addition of β1-42, at concentrations as low as 1 μg/ml, caused an increase in the release of bFGF into the cell culture media within 3 hours. A cascade may be initiated by elevations in bFGF. In vitro addition of bFGF yields a twofold elevation in astrocytic secretion of another potent trophic substance, nerve growth factor (NGF) (80); NGF has been reported to potentiate amyloid toxicity (70). Additionally, NGF can increase APP secretion (81). Finally, both bFGF and APP show a high binding affinity for HS (14, 82–84), which may increase their potency. Thus, the relationship among bFGF, NGF, and APP in AD may represent another example of a shift toward toxicity in the delicate degenerative/regenerative balance. These responses may be complementary, resulting in positive feedback cycles.

Taken together with the demonstration of bFGF and HS localization in senile plaques, these findings support a potential recursive cycle of plaque formation: β-amyloid accumulations stimulate bFGF production and bind to HS, elevations of bFGF, possibly made resistant to degradation by binding to HS, increase NGF levels, which in turn enhance APP release. Basic FGF could also directly increase APP secretion, which feeds back on bFGF regulation. These positive feedback cascades have the potential to accelerate senile plaque formation and potentiate the associated neuritic and toxic responses.

ORGANIZATION AND DISTRIBUTION OF APP IN VIVO: IMPLICATIONS FOR APP PROCESSING AND FORMATION OF β-AMYLOID

The cell culture experiments and preliminary data from in vivo injections of β-amyloid described above implicate a pivotal role for β-amyloid in AD pathology. β-amyloid is generally believed to be derived from APP by abnormal proteolytic processing. At present, however, the exact cellular origin of the APP that contributes to plaque formation is unknown. Recent cell culture and in situ hybridization studies suggest that APP may be produced by microglia, astrocytes, and/or neurons; in fact, nearly all cells in the body produce some amount of APP (for example, see refs. 85,86).

In order to understand the origin of the APP that leads to insoluble extracellular deposits, we have analyzed AD tissue in order to determine the characteristics of APP deposition in plaques and its possible relationship to bFGF and HS accumulations. Using an monoclonal antibody to protease nexin-2, which is homologous to the N-terminus of the APP molecule (87,88), we found only light staining of neuronal cytoplasm in control brains and no neuritic APP staining. In contrast, we detected strong APP-immunopositive neurons in select regions of the AD brain, many of which contained discrete granular intracellular deposits of APP (89).

Pyramidal neurons were seen completely filled with APP granules, and some even appeared to be bursting open (see Fig. 9C). We also detected the presence of fine, APP-immunopositive neurites surrounding and entering plaques, many with swollen varicosities along their length or ending in bulbous tips (see Fig. 9B). In addition, APP-immunoreactivity was present as granular

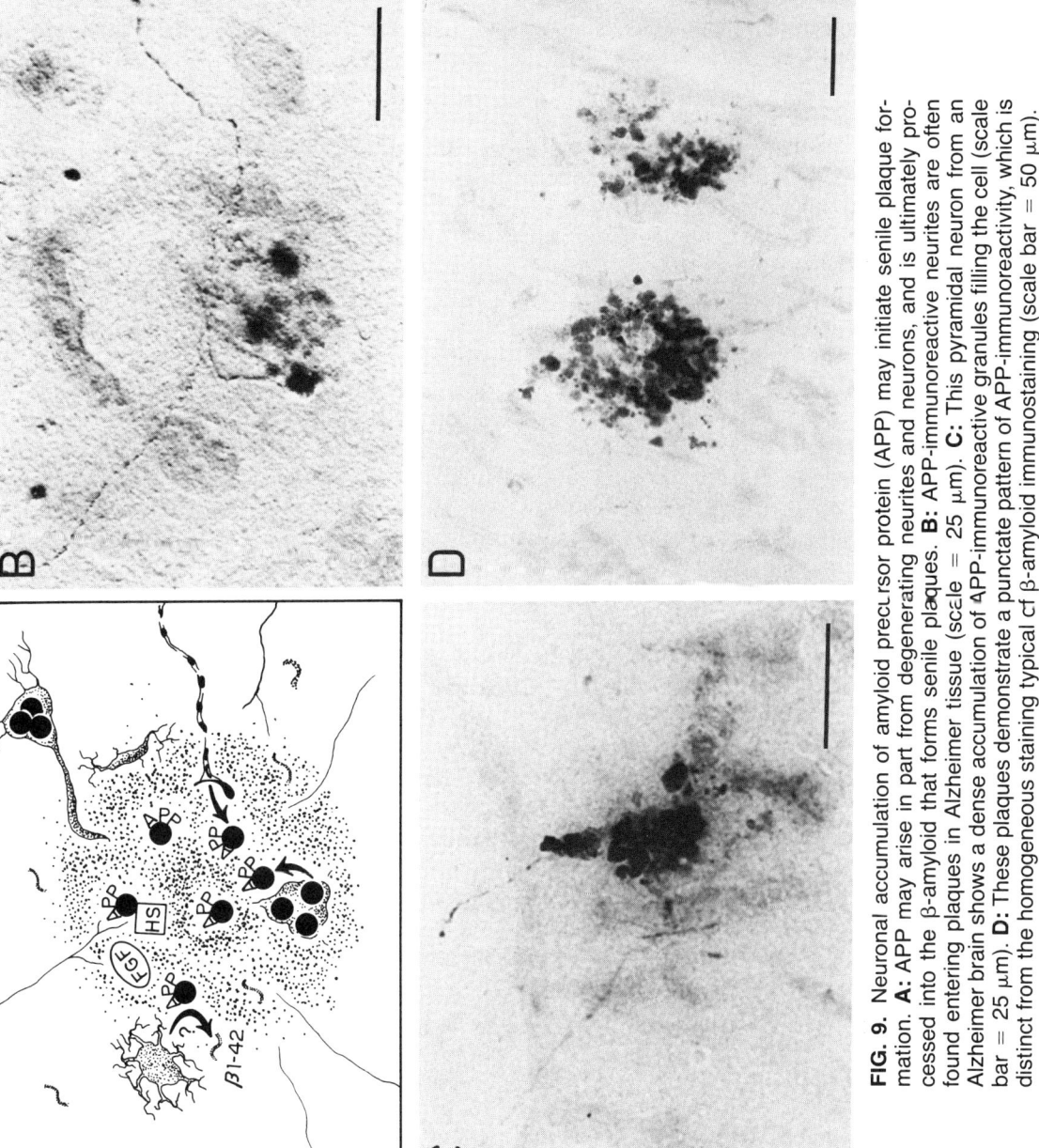

FIG. 9. Neuronal accumulation of amyloid precursor protein (APP) may initiate senile plaque formation. **A:** APP may arise in part from degenerating neurites and neurons, and is ultimately processed into the β-amyloid that forms senile plaques. **B:** APP-immunoreactive neurites are often found entering plaques in Alzheimer tissue (scale = 25 μm). **C:** This pyramidal neuron from an Alzheimer brain shows a dense accumulation of APP-immunoreactive granules filling the cell (scale bar = 25 μm). **D:** These plaques demonstrate a punctate pattern of APP-immunoreactivity, which is distinct from the homogeneous staining typical of β-amyloid immunostaining (scale bar = 50 μm).

deposits within plaques and could occasionally be detected in blood vessels in AD brains (see Fig. 9D).

In order to further determine the locus of the distinctive APP-positive granules, we used double-labeling immunohistochemistry with the APP antibody versus antibodies β-amyloid, glial fibrillary acidic protein (GFAP), and leucocyte common antigen (LCA) or *Rinucus cummunicus* agglutin lectin (RCA I). We found that APP granules did not co-localize within either astrocytes or microglia, but were often co-localized with HS deposits.

In summary, the predominantly neuronal and neuritic localization of APP-immunoreactivity suggests a neuronal source for much of the APP observed in AD pathology (89). The aggregation of β-amyloid could arise from abnormal APP processing or its interaction with other components such as HS-rich molecules. In either case, we suggest the end result is that the neurons degenerate or are placed at risk to injury from other factors.

EXACERBATION OF NEURONAL DYSFUNCTION BY EXCITOTOXICITY

Products that accumulate in AD may interact with various bioactive substances to alter the balance between adaptive plasticity and pathology. The brain's major excitatory neurotransmitter, glutamate, in elevated concentrations is known to cause neurotoxicity both in vitro and in vivo (90). Since β-amyloid is known to accumulate within aged and AD brains, we sought to determine if neurons pre-exposed to β-amyloid have an altered vulnerability to glutamate-mediated toxicity.

We found that following exposure to soluble, nonaggregated β-amyloid, administration of sublethal doses of glutamate causes massive toxicity in cortical cultures (69). Cortical neurons grown in culture for 14 days and then exposed to β1-42 for 2–4 days appear not to degenerate as demonstrated both by their morphological appearance and their release of lactic acid dehydrogenase. Similarly, when these cultures are exposed to subthreshold levels of glutamate, little cell death is observed. However, when cells treated with β1-42 are subsequently exposed to subthreshold levels of glutamate, neuronal death increases (see Fig. 8E).

AD patients early in the disease appear to show decreases in glucose utilization that increase in severity as the disease progresses (91). Such deficiency in energy metabolism may also serve as a risk factor when combined with amyloid accumulation. To test this possibility, we treated cultures with β1-42 and a normally nontoxic episode of glucose deprivation (92). Although the glucose deprivation by itself was not neurotoxic, in combination with β1-42 it caused nearly complete neuronal degeneration. Glutamate excitotoxicity appears to be involved since these neurons were protected by the addition of glutamate receptor antagonists such as MK-801 (92).

These findings are especially relevant to understanding the progression of AD since senile plaque distribution often corresponds to the terminals of glutamate pathways (93) and since many of these neurons show an increase in APP and may accumulate β-amyloid. Because early AD patients often show signs of a metabolic deficiency (91), neurons in the AD brain may be placed at greater risk.

AD neurodegeneration may be instigated by a misdirected plasticity cycle and ultimately concluded by various mechanisms related to glutamate receptors. While the accumulation of β-amyloid may be a risk factor in AD, other molecules, such as bFGF at the proper levels, have been reported to protect neurons (8). It may be that the overall balance and availability of these factors to the proper target is what is critical. In this way, glutamate and β-amyloid constitute risk factors that may converge on some final common pathway that causes degeneration.

THE AGED BRAIN: A BALANCE BETWEEN ADAPTIVE AND PATHOLOGICAL PLASTICITY

In the healthy brain, both regeneration and plasticity can function in a generally compensatory manner, enhancing neuritic sprouting and facilitating synaptic reestablishment in response to cell loss brought about by minor injuries or by normal aging. This plasticity and regeneration can help maintain function or restore function after trauma in many cases (see Fig. 10A). A variety of growth factors and substrate components, including bFGF and HS, are probably necessary to stimulate and maintain such responses. In the case of AD, it appears that the effective coordination of these interactive pathways is compromised, creating a progressive neurodegenerative cycle (see Fig. 10B).

As suggested in the opening section, multiple molecular events arise as a function of plasticity or aging, which may interact negatively with the primary and secondary factors in degenerative conditions (see Fig. 10C). Individually each event may be well within the tolerance range of the brain, particularly early in their time course. However, some combination of these processes, over time, may cause pathology. In the previous sections, we discussed several examples of such molecular cascades that may divert regenerative growth into plaques. We noted how the accumulation of growth factors and substrates may promote such sprouting. This aberrant growth may result in an abnormal circuitry with fewer functional connections in the affected vicinity. It would also create an imbalance in the fragile trophic interactions between neurons, making them more vulnerable. Further, we noted that the amyloid precursor protein in AD is expressed at high levels in neurons, that β-amyloid and/or its precursor protein accumulate in and around plaques, and that β-amyloid may promote toxicity in an "aged" aggregated state. We also noted that several recursive cycles may exist involving amyloid and growth factors. For example, bFGF promotes the production of the amyloid precursor protein and β-amyloid in turn stimulates the production of bFGF by astrocytes. Such cycles may contribute to plaque growth and place neurons at risk. The major excitatory neurotransmitter glutamate, somewhat ironically, may represent another risk factor. Excitotoxic-mediated neuronal death is exacerbated by β-amyloid. Thus, neurons that accumulate β-amyloid may be especially vulnerable to excitotoxicity. Together, these series of events appear to promote neuropathology, placing neurons at risk and even causing degeneration. Thus, rather than ameliorating the existing atrophy, AD regeneration compounds the condition and facilitates a cycle of progressive neurodegeneration.

There are several implications regarding the mechanisms of molecular cascades. In principle, molecular cascades can be arrested at any point. Since they often amplify as they progress, intervention early in the cascade is probably more effective than later. Early interference at one or more points may not stop the progression of the disease completely, but may slow its course. Finally, this notion of multiple molecular cascades may help provide a better understanding of the high and increasing prevalence of AD with age. As the brain ages, it becomes subject to multiple adaptive mechanisms, injuries, and compensations, all of which take some toll and may trigger molecular cascades like those described in this chapter. Some of these are beneficial, but others lead to enhanced risk of pathology and degeneration. According to this reasoning, AD is not caused by a single aberrant mechanism, but rather by a series of them, each of which carries probable

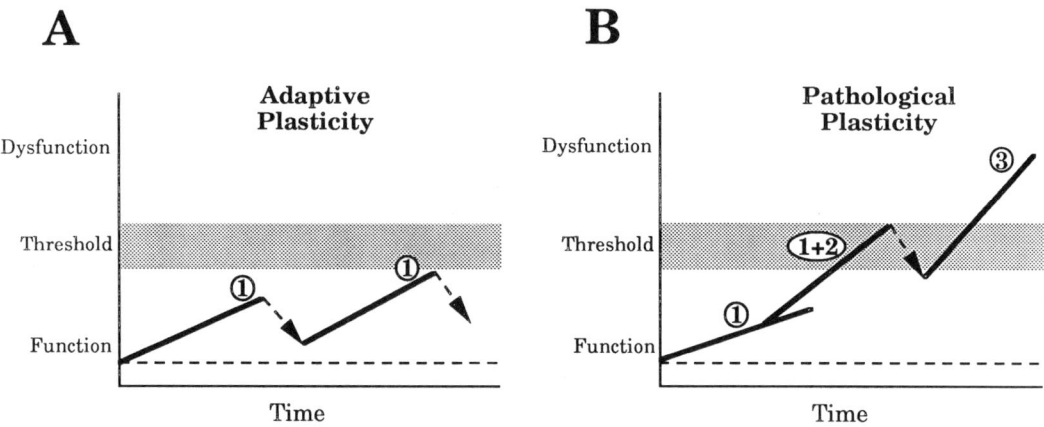

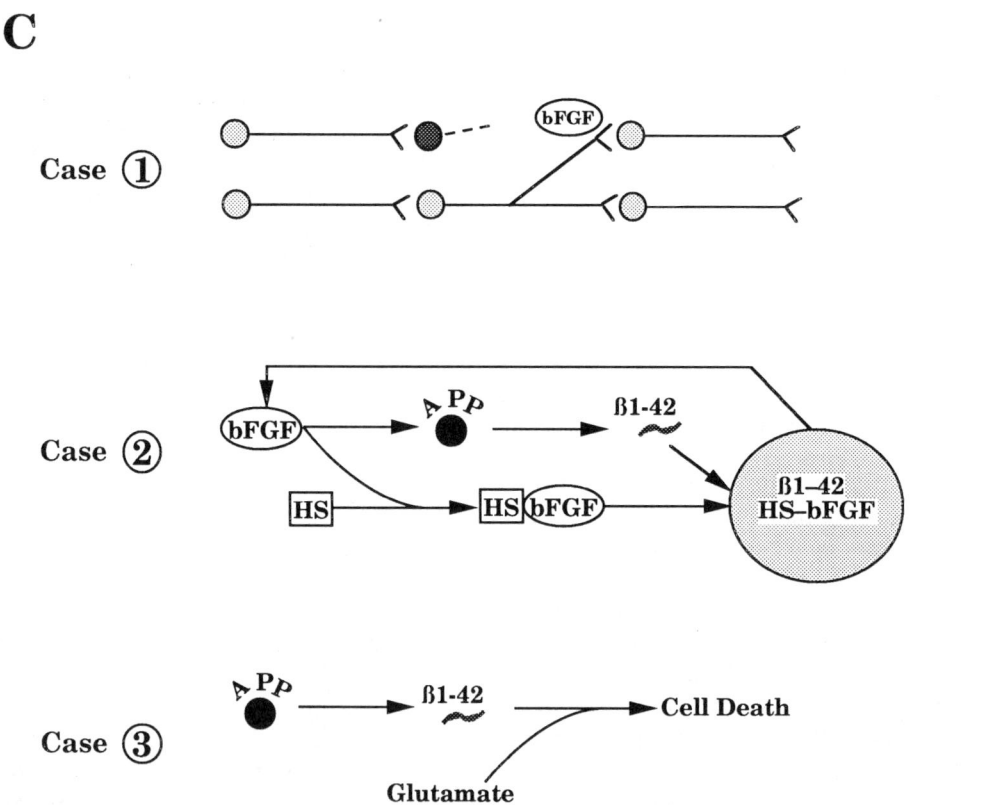

FIG. 10. Although normally compensatory in function, plasticity mechanisms may interact in an aberrant manner and lead to pathology. Cellular events and molecular cascades associated with plasticity form a delicate balance. **A:** Adaptive plasticity. Minor disturbances of this balance are tolerated by the healthy brain, with normal function being maintained by compensatory plasticity mechanisms (e.g., case 1). Over time, even a series of these disturbances would not reach a critical threshold in a healthy brain. **B:** Pathological plasticity. However, when β-amyloid deposition and/or aberrant plasticity events co-occur with normal regenerative mechanisms, synergistic interactions

risks and benefits. Identifying the primary aberrant mechanisms and finding ways to slow their course could help stabilize the relentless degeneration of the disease.

ACKNOWLEDGMENTS

The authors thank K. Christensen for her work on the illustrations and A. Copani for many helpful discussions. This work was supported by the NIA and the MacArthur Foundation. C.J.P. was supported by NIMH grant MH14599.

REFERENCES

1. Matthews D, Cotman CW, Lynch G. An electron microscopic study of lesion-induced synaptogenesis in the dentate gyrus of the adult rat. I. Magnitude and time course of degeneration. *Brain Res* 1976;115:1-21.
2. Matthews D, Cotman CW, Lynch G. An electron microscopic study of lesion-induced synaptogenesis in the dentate gyrus of the adult rat. II. Reappearance of morphologically normal synaptic contacts. *Brain Res* 1976;115:23-41.
3. Mattson M, Rychlik B. Cell culture of cyropreserved human fetal cerebral cortical and hippocampal neurons: neuronal development and responses to trophic factors. *Brain Res* 1990;522:204-214.
4. Morrison RS. Basic fibroblast growth factor supports the survival of cerebral cortical neurons in primary culture. *Proc Natl Acad Sci USA* 1986;83:7537-7541.
5. Walicke PA. Basic and acidic fibroblast growth factors have trophic effects on neurons from multiple CNS regions. *J Neurosci* 1988;8:2618-2627.
6. Walicke P, Cowan W, Ueno N, Baird A, Guillemin R. Fibroblast growth factor promotes survival of dissociated hippocampal neurons and enhances neurite extension. *Proc Natl Acad Sci USA* 1986;83:3012-3016.
7. Needles DL, Cotman CW. Basic fibroblast growth factor increases the survival of rat dentate granule cells in culture. *Soc Neurosci Abstr* 1988;14:363.
8. Mattson MP, Murrain M, Guthrie PB, Kater SB. Fibroblast growth factor and glutamate: opposing roles in the generation and degeneration of hippocampal neuroarchitecture. *J Neurosci* 1989;9:3728-3740.
9. Bähr M, Vanselow J, Thanos S. Ability of adult rat ganglion cells to regrow axons in vitro can be influenced by fibroblast growth factor and gangliosides. *Neurosci Lett* 1989;96:197-201.
10. Seifert W, Förster F, Flott B, Terlau H. Effects of a neurotrophic factor (FGF) on development, regeneration and synaptic plasticity of central neurons, In: Ben-Ari Y, ed. *Advances in experimental medicine and biology*, vol 268. New York: Plenum Press; 1990:395-399.
11. Sanes JR. Extracellular matrix molecules that influence neuronal development. *Annu Rev Neurosci* 1989;12:491-516.
12. Höök M, Robinson J, Kjellén L, Johansson S, Woods A. Heparan sulfate: On the structure and function of the cell-associated protcoglycans. In: Hawkes S, Wang JL, eds. *Extracellular matrix*. New York: Academic Press; 1982;15-23.
13. Toole BP. Glycosaminoglycans in morphogenesis. *Cell Biology of the Extracellular Matrix*. In: Hay ED ed., New York: Plenum Press; 1981;259-294.
14. Gospodarowicz D, Cheng J, Lui G, Baird A, Böhlent P. Isolation of brain fibroblast growth factor by heparin-Sepharose affinity chromatography: identity with pituitary fibroblast growth factor. *Proc Natl Acad Sci USA* 1984;81:6963-6967.
15. Baird A, Schubert D, Ling N, Guillemin R. Receptor and heparin binding domains of basic fibroblast growth factor. *Proc Natl Acad Sci USA* 1988;85:2324-2328.
16. Flaumenhaft R, Moscatelli D, Rifkin DB. Heparin and heparan sulfate increase the radius of

---

may result which breach the brain's tolerance threshold, causing dysfunction and pathology (e.g., cases 2 and 3). **C:** There are many possible scenarios of molecular cascades which would precipitate adaptive and/or pathological plasticity responses, including the cases outlined below. *Case 1:* Localized, age-related neuronal loss may be compensated for by reactive synaptogenesis, which is facilitated by growth factors such as bFGF. *Case 2:* Aberrant molecular cascades may misdirect otherwise beneficial plasticity. For example, bFGF, HS, APP, and β1-42 may interact in a recursive cycle; bFGF, facilitated by HS, induces APP production and ultimately the formation of β1-42. In turn, β1-42 feeds back on bFGF pathways by up-regulating its production. The end result is misdirected plasticity responses and an enhancement of neuronal vulnerability. *Case 3:* Additional pathways can exacerbate existing misdirected plasticity and injure susceptible cells, resulting in pronounced dysfunction and cell loss. Subtoxic levels of glutamate, in combination with the deposited amyloid, are theorized to operate in the neurodegeneration of Alzheimer's disease.

diffusion and action of basic fibroblast growth factor. *J Cell Biol* 1990;111:1651–1659.
17. Gospodarowicz D, Cheng J. Heparin protects basic and acidic FGF from inactivation. *J Cell Physiol* 1986;128:475–484.
18. Saksela O, Moscatelli D, Sommer A, Rifkin D. Endothelial cell-derived heparan sulfate binds basic fibroblast growth factor and protects it from proteolytic degradation. *J Cell Biol* 1988;107:743–751.
19. Ruoslahti E, Yamaguchi Y. Proteoglycans as modulators of growth factor activities. *Cell* 1991;64:867–869.
20. Walicke P. Interactions between basic fibroblast growth factor (FGF) and glycosoaminoglycans in promoting neurite outgrowth. *Exp Neurol* 1988;102:144–148.
21. Neufeld G, Gospodarowicz D, Dodge L, Fujii DK. Heparin modulation of the neurotropic effects of acidic and basic fibroblast growth factors and nerve growth factor on PC12 cells. *J Cell Physiol* 1987;131:131–140.
22. Williams LR, Varon S, Peterson GW, et al. Continuous infusion of nerve growth factor prevents basal forebrain neuronal death after fimbria-fornix transection. *Proc Natl Acad Sci USA* 1986;83:9231–9235.
23. Hefti F. Nerve growth factor (NGF) promotes survival of septal cholinergic neurons after fimbrial section. *J Neurosci* 1986;6:2155–2162.
24. Anderson KJ, Dam D, Lee S, Cotman CW. Basic fibroblast growth factor prevents death of lesioned cholinergic neurons in vivo. *Nature* 1988;332:360–361.
25. Cummings BJ, Yee GJ, Cotman CW. Basic fibroblast growth factor (bFGF) promotes entorhinal layer II cell survival after perforant path axotomy. (Submitted.)
26. Nieto-Sampedro M, Lewis ER, Cotman CW, et al. Brain injury causes a time-dependent increase in neurotrophic activity at the lesion site. *Science* 1982;217:860–861.
27. Cotman C, Matthews D, Taylor D, Lynch G. Synaptic rearrangement in the dentate gyrus: histochemical evidence of adjustments after lesions in immature and adult rats. *Proc Natl Acad Sci USA* 1973;70:3473–3477.
28. Gómez-Pinilla F, Cotman CW. Basic FGF in adult rat brain: Cellular distribution and response to entorhinal lesions and fimbria-fornix transaction. *J Neurosci* 1992; 12:345–355.
29. Almeric F, Baldin V, Bose-Bierne I, et al. Nuclear translocation of basic fibroblast growth factor. *Ann NY Acad Sci* (in press).
30. Florkiewicz RZ, Baird A, Gonzalez AM. Multiple forms of bFGF: differential nuclear and cell surface localization. *Growth Factors* 1991; 4:265–275.
31. Werz W, Fischer G, Schachner M. Glycosaminoglycans of rat cerebellum: II. A developmental study. *J Neurochem* 1985;44:907–910.
32. Mescher AL, Cox CA. Hyaluronate accumulation and nerve-dependent growth during regeneration of larval *Ambystoma* limbs. *Differentiation* 1988;38:161–168.
33. Margolis RU, Margolis RK, Chang LB, Preti C. Glycosaminoglycans of brain during development. *Biochemistry* 1975;14:85–88.
34. Bronner-Fraser, Lallier. A monoclonal antibody against a laminin-heparan sulfate proteoglycan complex perturbs cranial neural crest migration in vivo. *J Cell Biol* 1988;106:1321–1329.
35. Yayon A, Klagsbrun M, Esko JD, Leder P, Ornitz DM. Cell surface, heparin-like molecules are required for binding of basic fibroblast growth factor to its high affinity receptor. *Cell* 1991;64:841–848.
36. Buell SJ, Coleman PD. Dendritic growth in the aged human brain and failure of growth in senile dementia. *Science* 1979;206:854–856.
37. Buell SJ, Coleman PD. Quantitative evidence for selective dendritic growth in normal human aging but not in senile dementia. *Brain Res* 1981;214:23–41.
38. Coleman PD, Flood DG. Neuron numbers and dendritic extent in normal aging and Alzheimer's disease. *Neurobiol Aging* 1987;8:521–545.
39. Ben-Ari Y, Represa A. Brief seizure episodes induce long-term potentiation and mossy fibre sprouting in the hippocampus. *Trends Neurosci* 1990;13:312–318.
40. Hyman BT, Van Hoesen GW, Kromer LJ, Damasio AR. Perforant pathway changes and the memory impairment of Alzheimer's disease. *Ann Neurol* 1986;20:472–481.
41. Hyman BT, Kromer LJ, Van Hoesen GW. Reinnervation of the hippocampal perforant pathway zone in Alzheimer's disease. *Ann Neurol* 1987;21:259–267.
42. Hyman BT, Van Hoesen GW, Damasio AR, Barnes CL. Alzheimer's disease: cell-specific pathology isolates the hippocampal formation. *Science* 1984;225:1168–1170.
43. Cotman CW, Anderson KJ. Synaptic plasticity and functional stabilization in the hippocampal formation: possible role in Alzheimer's disease. *Adv in Neurol,* 1988;47:313–335.
44. Mann DM, Yates PO, Marcyniuk B. Correlation between senile plaque and neurofibrillary tangle counts in cerebral cortex and neuronal counts in cortex and subcortical structures in Alzheimer's disease. *Neurosci Lett* 1985;56:51–55.
45. Davies L, Wolska B, Hilbich C, et al. A4 amyloid protein deposition and the diagnosis of Alzheimer's disease: Prevalence in aged brains determined by immunocytochemistry compared with conventional neuropathologic techniques. *Neurology* 1988;38:1688–1693.
46. Geddes JW, Anderson KJ, Cotman CW. Senile plaques as aberrant sprout-stimulating structures. *Exp Neurol* 1986;94:767–776.
47. Cotman CW, Cummings BJ, Whitson JS. The role of misdirected plasticity in plaque biogenesis and Alzheimer's disease pathology, In: Hefti F, Brachet P, Will B, Christen Y, eds. *Growth factors and Alzheimer's disease.* Berlin: Springer-Verlag;1991:222–233.
48. Ramón y Cajal S. *Degeneration and regenera-*

tion of the nervous system, vol II. London: Hafner Publishing Company, 1928.
49. Ihara Y. Massive somatodendritic sprouting of cortical neurons in Alzheimer's disease. *Brain Res* 1988;459:138–144.
50. Geddes JW, Wong J, Choi BH, Kim RC, Cotman CW, Miller FD. Increased expression of the embryonic form of a developmentally regulated mRNA in Alzheimer's disease. *Neurosci Lett* 1990;109:54–61.
51. Kosik KS, Joachim CL, Selkoe DJ. Microtubule-associated protein tau (τ) is a major antigenic component of paired helical filaments in Alzheimer disease. *Proc Natl Acad Sci USA* 1986;83:4044–4048.
52. Dickson DW, Farlo J, Davies P, Crystal H, Fuld P, Yen SC. A double-labeling immunohistochemical study of senile plaques. *Am J Pathol* 1988;132:86–101.
53. Geddes JW, Wilson MC, Miller FD, Cotman CW. Molecular markers of reactive plasticity. In: Ben-Ari Y ed. *Excitatory amino acids and neuronal plasticity.* New York: Plenum Press; 1990:425–432.
54. Cotman CW, Geddes JW, Kahle JS. Axon sprouting in the rodent brain and Alzheimer's disease brain: a reactivation of developmental mechanisms? In: Strom-Mathisen J, Zimmer J, Ottersen OP, eds. *Progress in Brain Research.* vol 83. Amsterdam: Elsevier Science Publishers BV;1990:427–434.
55. Masliah E, Mallory M, Hansen L, et al. Patterns of aberrant sprouting in Alzheimer's disease. *Neuron* 1991;6:729–739.
56. Uchida Y, Ihara Y, Tomonaga M. Alzheimer's disease brain extract stimulates the survival of cerebral cortical neurons from neonatal rats. *Biochem Biophys Res Commun* 1988;150:1263–1267.
57. Gómez-Pinilla F, Cummings BJ, Cotman CW. Induction of basic fibroblast growth factor in Alzheimer's disease pathology. *NeuroReport* 1990;1:211–214.
58. Stopa EG, Gonzalez A, Chorsky R, et al. Basic fibroblast growth factor in Alzheimer's disease. *Biochem Biophys Res Commun* 1990;171:690–696.
59. Kato T, Sasaki H, Katagiri T, et al. The binding of basic fibroblast growth factor to Alzheimer's neurofibrillary tangles and senile plaques. *Neurosci Lett* 1991;122:33–36.
60. Perry G, Siedlak SL, Richey P, et al. Association of heparan sulfate proteoglycan with the neurofibrillary tangles of Alzheimer disease. *J Neurosci* 1991;11:3679–3683.
61. Suzuki K, Katzman R, Korey S. Chemical studies on Alzheimer's disease. *J Neuropathol Exp Neurol* 1965;24:211–224.
62. Snow AD, Wight TN. Proteoglycans in the pathogenesis of Alzheimer's disease and other amyloidoses. *Neurobiol Aging* 1989;10:481–497.
63. Snow AD, Kisilevsky R. Temporal relationship between glycosaminoglycan accumulation and amyloid deposition during experimental amyloidosis: A histochemical study. *Lab Invest* 1985;53:37–44.
64. Snow AD, Mar H, Nochlin D, et al. Early accumulation of heparan sulfate in neurons and in the beta-amyloid protein-containing lesions of Alzheimer's disease and Down's syndrome. *Am J Pathol* 1990;137:1253–1270.
65. Su JH, Cummings BJ, Cotman CW. Localization of heparan sulfate glycosaminoglycan and proteoglycan in Alzheimer's disease. *Neurosci* (in press).
66. Whitson JS, Selkoe DJ, Cotman CW. Amyloid β protein enhances the survival of hippocampal neurons in vitro. *Science* 1989;243:1488–90.
67. Whitson JS, Glabe CG, Shintani E, Abcar A, Cotman CW. β-amyloid protein promotes neuritic branching in hippocampal cultures. *Neurosci Lett* 1990;110:319–24.
68. Pike CJ, Walencewicz AJ, Glabe CG, Cotman CW. In vitro aging of β-amyloid protein causes peptide aggregation and neurotoxicity. *Brain Res* 1991;563:311–314.
69. Koh JY, Yang LL, Cotman CW. β-amyloid protein increases the vulnerability of cultured cortical neurons to excitotoxic damage. *Brain Res* 1990;533:315–320.
70. Yankner BA, Caceres A, Duffy LK. Nerve growth factor potentiates the neurotoxicity of β-amyloid. *Proc Natl Acad Sci USA* 1990;87:9020–9023.
71. Yankner BA, Duffy LK, Kirschner DA. Neurotrophic and neurotoxic effects of amyloid β-protein: reversal by tachykinin neuropeptides. *Science* 1990;250:279–282.
72. Yankner BA, Dawes LR, Fisher S, Villa KL, Oster GML, Neve RL. Neurotoxicity of a fragment of the amyloid precursor associated with Alzheimer's disease. *Science* 1989;245:417–420.
73. Kowall NW, Beal MF, Busciglio J, Duffy LK, Yankner BA. An in vivo model for the neurodegenerative effects of β amyloid and protection by substance P. *Proc Natl Acad Sci USA* 1991;88:7247–7251.
74. Hilbich C, Kisters-Woike B, Reed J, Masters CL, Beyreuther K. Aggregation and secondary structure of synthetic amyloid βA4 peptides of Alzheimer's disease. *J Mol Biol* 1991;218:149–163.
75. Barrow CJ, Zagorski MG. Solution structures of β peptide and its constituent fragments: relation to amyloid deposition. *Science* 1991;253:179–182.
76. Burdick D, Soreghan B, Kosmoski J, et al. Assembly and aggregation properties of synthetic Alzheimer's A4/β amyloid peptide analogs. *J Biol Chem* 1992;267:546–554.
77. Pike CJ, Walencewicz AJ, Glabe CG, Cotman CW. Aggregation-related toxicity of synthetic β-amyloid protein in hippocampal cultures. *Eur J Pharm* 1991;207:367–368.
78. Quon D, Catalano R, Cordell B. Fibroblast growth factor induces beta-amyloid precursor mRNA in glial but not neuronal cultured cells. *Biochem Biophys Res Commun* 1990;167:96–102.

79. Araujo DM, Cotman CW. β-Amyloid stimulates glial cells in vitro to produce growth factors that accumulate in senile plaques in Alzheimer's disease. *Brain Res* (in press).
80. Yoshida K, Gage FH. Fibroblast growth factors stimulate nerve growth factor synthesis and secretion by astrocytes. *Brain Res* 1991;538:118–126.
81. Schubert D, Jin L, Saitoh T, Cole G. The regulation of amyloid beta protein precursor secretion and its modulatory role in cell adhesion. *Neuron* 1989;3:689–694.
82. Klier FG, Cole G, Stallcup W, Schubert D. Amyloid beta-protein precursor is associated with extracellular matrix. *Brain Res* 1990;515:336–342.
83. Schubert D, LaCorbiere M, Saitoh T, Cole G. Characterization of an amyloid beta-precursor protein that binds heparin and contains tyrosine sulfate. *Proc Natl Acad Sci USA* 1989;86:2066–2069.
84. Van Nostrand WE, Wagner SL, Farrow JS, Cunningham DD. Immunopurification and protease inhibitory properties of protease nexin-2/amyloid beta-protein precursor. *J Biol Chem* 1990;265:9591–9594.
85. Selkoe DJ, Podlisny M, Joachim C, et al. Beta-amyloid precursor protein of Alzheimer disease occurs as 110- to 135-kilodalton membrane-associated proteins in neural and nonneural tissues. *Proc Natl Acad Sci USA* 1988;85:7341–7345.
86. Tanzi RE, Gusella JF, Watkins PC, et al. Amyloid β protein gene: cDNA, mRNA distribution, and genetic linkage near the Alzheimer locus. *Science* 1987;235:880–884.
87. Van Nostrand WE, Wagner SL, Suzuki M, et al. Protease nexin-2, a potent anti-chymotrypsin, shows identity to amyloid β-protein precursor. *Nature* 1989;341:546–549.
88. Olsterdof T, Fritz LC, Schenk DB, et al. The secreted form of the Alzheimer's amyloid precursor protein with the Kunitz domain is protease nexin-2. *Nature* 1989;341:144–147.
89. Cummings BJ, Su JH, Geddes JW, et al. Aggregation of the amyloid precursor protein (APP) within degenerating neurons and dystrophic neurites in Alzheimer's disease. *Neurosci* 1992;48:763–777.
90. Choi DW. Glutamate neurotoxicity and diseases of the nervous system. *Neuron* 1988;1:623–634.
91. Hoyer S, Oesterreich K, and Wagner O. Glucose metabolism as the site of the primary abnormality in early-onset dementia of Alzheimer type? *J Neurol* 1988;235:143–148.
92. Copani A, Koh J, Cotman CW. β-amyloid increases neuronal susceptibility to injury by glucose deprivation. *Neuro Report* 1991;2:763–765.
93. Maragos WF, Greenamyre JT, Penney JB, Young AB. Glutamate dysfunction in Alzheimer's disease: an hypothesis. *Trends Neurosci* 1987;10:65–68.
94. Pike CJ, Cummings BJ, Cotman CW. β-amyloid induces neurotic dystrophy in vitro: Similarities with alzheimer pathology. *Neuro Report* (in press).

12

Sprouting and Regeneration in the Spinal Cord

Their Roles in Recovery of Function After Spinal Injury

Michael M. Goldberger, Marion Murray, and Alan Tessler

Department of Anatomy and Neurobiology, The Medical College of Pennsylvania, Philadelphia, Pennsylvania 19129

Injury to the brain or spinal cord is followed by a period of severe depression of function which is then succeeded by some recovery of function. The mechanisms underlying both the loss of function and the recovery of function are incompletely understood. After spinal transection in adult cats, there is complete loss of descending control of motor function owing to interruption of the descending motor pathways (1). This effect of the transection is permanent. There is also a depression of reflex function caudal to the lesion, the reasons for which are not yet evident. This reflex depression is not permanent; most reflexes show recovery and some may become hyperactive (2). Eventually, recovery of reflex locomotion, as elicited by a treadmill, can be demonstrated (3,4). The mechanisms underlying the remarkable recovery of reflex behavior remain unidentified although there are changes within the spinal cord caudal to the transection that may contribute to recovery and indeed are suspected of doing so (see ref. 5 for review). Thus a permanent loss of voluntary movement and a transient loss of reflex function are seen after the same lesion. The permanence of the loss of descending control is due to the failure of descending pathways to regenerate. The recovery of reflex behavior implies plasticity in spinal segments below the lesion that have been indirectly affected by the transection. Identification of the loci of the impairment and particularly of the nature of the recovery is useful as a guide to which systems should be examined further to reveal the nature of that plasticity that leads to recovery of function. One naturally occurring anatomical mechanism that can account for recovery of function is collateral sprouting. New studies using fetal transplants into injured spinal cord offer the possibility of enhancing this naturally occurring plasticity and achieving greater recovery of function.

PLASTICITY IN THE INJURED SPINAL CORD

Collateral Sprouting

Definition and Demonstration

Collateral sprouting (reactive reinnervation) refers to an expansion of the terminal field of undamaged axons in response to partial denervation of target neurons by removal of converging systems. In adults, the amount of growth is generally limited and is demonstrable only within the normal terminal field as an increase in density of the projection. The absence of extension of a projection beyond its normal limits in the adult has been frequently confirmed, although it has sometimes been interpreted as indicating an absence rather than a limitation on sprouting (6). Sprouting appears to be a regulated rather than a random occurrence so that certain systems are more likely to increase their projections in response to a specific lesion than others. There are also conditions under which sprouting of a specific pathway does not occur subsequent to a lesion that appears to denervate its target (7–11). In at least some of these cases, these results suggest a target regulation of sprouting.

If lesions are made in developing animals before the adult patterns of axonal projections and synaptic contacts are established, the sprouting response may include extension of the projection to regions normally not supplied or only poorly supplied by the undamaged system. Another form of plasticity, compensatory sprouting or pruning, refers to the proliferation of collaterals located proximal to the site of axotomy (12). To elicit this form of sprouting, the neuron must be damaged. This form of plasticity, which sometimes results in aberrant projections, has been shown most clearly in developing neurons.

The controversies that have arisen over the truth and consequences of sprouting in spinal cord are in part due to unappreciated methodological difficulties in demonstrating differences in densities of projections. Detection of an increased density in a normal projection requires quantitative methods sufficiently sensitive to reveal a difference between the experimental and control projections. In most cases, sprouting has been examined using light microscopic tract tracing methods, and the contralateral projection is frequently used as the control. Intra-animal comparisons of density of the control and sprouted projections may be the most sensitive way to determine the extent of modification of an afferent projection, but this requires establishing that the ipsilateral and contralateral projections are normally comparable in size and that the projections are uncrossed; if either of these requirements is unfulfilled, the appropriate corrections must be made. If axonal transport methods are used to identify the projection, e.g., HRP labeling, then comparable supply of the label to the control and the sprouting projections must be demonstrated. These methods used with interanimal comparisons are too insensitive to recognize differences in density if there is considerable normal interanimal variability in the density of projections. The interpretation of the results will be additionally confounded by the difficulty of demonstrating comparable delivery of the label to the test and experimental projections in different animals. Immunocytochemical staining of specific pathways is another light microscopic method that has been used to demonstrate sprouting. Differences in the apparent density of projections can, however, be attributable to increased synthesis or transport of the labeled substance. No control for this possibility has been devised as yet.

Quantitative electron microscopy has also been used to study sprouting (reactive reinnervation). Changes in the synaptic complement in terminal fields of target nuclei with recovery of terminal number toward normal levels can be shown after lesions. These changes indicate proliferation of terminals by undamaged systems leading to reinnervation of the denervated targets. The major procedural problem in these ultrastructural studies is dealing with the limited sample size and the requirement for methods to assess the extent of shrinkage and other changes in neuropil.

It is considerably easier to demonstrate sprouting of axonal projections in neonatal animals. In addition to the increased projection density found in normal targets, the axons may also follow an aberrant course and form projections to inappropriate targets. Qualitative methods may therefore be sufficient to demonstrate aberrant projections. On the other hand, changes in the target (atrophy or cell death) are more likely to occur in a developing system following a lesion and compensation for these changes is required in order to interpret the results.

It should be noted that there are alternative interpretations of the increased density of projections seen after partial denervation. For example, projections normally not revealed, perhaps because the axons and terminals are below light microscopic resolution or because they contain inadequate amounts of label or immunoreactive material, may become demonstrable only under conditions of increased activity, without an actual increase in the number of contacts that are made. Such a possibility cannot be easily ruled out although there is relatively little evidence in support of this interpretation (45) and it is not supported by ultrastructural data.

Evidence for Plasticity Induced by Lesions in the Adult Spinal Cord

A considerable body of evidence has accumulated both supporting and questioning collateral sprouting after lesions in the adult and neonatal spinal cord since the first report in 1958 (13). The source of many of the controversies now appears to be accounted for by the methodological difficulties associated with demonstrating sprouting in the adult spinal cord.

Sprouting of Dorsal Root Axons

The Spared Root Preparation. This preparation is the classic model for demonstrating dorsal root sprouting (8,13–16). Several dorsal roots are cut rostral and caudal to the test dorsal root. After survival times adequate to permit sprouting by the central processes of the spared root and disappearance of the degeneration products from the cut roots, test lesions are made of the spared root and the contralateral control root. Using a newly developed method for identifying degenerating axons, Liu and Chambers (13) described an increased density of projection by the spared root axons on the experimental side, which they interpreted as sprouting of the spared root. They also described an extension of the projection of lumbar dorsal root axons to levels of Clarke's nucleus several segments rostral to the level at which control axons terminated, an increased projection which would be considered an aberrant projection. Their results were largely confirmed by Goldberger and Murray (8), with the exception of the aberrant extended projection. This disparity in results can probably be accounted for by methodological problems associated with the suppression step used in this procedure. These results have been criticized recently by Kruger and his colleagues (17–19) who attributed the apparent sprouting to inadequate controls. Rodin et al. (17) attempted to replicate the Liu and Chambers model but used transganglionic labeling with HRP instead of degeneration stains to compare the projections of test and experimental roots. They were unable to identify a difference in density of projection between a spared root in an experimental animal and the comparable root in another unoperated animal and therefore concluded that sprouting did not occur. Since the spared root projection was determined in one series of animals, and compared to the projection of a root at the same level in another group of animals, these authors were unable to make appropriate compensations for the very large differences between animals in numbers of dorsal root ganglion (DRG) cells and therefore numbers of centrally projecting axons at the lumbar levels. Since the number of DRG cells may vary as much as 50% from one animal to another (20), the sensitivity of their method was too low to support their conclusions. Polistina et al. (21) took advantage of the fact that the number of DRG cells in a lumbar ganglion does not vary greatly between the two sides of the same animal (20,22,23) and therefore used intra-animal comparisons supported by an internal control (counting the number of labeled neurons) to demonstrate comparable labeling of the test and control projections. Their results showed increased densities of the spared root projections that were statistically significant but no evidence of extension of projections to aberrant targets. They also showed that the normal interanimal variability is sufficient to mask these differences when uncontrolled interanimal comparisons are used.

Histochemical and immunocytochemical methods were used by McNeill and colleagues (15,16) to examine the density of projections of the spared T9 root in rat. Fluoride-resistant acid phosphatase (FRAP), a marker for axons originating from a class of small DRG neurons, was shown to increase in density in the superficial layers of the dorsal horn on the spared root side compared to the control side while calcitonin gene-related peptide (CGRP), a marker for terminals originating from other classes of dorsal root ganglion neurons, was shown to label approximately twice as many terminals in the dorsal horn at levels near the spared root compared to the control side. Further ultrastructural evidence supporting plasticity in dorsal root terminals of the spared root is provided by Zhang et al. (unpublished results), who have shown increased numbers of terminal contacts and increased lengths of postsynaptic densities associated with complex terminals arising from small DRG neurons on the spared root side. Thus the immunocytochemical studies of specific populations of dorsal root axons support the results from controlled horseradish peroxidase (HRP) and degeneration methods, all indicating increased densities of dorsal root projections in the spared root preparation. The electron microscopic (EM) studies further suggest that the sprouting is associated with terminal proliferation.

A variation of the spared root preparation has been used in two studies in which neurotoxic compounds, injected into the peripheral fields of spinal nerves, are transported to the DRG. A proportion of DRG cells are killed, but those spared can be examined for evidence of sprouting. Pubols and Bowen (24) injected ricin, a compound that kills a variable number of DRG cells, into sciatic nerves 2 weeks to 2 months before sacrifice. Six days prior to sacrifice they injected ricin into the contralateral (control) sciatic nerve. HRP injections into dorsal rootlets were then used to compare labeling on the two sides. These authors found considerable variability in labeling of the projections between the two sides, which appeared to be a function of variations in the amounts of HRP injected, but failed to find consistent differences between control and experimental sides. They interpreted this finding as absence of evidence for sprouting. The crucial controls in these experiments would have been first to demonstrate loss of axons after ricin injection on the two sides and then to compare projections in animals in which they could demonstrate comparable HRP uptake by dorsal roots of the two sides. Their interpretation is further complicated by the fact that sprouting is likely to have occurred on the control side at the 6 day postinjection survival time used (25) so that comparable labeling of the two sides might have been expected under well-controlled conditions. Lamotte et al. (26), using a similar paradigm, injected pronase, a combination of proteolytic enzymes, into the sciatic nerve. Pronase is also transported to the DRG where it kills ganglion cells. They later injected HRP and wheat germ agglutinin (WGA)-HRP into the cut saphenous nerves and measured the area in dorsal horn supplied by labeled axons. Controls showed evidence for comparable and symmetrical labeling in normal animals using their HRP methods, and demonstrate loss of unmyelinated axons in the dorsal roots caused by the pronase treatment. These workers found an increase in area labeled with HRP and an increase in the number of labeled terminals on the experimental side which they interpreted as evidence for sprouting by central processes of saphenous axons in response to loss of central processes of the sciatic axons. Whether the sprouting from the saphenous nerve extended into novel territories or simply increased within its normal territory is difficult to resolve given the unknown extent of overlap of the two projections in the dorsal horn (27,28,29a).

Lesions within the CNS that partially denervate targets of dorsal root axons can also elicit sprouting of dorsal roots. This was first reported using hemisection in the cat (29) and more recently was confirmed with immunocytochemical methods (30), although the same lesion in rats elicited clear evidence of dorsal root sprouting only in young animals (31a). Rodin and Kruger (18) again used transganglionic transport of HRP to look for differences in dorsal root projections ipsilateral and contralateral to a thoracic hemisection. They reached the conclusion that sprouting does not occur because they could find no consistent differences between projections of experimental or control roots; as in their previous study, they used interanimal comparisons and did not control for differences in amount of HRP transported, an approach that is not likely to be sensitive to differences in the projections between animals or technical differences in delivery of the label. More recently anterolateral cordotomy in the monkey has been shown to produce rearrangement of primary afferents within but not outside of regions of normal termination, a change consistent with denervation-induced sprouting (31).

Peripheral Nerve Lesions. It is well known that peripheral nerve lesions are often followed by regeneration of the cut axons. It has more recently been shown that these lesions also cause death of some DRG neurons (20) and degeneration of their central processes (32). These lesions also evoke a variety of changes in the surviving ganglion cells that appear to be reversed after regeneration of the peripheral process occurs (33). These changes include decreased synthesis of some peptide transmitters (34–36); up-regulation of synthesis of other peptides (37,38); increased synthesis of growth-associated proteins (39) and cytoskeletal proteins (40); and changes in morphology of the central terminals (41). Resection of the sciatic nerve, which prevents regeneration and partially denervates central targets, combined with crush of saphenous nerve, which stimulates saphenous regeneration, elicited central sprouting by the saphenous dorsal root afferents, which appeared to exceed the normal central projection of the saphenous nerve (42). These studies suggest that the changes in DRG neurons associated with the regenerative responses to peripheral nerve lesion can enhance the growth responses of the axons within the CNS (43). McMahon and Kett-White (44) tested this hypothesis more directly in adults by cutting the peripheral nerve of the spared root. This combined lesion enhanced sprouting by axons in the spared root and also increased the area supplied by the spared root. This important observation indicates that the usual spatial limitation of sprouting in the adult can be overridden by an additional manipulation that increases the growth potential of the adult axon.

Of particular interest in considering plasticity associated with peripheral lesions is the evidence that very marked and long lasting modifications of central pathways within the spinal cord (45,46) and extending to changes in cortical representations (47–49) occur after peripheral nerve lesions.

Sprouting of Central Pathways

Central pathways have also been shown to sprout. Most of the evidence in favor of central sprouting in the adult spinal cord comes from studies in which the cord has been deafferented by dorsal rhizotomies. Tessler et al. (50–52) first used immunocytochemistry and radioimmunoassay to demonstrate, in the cat, that deafferentation, which eliminates the major SP input to laminae I and II of the dorsal horn, elicits a recovery of SP, but not somatostatin. They interpreted these data as indicating sprouting by intraspinal SP-containing neurons. These observations were subsequently confirmed in the cat (19) and rat (11). The population of synaptic terminals in lamina II also changes following deafferentation, with a loss of all of the characteristic scalloped terminals and some of the simple terminals, but with no loss in total number of terminals (25). This observation suggests that complete deafferentation evoked rapid replacement of lost dorsal root terminals by simple terminals from intrinsic sources. Recent quantitative analyses by Zhang et al. have shown that the number of simple SP-labeled terminals increases after deafferentation, a finding consistent with the interpretation of reactive reinnervation (Fig. 1). Beattie et al. (10) compared synaptic input after transection to two nuclei in sacral spinal cord, Onuf's nucleus, and the sacral

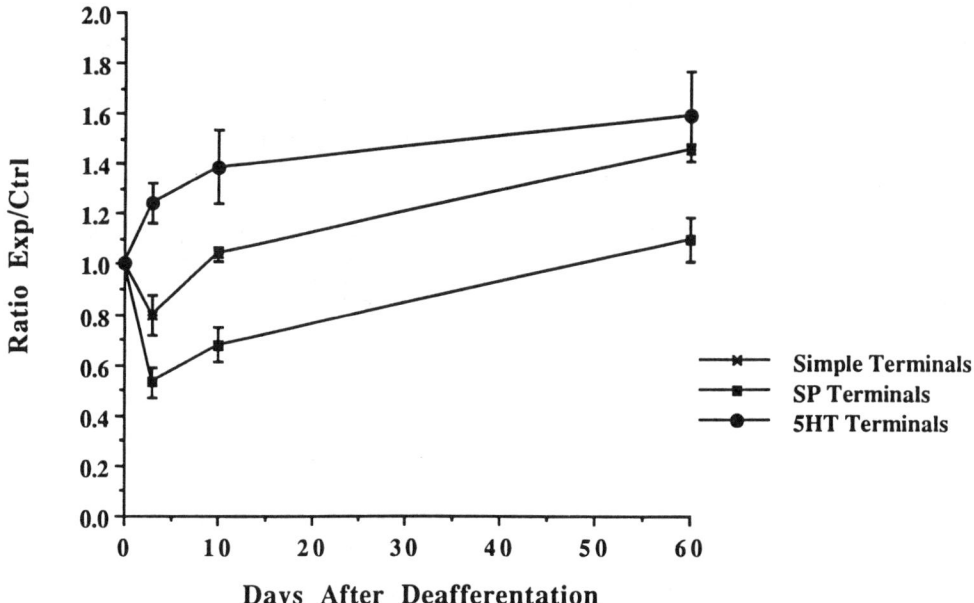

FIG. 1. Changes in the total number of simple terminals, number of simple terminals immunoreactive for SP, and number of simple terminals immunoreactive for 5HT in lamina II after unilateral lumbosacral deafferentation in the rat. The results are expressed as a ratio of counts on the control lamina II to counts in the deafferented lamina II. Postembedding immunocytochemical methods were used to identify SP and 5HT terminals. Note that the number of simple terminals decreased postoperatively and then increased to above normal levels, indicating proliferation in response to deafferentation. Immunocytochemical analyses indicated that part of the increase can be attributed to increased number of SP-containing terminals, which show a time course of change similar to that for total simple terminals, and part can be attributed to 5HT-containing terminals, which show a different time course. The time course of change of number of terminals parallels the time course of change of density of immunocytochemical reaction, shown light microscopically (11).

parasympathetic nuclei. They found evidence for synaptic replacement in Onuf's nucleus but permanent denervation in the sacral parasympathetic nucleus, suggesting that sprouting may be regulated differently in these two nuclei. Different results were reported by Chung (53), however, who counted synaptic thickenings in the sacral dorsal horn after unilateral deafferentation in the rat. They found a decrease in numbers of contacts compared to control animals on both operated and unoperated sides during the first postoperative week.

Serotonergic pathways that descend from the brainstem also sprout in response to deafferentation. Wang (11), using a complete lumbosacral deafferentation model, showed a twofold increase in density of 5-hydroxytryptamine (5HT) immunoreactivity in lamina I and II. Polistina (21) showed in a spared root preparation that the density of the 5HT projections increases at denervated spinal levels rostral to the zone where the spared root axons have increased their projections. These studies indicate that the descending serotonergic pathway will increase its projection density in response to removal of convergent dorsal root projections to the dorsal horn. EM-immunocytochemical studies by Zhang et al. indicate that serotonergic-containing terminals also increase in lamina II after deafferentation (Fig. 1). Interestingly, in the same preparation, the descending noradrenergic projection to the dorsal horn showed no change in density indicating a selectivity in which systems sprout in response to deafferentation (11).

Finally, hemisection lesions have also been shown to modify the projections of corticospinal neurons in the adult monkey (54). In this study HRP was injected into the spinal cord contralateral to a hemisection and increased numbers of labeled neurons were found in the cortex ipsilateral to the lesion, suggesting sprouting of projections across the midline or by ipsilaterally projecting corticospinal axons.

Evidence for Plasticity Induced by Lesions in Neonatal Animals

Lesions in neonatal animals often result in greater sprouting than in adults and as a result the issue of neonatal sprouting seems less controversial. This increased plasticity may account for the greater recovery of function associated with lesions in developing animals. Usually the extent of plasticity which can be evoked by lesions made in the neonate declines toward adult levels during the postnatal period.

Sprouting of Dorsal Root Axons

The classic spared root preparation has not been studied in neonatal animals. A similar paradigm is however provided by experiments in which capsaicin is injected (55,56). Capsaicin, when injected in neonatal rat, destroys most of the small DRG cells, eliminating about 90% of the unmyelinated axonal input to the dorsal horn. The spared large DRG cells, which normally project to deeper layers of the dorsal horn, develop aberrant projections into the denervated superficial layers as well and form terminals there.

Hulsebosch and colleagues (57,58) have shown that administration of antibodies to NGF to otherwise normal neonatal rats had the unexpected effect of eliciting sprouting of unmyelinated axons in the dorsal root and in Lissauer's tract. Administration of anti-NGF antibody results in the death of some DRG cells (59) with the possibility that small DRG cells are more vulnerable than the large cells. The surviving DRG cells appear to emit greater numbers of axonal collaterals in response to the loss of other DRG cells, and this form of sprouting was clearly demonstrable by axon counts both in the dorsal root and intraspinally (57,58). The mechanism by which this sprouting is elicited is likely to be neutralization of the nerve growth factor (NGF) necessary for the survival of small DRG cells and which is normally supplied to them by axonal transport from the periphery. The loss of this class of dorsal root ganglion cells thus elicits a response similar to that achieved by capsaicin delivered neonatally. As in the capsaisin studies, the surviving large DRG cells appear to project into aberrant regions of the spinal cord, i.e., Lissauer's tract.

The effects of peripheral nerve lesions in neonates have been compared with the same lesion in adults. Peripheral nerve section in neonates, in contrast to adults, produces massive DRG cell death, resulting in a much greater denervation of the dorsal horn. The neonatal lesion therefore provides a greater stimulus for sprouting by the spared ganglion cells than the adult lesion (20,59). Peripheral nerve section leads to loss of FRAP staining in the part of the dorsal horn supplied by the injured ganglion cells. In neonates, but not in adults, the area of depletion in the dorsal horn is rapidly filled in by the sprouting of FRAP-containing afferents from adjacent intact ganglion cells (60). Similarly, neonatal sciatic nerve lesions elicit an expansion in the saphenous terminal field in the dorsal horn. This sprouting is less extensive in animals more than 5 days old, indicating the postnatal critical period for this form of plasticity (61). Fitzgerald et al. (62) used physiological methods supported by HRP labeling to demonstrate sprouting of specific types of dorsal root afferents into inappropriate central fields as a result of neonatal sciatic nerve lesion. The terminals formed by the aberrant projections were appropriate to the new target areas, suggesting target regulation of terminal morphology.

Sprouting of Central Pathways

Neonatal deafferentation by rhizotomy (63) or by administration of capsaicin (64) has been used to demonstrate sprouting by serotonergic axons in the dorsal horn. Capsaicin injections on the day of birth, eliminating most of the central projections of the small DRG cells, elicited sprouting by descending 5HT axons into aberrant regions of the dorsal horn. Dorsal rhizotomy on postnatal day 5 evoked increased 5HT densities comparable to the twofold increase shown after deafferentation in adults (11). However, the sprouting in neonates extends into deeper layers of the dorsal horn than in the adult. These studies taken together suggest a critical period within the first 5 days postnatal that limits the extent of aberrant sprouting of the serotonergic fiber systems in response to rhizotomy.

Pyramidal lesions interrupt the corticospinal pathway and evoke sprouting of corticospinal axons to the contralateral spinal cord (65). Cerebral hemispherectomy also evokes sprouting to spinal areas (66). Both studies report greater effects when the lesions are made in the neonate than in the adult.

In summary, there is convincing anatomical evidence for sprouting in the spinal cord. Dorsal roots have been shown to increase their terminal density in adult spinal cord in a variety of experimental paradigms. In most of the experiments in which sprouting could not be demonstrated, methods were used that did not take into account normal variability either between animals or in the methods used to test sprouting. Similarly there is generally consistent evidence of sprouting by central systems in response to partial deafferentation. Most quantitative studies at both EM and light microscopic levels indicate that sprouting is associated with marked, not trivial, increases in projection densities, which may be sufficient to restore numbers of terminals on partially denervated targets to close to normal levels. Expansion of terminal fields into novel territories in adults has been demonstrated most convincingly in cases where additional manipulations are made, e.g., addition of peripheral nerve injury to the lesion paradigm. This suggests that the limitation on sprouting in adults can be overridden by increasing the metabolic drive of the sprouting neurons. In general, greater sprouting is seen when lesions are made before development has ceased, and this neonatal sprouting may include expansion into areas not normally supplied without additional manipulations. Naturally occurring plasticity in adults as well as in neonates represents a major compensatory response to CNS lesions, which needs to be taken into account in considering the consequences of CNS lesions, the extent of recovery of function, and ways of improving the extent of recovery of function.

Functional Recovery

Each of the three classical preparations that has been used to study sprouting in the spinal cord, i.e., hemisection, spared root, and deafferentation, has also been studied behaviorally to determine whether recovery of function can be observed. Not only is recovery of motor behavior documented but, in each case, the pathways that show sprouting have also been shown to have major roles in mediating recovery.

Spinal Cord Hemisection

Hemisections were made in the lower thoracic cord of the cat, sparing the dorsal columns so that motor impairments resulting from loss of the major ascending pathway would not be confused with those associated with loss of descending input (30). The animals had been preoperatively trained to walk on a 30 cm wide "simple" runway as well as on more challenging runways, including a horizontal ladder, a grid, and a narrow runway; the time to cross and number of errors were recorded and a kinematic analysis of joint angle excursions carried out. The threshold for placing, the force of the positive supporting reaction, and the kinematics of placing and hopping reactions were measured. Recovery of basic locomotion could therefore be compared with recovery of locomotion requiring accurate placement of the hindlimb. Careful analysis shows a predictable pattern of recovery of function. For a brief period, the hindlimb on the hemisected side is severely paralyzed both for locomotion and for postural reflexes but by the end of the first week considerable recovery occurs. During the first week, basic locomotion on the wide runway and also reflex locomotion on a treadmill recover. Measurement of joint angle excursions during the step cycle, however, reveals a kinematic pattern that is clearly abnormal; furthermore, the animals frequently walk on the dorsum of the toes on the hemisected side. Postural reflexes also show an early stage of recovery. Although contact (hair-bend) placing never recovers, proprioceptive placing (placing in response to bending of some part of the limb) does recover. The amount of bending required to elicit placing, i.e., the threshold, is considerable and the response is clearly hypermetric. Similar effects are seen when the monopedal hopping response is elicited; the amount of passive displacement on the treadmill is exaggerated compared to normal and the response is hypermetric. The positive supporting response is also deficient compared to the intact side.

During the second postoperative week, another phase of recovery begins. The thresholds for placing and hopping decrease although not to normal values (Fig. 2). Hypermetria is also reduced. The force of the positive supporting response recovers to normal. Most dramatic, however, is the recovery of accurate limb placement during locomotion, which begins to occur at this time. Initially, many errors in foot placement are observed and this slows the animal's crossing of the runway. In time, the number of errors decreases and speed increases, but normal values are not attained. During this period, the kinematic pattern returns almost to normal and the animals stop walking on the dorsum of the foot.

Therefore the first phase of recovery con-

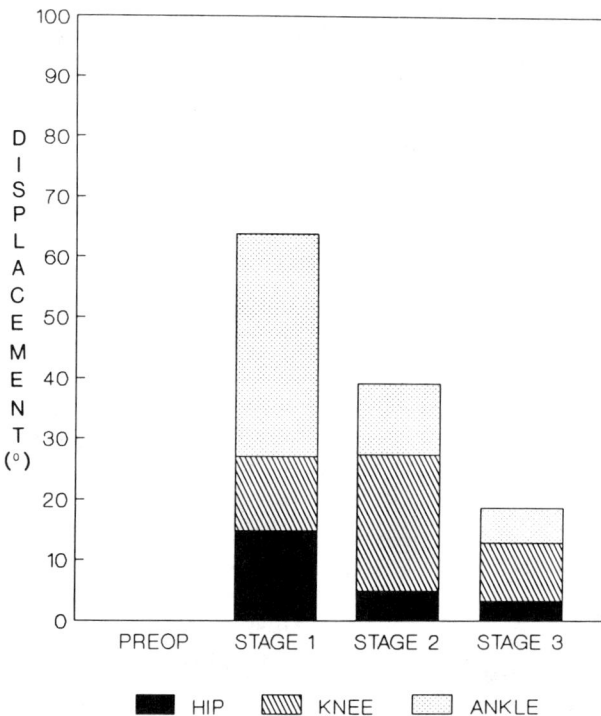

FIG. 2. This figure shows the amount of limb displacement required to elicit a placing response after spinal cord hemisection. The height of each bar corresponds to the total limb displacement, and the individual compartments correspond to the displacement of the hip, knee, and ankle. Preoperatively no displacement is required since the animals respond to hair stimulation. Immediately postoperatively, the amount of displacement is very large, especially at the ankle, but partial recovery takes place and becomes stable *(STAGE 3).*

sists of recovery of basic locomotion and of crudely performed, high threshold postural reflexes. The second phase consists of refinement of the postural reflexes including lowering of their thresholds. The change in threshold may be due to a compensatory increase in afferent control of movements when descending control has been interrupted. Collateral sprouting of dorsal root afferents has been demonstrated after hemisection of the cat spinal cord by degeneration methods (29,30) and by immunocytochemistry (30). This sprouting of dorsal root terminals may represent a mechanism underlying the increase in reflex control.

Physiological changes have been observed after hemisection that are consistent with the notion of a compensatory increase in afferent control after a loss of descending input. Hultborn and Malmsten (67,68) demonstrated an increase in the strength of the monosynaptic stretch reflex and also in the cutaneous flexor reflex by using ventral root response to these different inputs. More recently, Pubols and her colleagues (69–71) have shown that the number of spinal cord neurons responding to cutaneous (sural nerve) inputs increases substantially after damage to descending pathways on one side of the cat spinal cord. Interestingly, the magnitude of the increase is similar to the number of neurons that possess subliminal sural nerve inputs in normal cats (72). These neurons produce EPSPs but not impulses upon sural nerve stimulation suggesting that the increase after the lesion is due not to the formation of new aberrant connections but rather to the strengthening of already existing but weak connections. The strengthening of these connections could be mediated by sprouting of dorsal root terminals in the regions denervated by the lesion, denervation supersensitivity of neurons in such regions, or other unidentified mechanisms.

Spared Root Preparation

Since the spared root preparation was the first to be used to study sprouting (13), it is important to determine whether or not recovery of function can be demonstrated in this model. We have studied a group of cats with unilateral deafferentation, sparing the L6 root (73). Initially, the effect of the spared root deafferentation is quite marked. Locomotion is impaired, the partially deafferented limb is dragged, contact placing and the monopedal hopping reaction are abolished, and the positive supporting reaction is considerably weakened. These severe impairments are transient, however, and recovery begins during the first postoperative week. Basic locomotion, performed on a wide runway or a treadmill, returns, although the kinematic pattern used for locomotion is abnormal. Proprioceptive placing can be elicited, high threshold monopedal hopping responses return, and weight support begins to recover. There is thus an early recovery of basic locomotion and crudely executed postural reflexes. During the second week, a recovery of accurate limb placement on the complex runways is observed. Initially the animals make considerable numbers of misplacements but the errors decrease with time and the speed of crossing increases. There is continued recovery of the postural reflexes; contact placing returns, the frequency of placing to the lowest stimulus increases, the threshold for monopedal hopping decreases, and weight support increases. A normal kinematic pattern during locomotion is reestablished.

Thus the pattern of recovery is similar after hemisection and after spared root deafferentation: a lowering of the threshold for postural reflexes is associated with recovery of accurate limb placement and the return of a normal kinematic pattern used in locomotion. It is reasonable to hypothesize in both preparations that dorsal root sprouting increases the afferent control of movement and that this is responsible for the recovery of motor behavior. In both cases, there are alternative possibilities due to sparing of some of the descending pathways. After hemisection, the contralateral descending pathways are spared, and in spared root preparations the ipsilateral (as well as contralateral) descending pathways are available to mediate recovery. This possibility was tested by making contralateral hemisections in the hemisected animals and ipsilateral hemisections in the spared root animals after recovery had taken place. In both cases, most of the recovered behavior remained after the second lesion suggesting that it was the primary afferent control that was largely responsible for the recovery. This suggests that there may be a competitive interaction among the spared pathways after a lesion and they do not contribute equally to the recovery process.

There are physiological changes after partial spinal cord deafferentation which are consistent with the idea of increased afferent control mediated by the spared root in response to partial denervation of its terminal field. Pubols and Goldberger (74) found that there was a loss of responsiveness in the lateral dorsal horn acutely after spared root deafferentation sparing L6. There was then a recovery of responsiveness but the receptive field organization had changed in this portion of the dorsal horn. A permanent loss of proximal receptive fields was found, and this loss was compensated for by an increase of mixed receptive fields. This suggested the strengthening of weak afferent input, which might be mediated by sprouting or other mechanisms. Mendell et al. (75) made similar observations when they recorded from spinocervical tract cells after L7 spared root deafferentation. They also found a loss of responsiveness when peripheral areas supplied by the spared root were stimulated. There was a subsequent recovery of responsiveness owing to an increase in high threshold mechanoreceptive input. Thus although there was recovery, the recovered input was not the same, or in the same proportions, as the original normal input.

Hindlimb Deafferentation

To study the effect of dorsal rhizotomy on loss and recovery of motor function, the dorsal roots L_1–S_2 were cut on one side of the spinal cord (76). Reflex and overground locomotion were studied as in the other models. The initial deficit is more severe than after the other lesions described above. The deafferented limb is not used in locomotion but is dragged behind the animal as it walks on three legs. The descending reflexes, including the scratch and vestibular placing reflexes, are eliminated. All segmental reflex behavior, including crossed reflexes from the contralateral hindlimb, is abolished. Recovery begins soon, on the second postoperative day, and consists of participation of the deafferented limb in the step cycle for overground locomotion. The frequency of stepping is reduced from normal, i.e., the deafferented limb does not step each time the contralateral hindlimb steps. The kinematic pattern is clearly abnormal and the steps of the deafferented limb are sometimes hypermetric and sometimes hypometric. There is also some recovery of the descending scratch and vestibular reflexes during the first postoperative week. During the second postoperative week a marked change is seen in the use of the deafferented hindlimb. The limb can now be used for accurate placement on a narrow (5 cm) runway. Although weight-bearing is somewhat deficient, the animals can place the limbs under the center of gravity and bear weight. Initially there are many errors, but the number of errors decreases and the speed of crossing increases.

In the other two models, hemisection and spared root, the relationship between postural reflex recovery and recovery of locomotion could be examined. Since all afferent input has been eliminated on one side, a similar analysis cannot be carried out in this model. However, it is possible to compare descending control of locomotor recovery and reflex control (Fig. 3). Overground locomotion depends on the presence of descending input; since it is conditioned, it presumably requires input from the brain. Quadrupedal treadmill locomotion requires descending input of the propriospinal system but does not require supraspinal control. Bipedal hindlimb locomotion requires only segmental systems since it recovers after complete spinal transection. When these three types of locomotion are examined after deafferentation, it becomes clear that the recovery is selective. Overground locomotion on the runway begins to recover during the first week. Quadrupedal locomotion on the treadmill begins to recover during the second week and the frequency of stepping of the deafferented limb is permanently reduced. Bipedal locomotion on the treadmill does not recover at all. This implies that activation of the deafferented limb requires descending supraspinal or propriospinal input but that segmental input activated by the contralateral hindlimb is inadequate. Thus recovery of locomotion is mediated by descending systems but not by segmental systems, or segmental systems by themselves cannot mediate locomotion after deafferentation.

This result was surprising considering that the spinal pattern generator for locomotion remained intact. We considered that after deafferentation, the deafferented limb might be dominated by some descending inhibitory system. If this were true, then removal of descending input after recovery from deafferentation might release the deaf-

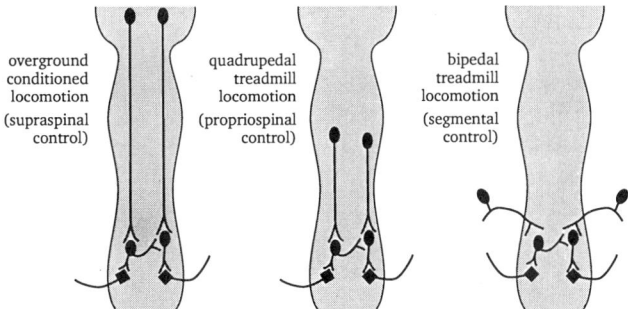

FIG. 3. These diagrams indicate pathways required for the three types of locomotion tested. Conditioned overground locomotion requires the presence of descending supraspinal pathways. Quadrupedal locomotion on a treadmill requires descending propriospinal connections between the forelimb and hindlimb segments of the spinal cord. In contrast, bipedal treadmill locomotion requires only the local spinal pattern generators in the lumbosacral segments.

ferented limb from inhibition and permit the return of bipedal hindlimb stepping. Therefore the spinal cord was transected after the recovery from deafferentation had reached a plateau. There was no subsequent recovery of locomotion in the deafferented limb and even the recovery of locomotion on the other side was slower and less extensive than in otherwise intact spinal cats. An alternative explanation for the results is that there is simply inadequate facilitation, after deafferentation, to activate locomotor circuits on the deafferented side when descending pathways are inactivated by the behavioral conditions (i.e., when bipedal rather than quadrupedal locomotion is tested) or by transection.

These behavioral observations cannot completely define the mechanisms underlying recovery. The anatomical patterns seen after chronic deafferentation are, however, consistent with the pattern of recovery. First, there is a complete recovery of terminal number in major target areas of the dorsal roots (25). Second, when the distribution of staining using a monoclonal antibody specific to dorsal roots is examined, it is clear that the deafferented side remains depleted of dorsal root input and that dorsal roots from the intact side do not invade deafferented regions (30). This is consistent with the observation that recovery does not depend on contralateral systems. Third, an interneuronal system containing substance P and a descending system containing serotonin both exhibit increases in transmitter content in the dorsal horn after deafferentation (11). This is consistent with the idea that descending control is important in mediating recovery of locomotion after deafferentation.

Mechanisms of Sprouting

There are two classes of hypotheses for mechanisms that may regulate sprouting: 1) receptor modification secondary to denervation, which promotes formation and stabilization of new synaptic terminals, and 2) release of growth factors in the environment that can stimulate neurite outgrowth and synaptogenesis. There is as yet relatively little direct evidence that any of these factors contribute to sprouting in vivo.

Receptor Modification

A lesion partially denervates its target neuron and creates vacant synaptic sites, which may evoke denervation supersensitivity on the target neuron. The experiments to relate vacated sites or receptor modification to the formation of new synaptic terminals by intact neurons have not yet been done. There is, however, evidence that dorsal rhizotomy which modifies both the SP and the 5HT projections within the dorsal horn (11,19,21,50–52) is also associated with an increase in the density of tachykinin receptors (77–79) and a down-regulation of 5HT receptors (80). These events may be related to sprouting, as elsewhere in the CNS. The N-methyl-D-aspartate (NMDA) receptor-mediated portion of the excitatory amino acid system, for example, has been shown to play an important role in activity-dependent mechanisms associated with synaptic plasticity and stabilization in other CNS systems (81,82). In the denervated hippocampus, the NMDA receptor density increases transiently, a phenomenon that might promote stabilization of newly formed synapses from sprouting afferents (84). It is therefore of interest both that DRG cells contain excitatory amino acids and that NMDA-binding sites (83) are present in high densities in regions of the dorsal horn where plasticity has been demonstrated. Surprisingly, blockade of the NMDA receptor has been reported to induce sprouting of undamaged dorsal root afferents in adult spinal cord (85). It is likely that new information on the role of receptor changes in sprouting response will be forthcoming.

Growth Factors

Peripheral sprouting and regeneration are known to be regulated by growth factors although the regulation of these two processes may be different (86). There is considerable evidence that polypeptide growth factors are secreted by target or supporting cells, bind to receptors on axons, become internalized, and are transported retrogradely to the cell body where they activate genes whose expression leads to synthesis of proteins necessary for neurite outgrowth (87). Both NGF and insulin-like growth factors promote sprouting from sensory neurons both in vitro and in vivo (88–90), and NGF administration will prevent some effects of peripheral nerve section (91,92). These studies suggest that one stimulus for plasticity at least of DRG neurons is the elimination of NGF, which is normally supplied to the DRG neurons. Synthesis of growth-associated proteins, but not of cytoskeletal elements (92), is stimulated by NGF, and increased synthesis of GAP43 is associated with central sprouting (39, 92). The identification, isolation, and function of growth factors in regulation of central sprouting in vivo remains a challenge.

INTRASPINAL TRANSPLANTS

In the previous sections we have documented the considerable plasticity of the spinal cord after injury in the adult or neonatal mammal. A next step is to attempt to extend or enhance the naturally occurring plasticity of spinal neurons by introducing transplants into damaged spinal cord.

One strategy for promoting recovery after spinal cord injury is to transplant brainstem monoaminergic neurons that can restore function without reconstituting damaged neuronal circuits (93,94). The rationale for this approach is based on the results of experiments suggesting that monoamines administered systemically after spinal cord transection can activate the intrinsic spinal cord circuitry that mediates locomotor (95) or autonomic (96) function. Both brainstem catecholaminergic neurons important for locomotion and serotonergic neurons important for autonomic function have been transplanted into the caudal region of transected spinal cord (97). The transplanted noradrenergic locus coeruleus and serotonergic mesencephalic or medullary raphe neurons extend axons for up to 1–2 cm into host spinal cord (94,98–101), restore levels of neurotransmitter depleted by the transection (102,103), and terminate in the same regions as in normal spinal cord (101–103). Transplanted serotonergic axons establish synapses on host motoneurons and neurons in the host intermediolateral column that are similar to those formed by brainstem serotoninergic axons in normal spinal cord (102,103). The projections of transplanted locus coeruleus neurons have not yet been studied with the electron microscope.

Both types of transplanted brainstem monoaminergic neurons contribute to recovery in experimental models of spinal cord injury. Rats with spinal cord transections recover reflex ejaculation if they receive transplants of embryonic raphe serotonergic neurons, but rarely if they receive no transplant or a transplant that does not contain serotonergic cells (102,103). Transplanted noradrenergic locus coeruleus neurons are thought to account for the recovery of hindlimb flexion reflexes in rats whose catecholamines have been chemically depleted (104) and for the recovery of reflex stepping activity in rats whose spinal cord has been transected (105). These embryonic transplants therefore contribute to behavioral recovery although they have been placed in the spinal cord caudal to transection and cannot be regulated normally by the host or restore the damaged neuronal circuits. The activation of intrinsic spinal cord networks by the release of transmitter onto or in the vicinity of the normal targets of these neurons appears to be adequate to account for the recovery of these behaviors.

The recovery of other types of behavior lost after spinal cord injury is likely to require more faithful reconstruction of the damaged neuronal circuits. Additional strategies using peripheral nerve grafts or embryonic spinal cord transplants have therefore been developed. Such transplants may contribute to the restoration of function in at least three ways (Fig. 4): 1) by

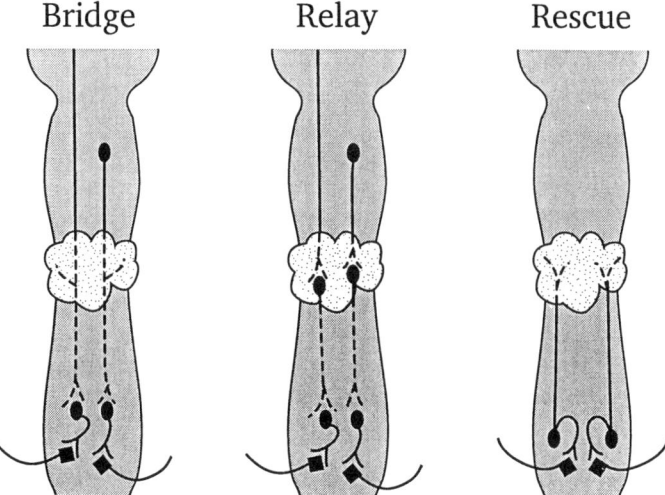

FIG. 4. Diagram illustrating three possible mechanisms by which intraspinal transplants can enhance locomotor function after spinal cord injury. The transplant *(pale area)* is shown at the site of spinal transection. The four neurons in the lower portion of each diagram represent the lumbar spinal pattern generator for locomotion. The vertical lines in the left and middle diagrams represent the axons of supraspinal and propriospinal neurons or of neurons within the transplant and in the third diagram the axons of neurons within the lumbar pattern generator. *Bridge* shows axons of host neurons traversing the transplant. *Relay* shows the establishment of connections within the transplant between the axons of host and transplant neurons. *Rescue* shows the survival of axotomized host pattern generator neurons that would otherwise die. (Reproduced by permission from ref. 30.)

rescuing axotomized neurons that would otherwise die; 2) by serving as a conduit for the regrowth of damaged host axons directly across an area of damage; 3) by serving as a site in which relays are established between neurons in host spinal cord and neurons in the transplant that may project to host neurons.

Segments of peripheral nerve rescue axotomized retinal ganglion cells (106) and when inserted into the spinal cord support the elongation of intraspinal axons (107–109). The axons of DRG neurons and those that originate from neurons whose perikarya are located close to the site of insertion appear favored to grow. The axons of supraspinal neurons that have been injured farther from their perikarya are less likely to project into the grafts (108). CNS axons can grow within the peripheral nerve graft for distances that exceed their normal length, and retinal axons establish synapses on normal target neurons that retain the normal morphological features and activate the target neurons (reviewed in 110). After leaving the peripheral nerve graft, however, the CNS axons show very limited growth within the host parenchyma and terminate within 1–2 mm of the end of the graft (111). Peripheral nerve grafts have contributed a great deal to our understanding of the importance of the neuron's environment for regeneration, but their contribution to functional recovery after spinal cord injury has received little attention.

Eighty to 90% of embryonic spinal cord transplants now survive in the acutely injured spinal cord of adult and newborn rats (112,113) and in the chronically injured spinal cord of adult rats (114). Transplants also survive in the completely severed spinal cord (115,116). Although they lack the characteristic butterfly shape of normal spinal cord gray matter, several morphological features of these transplants encourage the expectation that transplants can contribute to the reconstruction of interrupted neuronal circuits and replace damaged populations of spinal cord neurons. For example, areas develop within transplants that resemble substantia gelatinosa (117), supporting the hypothesis that transplants might function as relays. The astrocytic reaction that develops between transplant and host is interrupted by regions in which the tissues are apposed and processes pass from one to the other (113). Transplants may also reduce the extent of the astrocytic scarring that follows spinal cord injury (114,118), which is thought to represent an obstacle to regeneration.

The connectivity between transplants and adult hosts has been studied by tract tracing and immunocytochemical techniques, and electrophysiological methods are beginning to be employed. Fetal spinal cord neurons transplanted into adult spinal cord form an extensive network of connections with one another; however, few donor neurons extend processes into host spinal cord, and most of these terminate near the interface between transplant and host (119). The number of host spinal neurons that extend processes into transplants is also limited, and the perikarya of most of these are located within 0.5 mm of the interface (119). Only a few corticospinal (120,121) or serotonergic brainstem (113) axons are found within transplants placed into aspiration cavities made in adult spinal cord, and these axons also penetrate only a short distance into the transplants. In adult hosts, therefore, it seems unlikely that transplants can function as conduits that will allow regenerating axons to traverse a region of injury. When transplants are placed into excitotoxic rather than aspiration lesions where cells are killed but axons spared and the observed growth represents axonal sprouting rather than regeneration, central monoaminergic axons grow more robustly than corticospinal or rubrospinal axons (122).

The possibility that embryonic spinal cord transplants might function as the site of relays between sets of injured adult axons has been tested by studying the ability of cut dorsal roots to regenerate into transplants (123). The cut central processes of DRG neurons cannot regenerate into adult spinal cord in the absence of a transplant, but, when provided with a transplant, at least the subset of dorsal roots that contains CGRP grows in sufficient numbers to allow features of their growth to be analyzed quantitatively (123–126). The terminals of regenerated CGRP-containing dorsal roots form synapses with transplant neurons; as in lamina I of normal dorsal horn, most of these are axodendritic and simple and complex synaptic contacts are present in proportions similar to normal (125). Differences between the synapses formed in transplants and normal lamina I are also found. For example, regenerated CGRP-containing axons are significantly more likely to form axoaxonic synapses than normal. Nevertheless, the presence within transplants of regenerated primary afferent synapses with normal features supports the notion that transplants can support or encourage the formation of relays across regions of damaged spinal cord. Our observation that the axons of donor neurons grow into host sciatic nerve at least raises the possibility that transplants can contribute to reestablishing a damaged segmental reflex arc (123).

The possibility that fetal spinal cord transplants might rescue axotomized neurons that would otherwise die was first confirmed in newborn rats (127). Rubrospinal neurons were permanently rescued by transplants of embryonic spinal cord, a normal target of rubrospinal axons, but not by hippocampus, suggesting that survival after injury depended on target-specific factors. We have subsequently found that the neurons of Clarke's nucleus are rescued in newborn rats not only by fetal transplants of their normal targets, cerebellum and spinal cord, but also by transplants of embryonic neocortex (128). The axons of Clarke's nucleus neurons do not normally encounter neocortex, which is therefore an inappropriate target for these neurons. This result suggests that the neurons of Clarke's nucleus can be rescued by several different factors or by a single factor that is produced in several regions of the embryonic CNS. This factor has not yet been identified. It appears not to be produced ubiquitously in the fetal CNS, however, because axotomized Clarke's nucleus neurons die in spite of the presence of embryonic striatum transplants (129). Embryonic CNS transplants also rescue Clarke's nucleus neurons after axotomy in adult rats (128), suggesting that transplants can contribute to recovery in adult as well as in newborns.

When placed into the spinal cord of newborn rats, embryonic spinal cord transplants function as conduits that stimulate or allow the axons of supraspinal neurons to grow across the site of injury. The axons of corticospinal neurons (121) and of serotonergic (130) and other brainstem neurons (131) traverse transplants placed in the injured thoracic spinal cord of newborn rats and extend into their normal regions of termination as far caudal as the lower lumbar segments of host spinal cord. In part the greater growth of newborn axons is due to the continued elongation of developing axons that have not reached thoracic levels at the time of transplantation and therefore have not been axotomized. At least some of those axons that reach the lumbar segments, however, were interrupted by the spinal cord lesion and then regenerated (131).

The idea has been tested that the axons that have traversed the site of spinal cord injury and transplantation alter the development or recovery of locomotor function (132). Newborn rats that received subtotal thoracic spinal cord injuries and transplants of embryonic spinal cord were examined with a battery of tests and compared to rats that received lesions but no transplant. Rats with transplants performed better than rats with thoracic spinal cord lesions alone. For example, when examined 8–12 weeks postoperatively, rats with transplants crossed a mesh runway more quickly and made fewer errors in foot placement than the group with lesion only. They also recovered more quickly from their errors. The results of this study therefore support the notion that axons that traverse the transplant and grow into caudal host spinal cord are responsible for the improved performance. Because the spinal cord lesion was incomplete, however, other mechanisms for the improved performance are possible. One possibility is that the transplants have changed the response to injury of the residual host spinal cord adjacent to the transplant and allowed axons of supraspinal neurons to grow through host spinal cord rather than through the transplant. The axons of corticospinal neurons are known to grow through regions of newborn spinal cord adjacent to injury (133), and transplants of DRG neurons and Schwann cells have been shown to enhance this response (134). Therefore, supraspinal axons that have traversed host spinal cord rather than the transplant may account for the improved locomotor function or may have contributed to the improved performance.

Locomotor function is also being evaluated by Howland in newborn cats that received a transplant into the site of a complete spinal cord transection. These experiments complement those in rat because the spinal cord lesion is complete rather than subtotal, locomotor function can be analyzed in greater detail in the cat than in rat, and because the anatomical pathways that account for various types of locomotor performance are better defined in cat than in rat. Three types of locomotion, which are mediated by three different types of spinal systems, have been analyzed in the cat (reviewed in 30). Hindlimb motion on a moving treadmill (bipedal reflex locomotion) requires only that the spinal pattern generators for each hindlimb and the connections between them remain intact. Reflex locomotion on a treadmill that requires coordination between forelimbs and hindlimbs (quadrupedal reflex locomotion) depends on propriospinal connections between forelimb and hindlimb pattern generators in the cervical and lumbar spinal cord as well as on the pattern generators themselves. Conditioned (voluntary) overground locomotion for a food reward depends on intact pathways descending from brain as well as on intact segmental and intersegmental connections. In cats with thoracic spinal cord transections that have received a transplant on the day after birth, performance of quadrupedal reflex locomotion will, therefore, suggest that propriospinal connections have grown across the transplant either directly or via relays. In these animals, the presence of conditioned overground locomotion will suggest the growth of axons with perikarya in the brain.

The locomotor function of two cats that received transplants of E26 spinal cord into T12 transections on the day after birth has been examined for periods of 6 weeks and 5 months (115,135). These cats were compared to two cats with transections on the day after birth that did not receive transplants. Both groups developed quadrupedal locomotion in addition to bipedal locomotion, but the group with transplants achieved overground locomotion approximately 6 weeks earlier than the group with transection alone. The preliminary results also indicate that the performance of animals with transplants is far superior to those with transection alone in the ability of the animals to support their weight, to maintain postural stability, and to coordinate the movement of forelimbs and hindlimbs. Even in animals with transplants, however, the coordination is only sometimes similar to that of normal cats, and overground locomotion is abnormal. The postural stability of the hindlimbs, for example, is impaired, the step cycle is prolonged, and the normal 1:1 pairing of forelimb and hindlimb step cycles is inconsistent. In both cats that received transplants and were studied behaviorally, histological evaluation revealed transplants to be present.

Preliminary studies are also being carried

out to identify the anatomical connections in these cats (135). One animal that received a transplant of E21 spinal cord has so far been studied. Descending serotonergic and noradrenergic axons whose cell bodies are in the brainstem grow extensively in this transplant and enter host spinal cord caudal to the transplant. Serotonergic axons grow as far caudally as the host L6 segment. Regenerated CGRP-immunoreactive host dorsal roots and substance P-containing processes that arise from multiple sources are also found throughout the transplants, where they are accumulated in some areas that resemble the substantia gelatinosa and superficial dorsal horn of normal spinal cord. These preliminary results indicate that transplants enhance the development of locomotor function in newborn cats with complete spinal cord transections and suggest that this effect is mediated by descending axons that grow into the transplants. Whether these axons alone account for the enhanced locomotor function remains to be determined.

SUMMARY

Plasticity of undamaged projections in the adult mammalian spinal cord has been documented many times and by a number of different methods, including degeneration techniques, tract tracing, immunocytochemistry, and quantitative electron microscopy.

Sprouting in the adult appears to be spatially limited and regulated rather than random. When damage is made in the neonate, the amount of sprouting or the distance over which sprouting takes place is usually, but not always, greater than in the adult. In some paradigms, the sprouting has been associated with recovery of motor behavior, and specific systems that sprout can be related to recovery of specific functions. This normally occurring plasticity may be enhanced by the use of embyronic CNS or peripheral nerve transplants; furthermore, transplants can encourage axonal growth. For example, cut dorsal root fibers will grow into a spinal cord transplant and make connections that appear morphologically similar to normal. Descending projections can also grow into the transplant and, in the neonate, these axons grow not only into the transplants but also extend caudal to the transplants and into the host spinal cord. These animals display greater and qualitatively different recovery of function than those with lesions but not transplants. At the present time, the mechanisms underlying transplant-mediated recovery are unclear. For example, we do not know whether transplanted tissue acts as a bridge or as a relay in order to mediate recovery. The anatomical and functional analyses that have been carried out in sprouting systems have not yet been applied to transplants. Such studies will undoubtedly contribute to our understanding of the mechanisms by which transplants can contribute to enhanced recovery of function after spinal injury.

ACKNOWLEDGMENTS

This work was supported by NS24707-05 (M.G., M.M., A.T.), ARMY DAMD17-87-C-7117 (A.T.), and the Research Service of the Veteran's Administration.

We are happy to acknowledge the comments and contributions of Sid Croul, Tim Himes, Dena Howland, Fatiha Nothias, and Bin Zhang.

REFERENCES

1. Sherrington CS. Experiments in the examination of the peripheral distribution of the fibers of the posterior roots of some spinal nerves. *Philos Trans R Soc Lond [Biol]* 1898; 190B: 45–186.
2. Chambers WE, Liu CN, McCouch GP, D'Aquili E. Descending tracts and spinal shock in the cat. *Brain* 1966; 89: 337–390.
3. Forssberg H, Grillner S, Halbertsma J. The locomotion of the low spinal cat. I. Coordination

within a hindlimb. *Acta Physiol Scand* 1980; 108: 269–281.
4. Forssberg H, Grillner S, Halbertsma J. The locomotion of the low spinal cat. II. Interlimb coordination. *Acta Physiol Scand* 1980; 108: 281.
5. Goldberger ME, Murray M. Patterns of sprouting and implications for recovery of function. In: Waxman SG, ed. *Physiologic basis for functional recovery in neurological disorder.* New York: Raven Press; 1988: 361–385.
6. Hallas BH, Renehan WE, Klein BG, Jacquin MF. Absence of intramedullary sprouting in trigeminal primary afferent axons caudal and rostral to a partial medullary hemisection. In: Pubols LM, Sessle BJ, eds. *Effects of injury on trigeminal and spinal somatosensory systems.* New York: Alan R. Liss, Inc.; 1987: 205–214.
7. Goldberger ME, Murray M. Recovery of movement and axonal sprouting may obey some of the same laws. In: Cotman C, ed. *Neuronal plasticity.* New York: Raven Press; 1978: 73–96.
8. Goldberger ME, Murray M. Lack of sprouting and its presence after lesion of the cat spinal cord. *Brain Res* 1982; 241: 227–239.
9. Battisti WP, Artymyshyn R, Murray M. β1 and β2 adrenergic ^{125}I-pindolol binding sites in the interpeduncular nucleus of the rat. *J Neurosci* 1989; 9: 2509–2518.
10. Beattie MS, Breshnahan JC, Leedy MG. Synaptic plasticity in the adult sacral spinal cord. In: Horracks LA, ed. *Trophic factors and the nervous system.* New York: Raven Press; 1990: 263–276.
11. Wang SD, Goldberger ME, Murray M. Plasticity of spinal systems after unilateral lumbosacral dorsal rhizotomy in the adult rat. *J Comp Neurol* 1991; 304: 555–568.
12. Schneider GE. Early lesions of superior colliculus factors affecting the formation of abnormal retinal projections. *Brain Behav Evol* 1973; 8: 73–109.
13. Liu CN, Chambers WW. Intraspinal sprouting of dorsal root axons. *Arch Neurol Psychiatry* 1958; 79: 46–61.
14. Murray M, Wu LF, Goldberger ME. Spared root deafferentation of cat spinal cord. In: Pubols LM, Sessle BJ, eds. *Effects of injury on trigeminal and spinal somatosensory systems.* New York: Alan R. Liss, Inc.; 1987: 261–271.
15. McNeill DL, Hulsebosch CE. Intraspinal sprouting of rat primary afferents after deafferentation. *Neurosci Lett* 1987; 81: 57–62.
16. McNeill DL, Carlton SM, Coggeshall RE, Hulsebosch CE. Denervation-induced intraspinal synaptogenesis of calcitonin gene-related peptide containing primary afferent terminals. *J Comp Neurol* 1990; 296: 263–268.
17. Rodin BE, Sampogna SL, Kruger L. An examination of intraspinal sprouting in dorsal root axons with the tracer horseradish peroxidase. *J Comp Neurol.* 1983; 215: 187–198.
18. Rodin BE, Kruger L. Absence of evidence for intraspinal sprouting in dorsal root axons caudal to a partial spinal hemisection. *Somatosens Res* 1984; 2: 171–192.
19. Micevych PE, Stroink A, Yaksh T, Go VLW. Immunochemical studies of substance P and cholecystokinin octapeptide recovery in dorsal horn following unilateral lumbosacral ganglionectomy. *Somatosens Res* 1986; 3: 239–260.
20. Himes BT, Tessler A. Death of some dorsal root ganglion neurons and plasticity of others following sciatic nerve section in adult and neonatal rats. *J Comp Neurol* 1989; 284: 215–230.
21. Polistina DC, Murray M, Goldberger ME. Plasticity of dorsal root and descending serotoninergic projections after partial deafferentation of the adult rat spinal cord. *J Comp Neurol* 1990; 299: 349–363.
22. Ygge J, Aldskogius H, Grant G. Asymmetries and symmetries in the number of thoracic dorsal root ganglion cells. *J Comp Neurol* 1981; 202: 365–372.
23. Molander C. *On the organization of spinal cord projections from hindlimb sensory nerves.* GOTAB Stockholm: ISBN.
24. Pubols LM, Bowen D. Lack of central sprouting of primary afferent fibers after ricin deafferentation. *J Comp Neurol* 1988; 275: 282–287.
25. Murray M, Goldberger ME. Replacement of synaptic terminals in lamina II and Clarke's nucleus after unilateral dorsal rhizotomy in adult cats. *J Neurosci* 1986; 6: 3205–3218.
26. LaMotte C, Kapadia SE, Kocol CM. Deafferentation-induced expansion of saphenous terminal field labelling in the adult rat dorsal horn following pronase injection of the sciatic nerve. *J Comp Neurol* 1989; 288: 311–325.
27. Swett JE, Woolf CJ. Somatotopic organization of primary afferent terminals in the superficial dorsal horn of the rat spinal cord. *J Comp Neurol* 1985; 231: 66–71.
28. Molander CE, Grant G. Laminar distribution and somatotopic organization of primary afferent fibers from hindlimb nerves to the dorsal horn. *Neuroscience* 1986; 19: 287–312.
29. Murray M, Goldberger ME. Restitution of function and collateral sprouting in cat spinal cord: the partially hemisected animal. *J Comp Neurol* 1974; 158: 19–36.
29a. Shortland P, Woolf CJ, Fitzgerald M. Morphology and somatotopic organization of the central terminals of hindlimb hair follicle afferents in the rat lumbar spinal cord. *J Comp Neurol* 1989; 289: 416–433.
30. Goldberger ME. The use of behavioral methods to predict spinal cord plasticity. *Rest Neurol Neurosci* 1991; 2: 339–350.
31. Bullitt E, Stofer WD, Vierck CJ, and Perl ER. Reorganization of primary afferent nerve terminals in the spinal dorsal horn of the primate caudal to anterolateral chordotomy. *J Comp Neurol* 1988; 270: 549–558.
31a. Stelzner DJ, Weber ED, Prendergast J. A comparison of the effects of mid-thoracic hemisection in the neonatal or weanling rat on the distribution and density of dorsal root axons in the

lumbosacral spinal cord of the adult. *Brain Res* 1979; 172: 407–426.
32. Arvidsson J, Ygge J, Grant G. Cell loss in the lumbar dorsal root ganglion and transganglionic degeneration after sciatic nerve resection in the rat. *Brain Res* 1986; 373: 15–21.
33. Knyihar-Csillik E, Torok A, Csillik B. Primary afferent origin of substance P-containing axons in the superficial dorsal horn of the rat spinal cord: depletion, regeneration and replenishment of presumed nociceptive central terminals. *J Comp Neurol* 1990; 297: 594–612.
34. Barbut D, Polak JM, Wall PD. Substance P in the spinal cord dorsal horn decreases following peripheral nerve injury. *Brain Res* 1981; 205: 289–298.
35. Jessell T, Tsunoo A, Kanazawa I, Otsuka M. Substance P depletion in the dorsal horn of rat spinal cord after section of the peripheral processes of primary sensory neurons. *Brain Res* 1979; 168: 249–259.
36. Kar S, Gibson SJ, Scaravilli F, Jacobs JM, Aber VR, Pola JM. Reduced numbers of calcitonin gene-related peptide- (CGRP-) and tachykinin-immunoreactive sensory neurones associated with greater enkephalin immunoreactivity in the dorsal horn of a mutant rat with hereditary sensory neuropathy. *Cell Tissue Res* 1989; 225: 451–466.
37. McGregor GP, Gibson SJ, Sabatge IM, Blank MA, Cristofides ND, Wall PD, Polak JM, Bloom SR. Effect of peripheral nerve section and nerve crush on spinal cord neuropeptides in the rat; increased VIP and PHI in the dorsal horn. *Neuroscience* 1984; 13: 207–216.
38. Shehab SAS, Atkinson M. Vasoactive intestinal polypeptide increases in areas of the dorsal horn of the spinal cord from which other neuropeptides are depleted following peripheral axotomy. *Exp Brain Res* 1986; 62: 422–430.
39. Woolf CJ, Reynolds ML, Molander C, O'Brien C, Lindsay RM, Benowitz LI. The growth-associated protein GAP-43 appears in dorsal root ganglion cells and in the dorsal horn of the rat spinal cord following peripheral nerve injury. *Neuroscience* 1990; 34: 465–478.
40. Wong J, Oblinger M. A comparison between peripheral and central axotomy effects on neurofilament and tubulin gene expression of rat DRG neurons. *J Neurosci* 1990; 10: 2215–2222.
41. Knyihar-Csillik E, Kreutzberg GW, Csillik B. Enzyme translocation in the course of regeneration of central primary afferent terminals in the substantia gelatinosa of the adult rodent spinal cord. *J Neurosci Res* 1989; 22: 74–82.
42. Molander C, Kinnman E, Aldskogius H. Expansion of spinal cord primary sensory afferent projection following combined sciatic nerve resection and saphenous nerve crush: a horseradish peroxidase study in the adult rat. *J Comp Neurol* 1988; 276: 436–441.
43. Richardson PM, Issa VMK. Peripheral injury enhances central regeneration of primary sensory neurones. *Nature* 1984; 309: 781–793.
44. McMahon SB, Kett-White R. Sprouting of peripherally regenerating primary sensory neurones in the adult central nervous system. *J Comp Neurol* 1991; 304: 307–315.
45. Devor M, Wall PD. Plasticity in the spinal cord sensory map following peripheral nerve injury in rats. *J Neurosci* 1981; 7: 679–684.
46. DiGiulio AM, Tenconi B, Mannavola A, Mantegazza P, Schiavinato A, Gorio A. Spinal cord interneuron degenerative atrophy caused by peripheral nerve lesions is prevented by serotonin depletion. *J Neurosci Res* 1987; 18: 443–448.
47. Merzenich MM, Nelson RJ, Stryker MP, Cynader MS, Schoppmann A, Zook JM. Somatosensory cortical map changes following digit amputation in adult monkeys. *J Comp Neurol* 1984; 224: 591–605.
48. Wall JT, Kaas JH, Sur M, Nelson RJ, Felleman DJ, Merzenich MM. Functional reorganization in somatosensory cortical areas 3b and 1 of adult monkeys after median nerve repair: possible relationships to sensory recovery in humans. *J Neurosci* 1986; 6: 218–233.
49. Pons TP, Garraghty PE, Ommaya AK, Kaas JH, Taub E, Mishkin M. Massive cortical reorganization after sensory deafferentation in adult macques. *Science* 1991; 252: 1857–1860.
50. Tessler A, Glazer E, Artymyshyn R, Murray M, Goldberger ME. Recovery of substance P in the cat spinal cord after unilateral lumbosacral deafferentation of cat spinal cord. *Brain Res* 1980; 191: 459–470.
51. Tessler A, Himes BT, Artymyshyn R, Murray M, Goldberger ME. Spinal neurons mediate return of substance P following deafferentation of cat spinal cord. *Brain Res* 1981; 230: 263–281.
52. Tessler A, Himes BT, Soper K, Murray M, Goldberger ME, Reichlin S. Recovery of substance P but not somatostatin in the cat spinal cord after unilateral lumbosacral dorsal rhizotomy: a quantitative study. *Brain Res* 1984; 305: 95–102.
53. Chung K, McNeill DL, Hulsebosch CE, Coggeshall RE. Changes in dorsal horn synaptic disc numbers following unilateral dorsal rhizotomy. *J Comp Neurol* 1989; 283: 568–577.
54. Aoki M, Fujito Y, Satomi H, Kurosawa Y, Kasaba T. The possible role of collateral sprouting in the functional restitution of corticospinal connections after spinal hemisection. *Neurosci Res* 1986; 3: 617–627.
55. Nagy JI, Hunt SP. The termination of primary afferents within the rat dorsal horn: evidence for rearrangement following capsaicin treatment. *J Comp Neurol* 1983; 218: 145–158.
56. Rethelyi M, Salim MZ, Jancso G. Altered distribution of dorsal root fibers in the rat following neonatal capsaicin treatment. *Neuroscience* 1986; 18: 749–761.
57. Hulsebosch CE, Perez-Polo JR, Coggeshall RE. In vivo anti-NGF induces sprouting of sensory axons in dorsal roots. *J Comp Neurol* 1987; 259: 445–451.

58. Hulsebosch CE, Coggeshall RE. Intraspinal sprouting after administration of nerve growth factor antibodies to neonatal rats. *Brain Res* 1988; 461: 322–327.
59. Yip HK, Rich KM, Lampe PA, Johnson EM. The effects of nerve growth factor and its antiserum on the postnatal development and survival after injury of sensory neurons in rat dorsal root ganglia. *J Neurosci* 1984; 4: 2986–2992.
60. Fitzgerald M, Vrbova G. Plasticity of acid phosphatase (FRAP) afferent terminal fields and of dorsal horn cell growth in the neonatal rat. *J Comp Neurol* 1985; 240: 414–422.
61. Fitzgerald M. The sprouting of saphenous nerve terminals in the spinal cord following early postnatal sciatic nerve section in the rat. *J Comp Neurol* 1985; 240: 407–413.
62. Fitzgerald M, Woolf CJ, Shortland P. Collateral sprouting of the central terminals of cutaneous primary afferent neurons in the rat spinal cord: pattern, morphology, and influence of targets. *J Comp Neurol* 1990; 300: 370–385.
63. Wang SD, Goldberger ME, Murray M. Normal development and the effects of early rhizotomy of spinal systems in the rat. *Dev Brain Res* 1991; 64:57–69.
64. Marlier L, Rajaofetra N, Poulat P, Privat A. Modification of serotonergic innervation of the rat spinal cord dorsal horn after neonatal capsaicin treatment. *J Neurosci Res* 1990; 25: 112–118.
65. Kuang RZ, Kalil K. Specificity of corticospinal axon arbors sprouting into denervated contralateral spinal cord. *J Comp Neurol* 1990; 302: 461–472.
66. Gomez-Pinilla F, Villablanca JR, Sonnier BJ, Levine MS. Reorganization of pericruciate cortical projections to the spinal cord and dorsal column nuclei after neonatal or adult cerebral hemispherectomy in cats. *Brain Res* 1986; 385: 343–355.
67. Hultborn H, Malmsten J. Changes in segmental reflexes following chronic spinal cord hemisection in the cat. I. Increased monosynaptic and polysynaptic ventral root discharges. *Acta Physiol Scand* 1983a; 119: 405–422.
68. Hultborn H, Malmsten J. Changes in segmental reflexes following chronic spinal cord hemisection in the cat. II. Conditioned monosynaptic test reflexes. *Acta Physiol Scand* 1983b; 119: 423–433.
69. Brenowitz GL, Pubols LM. Increased response to sural nerve input in the dorsal horn following chronic spinal cord hemisection. *Brain Res* 1981; 208: 421–425.
70. Brenowitz GL, Pubols LM. Increased receptive field size of dorsal horn neurons following chronic spinal cord hemisection in cats. *Brain Res* 1981; 216: 45–59.
71. Pubols LM, Hirata H, Brown PB. Temporally dependent changes in response properties of dorsal horn neurons after dorsolateral funiculus lesions. *J Neurophysiol* 1988; 60: 1253–1267.
72. Pubols LM. Characteristics of dorsal horn neurons expressing subliminal responses to sural nerve stimulation. *Somatosens Res* 1990; 7: 137–151.
73. Goldberger ME. Spared root deafferentation of a cat's hindlimb: hierarchical regulation of pathways mediating recovery of motor behavior. *Exp Brain Res* 1988; 73: 329–342.
74. Pubols LM, Goldberger ME. Recovery of function in dorsal horn following partial deafferentation. *J Neurophysiol* 1980; 43: 102–117.
75. Mendell LM, Sedivec MJ, Traub RJ. Response of an identified population of spinal cord neurons to partial deafferentation. In: Goldberger ME, Gorio A, Murray M, eds. *Development and plasticity of the mammalian spinal cord*, New York: Liviana Press and Springer-Verlag; 1986: 111–121.
76. Goldberger ME. Partial and complete deafferentation of cat hindlimb: the contribution of behavioral substitution to recovery of motor function. *Exp Brain Res* 1988b; 73: 343–353.
77. Mantyh PW, Hunt SP. The autoradiographic localization of SP receptors in rat and bovine spinal cord and the effects of neonatal capsaicin. *Brain Res* 1985; 332: 315–324.
78. Massari VJ, Shults CW, Park CW, Tizabi Y, Moody TW, Chronwall BM, Culber M, Chase TN. Deafferentation causes a loss of presynaptic bombesin receptors and supersensitivity of SP receptors in dorsal horn of cat. *Brain Res* 1985; 343: 268–274.
79. Helke CJ, Charlton G, Wiley RG. Studies on the cellular localization of spinal cord SP receptors. *J Neurosci* 1986; 19: 523–533.
80. Daval G, Verge D, Bashaum AI, Bourjour S, Hamon M. Autoradiographic evidence of 5HT-1 binding sites on primary afferent fibers in the dorsal horn of the rat spinal cord. *Neurosci Lett* 1987; 83: 71–76.
81. Desmond NL, Levy WB. Anatomy of associative long-term synaptic modification. In: Landfield PW, Deadwyler SA, eds. *Long-term potentiation. from biophysics to behavior.* New York: Alan R. Liss, Inc.; 1987: 265–305.
82. Constantine-Paton M, Cline HT, Debski E. Patterned activity, synaptic convergence and the NMDA receptor in developing visual pathways. *Annu Rev Neurosci* 1990; 13: 129–154.
83. Monaghan DT, Cotman CW. Distribution of n-methyl-d-aspartate sensitive l-3H glutamate binding sites in rat brain. *J Neurosci* 1985; 5: 2009–2919.
84. Ulas J, Monaghan DT, Cotman CW. Plastic response of hippocampal excitatory amino acid receptors to deafferentation and reinnervation. *Neuroscience* 1990; 34: 9–17.
85. Harris CH, Fagan EL, Shew RL, Kammerlocher TC, McNeill DL. MK-801 induced sprouting by CGRP immunoreactive primary afferent fibers in the dorsal spinal cord of the rat. *Neurosci Lett* 1990; 115: 24–28.
86. Diamond J, Coughlin M, Macintyre L, Holmes

M, Bisheau B. Evidence that endogenous β nerve growth factor is responsible for the collateral sprouting, but not the regeneration, of nociceptive axons in adult rats. *Proc Natl Acad Sci USA* 1987; 84: 6596–6600.
87. Murray M. In situ hybridization as a means of studying the role of growth factors, oncogenes and proto-oncogenes in the nervous system. In: Chesselet M-F, ed. *In situ hybridization histochemistry*. CRC Press; A. 1990: 111–140.
88. Levi-Montalcini R. Developmental neurobiology and the natural history of nerve growth factor. *Annu Rev Neurosci* 1982; 5: 341–362.
89. Caroni P, Grandes P. Nerve sprouting in innervated adult skeletal muscle induced by exposure to elevated levels of insulin-like growth factors. *J Cell Biol* 1990; 110: 1307–1317.
90. Helper JE, Lund PK. Molecular biology of the insulin-like growth factors. In: Bazan N, ed. *Molecular neurobiology* vol 4. New York: The Humana Press; 1990: 93–127.
91. Fitzgerald M, Wall PD, Goedert M, Emson PC. Nerve growth factor counteracts the neurophysiological and neurochemical effects of chronic sciatic nerve section. *Brain Res* 1985; 332: 1313–1341.
92. Wong J, Oblinger M. NGF rescues substance P expression but not neurofilament or tubulin gene expression in axotomized sensory neurons. *J Neurosci* 1991; 11: 543–552.
93. Björklund A, Stenevi U, Dunnett SB. Transplantation of brainstem monoaminergic "command" systems: models for functional reactivation of damaged CNS circuitries. In: Kao CC, Bunge RP, Reier PJ, eds. *Spinal cord reconstruction*. New York: Raven Press; 1983: 397–413.
94. Nornes H, Björklund A, Stenevi U. Transplant strategies in spinal cord regeneration. In: Sladek JR, Gash DM, eds. *Neural transplants: development and function*. New York: Plenum Press; 1984: 407–421.
95. Forssberg H, Grillner S. The locomotion of the acute spinal cat injected with clonidine i.v. *Brain Res* 1973; 50: 184–186.
96. Mas M, Zahradnik MA, Martino V, Davidson JM. Stimulation of spinal serotonergic receptors facilitates seminal emission and suppresses penile erectile reflexes. *Brain Res* 1985; 342: 128–134.
97. Nygren L-G, Olson L, Seiger A. Monoaminergic reinnervation of the transected spinal cord by homologous fetal brain grafts. *Brain Res* 1977; 29: 227–235.
98. Björklund A, Nornes H, Gage FH. Cell suspension grafts of noradrenergic locus coeruleus neurons in rat hippocampus and spinal cord: reinnervation and transmitter turnover. *Neuroscience* 1986; 18: 685–698.
99. Commissiong JW. Fetal locus coeruleus transplanted into the transected spinal cord of the adult rat. *Brain Res* 1984; 271: 174–179.
100. Commissiong JW. Fetal locus coeruleus transplanted into the transected spinal cord of the adult rat: some observations and implications. *Neuroscience* 1984; 12: 839–853.
101. Nornes H, Björklund A, Stenevi U. Reinnervation of the denervated adult spinal cord of rats by intraspinal transplants of embryonic brain stem neurons. *Cell Tissue Res* 1983; 230: 15–35.
102. Privat A, Mansour H, Rajaofetra N, Geffard M. Intraspinal transplants of serotonergic neurons in the adult rat. *Brain Res Bull* 1989; 22: 123–129.
103. Privat A, Mansour H, Geffard M. Transplantation of fetal serotonin neurons into the transected spinal cord of adult rats: morphological development and functional influence. In: Gash DM, Sladek JR, Jr., eds. *Progress in Brain Research* 1988; 78: 155–166.
104. Buchanan JT, Nornes HO. Transplants of embryonic brainstem containing the locus coeruleus into spinal cord enhance the hindlimb flexion reflex in adult rats. *Brain Res* 1986; 381: 225–236.
105. Yakovleff A, Roby-Brami A, Guezard B, Mansour H, Bussel B, and Privat A. Locomotion in rats transplanted with noradrenergic neurons. *Brain Res Bull* 1989; 22: 115–121.
106. Villegas-Perez MP, Vidal-Sanz M, Bray GM, Aguayo AJ. Influences of peripheral nerve grafts on the survival and regrowth of axotomized retinal ganglion cells in adult rats. *J Neurosci* 1988; 8: 265–280.
107. Richardson PM, McGuinness UM, Aguayo A. Axons from CNS neurones regenerate into PNS grafts. *Nature* 1980; 284: 264–265.
108. Richardson PM, Issa VMK, Aguayo AJ. Regeneration of long spinal axons in the rat. *J Neurocytol* 13: 165–182.
109. Houle JD. Demonstration of the potential for chronically injured neurons to regenerate axons into intraspinal peripheral nerve grafts. *Exp Neurol* 1991; 113: 1–9.
110. Aguayo AJ, Bray GM, Rasminsky M, Zwimpfer T, Carter D, Vidal-Sanz M. Synaptic connections made by axons regenerating in the central nervous system of adult mammals. *J Exp Biol* 1990; 153: 199–224.
111. Aguayo AJ. Axonal regeneration from injured neurons in the adult mammalian central nervous system. In: Cotman CW, ed. *Synaptic plasticity*. New York: Guilford Press; 1985: 457–484.
112. Bernstein JJ, Patel U, Kelemen M, Jefferson M, Turtil S. Ultrastructure of fetal spinal cord and cortex implants into adult rat spinal cord. *J Neurosci Res* 1984; 11: 359–372.
113. Reier PJ, Bregman BS, Wujek JR. Intraspinal transplantation of embryonic spinal cord tissue in neonatal and adult rats. *J Comp Neurol* 1986; 247: 275–296.
114. Houle JD, Reier PJ. Transplantation of fetal spinal cord tissue into the chronically injured adult rat spinal cord. *J Comp Neurol* 1988; 269: 535–547.
115. Howland DR, Bregman BS, Tessler A, Gold-

berger ME. Transplants alter the motor development of kittens after neonatal spinal cord transection. *Soc Neurosci Abstr* 1990; 16: 37.
116. Pallini R, Fernandez E, Gangitano C, Del Fa A, Olivieri-Sangiacomo C, Sbriccoli A. Studies on embryonic transplants to the transected spinal cord of adult rats. *J Neurosurg* 1989; 70: 454–462.
117. Jakeman LB, Reier PJ, Bregman BS, Wade EB, Dailey M, Kastner RJ, Himes BT, Tessler A. Differentiation of substantia gelatinosa-like regions in intraspinal and intracerebral transplants of embryonic spinal cord tissue in the rat. *Exp Neurol* 1989; 103: 17–33.
118. Kao CC. Comparison of healing process in transected spinal cords grafted with autogenous brain tissue, sciatic nerve, and nodose ganglion. *Exp Neurol* 1974; 44: 424–439.
119. Jakeman LB, Reier PJ. Axonal projections between fetal spinal cord transplants and the adult spinal cord: a neuroanatomical tracing study of local interactions. *J Comp Neurol* 1991; 307: 311–334.
120. Jakeman LB, Reier, PJ. Regeneration of sprouting of corticospinal tract axons into fetal spinal cord transplants in the adult rat. *Soc Neurosci Abstr* 1989; 15: 1242.
121. Bregman BS, Kunkel-Bagden E, McAtee M, O'Neill A. Extension of the critical period for developmental plasticity of the corticospinal pathway. *J Comp Neurol* 1989; 282: 355–370.
122. Nothias F, Peschanski M. Homotypic fetal transplants into an experimental model of spinal cord neurodegeneration. *J Comp Neurol* 1990; 301: 520–534.
123. Tessler A, Himes BT, Houle J, Reier PJ. Regeneration of adult dorsal root ganglion axons into transplants of embryonic spinal cord. *J Comp Neurol* 1988; 270: 537–548.
124. Houle JD, Reier PJ. Regrowth of calcitonin gene-related peptide (CGRP) immunoreactive axons from the chronically injured rat spinal cord into fetal spinal cord tissue in the rat. *Neurosci Lett* 1989; 103: 17–23.
125. Itoh Y, Tessler A. Ultrastructural organization of adult dorsal root ganglion neurons regenerated into transplants of fetal spinal cord. *J Comp Neurol* 1990; 292: 396–411.
126. Itoh Y, Tessler A. Regeneration of adult dorsal root axons into transplants of fetal spinal cord and brain: a comparison of growth and synapse formation in appropriate and inappropriate targets. *J Comp Neurol* 1990; 302: 272–293.
127. Bregman BS, Reier PJ. Neural tissue transplants rescue axotomized rubrospinal cells from retrograde death. *J Comp Neurol* 1986; 244: 86–95.
128. Himes BT, Goldberger ME, Tessler A. Grafts of fetal CNS tissue rescue axotomized Clarke's nucleus neurons in adult and neonatal operates. *Soc Neurosci Abstr* 1990; 16: 818.
129. Himes BT, Baker P, Goldberger ME, Tessler A. Not all CNS transplants can rescue axotomized Clarke's nucleus neurons. *Soc Neurosci Abstr* 1991; 17:1499.
130. Bregman BS. Spinal cord transplants permit the growth of serotonergic axons across the site of neonatal spinal cord transection. *Dev Brain Res* 1987; 34: 265–279.
131. Bregman BS, Bernstein-Goral H. Both regenerating and late developing pathways contribute to transplant-induced anatomical plasticity after spinal cord lesions at birth. *Exp Neurol* 1991; 112: 49–63.
132. Kunkel-Bagden E, Bregman BS. Spinal cord transplants enhance the recovery of locomotor function after spinal cord injury at birth. *Exp Brain Res* 1990; 81: 25–34.
133. Bregman BS, Goldberger ME. Infant lesion effect. II. Anatomical correlates of sparing and recovery of function after spinal cord damage in newborn and adult cats. *Dev Brain Res* 1983; 9: 137–154.
134. Kuhlengel KR, Bunge MB, Bunge RP, Burton H. Implant of cultured sensory neurons and Schwann cells into lesioned neonatal rat spinal cord. II. Implant characteristics and examination of corticospinal tract growth. *J Comp Neurol* 1989; 293: 74–91.
135. Howland DR, Bregman BS, Tessler A, Goldberger ME. Anatomical and behavioral effects of transplants in spinal kittens. *Soc Neurosci Abstr* 1991; 17:236.

13

Neurotrophic Factors and CNS Regeneration

Theo Hagg, Jean-Claude Louis, and Silvio Varon

Department of Biology, 0601, University of California, San Diego, La Jolla, California 92093

It has long been recognized that regeneration in the adult mammalian CNS may be restricted by properties of the CNS tissue environment. This concept, first postulated around the turn of the century by Cajal and Tello (1,2) and later expanded by others (3), was mainly supported by the findings that CNS axons can regrow over long distances into peripheral nerve grafts. Over the past decade, the molecular basis for the difference between CNS and PNS with regard to regeneration has been further investigated. It has become clear that one of the mechanisms contributing to successful regeneration into the PNS environment may be the availability of "neuronotrophic" or "neurotrophic" factors (NTFs).

From experiments initiated in the 1940s by Hamburger, NTFs were recognized as target-derived proteins essential for the development, maintenance, growth and functional performances of selected populations of neurons (4–8). During development, a large proportion of neurons die at the stage when their axons reach the innervation territory. The remaining neurons apparently survive this "developmental neuronal death" by acquiring NTFs from the postsynaptic elements and/or neighboring glial cells. The prototype and best-characterized NTF is nerve growth factor (NGF), a 26 kD dimer protein essential for the survival and function of developing peripheral sympathetic and dorsal root sensory ganglionic neurons (6). In fact, the very name "nerve growth factor" refers to its neurite-promoting effects both in vivo and on cultured peripheral ganglia, a method by which its biological activity was initially followed. During the last half of the 1980s NGF has been recognized as a putative NTF for certain adult CNS neurons as well, in particular the cholinergic ones of the basal forebrain (9,10), and from its investigation have emerged the relations between NTF and CNS regeneration. The importance of the concept that special proteins are in control of cellular development and function was acknowledged by the 1986 Nobel prize for Medicine to Levi-Montalcini and Cohen for their discovery and further investigation of NGF and epidermal growth factor (EGF). During the late 1980s a few more NTFs such as the NGF family members, brain derived neurotrophic factor (BDNF) and neurotrophin-3 (NT-3), and ciliary neurotrophic factor (CNTF) have been purified and their availability will allow their testing for in vivo regeneration-related activities.

In this chapter we shall review some of the advances made during the 1980s in the understanding of the role of NTFs in neurite outgrowth in vitro and for axonal regeneration in vivo. Discussion of the latter will focus on the effects of NGF on the cholinergic basal forebrain neurons of the adult rat, since most insights have been derived from such studies.

IN VITRO NEURITE-PROMOTING EFFECTS OF NTFs

The establishment of functional neuronal circuits in the brain is dependent on the specification of connections between neurons during various phases of their development. The specificity of these connections requires axonal elongation along defined routes and recognition of the appropriate partner cells to form synaptic contacts. Similarly, the success of axonal regeneration after injury is determined by the ability to extend axons and to reconnect to a proper target. The development of neurons depends on their dialogue with extracellular signaling molecules. These molecules belong to various classes of agents including trophic factors (e.g., NGF, BDNF, CNTF), growth factors (e.g., FGF, EGF, PDGF), cell-adhesion molecules (e.g., N-CAM, cadherins), and components of the extracellular matrix (e.g., fibronectin, laminin, collagens, thrombospondin, tenascin). Each class of molecule has been shown to influence major events in the development of the nervous system, including neuronal survival, migration, and differentiation, axonal extension and guidance, and formation of specific synaptic circuits. For a detailed account of the role of extracellular matrix and cell-adhesion molecules in neuronal development and axonal outgrowth, the reader is directed to recent reviews (11,12). In this section, we shall address the role of neurotrophic factors on neurite extension in vitro. Although stimulation of neuritic growth by the more recently identified NTFs, such as BDNF, NT-3, or CNTF, as well as by growth factors such as FGF, EGF, and insulin-like growth factors have been reported, this section will deal only with the neurite-promoting effects of NGF.

As indicated by its name, nerve growth factor was first recognized for its stimulation of the growth of neuronal fibers (neurites). Explant cultures of dorsal root ganglia (DRG) or sympathetic ganglia (SG) respond to NGF with a dose-dependent growth of neurites and, therefore, have been used in the early studies as a semiquantitative assay for NGF activities (reviewed in ref. 6). The effect of NGF was later also observed on dissociated neuronal cultures of chick SG and DRG. These cultures were used for quantitative determinations of NGF concentrations in terms of survival and neuritic outgrowth responses (13). In addition to its neurite-promoting action, NGF also stimulates the differentiation of sensory and sympathetic neurons, by increasing the synthesis of their respective neurotransmitters, e.g., noradrenaline and neuropeptides. The neurite-promoting activity of NGF seems to be distinct from its trophic effect, since NGF has been shown to enhance neurite outgrowth under conditions where the test neurons (DRG and SG) did not depend on it for their survival (14,15).

The extension and maintenance of neurites by NGF requires the direct exposure of the growth cone, the elongating end of a neurite, to NGF (16–18). Neuronal survival, in contrast, can be achieved by presenting NGF to either the soma or the nerve ending (16). In vitro experiments revealed another important property of NGF on neuritic outgrowth—its neurotropic action. Neurites of NGF target cells can be guided along an NGF concentration gradient, and the direction of the neuritic growth can be deflected by the position of the NGF source (19,20). These actions of NGF, neuritic stimulation and neurite guidance, together with its trophic action are key elements of axonal regeneration by its PNS and CNS target neurons.

The neural crest-derived chromaffin cells of the adrenal medulla are induced by NGF to differentiate into neurons with characteristics similar to SG neurons, including neurite extension, noradrenaline synthesis, and electrical excitability (21,22). Most of the studies on the molecular mechanisms of neuritic extension by NGF have been made possible by the establishment of the adrenal medulla-derived pheochromocytoma PC12 cell line, which, like their normal counterparts, responds to NGF by extending neurites and acquiring a neuronal phenotype (23,24). The cellular process of neurite extension by NGF involves the combined operation of two components, one that requires synthesis of the proteins involved in the fiber-outgrowth (priming) and another that is transcription independent (25).

The initiation and elongation of neurites requires the organization of tubulin into microtubules and involves their interaction with a set of proteins known as the microtubule-associated proteins or MAPs. NGF has been shown to enhance the polymerization of tubulin into microtubules and to stabilize the microtubules (26). The increase in polymerized tubulin causes a secondary increase in tubulin synthesis (27). Moreover, NGF strongly stimulates the synthesis of several of the MAPs (26,28). NGF also causes the rapid phosphorylation of MAPs, which results in an increase interaction with the microtubules (29). The phosphorylation of MAPs by NGF has recently been attributed to the selective activation of an NGF-sensitive protein kinase (30).

The modulation of the cytoskeleton by its effect on the synthesis of tubulin and MAPs and on the stability of the microtubules need, however, not be the sole mechanism by which NGF influences neuritic extension. In fact, NGF has been shown to act locally at the level of the growth cone (16–18). This effect may involve the described actions at the level of proteins involved in growth cone motility, such as actin, vimentin, vincullin, neurofilament proteins and GAP-43 (31–36). Furthermore, NGF may modify the interaction of the growth cone with the extracellular matrix components and cell-adhesion molecules (11,12,37), two other classes of molecules known to play a key role in neuritic extension. Finally, in addition to these effects on the cytoskeleton, several of the many signals elicited by NGF might contribute to the modulation of neuritic elongation. These responses include early gene expression, changes in ion fluxes, production of second messengers such as cAMP, inositol phosphates, or diacylglycerols, increase in intracellular calcium concentrations, and activation of various protein kinases (cf. reviews in refs. 38,39).

NTFS AND REGENERATION IN THE ADULT MAMMALIAN CNS

NGF and Normal Cholinergic CNS Neurons

The recognition and further understanding of a role of NTFs in the adult CNS evolved through a number of observations during the 1980s. Fetal CNS tissue transplants survived and grew neurites increasingly better when implanted with longer delays after a mechanical or chemical lesion of the neonate or adult rat cortex (40). This phenomenon correlated in time with the accumulation of NTF activity in fluid and tissue adjacent to the lesion as measured by in vitro biological assays (41,42). The next critical step was the identification of an NTF acting on adult CNS neurons, namely the evidence for a potential physiological role of NGF for the normal cholinergic basal forebrain neurons: 1) NGF and its mRNA are present in the hippocampal formation and the neocortex (43–46), the innervation territories of cholinergic neurons of the medial septum/diagonal band and of the nucleus basalis, respectively; 2) these cholinergic neurons have high-affinity transducing NGF receptors (47,48); 3) radiolabeled NGF injected in their territories is retrogradely transported to and selectively accumulated in their cell bodies (49,50); 4) in the basal forebrain NGF immunoreactivity is exclusively localized in the cholinergic neurons (51,52); 5) NGF administration in vivo causes increased activity of choline acetyltransferase (ChAT), the acetylcholine-synthesizing enzyme (53,54), but see (55); 6) administration in normal neonatal rats of Fab fragments of antibodies to NGF results in reductions of ChAT in the cholinergic systems (56) and can impair cholinergic memory-related behaviors in adult rats (57); 7) NGF treatments also result in an increased expression of mRNA and immunoreactivity for low-affinity NGF receptors (LNGFR) (58,59), which in the basal forebrain are exclusively present on the cholinergic neurons (60). In addition, NGF also may be an NTF for neostriatal cholinergic neurons, which express high-affinity NGF receptors (47,48), and respond to NGF with an increase in ChAT (55,61,62), LNGFR immunoreactivity (63,64), LNGFR mRNA (65), and cell body size (66).

Protective and Restorative Effects of NGF on Cholinergic CNS Neurons

Septohippocampal System

An earlier speculation of a physiological role of endogenous NTFs for maintenance and performance of adult CNS neurons (7) (Fig. 1A) had included the notion that 1) NTF deficits may result in neuronal dysfunction and/or degeneration and may also prohibit axonal regeneration (Fig. 1B), and 2) treatments with NTFs may project injured neurons against degeneration (Fig. 1C) and may promote axonal regeneration (Fig. 1D and E). The septohippocampal and nucleus basalis-cortex cholinergic systems of the adult rat have proven to be very useful models to test this NTF hypothesis. In the septohippocampal system, cholinergic neurons of the medial septum and vertical limb of the diagonal band nucleus of Broca project their axons predominantly to the ipsilateral dorsal hippocampal formation through the fimbria-fornix and supracallosal stria (67).

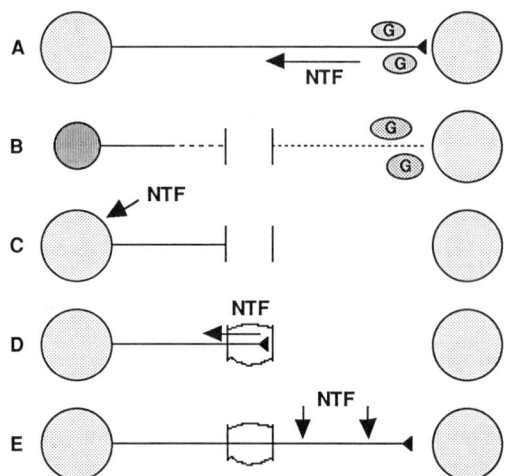

FIG. 1. Potential NTF involvements in neuronal degeneration and regeneration. **A:** In the normal adult CNS target-derived NTFs (from postsynaptic neurons or glial cells, G may be essential for the function and maintenance of the neurons. **B:** If so, NTF interruption/deficits would result in dysfunction and degeneration. **C:** Administration of exogenous NTF may substitute for the "lost" NTF and thus prevent degeneration. **D:** NTFs may play a role in the recruitment of regrowing axons into grafts as well as **(E)** promote regeneration into the original innervation territory or other host CNS tissues.

NGF Prevents Degeneration of Cholinergic Neurons

Interruption of retrograde delivery of the putative hippocampal NGF should have recognizable effects on the septal cholinergic neurons (Fig. 1B). In fact, a fimbria-fornix transection results over a 2 week postlesion period in the loss of 60–80% of the medial septum and about half of the vertical diagonal band cholinergic cell bodies (Fig. 2A), recognizable by their markers acetylcholinesterase (AChE) (68), ChAT (69) or LNGFR (70) immunostaining. Conversely, if the interruption of endogenous NGF was a critical component for the neuronal degeneration, substitution with exogenous NGF may prevent such changes. In fact, intraventricular administration (injec-

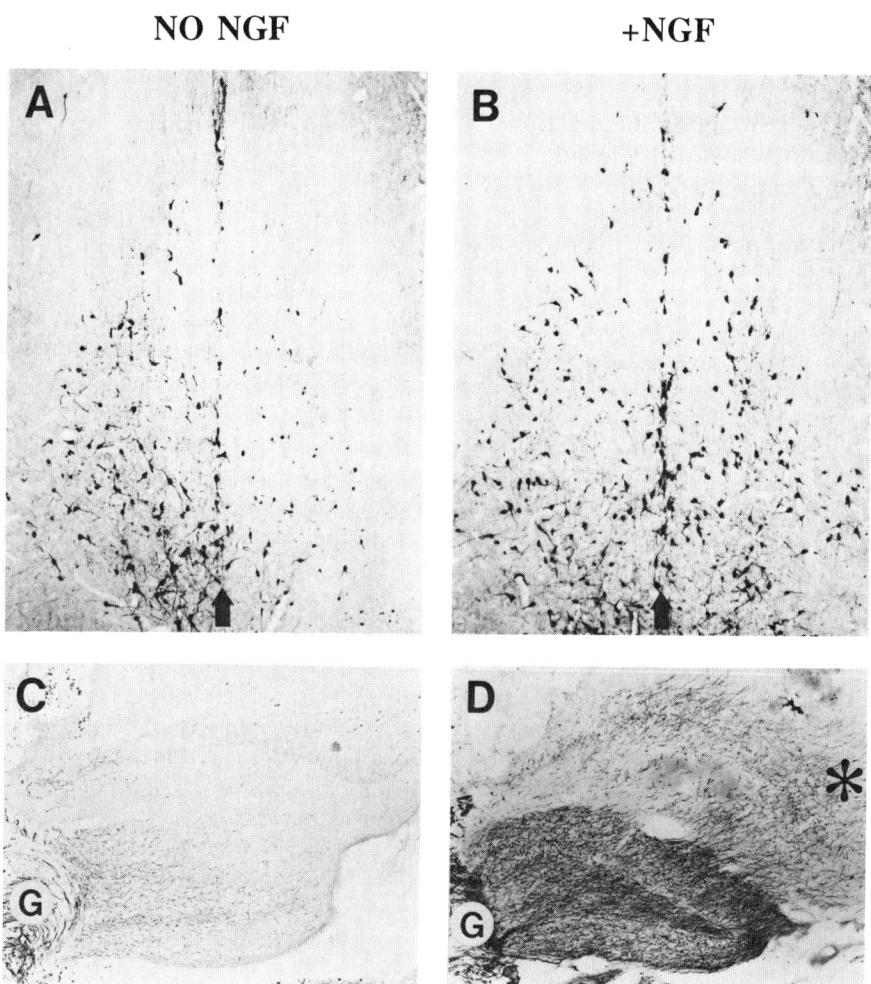

FIG. 2. NGF prevents degeneration and promotes regeneration of cholinergic neurons in the adult rat CNS. **A:** After a fimbria-fornix transection the number of axotomized medial septum cholinergic neurons (here immunostained for ChAT) is reduced compared to the nontransected control side (*left*). *Arrows* in A and B indicate the midline of the medial septum. **B:** With a 14 day intraventricular NGF infusion, starting immediately after the lesion, all axotomized ipsilateral cholinergic neurons are detectable. **C:** One month after a bilateral fimbria-fornix transection and implantation of a peripheral nerve graft, a modest number of cholinergic fibers (stained for AChE) have again entered the denervated dorsal hippocampal formation through the graft *(G)*. **D:** In contrast, with a 1 month infusion of NGF into the hippocampal tissue *(asterisk)*, about 2 mm from the nerve graft, dramatically more cholinergic fibers have entered the hippocampal CNS tissue.

tion or infusion) of NGF starting immediately after the lesion can prevent the disappearance of all the lesioned cholinergic neurons (Figure 2B) (59,71–74), as well as preserve their normal size and morphometric features (59,74). Exogenous NGF treatments after axotomy may have to persist until sufficient endogenous sources may be reacquired by the cholinergic neurons/axons, locally or through regeneration back to the hippocampal formation (75). The lesioned septal cholinergic neurons have been similarly protected by NGF from implanted slow-release materials (76) and NGF-producing fibroblasts (77,78) and putatively by NGF from implanted peripheral nerve grafts (79) whose cells are induced by the nerve transection to produce more NGF (80,81). In the forebrain, NGF may be a specific NTF for cholinergic neurons since only these cells express detectable levels of high-affinity NGF receptors. Furthermore, NGF only protects the cholinergic and not the other axotomized (mostly GABAergic) neurons after a fimbria-fornix transection (63,75,82) (but also see ref. 72). From these several studies it was concluded that the exogenous NGF could specifically prevent the axotomy-induced neuronal death and that, therefore, endogenous hippocampal-derived NGF might act normally as a survival-promoting NTF for the cholinergic neurons. More recently, another study (83) showed that the septal cholinergic neurons did not disappear after chemical destruction by N-methyl-D-aspartic acid of almost the entire hippocampal formation, but were "lost" after a subsequent fimbria-fornix transection. Thus, normal nonaxotomized adult septal cholinergic neurons either do not depend on hippocampal-derived NGF or can obtain another NTF source (e.g., from reactive astroglia in the fimbrial tissue) after removal of their target territory.

NGF Reverses Degeneration of Cholinergic Neurons

A further speculation is that the dependence on NTFs by adult CNS neurons may not concern their survival but the expression of functional properties. This appears to be the case with adult PNS neurons (14), which upon axotomy undergo NGF-sensitive changes, including reductions in transmitter enzyme and NGF receptor expression (84–87). In fact, a loss of transmitter enzyme without cell degeneration has been described for a number of other CNS neurons (88–91). Thus, the axotomy-induced "loss" of medial septum cholinergic neurons could have resulted from losses of their cholinergic markers (AChE, ChAT, LNGFR) by which they are detectable, rather than of the cells themselves. This possibility was tested (59,92,93) by delaying the start of intraventricular NGF infusions until later postlesion times when the number of cholinergic medial septum neurons, detectable by ChAT and LNGFR, had been reduced to 50% (7 days) or 35% (14 day onward). With NGF treatments delayed up to 7 days, the already incurred loss was rapidly (3–7 days) and completely reversed and even after 95 days, the number of detectable ChAT-positive neurons was restored to about 60% of the original population (more recently up to 80%, unpublished observations). Delayed NGF not only reversed marker-related losses (i.e., several "functional" competences), but also reversed the axotomy-induced atrophy (signifying a general trophic effect) (59). Others (75) were not able to reverse the neuronal "loss" after a partial fimbria-fornix transection with intermittent biweekly NGF injections, raising the possibility that continuous and high doses of NGF may be necessary to achieve restoration. By retrograde tracer labeling of the septal neurons before the fimbria-fornix transection, one investigator (94) found shrinkage but persistence of the axotomized neurons, whereas others (95,96) showed a loss of ChAT that precedes by 2 weeks the disappearance of fluoro-labeled medial septum neurons. The tracing technique has inherent problems. The tracer could add a toxic component to the axotomy insult and thus lead to cell death (97). Also, retention of the tracer may be reduced by the axotomy even in neurons that do not die. Third, the retrolabeling does not discriminate between the cholinergic and more numerous GABAergic neurons, making exact calculations difficult. Thus, definite evidence may still have to be secured as to whether all adult septal cholinergic neurons need not be lost after their axotomy, can persist in an atrophic state, and are amenable to subsequent treatment and restoration with NGF. The possibility of a "grace" period between the time of acute injury (or onset of more chronic degenerative disease) and the start of NTF treatment has obvious implications for future clinical applications.

Nucleus Basalis-Cortex System

The cholinergic neurons of the nucleus basalis of Meynert project extensively to the cortex. These neurons undergo atrophy, but do not disappear after removal of their target territory by aspiration or ischemia (98,99). As in the septum, intraventricular infusion with NGF can prevent the lesion-induced cholinergic cell body atrophy (100,101). Moreover, co-treatment with NGF and gangliosides (intraventricularly infused or peripherally injected) leads to an improved protection of these neurons (100,101). NGF administration also results in an increased level of ChAT in the regions around the cortical lesion (102,103), suggesting that the remaining cholinergic projections function at a higher level or have sprouted (see also "Effects of NGF on Regeneration of Cortical Cholinergic Fibers" below). A similar mechanism may explain the NGF-induced improvement of cortical ChAT levels of animals with excitotoxic lesions of parts of the nucleus basalis (104). In those basalis-lesioned animals, NGF could improve their impaired water maze memory-related behaviors. A proportion of naturally aging rats exhibits atrophy of their cholinergic nucleus basalis neurons (as well as those of the neostriatum) in correlation with impairments of their water-maze behavior. When infused with NGF, the neuronal atrophy is partially reversed (both basalis and neostriatum) and in parallel these animals show a remarkably improved maze performance (105)—a finding that may be relevant to Alzheimer disease, where cholinergic deficits are part of the pathology.

NGF and Cholinergic Axonal Regeneration

Beside the role of NGF in the protection against and restoration from injury-induced damage, its role in axonal regeneration has also become clear over the last decade. Most information was again gained from studies of the cholinergic septohippocampal system.

Septohippocampal Regeneration

Regeneration Models

The study of the role of NTFs in CNS regeneration has been facilitated by the use of the cholinergic septohippocampal system. In most studies the septum was separated from the hippocampal formation by aspirative lesions of the fimbria-fornix tract, resulting in a cholinergic denervation of the hippocampal terrain, while creating a lesion cavity for the placement of a variety of "bridges." The host septal cholinergic axons could invade, traverse, and again leave these grafts to re-enter their original territory. Such grafts have included fetal hippocampal tissue (106–109), which, when fused with the host hippocampal formation, theoretically provides a continuous innervation territory. Peripheral nerve grafts have been used (110,111), in the knowledge that they can promote regeneration from a variety of CNS regions (3). The evaluation of cholinergic axonal regeneration in the septohippocampal system has been facilitated by establishing a quantitative temporal baseline of regrowth from the septum into the denervated hippocampal tissue through segments of autologous sciatic nerve (111). In general, the septal cholinergic fibers enter the fetal or nerve grafts after 3–7 days and reach a substantial and maximal number at the bridge's end between 2 and 4 weeks. However, entry and further elongation into the dorsal hippocampal formation is much less vigorous and progressively less rapid. Although after 6–9 months a nearly normal density and pattern of cholinergic innervation is again seen in the most rostral 1–2 mm, only a very limited number of fiber regrow back into deeper hippocampal regions.

Cell Atrophy and NGF Treatments

A prerequisite for successful regeneration is the availability of neurons capable of regrowing their axons. In the grafted animals, the disappearance of ChAT-positive medial septum neurons, resulting from the fimbria-fornix transection, was not prevented by the presence of the nerve bridges (111), although putative nerve-derived NGF may delay such reductions by 2 weeks (79,81). The atrophic septal cholinergic neurons are presumably unable to initiate the biosynthetic processes necessary for growth cone formation and axonal elongation, leaving only the spared neurons to contribute fibers into the graft. Concurrent infusion for 1 month with NGF into the ventricle (i.e., proximal to the lesion) fully protected the ChAT-positive neurons and induced the appearance of a cholinergic fiber plexus in the dorso-lateral septum oriented toward the NGF-infused ventricle (63,66,72,74,93). Even so, the number of cholinergic fibers in the graft and hippocampal formation was in fact reduced compared to grafted animals not infused with NGF (230). It appears that the high periventricular NGF can induce local sprouting, but diverts regrowing fibers away from the nerve graft, an effect similar to the in vitro neurite-promoting and guidance action of NGF (see "In Vitro Neurite-Promoting Effects of NTFs" above). This phenomenon is also in agreement with the incompetence of NGF applied to the cell bodies in vitro to induce neurite outgrowth into an environment relatively devoid of NGF (see same section above). Others have shown that intraventricular NGF infusion during the first 2 weeks after implantation of a fetal hippocampal tissue graft enhances the long-term preservation of the cholinergic cell bodies and the regeneration of cholinergic fibers into the graft and hippocampal formation (109). This suggests that an early (and temporary) protection of the cholinergic neurons allows more of them to participate in the regeneration process, i.e., a greater number of axons become available to enter the grafted and host hippocampal tissue. It also suggests that the fetal graft becomes an available source of NGF for the cholinergic septal neurons.

Grafts and NTFs

The success of nerve or fetal CNS grafts (fetal innervation territory) to recruit regenerating CNS axons may reflect the ability of the living cells in the graft to produce and release NTFs into the CNS environment (108,112,113). Conversely, the failure of freeze-thawed nerves to do so may result from a lack of viable cells (114,115). Schwann cells can produce NGF in vitro (116,117) and NGF levels in the peripheral nerve increases after its transection in vivo (80,118). To address this issue an "acellular" nerve was prepared (119) by in situ degeneration of a transected distal nerve segment, freeze-thawing, and in vitro removal of the debris by rat peritoneal macrophages. The final preparation was completely devoid of myelin, axons, and intact cells and consisted of longitudinally arranged basal lamina tubes essentially free of debris. Such preparations are rich in laminin and collagen, extracellular matrix glycoproteins, both known for their in vitro neurite-promoting activities (120). One month after implantation in the septo-hippocampal model (119), essentially no cholinergic fibers were detectable in the acellular nerve. In marked contrast, acellular nerves that had been soaked in purified NGF overnight prior to their implantation contained nearly as many cholinergic fibers as the standard fresh nerve grafts. Thus, it appears that the availability of NGF in or from the nerve bridge is essential for regeneration of cholinergic axons into the bridge. Furthermore, exogenous NGF may replace the putative endogenous NGF produced and supplied by the living nerve cells. These results also showed that the mechanochemical scaffold of the acellular nerve remains competent to support regeneration of cholinergic axons (if appropriately stimulated by NGF), facilitating further development of artificial regeneration bridge materials. Such materials, when combined with neuron-selective NTFs, may be able to recruit and promote the regeneration of specific sets of CNS neurons.

CNS Tissue Environment and NTFs

The exogenous NGF, or putative nerve or fetal graft-derived NTFs, while promoting regeneration into the grafts themselves, failed to stimulate regeneration with a similar magnitude into the hippocampal CNS tissue. In fact, less than one-third of the fibers that at 1 month were already maximally available at the hippocampal end of a fresh nerve bridge had entered the hippocampal tissue (111,119). Apparently, restrictions on hippocampal entry and penetration by cholinergic axons are defined by properties intrinsic to the hippocampus. One of the main "restrictions" may be the absence of sufficient levels of local NGF, the requirement recognized for the nerve grafts. The temporal and/or spatial gradient observed for the cholinergic fiber invasion of hippocampal tissue could thus potentially result from a correspondingly graded availability of hippocampal NGF. Such NGF could be supplied by the nerve graft (see previous paragraph), by astroglial cells at the lesion site (41,42), or by the denervated hippocampal formation itself (121–123). Thus, the hypothesis was formulated (111,124) that 1) the hippocampal CNS tissue properties that restrict cholinergic regeneration in the adult are dynamic and not immutable; 2) a localized or transient availability of NTFs such as NGF may be responsible for the initial successful regeneration; 3) failure of sustained regeneration may result primarily from an insufficient availability of such NTFs; and 4) supplying NTFs may promote further CNS regeneration. In fact, infusion with NGF for 1 month directly into the dorsal hippocampal formation itself (2 mm from implanted fresh nerve grafts) enhanced severalfold the number of cholinergic fibers entering and further penetrating the hippocampal CNS tissue over those seen in control-infused animals (124) (compare Fig. 2C and D). Fiber numbers and distances reached by them after 1 month were nearly equal to those seen previously at 6 months without NGF infusions (111). The enhanced presence of fibers did not result from recruitment of more cholinergic neurons or an increased availability of fibers at the nerve end, i.e., represented better penetration of the hippocampal tissue. Subsequent analyses (63,124) showed that the NGF-induced increase of cholinergic fibers represents genuine axonal elongation, rather than an increase in the marker molecules by which they are detected. Thus, supplementation of NGF in the hippocampal formation can overcome the "resistances" or "deficiencies" of this CNS tissue environment for cholinergic reinnervation.

Of interest is the possibility that exogenous NGF only promotes the outgrowth of axotomized neurons in the adult brain. NGF infusions into the ventral hippocampal tissue, which promoted axonal regeneration from the septum into the dorsal hippocampal formation, did not induce sprouting of the nonlesioned cholinergic pathway to the ventral hippocampal formation (124). Also, intraventricular NGF infusions induce sprouting of cholinergic fibers into the dorsolateral septum only after a fimbria-fornix transection (66). In vitro, NGF has also been shown to promote neurite outgrowth in cholinergic septal/basal forebrain neurons only after their axotomy (125). Another important question will be whether the NGF treatment would promote, or at least respect, a normal distribution pattern of reinnervation such as is achievable after long postimplantation times without NGF (107,111) and allow appropriate synaptic reconnections.

NGF and Intrahippocampal Sprouting

When the afferents from the entorhinal cortex to the dentate gyrus are removed by transection of the perforant pathway or by destruction of the entorhinal cortex, cholinergic axons from the septum sprout into the denervated molecular layer of the dentate gyrus (126,127). In parallel with the appearance of cholinergic sprouts, microglia/macroglia become immunoreactive for interleukin-1 (IL-1) (128), an increase in immunostainable NGF appears in the denervated dentate tissue (129), and hippocampal NGF activity levels increase (130). Macrophage-derived IL-1 can promote the synthesis of NGF by sciatic nerve cells (131), and purified IL-1 can induce NGF production in cultured astrocytes (132). Thus, a cascade of growth and trophic factor production and release (see also 41,42,133) may be part of the response to injury by neural tissues and may play important roles in the ensuing compensatory repair processes.

Another model for intrahippocampal sprouting involves the ingrowth into the hippocampal formation of peripheral noradrenergic sympathetic axons after removal of the septohippocampal innervation (134–136). Since hippocampal NGF levels increase after septohippocampal lesions (121–123) and sympathetic neurons are responsive to NGF (6), the role of NGF in sympathetic sprouting is possible (136). In an attempt to address this issue, intraventricular NGF infusions into the normal adult rat failed to elicit sympathetic ingrowth into the hippocampal formation, even though it caused the hypertrophy of sympathetic innervation of cerebrovascular targets (137). These results suggest that simple elevation of brain NGF, while perhaps necessary, is insufficient to induce sympathetic axonal outgrowth into the mature mammalian CNS.

Effects of NGF on Regeneration of Cortical Cholinergic Fibers

Axonal regeneration of the cholinergic neurons of the adult rat nucleus-basalis has been studied in a model that utilizes a knife-cut across the cortex and deprives the region caudal to the lesion from cholinergic innervation (138–140). After several weeks of twice-weekly injections with NGF into the lateral ventricle a much more extensive AChE-positive fiber plexus had developed both proximal and distal to the lesion (138). Whether this enhanced presence of fibers resulted from collateral sprouting or from genuine regeneration is unknown. In another study (141), proliferating fibroblasts were transfected in vitro with the NGF gene, resulting in fibroblasts capable of producing large amounts of NGF. Such cells were implanted into the cortex of adult rats in combination with fetal septal grafts (containing cholinergic neurons). Both grafted and host cholinergic neurons were induced to regrow their axons into the cholinergically denervated cortex.

The role of NGF in the preservation and remodeling of cholinergic synaptic connections has recently been evidenced. After ischemic decortication in adult rat, the remaining cortex shows substantial reductions in ChAT enzymatic activity levels, number of cholinergic fibers, and size of the cholinergic boutons (101,142). These "degenerative" changes could all be prevented by intraventricular infusion of NGF started immediately after the lesion. In fact, NGF induced modification of the shape, size, breadth, and width of the cholinergic boutons and resulted in their hypertrophy.

NGF Effects on Noncholinergic CNS Neurons

Besides the cholinergic neurons of the CNS, which are clearly responsive to and protected by NGF, the repair-related role of NGF has been investigated in a few other systems after their injury.

Visual System

The well-defined properties of the adult rat visual system, i.e., a relatively homogeneous population of retinal ganglion cells (RGCs) projecting through the optic nerve to the tectum, have made it a convenient model for regeneration research (3). However, only recently has investigation of NTFs begun in this model. Transection of the optic tract (either intracranial, leaving intact a moderate length of axons, or intraorbital, close to the retina) results after several weeks in an 80% "loss" of RGCs. NGF, when injected repeatedly into the eye at high doses, was shown to prevent about 20% of the otherwise occurring loss (143). Furthermore, peripheral nerve grafts, potentially producing and releasing NTFs such as NGF (see "Septohippocampal Regeneration" above), can prevent/delay axotomy-induced RGC degeneration (144). These nerve grafts can also promote regeneration of a small proportion of RGC axons over very long distances to reach the tectum, their original target territory, and form functional synapses (145–147). Thus, a subset of RGCs appears responsive to NGF, a finding that would fit with their immunoreactivity and expression of mRNA for LNGFR (148).

Another useful visual regeneration model involves the intraretinal transection of part of the retina (through the front of the eye), denervating the peripheral retina beyond the lesion. When injected into the eye, NGF promoted a substantial regrowth of substance P-positive fibers into the denervated part of the retina (149).

Red Nucleus and Corticospinal Motor Neurons

Neurons of the red nucleus project to the spinal cord and direct motor functions in concert with the corticospinal neurons. In the neonate rat, spinal cord transection results in the degeneration of red nucleus neurons over a 5 day period but concurrent daily injections with NGF into the ventricle can prevent the axotomy-induced neuronal loss (150). Transection of the adult rat spinal cord at a low thoracic level results in the atrophy, but not the loss of red nucleus neurons (151). These neurons can be retrogradely traced from a higher spinal level with fluorogold, but not with HRP, even 10 weeks after the lesion. Intraventricular NGF infusion apparently can improve the HRP transport capability of these lesioned neurons (152), suggesting that also adult red nucleus neurons can respond to NGF.

Corticospinal motor neurons are not known to be responsive to NGF in vitro and do not exhibit NGF receptors (47,48). However, intraventricularly infusion with NGF reportedly improves their HRP transport capability, as it did for the red nucleus (153). Moreover, neonatal rat corticospinal motor axons can regenerate along Schwann cell grafts (154), which in vitro can produce NGF and other NTFs (116,117,155) and are thus potential sources of NTFs in vivo.

Intraspinal Sensory Regeneration

Regrowth of peripheral sensory DRG fibers after peripheral nerve injury is the prime example of successful regeneration in the mammalian nervous system. However, the central axons of adult DRG neurons regenerate poorly into their original spinal CNS territory after their ablation and reimplantation into the white matter (156,157). Developing as well as adult DRG neurons respond to NGF with increased neurite outgrowth (14,158), and regeneration of adult rat peripheral sensory fibers is enhanced into peripheral nerve chambers filled with NGF (159,160). Thus, it is likely that NGF would also play a beneficial role for the regeneration of central sensory DRG processes back into the spinal cord. In fact, NGF-coated nitrocellulose bridges can promote ingrowth of reimplanted dorsal root fibers over short distances into the spinal cord of neonatal rats (161). The neurite-promoting activity of nitrocellulose-bound NGF has also been demonstrated in vitro (162).

Other NTFs

NGF Family Members

Three other NTFs have recently been sequenced, i.e., brain derived neurotrophic factor (BDNF) (163), neurotrophin-3 (NT-3, also named HDNF and NGF2) (164–169) and neurotrophin-4 (NT-4) (170). These factors have a high degree of sequence homology with the NGF protein, overlap in biological activity and target cells with NGF, and are viewed as members of an NGF family. Gene expression for NGF, BDNF, and NT-3 (by in situ hybridizing techniques) is distributed in the rat hippocampal formation with only partly overlapping patterns (44,171,172). BDNF is also expressed in several CNS areas beside the hippocampal formation, e.g., cerebral cortex and amygdala. Both BDNF and NT-3 have trophic and neurite-promoting effects in vitro (164,165,167,168,173). Of particular interest is the recognition that BDNF can promote neuronal survival from mesencephalic (substantia nigra) dopaminergic neurons in vitro (174). The degeneration of these neurons is the main characteristic of Parkinson disease. When these factors become available in large enough quantities to a large enough number of investigators/laboratories their potential role in neuronal protection and regeneration is expected to become evident.

Ciliary Neuronotrophic Factor (CNTF)

CNTF was recognized and defined by its survival-promoting activity on developing ciliary ganglionic (CG) neurons (for a review, see ref. 175). Eye-derived CNTF protects CG neurons in vitro during a defined embryonic stage when their naturally occurring death takes place, suggesting that CNTF is their target-derived NTF (176, 177). A skeletal muscle-derived CNTF-like factor may similarly serve as an NTF for spinal motor neurons during development. CNTF promotes the survival and ChAT and neurofilament expression of spinal motor neurons in vitro from E6 chick (178) and E14 rat (179,180). Administration of CNTF to the chick in vivo can prevent 40% of the neuronal death of motor neurons (181). In the adult rat, CNTF mRNA has not been detected in skeletal muscle by Northern blot analysis (182). In contrast, both CNTF protein and mRNA are present in large amounts in the adult, but not the neonate, peripheral nerve (182). Almost all the CNTF of adult nerve is found immunohistochemically to be associated with the Schwann cells (183) and Schwann cells produce it in vitro (116). Thus, nerve-derived CNTF may play a crucial role in the protection of motor neurons against injury-induced degeneration. Transection of the facial nerve of 1 week old rats results in the degeneration of facial motor neurons, which coincides with the low levels of 1 week nerve CNTF (182). In sharp contrast, most of these lesioned motor neurons are protected by the application of CNTF to the proximal nerve stump (184). In the adult rat, where nerve CNTF is abundant, axotomy is not followed by motor neuron death.

In the CNS, CNTF mRNA has been extracted from whole spinal cord and detected by Northern blot analysis in several regions (182, 231), with the highest levels found in olfactory bulb and optic nerve. In the adult CNS, CNTF immunoreactivity has been shown in a subset of astrocytes (231). In vitro, type-1 astrocytes from neonatal rat cortex can produce CNTF activity (185–188) and neonatal astrocytes from the hippocampus express mRNA for CNTF as well as CNTF-immunoreactivity on their cell surface (189).

Infusion of CNTF into the lateral ventricles of adult rats after a fimbria-fornix transection can prevent the loss and atrophy of most medial septal neurons, i.e., both cholinergic and noncholinergic (63,82). Thus, CNTF may have protective (trophic) effects on a broad range of neurons in the adult CNS. In addition, CNTF prevents the axotomy-induced losses of LNGFR, but not of ChAT staining, in the septal cholinergic neurons. Furthermore, CNTF induces LNGFR (but not ChAT) staining in the neostriatal cholinergic neurons—both being markers also known to respond to NGF (55,66). In cultures from a variety of fetal CNS regions, CNTF is required for the survival of some neurons, while soliciting LNGFR (and in some cases ChAT) expression in others (179,190). However, it remains to be established whether CNTF acts directly on the neurons through their own receptors or indirectly by stimulating the production of NTFs by nonneuronal cells. Also yet to be investigated are any regeneration-promoting capabilities of CNTF, since neurite-promoting activity with identified/purified CNTF in vitro has been reported in some (180) but refuted by other (162) studies.

Fibroblast Growth Factor (FGF)

Acidic FGF (aFGF) and basic (bFGF) are two polypeptide factors belonging to a larger family of FGFs which have a well-documented mitogenic action on non-neuronal cells (191–193). These "growth factor" activities include the stimulation of proliferation, chemotaxis, differentiation, wound healing and tissue repair, angiogenesis, and fetal development. Since the brain has the highest concentrations of FGF (194,195), it is likely that it has important functions in the CNS. In the rat pup expression of mRNA for FGF receptor is found on cholinergic neurons of the basal forebrain, the brainstem reticular and motor nuclei, and cerebellar Purkinje and granule cells. In the adult rat, FGF receptor mRNA is found in hippocampal formation neurons, the pontine cholinergic neurons, the limbic system, the brainstem nuclei, spinal cord neurons, and cerebellar granule cells (196). However, the adult basal forebrain cholinergic nuclei do not express FGF receptor mRNA. In addition, labeled FGF is taken up by hippocampal neurons, but not by basal forebrain ones (197). bFGF injected into the adult rat eye is anterogradely transported to the lateral geniculate body and superior colliculus raising the possibility that bFGF may act as an anterograde trophic factor in the visual system, a system known to undergo anterograde transneuronal cell death (198). FGF is released after CNS injury (199) and increased bFGF-immunostaining has been detected in mechanically damaged brain (200).

Both aFGF and bFGF support in vitro survival and differentiation of primary cultures of neurons from cortex, hippocampus, striatum, septum, thalamus, and mesencephalon (reviewed in refs. 192,201). Basic FGF can also support cultured motor neurons from chick CG (202) and spinal cord (178). In vivo, application of aFGF to the stump of a transected adult rat optic nerve prevents the degeneration of RGCs (203). Injection of bFGF stimulates ChAT activity in the hippocampal formation following a partial fimbria-fornix transection in adult rats and enhances the astroglial reaction to injury (204). Moreover, administration of bFGF (via intraventricular infusion or implantation of a piece of FGF-soaked gelfoam) after a fimbria-fornix transection prevents the degeneration of a substantial number of medial septum cholinergic neurons in young adult animals (205, 206). However, since these cholinergic neurons neither transport FGF nor have FGF receptor mRNA (see above), this protective effect of bFGF may be mediated by other cell types, possibly astrocytes. In fact, bFGF can induce the production of NGF by rat astrocytes (207,208).

The angiogenic and mitogenic effects of FGF may or may not be beneficial in CNS regeneration. In vitro, bFGF can be a potent mitogen for oligodendrocytes (209,210) and oligodendrocyte-type-2 astrocyte progenitor cells (211) and can prevent their differentiation (212). This effect may be useful in substituting lost oligodendrocytes and for remyelination of regenerated central axons.

Epidermal Growth Factor (EGF)

EGF was purified from the mouse submaxillary gland shortly after NGF (213,214) and is the prototype growth factor, i.e., it has a mitogenic activity for a variety of epidermal cells (215). In vitro, EGF promotes survival and neurite outgrowth from embryonic neocortical neurons (216,217). Immunoreactivity for EGF and its receptor and the mRNA for a precursor of EGF have been found in the normal CNS (218–221). EGF-binding sites in the fetal and adult mouse CNS are particularly abundant in the substantia nigra (222). In fact, intraventricular infusion of EGF leads to improvements in dopaminergic functions in a mouse model for Parkinson disease (223). Furthermore, in response to brain injury EGF receptor immunoreactivity is increased in the reactive astroglial cells (221,224).

Lymphokines

Lymphokines may not be NTFs per se, but may be involved in the reaction to brain injury, which includes the promotion of NTF production by glial cells. In vitro, macrophage-derived interleukin-1 (IL-1) stimulates the production of NGF by Schwann cells and fibroblasts (131). IL-1 is a potent astroglial mitogen (225,226) and can induce an increased synthesis of NGF by cultured astrocytes (132). The synthesis of IL-1 and IL-2 is increased after injury to the CNS (133,225,227). The mRNA for IL-3 is abundantly expressed in neurons and glial cells of the adult mouse, especially in the hippocampal formation (228). Recently, IL-3 has been shown to increase neurite growth and ChAT levels in cultured mouse septal neurons and to protect a portion of the adult rat septal cholinergic neurons after a fimbria-fornix transection (229).

CONCLUSIONS

During the past decade the knowledge about NTFs and about adult mammalian CNS regeneration has rapidly evolved and has started to converge toward a common understanding. The primary thrust for this advance has been the recognition that NTFs are essential for the normal function and maintenance of adult CNS neurons and that, conversely, a deficiency of such NTFs can result in neuronal dysfunction and degeneration. An obvious next step, which has been supported by several studies from several research groups, was the application of exogenous NTFs to prevent and restore neuronal damages. In particular, NGF has been shown to have crucial roles for the repair of axotomized cholinergic neurons in the adult mammalian CNS. In the rat basal forebrain, NGF can protect and restore cholinergic cell body size and functional properties (e.g., AChE, ChAT, and LNGFR), and even improve behavioral deficits. Moreover, NGF can play a role in the recruitment and promotion of cholinergic fiber growth not only into grafts but also into the nonpermissive adult CNS environment. Thus, failure of CNS regeneration may result from an insufficient availability of

NTFs and treatment with such factors may lead to successful CNS repair. If generalizable to other CNS systems and other NTFs, these concepts may signify a new level of understanding about the mechanisms of neuroregeneration. However, one should guard against oversimplifications of the problem of CNS regeneration, which might lead to "heroic," but still unwarranted, attempts to apply these concepts in a clinical setting.

ACKNOWLEDGMENT

This study was supported by NINCDS grants NS-16349 and NS-27047.

REFERENCES

1. Ramón y Cajal S. *Degeneration and regeneration of the nervous system* (May RM, translator). New York: Oxford University Press; 1928.
2. Tello F. La influencia del neurotropismo en la generación de los centros nerviosos. *Trab Lab Invest Biol* 1911; 9: 123–159.
3. Aguayo AJ. Capacity for renewed axonal growth in the mammalian central nervous system. In: Bignami A, Bloom FE, Bolis CL, Adeloye A, eds. *Central nervous system plasticity and repair*. New York: Raven Press; 1985: 31–40.
4. Cowan WM, Fawcett JW, O'Leary DDM, Stanfield BB. Regressive events in neurogenesis. *Science* 1984: 225: 1258–1265.
5. Hamburger V. The journey of a neuroembryologist. *Annu Rev Neurosci* 1989; 12: 1–12.
6. Levi-Montalcini R. The nerve growth factor 35 years later. *Science* 1987; 237: 1154–1162.
7. Varon S, Manthorpe M, Williams LR. Neuronotrophic and neurite-promoting factors and their clinical potentials. *Dev Neurosci* 1984; 6: 73–100.
8. Oppenheim RW. Cell death during development of the nervous system. *Annu Rev Neurosci* 1991b; 14: 453–501.
9. Hefti F, Hartikka J, Knusel B. Function of neurotrophic factors in the adult and aging brain and their possible use in the treatment of neurodegenerative diseases. *Neurobiol Aging* 1989; 10: 515–533.
10. Whittemore SR, Seiger A. The expression, localization and functional significance of beta-nerve growth factor in the central nervous system. *Brain Res* 1987; 434: 439–464.
11. Sanes JR. Extracellular matrix molecules that influence neural development. *Annu Rev Neurosci* 1989; 12: 491–516.
12. Reichardt LF, Tomaselli KJ. Extracellular matrix molecules and their receptors: functions in neural development. *Annu Rev Neurosci* 1991; 14: 531–570.
13. Levi-Montalcini R, Angeletti PU. Essential role of the nerve growth factor in the survival and maintenance of dissociated sensory and sympathetic embryonic nerve cells in vitro. *Dev Biol* 1963; 7: 653–657.
14. Lindsay RM. Nerve growth factors (NGF, BDNF) enhance axonal regeneration but are not required for survival of adult sensory neurons. *J Neurosci* 1988; 8: 2394–2405.
15. Greene LA, Volonte C, Chalazonitis A. Purine analogs inhibit nerve growth factor-promoted neurite outgrowth by sympathetic and sensory neurons. *J Neurosci* 1990; 10: 1479–1485.
16. Campenot RB. Development of sympathetic neurons in compartmentalized cultures. I. Local control of neurite growth by nerve growth factor. *Dev Biol* 1982a; 93: 1–12.
17. Campenot RB. Development of sympathetic neurons in compartmentalized cultures. II. Local control of neurite survival by nerve growth factor. *Dev Biol* 1982b; 93: 13–21.
18. Seely JP, Greene LA. Short-latency local actions of nerve growth factor at the growth cone. *Proc Natl Acad Sci USA* 1983; 80: 2789–2793.
19. Gundersen RW, Barrett JN. Characterization of the turning response of dorsal root neurites toward nerve growth factor. *J Cell Biol* 1980; 87: 546–554.
20. Gundersen RW, Barrett JN. Neuronal chemotaxis: chick dorsal-root axons turn toward high concentrations of nerve growth factor. *Science* 1979; 206: 1079–1080.
21. Aloe L, Levi-Montalcini R. Nerve growth factor-induced transformation of immature chromaffin cells in vivo into sympathetic neurons: effects of antiserum to nerve growth factor. *Proc Natl Acad Sci USA* 1979; 76: 1246–1250.
22. Unsicker K, Krisch B, Otten J, Thoenen H. Nerve growth factor-induced fiber outgrowth from rat adrenal chromaffin cells: impairment by glucocorticoids. *Proc Natl Acad Sci USA* 1978; 75: 3498–3502.
23. Greene LA, Tischler AS. Establishment of a noradrenergic clonal cell line of rat adrenal pheochromocytoma cells which respond to nerve growth factor. *Proc Natl Acad Sci USA* 1976; 73: 2424–2428.
24. Greene LA. NGF prevents the death and stimulates the neuronal differentiation of clonal PC12 pheochromocytoma cells in serum-free medium. *J Cell Biol* 1978; 78: 747–755.
25. Greene LA. The importance of both early and delayed responses in the biological actions of NGF. *Trends Neurosci* 1984; 7: 91–94.
26. Black MM, Aletta JM, Greene LA. Regulation of MT composition and stability during NGF promoted neurite outgrowth. *J Cell Biol* 1986; 103: 545–557.
27. Drubin D, Kobayashi S, Kellogg D, Kirschner M. Regulation of microtubule protein levels during cellular morphogenesis in nerve growth factor-treated PC12 cells. *J Cell Biol* 1988; 106: 1583–1591.

28. Drubin DG, Kobayashi S, Kellogg D, Kirschner M. Nerve growth factor-induced neurite outgrowth in PC12 cells involves the coordinate induction of microtubule assembly and assembly-promoting factors. *J Cell Biol* 1985; 101: 1799–1807.
29. Aletta JM, Lewis SA, Cowan NJ, Greene LA. Nerve growth factor regulates both the phosphorylation and steady-state levels of microtubule-associated protein 1.2 (MAP1.2). *J Cell Biol* 1988; 106: 1573–1581.
30. Tsao H, Aletta JM, Greene LA. Nerve growth factor and fibroblast growth factor selectively activate a protein kinase that phosphorylates high molecular weight microtubule-associated proteins. Detection, partial purification, and characterization in PC12 cells. *J Biol Chem* 1990; 265: 15471–15480.
31. Federoff HJ, Grabczyk E, Fishman MC. Dual regulation of GAP-43 gene expression by nerve growth factor and glucocorticoids. *J Biol Chem* 1988; 263: 19290–19295.
32. Costello B, Meymandi A, Freeman JA. Factors influencing GAP-43 gene expression in PC12 pheochromocytoma cells. *J Neurosci* 1990; 10: 1398–1406.
33. Lee VM, Page C. The dynamics of NGF-induced neurofilament and vimentin expression and organization in PC12 cells. *J Neurosci* 1984; 4: 1705–1714.
34. Lindenbaum MH, Carbonetto S, Grosveld F, Flavell D, Mushynski WE. Transcriptional and post-transcriptional effects of nerve growth factor on expression of the three neurofilament subunits in PC12 cells. *J Biol Chem* 1988; 263: 5662–5667.
35. Dickson G, Prentice H, Julien J-P, Ferrari G, Leon A, Walsh FS. Nerve growth factor activates Thy-1 and neurofilament gene transcription in rat PC12 cells. *EMBO J* 1986; 5: 3449–3453.
36. Halegoua S. Changes in the phosphorylation and distribution of vinculin during nerve growth factor induced neurite outgrowth. *Dev Biol* 1987; 121: 97–104.
37. Takeichi M. Cadherin cell adhesion receptors as a morphogenetic regulator. *Science* 1991; 251: 1451–1455.
38. Levi A, Biocca S, Cattaneo A, Calissano P. The mode of action of nerve growth factor in PC12 cells. *Mol Neurobiol* 1988; 2: 201–226.
39. Hagg T, Louis JC, Varon S. Neurotrophic factors, growth factors and CNS trauma. In: Salzman SK, Faden AI, eds. *The neurobiology of central nervous system trauma*. New York: Oxford University Press; 1993; (in press).
40. Lewis ER, Cotman CW. Mechanisms of septal lamination in the developing hippocampus analyzed by outgrowth of fibers from septal implants: II. Absence of guidance by degenerative debris. *J Neurosci* 1982; 2: 66–77.
41. Manthorpe M, Nieto-Sampedro M, Skaper SD, et al. Neuronotrophic activity in brain wounds of the developing rat. Correlation with implant survival in the wound cavity. *Brain Res* 1983; 267: 47–56.
42. Nieto-Sampedro M, Manthorpe M, Barbin G, Varon S, Cotman CW. Injury-induced neuronotrophic activity in the adult rat brain. Correlation with survival of delayed implants in a wound cavity. *J Neurosci* 1983; 3: 2219–2229.
43. Ayer LC, Olson L, Ebendal T, Seiger A, Persson H. Expression of the beta-nerve growth factor gene in hippocampal neurons. *Science* 1988; 240: 1339–1341.
44. Ernfors P, Wetmore C, Olson L, Persson H. Identification of cells in the rat brain and peripheral tissues expressing mRNA for members of the nerve growth factor family. *Neuron* 1990a; 5: 511–526.
45. Shelton DL, Reichardt LF. Studies on the expression of the beta nerve growth factor (NGF) gene in the central nervous system: level and regional distribution of NGF mRNA suggest that NGF functions as a trophic factor for several distinct populations of neurons. *Proc Natl Acad Sci USA* 1986; 83: 2714–2718.
46. Korsching S, Auburger G, Heumann R, Scott J, Thoenen H. Levels of nerve growth factor and its mRNA in the central nervous system of the rat correlates with cholinergic innervation. *EMBO J* 1985; 4: 1389–1393.
47. Richardson PM, Issa VM, Riopelle RJ. Distribution of neuronal receptors for nerve growth factor in the rat. *J Neurosci* 1986; 6: 2312–2321.
48. Altar CA, Burton LE, Bennett GL, Dugich DM. Recombinant human nerve growth factor is biologically active and labels novel high-affinity binding sites in rat brain. *Proc Natl Acad Sci USA* 1991; 88: 281–285.
49. Seiler M, Schwab ME. Specific retrograde transport of nerve growth factor (NGF) from neocortex to nucleus basalis in the rat. *Brain Res* 1984; 300: 33–39.
50. Schwab ME, Otten U, Agid Y, Thoenen H. Nerve growth factor (NGF) in the rat CNS: absence of specific retrograde axonal transport and tyrosine hydroxylase induction in locus coeruleus and substantia nigra. *Brain Res* 1979; 168: 473–483.
51. Conner JM, Hagg T, Manthorpe M, Varon S. Nerve growth factor (NGF) and NGF receptor immunoreactivity in the adult rat CNS. *Soc Neurosci Abstr* 1990; 16: 480.
52. Conner JM, Muir D, Varon S, Hagg T, Manthorpe M. Immunohistochemical localization of nerve growth factor in the adult rat basal forebrain and hippocampal formation. *J Comp Neurol* 1991b; 319:454–462.
53. Mobley WC, Rutkowski JL, Tennekoon GI, Gemski J, Buchanan K, Johnston MV. Nerve growth factor increases choline acetyltransferase activity in developing basal forebrain neurons. *Brain Res* 1986; 387: 53–62.
54. Fusco M, Oderfeld NB, Vantini G, et al. Nerve growth factor affects uninjured, adult rat septohippocampal cholinergic neurons. *Neuroscience* 1989; 33: 47–52.
55. Williams LR, Jodelis KS, Donald MR. Axotomy-dependent stimulation of choline acetyltransferase activity by exogenous mouse nerve

growth factor in adult rat basal forebrain. *Brain Res* 1989; 498: 243–256.
56. Vantini G, Schiavo N, Di MA, et al. Evidence for a physiological role of nerve growth factor in the central nervous system of neonatal rats. *Neuron* 1989; 3: 267–273.
57. Nabeshima T, Ogawa S, Ishimaru H, et al. Memory impairment and morphological changes in rats induced by active fragment of anti-nerve growth factor-antibody. *Biochem Biophys Res Commun* 1991; 175: 215–219.
58. Cavicchioli L, Flanigan T, Vantini G, et al. NGF amplifies the expression of NGF receptor messenger RNA in mammalian forebrain cholinergic neurons. *Eur J Neurosci* 1989; 1: 258–262.
59. Hagg T, Fass HB, Vahlsing HL, Manthorpe M, Conner JM, Varon S. Nerve growth factor (NGF) reverses axotomy-induced decreases in choline acetyltransferase, NGF receptor and size of medial septum cholinergic neurons. *Brain Res* 1989a; 505: 29–38.
60. Bachelor PE, Armstrong DM, Blaker SN, Gage FH. Nerve growth factor receptor and choline acetyltransferase colocalization in neurons within the rat forebrain: response to fimbria-fornix transection. *J Comp Neurol* 1989; 284: 187–204.
61. Mobley WC, Rutkowski JL, Tennekoon GI, Buchanan K, Johnston MV. Choline acetyltransferase activity in striatum of neonatal rats increased by nerve growth factor. *Science* 1985; 229: 284–286.
62. Williams LR, Rylett RJ. Exogenous nerve growth factor increases the activity of high-affinity choline uptake and choline acetyltransferase in brain of Fisher 344 male rats. *J Neurochem* 1990; 55: 1042–1049.
63. Hagg T, Quon D, Higaki J, Varon S. Ciliary neurotrophic factor prevents neuronal degeneration and promotes low affinity NGF receptor expression in the adult rat CNS. *Neuron* 1992; 8:145–158.
64. Gage FH, Batchelor P, Chen KS, et al. NGF receptor reexpression and NGF-mediated cholinergic neuronal hypertrophy in the damaged adult neostriatum. *Neuron* 1989; 2: 1177–1184.
65. Higgins GA, Koh S, Chen KS, Gage FH. NGF induction of NGF receptor gene expression and cholinergic neuronal hypertrophy within the basal forebrain of the adult rat. *Neuron* 1989; 3: 247–256.
66. Hagg T, Hagg F, Vahlsing HL, Manthorpe M, Varon S. Nerve growth factor effects on cholinergic neurons of neostriatum and nucleus accumbens in the adult rat. *Neuroscience* 1989b; 30: 95–103.
67. Swanson LW, Köhler C, Björklund A. The limbic region. I: the septohippocampal system. In: Björklund A, Hökfelt T, Swanson LW, eds. *Handbook of Chemical Neuroanatomy*, vol. 5: *Integrated systems of the CNS*, Part I. Amsterdam: Elsevier; 1987: 125–277.
68. Gage FH, Wictorin K, Fischer W, Williams LR, Varon S, Björklund A. Retrograde cell changes in medial septum and diagnoal band following fimbria-fornix transection: quantitative temporal analysis. *Neuroscience* 1986; 19: 241–255.
69. Armstrong DM, Terry RD, Deteresa RM, Bruce G, Hersh LB, Gage FH. Response of septal cholinergic neurons to axotomy. *J Comp Neurol* 1987; 264: 421–436.
70. Springer JE, Koh S, Tayrien MW, Loy R. Basal forebrain magnocellular neurons stain for nerve growth factor receptor: correlation with cholinergic cell bodies and effects of axotomy. *J Neurosci Res* 1987; 17: 111–118.
71. Hefti F. Nerve growth factor promotes survival of septal cholinergic neurons after fimbrial transections. *J Neurosci* 1986; 6: 2155–2162.
72. Williams LR, Varon S, Peterson GM, et al. Continuous infusion of nerve growth factor prevents basal forebrain neuronal death after fimbria fornix transection. *Proc Natl Acad Sci USA* 1986; 83: 9231–9235.
73. Kromer LF. Nerve growth factor treatment after brain injury prevents neuronal death. *Science* 1987a; 235: 214–216.
74. Gage FH, Armstrong DM, Williams LR, Varon S. Morphological response of axotomized septal neurons to nerve growth factor. *J Comp Neurol* 1988; 269: 147–155.
75. Montero CN, Hefti F. Rescue of lesioned septal cholinergic neurons by nerve growth factor: specificity and requirement for chronic treatment. *J Neurosci* 1988; 8: 2986–2999.
76. Hoffman D, Wahlberg L, Aebischer P. NGF released from a polymer matrix prevents loss of ChAT expression in basal forebrain neurons following a fimbria-fornix lesion. *Exp Neurol* 1990; 110: 39–44.
77. Rosenberg MB, Friedmann T, Robertson RC, et al. Grafting genetically modified cells to the damaged brain: restorative effects of NGF expression. *Science* 1988; 242: 1575–1578.
78. Stromberg I, Wetmore CJ, Ebendal T, Ernfors P, Persson H, Olson L. Rescue of basal forebrain cholinergic neurons after implantation of genetically modified cells producing recombinant NGF. *J Neurosci Res* 1990; 25: 405–411.
79. Messersmith DJ, Kromer LF. Effects of sciatic nerve transplants on medial septal cholinergic cells after fornix/fimbria lesion. *Soc Neurosci Abstr* 1989; 15: 1093.
80. Heumann R, Korsching S, Bandtlow C, Thoenen H. Changes of nerve growth factor synthesis in nonneuronal cells in response to sciatic nerve transection. *J Cell Biol* 1987; 104: 1623–1631.
81. Messersmith DJ, Fabrazzo M, Mocchetti K, Kromer LF. Effects of sciatic nerve transplants after fimbria-fornix lesion: examination of the role of nerve growth factor. *Brain Res* 1991; 557:293–297.
82. Hagg T, Varon S. Ciliary neuronotrophic factor (CNTF) prevents neuronal degeneration and induces NGF receptors in the injured adult rat brain; comparison with NGF. *Soc Neurosci Abstr* 1991d; 17:1120.
83. Sofroniew MV, Galletly NP, Isacson O, Svend-

sen CN. Survival of adult basal forebrain cholinergic neurons after loss of target neurons. *Science* 1990; 247: 338–342.
84. Verge VM, Riopelle RJ, Richardson PM. Nerve growth factor receptors on normal and injured sensory neurons. *J Neurosci* 1989; 9: 914–922.
85. Lindsay RM, Lockett C, Sternberg J, Winter J. Neuropeptide expression in cultures of adult sensory neurons: modulation of substance P and calcitonin gene-related peptide levels by nerve growth factor. *Neuroscience* 1989; 33: 53–65.
86. Lieberman AR. Some factors affecting retrograde neuronal responses to axonal lesions. In: Bellairs R, Gray EG, eds. *Essays on the nervous system.* Oxford: Clarendon; 1974: 71–105.
87. Johnson EM, Rich KM, Yip HK. The role of NGF in sensory neurons in vivo. *Trends Neurosci* 1986; 9: 33–37.
88. Ross RA, Joh TH, Reis DJ. Reduced rate of biosynthesis of dopamine-beta-hydroxylase in the locus coeruleus during the retrograde reaction. *Brain Res* 1978; 160: 174–179.
89. Reis DJ, Ross RA, Gilad G, Joh TH. Reaction of central catecholaminergic neurons to injury: model systems for studying the neurobiology of central regeneration and sprouting. In: Cotman CW, ed. *Neuronal plasticity.* New York: Raven Press; 1978: 197–226.
90. Wood SJ, Pritchard J, Sofroniew MV. Re-expression of nerve growth factor receptor after axonal injury recapitulates a developmental event in motor neurons: differential regulation when regeneration is allowed or prevented. *Eur J Neurosci* 1990; 2: 650–657.
91. Armstrong DM, Brady R, Hersh LB, Hayes RC, Wiley RG. Expression of choline acetyltransferase and nerve growth factor receptor within hypoglossal motoneurons following nerve injury. *J Comp Neurol* 1991; 304: 596–607.
92. Hagg T, Manthorpe M, Vahlsing HL, Varon S. Delayed treatment with nerve growth factor reverses the apparent loss of cholinergic neurons after acute brain damage. *Exp Neurol* 1988; 101: 303–312.
93. Vahlsing HL, Hagg T, Spencer M, Conner JM, Manthorpe M, Varon S. Dose-dependent responses to nerve growth factor by adult rat cholinergic medial septum and neostriatum neurons. *Brain Res* 1991; 552:320–329.
94. Peterson GM, Lanford GW, Powell EW. Fate of septohippocampal neurons following fimbria-fornix transection: a time course analysis. *Brain Res Bull* 1990; 25: 129–137.
95. Tuszynski MH, Armstrong DM, Gage FH. Basal forebrain cell loss following fimbria/fornix transection. *Brain Res* 1990a; 508: 241–248.
96. O'Brien TS, Svendsen CN, Isacson O, Sofroniew MV. Loss of true labelling from the medial septum following transection of the fimbria-fornix: evidence for the death of cholinergic and non-cholinergic neurons. *Brain Res* 1990; 508: 249–256.
97. Garrett WT, McBride RL, Williams JK, Feringa ER. Prelabeling with true blue is superior to fluoro-gold in demonstrating the effect of hindlimb amputation on dorsal root ganglion neurons (DRGs). *Soc Neurosci Abstr* 1989; 15: 444.
98. Sofroniew MV, Pearson RCA, Eckenstein F, Cuello AC, Powell TPS. Retrograde changes in cholinergic neurons in the basal forebrain of the rat following cortical damage. *Brain Res* 1983; 289: 370–374.
99. Sofroniew MV, Pearson RC, Powell TP. The cholinergic nuclei of the basal forebrain of the rat: normal structure, development and experimentally induced degeneration. *Brain Res* 1987; 411: 310–331.
100. Casamenti F, Di PP, Milan F, Petrelli L, Pepeu G. Effects of nerve growth factor and GM1 ganglioside on the number and size of cholinergic neurons in rats with unilateral lesion of the nucleus basalis. *Neurosci Lett* 1989; 103: 87–91.
101. Cuello AC, Garofalo L, Kenigsberg RL, Maysinger D. Gangliosides potentiate in vivo and in vitro effects of nerve growth factor on central cholinergic neurons. *Proc Natl Acad Sci USA* 1989; 86: 2056–2060.
102. Haroutunian V, Kanof PD, Davis KL. Partial reversal of lesion-induced deficits in cortical cholinergic markers by nerve growth factor. *Brain Res* 1986; 386: 397–399.
103. Haroutunian V, Kanof PD, Davis KL. Attenuation of nucleus basalis of Meynert lesion-induced cholinergic deficits by nerve growth factor. *Brain Res* 1989; 487: 200–203.
104. Mandel RJ, Gage FH, Thal LJ. Spatial learning in rats: correlation with cortical choline acetyltransferase and improvement with NGF following NBM damage. *Exp Neurol* 1989; 104: 208–217.
105. Fischer W, Wictorin K, Björklund A, Williams LR, Varon S, Gage FH. Amelioration of cholinergic neuron atrophy and spatial memory impairment in aged rats by nerve growth factor. *Nature* 1987; 329: 65–68.
106. Kromer LF, Björklund A, Stenevi U. Innervation of embryonic hippocampal implants by regenerating axons of cholinergic septal neurons in the adult rat. *Brain Res* 1980; 210: 153–171.
107. Kromer LF, Björklund A, Stenevi U. Regeneration of the septohippocampal pathways in adult rats is promoted by utilizing embryonic hippocampal implants as bridges. *Brain Res* 1981; 210: 173–200.
108. Kromer LF, Cornbrooks CJ. Identification of trophic factors and transplanted cellular environments that promote CNS axonal regeneration. *Ann N Y Acad Sci* 1987b; 495: 207–224.
109. Tuszynski MH, Buzsaki G, Gage FH. Nerve growth factor infusions combined with fetal hippocampal grafts enhance reconstruction of the lesioned septohippocampal projection. *Neuroscience* 1990b; 36: 33–44.
110. Wendt JS, Fagg GE, Cotman CW. Regeneration of rat hippocampal fimbria fibers after fimbria transection and peripheral nerve or fetal hippocampal implantation. *Exp Neurol* 1983; 79: 452–461.
111. Hagg T, Vahlsing HL, Manthorpe M, Varon S.

Septohippocampal cholinergic axonal regeneration through peripheral nerve bridges: quantification and temporal development. *Exp Neurol* 1990a; 109: 153–163.
112. Gage FH, Björklund A. Trophic and growth-regulating mechanisms in the central nervous system monitored by intracerebral neural transplants. *Ciba Found Symp* 1987; 126: 143–159.
113. Olson L, Ayer LC, Ebendal T, et al. Grafts, growth factors and grafts that make growth factors. *Prog Brain Res* 1990; 82: 55–66.
114. Berry M, Rees L, Hall S, Yiu P, Sievers J. Optic axons regenerate into sciatic nerve isografts only in the presence of Schwann cells. *Brain Res Bull* 1988; 20: 223–231.
115. Smith GV, Stevenson JA. Peripheral nerve grafts lacking viable Schwann cells fail to support central nervous system axonal regeneration. *Exp Brain Res* 1988; 69: 299–306.
116. Muir D, Gennrich C, Varon S, Manthorpe M. Rat sciatic nerve Schwann cell microcultures: responses to mitogens and production of trophic and neurite-promoting factors. *Neurochem Res* 1989; 14: 1003–1012.
117. Varon S, Adler R. Trophic and specifying factors directed to neuronal cells. *Adv Cell Neurobiol* 1981; 2: 115–163.
118. Taniuchi M, Clark HB, Johnson EM. Expression of nerve growth factor receptors by Schwann cells of axotomized peripheral nerves: ultrastructural location, suppression by axonal contact, and binding properties. *J Neurosci* 1988; 8: 664–681.
119. Hagg T, Gulati AK, Behzadian MA, Vahlsing HL, Varon S, Manthorpe M. Nerve growth factor promotes CNS axonal regeneration into acellular peripheral nerve grafts. *Exp Neurol* 1991a; 112: 79–88.
120. Manthorpe M, Muir D, Hagg T, Varon S. Growth promoting and inhibiting factors for neurons. In: Seil F, ed. *Advances in neural regeneration research: The Third International Neural Regeneration Research Symposium*. New York: Alan R. Liss, Inc.; 1990, pp. 87–102.
121. Gasser UE, Weskamp G, Otten U, Dravid AR. Time course of the elevation of nerve growth factor (NGF) content in the hippocampus and septum following lesions of the septohippocampal pathway in rats. *Brain Res* 1986; 376: 351–356.
122. Korsching S, Heumann R, Thoenen H, Hefti F. Cholinergic denervation of the rat hippocampus by fimbrial transection leads to a transient accumulation of nerve growth factor (NGF) without change in mRNANGF content. *Neurosci Lett* 1986; 66: 175–180.
123. Larkfors L, Stromberg I, Ebendal T, Olson L. Nerve growth factor protein level increases in the adult rat hippocampus after a specific cholinergic lesion. *J Neurosci Res* 1987; 18: 525–531.
124. Hagg T, Vahlsing HL, Manthorpe M, Varon S. Nerve growth factor infusion into the denervated adult rat hippocampal formation promotes its cholinergic reinnervation. *J Neurosci* 1990b; 10: 3087–3092.
125. Schinstine M, Cornbrooks CJ. Effect of nerve growth factor on the elongation of neurites from axotomized rat embryonic septal-basal forebrain neurons: an in vitro analysis. *J Neurosci Res* 1989; 23: 371–383.
126. Cotman CW, Nieto-Sampedro M, Harris EW. Synapse replacement in the nervous system of adult vertebrates. *Physiol Rev* 1981; 61: 684–784.
127. Steward O. Lesion-induced synapse growth in the hippocampus: in search of cellular and molecular mechanisms. In: Isaacson RL, Pribam KH, eds. *The hippocampus*. New York: Plenum Press; 1986: 65–110.
128. Fagan AM, Gage FH. Cholinergic sprouting in the hippocampus: a proposed role for IL-1. *Exp Neurol* 1990; 110: 105–120.
129. Conner JM, Fass-Holmes B, Varon S. Time course of changes in nerve growth factor immunoreactivity (NGFi) in the dentate gyrus following entorhinal cortex lesion. *Soc Neurosci Abstr* 1991a; 17:139.
130. Crutcher KA, Collins F. Entorhinal lesions result in increased nerve growth factor-like growth-promoting activity in medium conditioned by hippocampal slices. *Brain Res* 1986; 399: 383–389.
131. Lindholm D, Heumann R, Meyer M, Thoenen H. Interleukin-1 regulates synthesis of nerve growth factor in non-neuronal cells of rat sciatic nerve. *Nature* 1987; 330: 658–659.
132. Carman-Krzan M, Vige X, Wise BC. Regulation by interleukin-1 of nerve growth factor secretion and nerve growth factor mRNA expression in rat primary astroglial cultures. *J Neurochem* 1991; 56: 636–643.
133. Nieto-Sampedro M, Berman MA. Interleukin-1-like activity in rat brain: sources, targets, and effect of injury. *J Neurosci Res* 1987a; 17: 214–219.
134. Loy R, Moore RY. Anomalous innervation of the hippocampal formation by peripheral sympathetic axons following mechanical injury. *Exp Neurol* 1977; 57: 645–650.
135. Crutcher KA, Brothers L, Davis JN. Sympathetic noradrenergic sprouting in response to central cholinergic denervation: a histochemical study of neuronal sprouting in the rat hippocampal formation. *Brain Res* 1981; 210: 115–128.
136. Crutcher KA. Sympathetic sprouting in the central nervous system: a model for studies of axonal growth in the mature mammalian brain [published erratum appears in *Brain Res* 1987 Nov; 434(4): 467]. *Brain Res* 1987; 434: 203–233.
137. Saffran BN, Woo JE, Mobley WC, Crutcher KA. Intraventricular NGF infusion in the mature rat brain enhances sympathetic innervation of cerebrovascular targets but fails to elicit sympathetic ingrowth. *Brain Res* 1989; 492: 245–254.
138. Butcher LL, Woolf NJ. Cholinergic neuronal regeneration can be modified by growth fac-

tors. In: Dowdall MJ, Hawthorne JN, eds. *Cellular and molecular basis of cholinergic function*, vol. Chichester, U.K.: Ellis Horwood; 1987: 395–402.
139. Farris TW, Butcher LL. Reinnervation of medial cortex by cholinergic projections from basal forebrain: an in vivo model to test hypothesis about regeneration with growth factors. *Soc Neurosci Abstr* 1990; 16: 1158.
140. Wendt JS, Ayyad KA. Is there regeneration of cholinergic axons through traumatic scar tissue in adult mammalian brain? *Exp Neurol* 1987; 95: 65–75.
141. Ernfors P, Ebendal T, Olson L, Mouton P, Stromberg I, Persson H. A cell line producing recombinant nerve growth factor evokes growth responses in intrinsic and grafted central cholinergic neurons. *Proc Natl Acad Sci USA* 1989; 86: 4756–4760.
142. Garofalo L, Ribeiro-da-Silva A, Cuello AC. Effect of decortication and trophic factor treatment on the ChAT immunoreactive fiber network of the adult rat cortex. *Soc Neurosci Abstr* 1990; 16: 296.
143. Carmignoto G, Maffei L, Candeo P, Canella R, Comelli C. Effect of NGF on the survival of rat retinal ganglion cells following optic nerve section. *J Neurosci* 1989; 9: 1263–1272.
144. Villegas PM, Vidal SM, Bray GM, Aguayo AJ. Influences of peripheral nerve grafts on the survival and regrowth of axotomized retinal ganglion cells in adult rats. *J Neurosci* 1988; 8: 265–280.
145. Carter DA, Bray GM, Aguayo AJ. Regenerated retinal ganglion cell axons can form well-differentiated synapses in the superior colliculus of adult hamsters. *J Neurosci* 1989; 9: 4042–4050.
146. Vidal SM, Bray GM, Villegas PM, Thanos S, Aguayo AJ. Axonal regeneration and synapse formation in the superior colliculus by retinal ganglion cells in the adult rat. *J Neurosci* 1987; 7: 2894–2909.
147. Aguayo AJ, Bray GM, Rasminsky M, Zwimpfer T, Carter D, Vidal SM. Synaptic connections made by axons regenerating in the central nervous system of adult mammals. *J Exp Biol* 1990; 153: 199–224.
148. Carmignoto G, Comelli MC, Candeo P, et al. Expression of NGF receptor and NGF receptor mRNA in the developing and adult rat retina. *Exp Neurol* 1991; 111: 302–311.
149. Ehrlich D, Keyser K, Manthorpe M, Varon S, Karten HJ. Differential effects of axotomy on substance P-containing and nicotinic acetylcholine receptor-containing retinal ganglion cells: time course of degeneration and effects of nerve growth factor. *Neuroscience* 1990; 36: 699–723.
150. Kunkel-Bagden E, Bregman BS. NGF prevents the retrograde cell loss of red nucleus neurons after spinal cord injury at birth. *Soc Neurosci Abstr* 1990; 16: 479.
151. Barron KD. Comparative observations on the cytological reactions of central and peripheral nerve cells to axotomy. In: Kao CC, Bunge RP, Reier PJ, eds. *Spinal cord reconstruction*. New York: Raven Press; 1983: 7–39.
152. Feringa E, McBride RL, Varon S, Manthorpe M. Continuous nerve growth factor (NGF) treatment normalizes HRP transport in axotomized rubrospinal neurons. *J Neuropathol Exp Neurol* 1989b; 48: 362.
153. Feringa E, McBride RL, Pruitt JN, et al. Intraventricular nerve growth factor (NGF) effect on axotomized cortico-spinal neurons in vivo. *Neurology* (suppl) 1989a: 39–426.
154. Kuhlengel KR, Bunge MB, Bunge RP, Burton H. Implantation of cultured sensory neurons and Schwann cells into lesioned neonatal rat spinal cord. II. Implant characteristics and examination of corticospinal tract growth. *J Comp Neurol* 1990; 293: 74–91.
155. Assouline JG, Bosch P, Lim R, Kim IS, Jensen R, Pantazis NJ. Rat astrocytes and Schwann cells in culture synthesize nerve growth factor-like neurite-promoting factors. *Brain Res* 1987; 428: 103–118.
156. Carlstedt T, Cullheim S, Risling M, Ulfhake B. Nerve fibre regeneration across the PNS-CNS interface at the root-spinal cord junction. *Brain Res Bull* 1989; 22: 93–102.
157. Siegal JD, Kliot M, Smith GM, Silver J. A comparison of the regeneration potential of dorsal root fibers into gray or white matter of the adult rat spinal cord. *Exp Neurol* 1990; 109: 90–97.
158. Yasuda T, Sobue G, Ito T, Mitsuma T, Takahashi A. Nerve growth factor enhances neurite arborization of adult sensory neurons; a study in single-cell culture. *Brain Res* 1990; 524: 54–63.
159. Da Silva CF, Langone F. Addition of nerve growth factor to the interior of a tubular prosthesis increases sensory neuron regeneration in vivo. *Braz J Med Biol Res* 1989; 22: 691–694.
160. Rich KM, Alexander TD, Pryor JC, Hollowell JP. Nerve growth factor enhances regeneration through silicone chambers. *Exp Neurol* 1989; 105: 162–170.
161. Houle JD, Johnson JE. Nerve growth factor (NGF)-treated nitrocellulose enhances and directs the regeneration of adult rat dorsal root axons through intraspinal neural tissue transplants. *Neurosci Lett* 1989; 103: 17–23.
162. Pettmann B, Manthorpe M, Powell JA, Varon S. Biological activities of nerve growth factor bound to nitrocellulose paper by Western blotting. *J Neurosci* 1988; 8: 3624–3632.
163. Leibrock J, Lottspeich F, Hohn A, et al. Molecular cloning and expression of brain-derived neurotrophic factor. *Nature* 1989; 341: 149–152.
164. Hohn A, Leibrock J, Bailey K, Barde YA. Identification and characterization of a novel member of the nerve growth factor/brain-derived neurotrophic factor family. *Nature* 1990; 344: 339–341.
165. Ernfors P, Ibanez CF, Ebendal T, Olson L, Persson H. Molecular cloning and neurotrophic activities of a protein with structural similarities to nerve growth factor: developmental and

topographical expression in the brain. *Proc Natl Acad Sci USA* 1990b; 87: 5454–5458.
166. Kaisho Y, Yoshimura K, Nakahama K. Cloning and expression of a cDNA encoding a novel human neurotrophic factor. *FEBS Lett* 1990; 266: 187–191.
167. Maisonpierre PC, Belluscio L, Squinto S, et al. Neurotrophin-3: a neurotrophic factor related to NGF and BDNF. *Science* 1990; 247: 1446–1451.
168. Rosenthal A, Goeddel DV, Nguyen T, et al. Primary structure and biological activity of a novel human neurotrophic factor. *Neuron* 1990; 4: 767–773.
169. Jones KR, Reichardt LF. Molecular cloning of a human gene that is a member of the nerve growth factor family. *Proc Natl Acad Sci USA* 1990; 87: 8060–8064.
170. Hallbook F, Ibanez CF, Persson H. Evolutionary studies of the nerve growth factor family reveal a novel member abundantly expressed in Xenopus ovary. *Neuron* 1991; 6: 845–858.
171. Hofer M, Pagliusi SR, Hohn A, Leibrock J, Barde YA. Regional distribution of brain-derived neurotrophic factor mRNA in the adult mouse brain. *Embo J* 1990; 9: 2459–2464.
172. Philips HS, Hains JM, Laramee GR, Rosenthal A, Winslow JW. Widespread expression of BDNF but not NT3 by target areas of basal forebrain cholinergic neurons. *Science* 1990; 250: 290–294.
173. Knusel B, Winslow JW, Rosenthal A, et al. Promotion of central cholinergic and dopaminergic neuron differentiation by brain-derived neurotrophic factor but not neurotrophin 3. *Proc Natl Acad Sci USA* 1991; 88: 961–965.
174. Hyman C, Hofer M, Barde YA, et al. BDNF is a neurotrophic factor for dopaminergic neurons of the substantia nigra. *Nature* 1991; 350: 230–232.
175. Manthorpe M, Louis JC, Hagg T, Varon S. The ciliary neuronotrophic factor. In: Fallon J, Loughlin S, eds. *Neurotrophic factors.* San Diego: Academic Press; 1992 (in press).
176. Adler R, Landa KB, Manthorpe M, Varon S. Cholinergic neuronotrophic factors: intraocular distribution of trophic activity for ciliary neurons. *Science* 1979; 204: 1434–1436.
177. Landa KB, Adler R, Manthorpe M, Varon S. Cholinergic neuronotrophic factors: III. Developmental increase of trophic activity for chick embryo ciliary ganglion neurons in their intraocular target tissues. *Dev Biol* 1980; 74: 401–408.
178. Arakawa Y, Sendtner M, Thoenen H. Survival effect of ciliary neurotrophic factor (CNTF) on chick embryonic motoneurons in culture: comparison with other neurotrophic factors and cytokines. *J Neurosci* 1990; 10: 3507–3515.
179. Magal E, Burnham P, Varon S. Effect of ciliary neuronotrophic factor on rat spinal cord neurons in vitro: survival and expression of choline acetyltransferase and low-affinity nerve growth factor receptors. *Dev Brain Res* 1991; 63:141–150.
180. Wong V, Arriaga R, Lindsay RM. Effects of ciliary neurotrophic factor (CNTF) on ventral spinal cord neurons in culture. *Soc Neurosci Abstr* 1990; 16: 384.
181. Oppenheim RW, Prevette D, Qin-Wei Y, Collins F, MacDonald J. Control of embryonic motoneurons survival in vivo by ciliary neurotrophic factor (CNTF). *Science* 1991a; 251: 1616–1618.
182. Stöckli KA, Lottspeich F, Sendtner M, et al. Molecular cloning, expression and regional distribution of rat ciliary neurotrophic factor. *Nature* 1989; 342: 920–923.
183. Rende M, Muir D, Ruoslahti E, Hagg T, Varon S, Manthorpe M. Immunolocalization of ciliary neurotrophic factor in adult rat sciatic nerve. *Glia* 1991; 5:25–32.
184. Sendtner M, Kreutzberg GW, Thoenen H. Ciliary neurotrophic factor prevents the degeneration of motor neurons after axotomy. *Nature* 1990; 345: 440–441.
185. Manthorpe M, Rudge J, Varon S. Astroglial cell contributions to neuronal survival and neuritic growth. In: Fedoroff S, Vernadakis A, eds. *Astrocytes,* vol 2. San Diego: Academic Press; 1986: 315–376.
186. Manthorpe M, Pettmann B, Varon S. Modulation of astroglial cell output of neuronotrophic and neurite promoting factors. In: Norenberg M, Hertz L, Schousboe A, eds. *The biochemical pathology of astrocytes,* vol 39. New York: Alan R. Liss, Inc.; 1988: 41–57.
187. Rudge JS, Manthorpe M, Varon S. The output of neuronotrophic and neurite-promoting agents from rat brain astroglial cells: a microculture method for screening potential regulatory molecules. *Dev Brain Res* 1985; 19: 161–172.
188. Rudge JS, Davis GE, Manthorpe M, Varon S. An examination of ciliary neuronotrophic factors from avian and rodent tissue extracts using a blot and culture technique. *Brain Res* 1987; 429: 103–110.
189. Rudge JS, Alderson RF, Ip N, Lindsay RM. Characterization of ciliary neurotrophic factor in rat astrocytes. *Soc Neurosci Abstr* 1990; 16: 484.
190. Magal E, Burnham P, Varon S. Effects of CNTF on low-affinity NGF receptor expression by cultured neurons from different rat brain regions. *J Neurosci Res* 1991; 30:560–566.
191. Gospodarowicz D, Neufeld G, Schweigerer L. Fibroblast growth factor. *Mol Cell Endocrinol* 1986; 46: 187–204.
192. Klagsbrun M. The fibroblast growth factor family: structural and biological properties. *Prog Growth Factor Res* 1989; 1: 207–235.
193. Baird A, Walicke PA. Fibroblast growth factors. *Br Med Bull* 1989; 45: 438–452.
194. Burgess WH, Maciag T. The heparin-binding (fibroblast) growth factor family of proteins. *Annu Rev Biochem* 1989; 58: 575–606.
195. Gonzalez AM, Buscaglia M, Ong M, Baird A. Distribution of basic fibroblast growth factor in

the 18-day rat fetus: localization in the basement membranes of diverse tissues. *J Cell Biol* 1990; 110: 753–765.
196. Wanaka A, Johnson EJ, Milbrandt J. Localization of FGF receptor mRNA in the adult rat central nervous system by in situ hybridization. *Neuron* 1990; 5: 267–281.
197. Ferguson IA, Wanaka A, Johnson EMJ. bFGF undergoes receptor-mediated transport in CNS neurons. *Soc Neurosci Abstr* 1990b; 16: 824.
198. Ferguson IA, Schweitzer JB, Johnson EJ. Basic fibroblast growth factor: receptor-mediated internalization, metabolism, and anterograde axonal transport in retinal ganglion cells. *J Neurosci* 1990a; 10: 2176–2189.
199. Nieto-Sampedro M, Lim R, Hicklin DJ, Cotman CW. Early release of glia maturation factor and acidic fibroblast growth factor after rat brain injury. *Neurosci Lett* 1988c; 86: 361–365.
200. Finklestein SP, Apostolides PJ, Caday CG, Prosser J, Philips MF, Klagsbrun M. Increased basic fibroblast growth factor (bFGF) immunoreactivity at the site of focal brain wounds. *Brain Res* 1988; 460: 253–259.
201. Walicke PA. Novel neurotrophic factors, receptors, and oncogenes. *Annu Rev Neurosci* 1989; 12: 103–126.
202. Eckenstein FP, Esch F, Holbert T, Blacher RW, Nishi R. Purification and characterization of a trophic factor for embryonic peripheral neurons: comparison with fibroblast growth factors. *Neuron* 1990; 4: 623–631.
203. Sievers J, Hausmann B, Unsicker K, Berry M. Fibroblast growth factors promote the survival of adult rat retinal ganglion cells after transection of the optic nerve. *Neurosci Lett* 1987; 76: 157–162.
204. Barotte C, Eclancher F, Ebel A, Labourdette G, Sensenbrenner M, Will B. Effects of basic fibroblast growth factor (bFGF) on choline acetyltransferase activity and astroglial reaction in adult rats after partial fimbria transection. *Neurosci Lett* 1989; 101: 197–202.
205. Anderson KJ, Dam D, Lee S, Cotman CW. Basic fibroblast growth factor prevents death of lesioned cholinergic neurons in vivo. *Nature* 1988; 332: 360–361.
206. Otto D, Frotscher M, Unsicker K. Basic fibroblast growth factor and nerve growth factor administered in gel foam rescue medial septal neurons after fimbria fornix transection. *J Neurosci Res* 1989; 22: 83–91.
207. Yoshida K, Gage FH. Fibroblast growth factors stimulate nerve growth factor synthesis and secretion by astrocytes. *Brain Res* 1991; 538: 118–126.
208. Fukumoto H, Kakihana M. Suno M. Recombinant human basic fibroblast growth factor (rhbFGF) induces secretion of nerve growth factor (NGF) in cultured rat astroglial cells. *Neurosci Lett* 1991; 122: 221–224.
209. Saneto RP, de Vellis J. Characterization of cultured rat olidodendrocytes proliferating in a serum-free, chemically-defined medium. *Proc Natl Acad Sci USA* 1985; 82: 3509–3513.
210. Besnard F, Perraud F, Sensenbrenner M, Labourdette G. Effects of acidic and basic fibroblast growth factors on proliferation and maturation of cultured rat oligodendrocytes. *Int J Dev Neurosci* 1989; 7: 401–409.
211. Noble M, Wolswijk G, Wren D. The complex relationship between cell division and the control of differentiation in oligodendrocyte-type-2 astrocyte progenitor cells isolated from perinatal and adult rat optic nerves. *Prog Growth Factor Res* 1989; 1: 179–194.
212. McKinnon RD, Matsui T, Dubois DM, Aaronson SA. FGF modulates the PDGF-driven pathway of oligodendrocyte development. *Neuron* 1990; 5: 603–614.
213. Cohen S. Isolation of a mouse submaxillary gland protein accelerating incisor eruption and eyelid opening in the newborn animal. *J Biol Chem* 1962; 237: 1555–1562.
214. Cohen S. Epidermal growth factor. *In vitro cell Dev Biol* 1987; 23: 239–246.
215. Stoscheck CM, King LEJ. Functional and structural characteristics of EGF and its receptor and their relationship to transforming proteins. *J Cell Biochem* 1986; 31: 135–152.
216. Kornblum HI, Raymon HK, Morrison RS, Cavanaugh KP, Bradshaw RA, Leslie FM. Epidermal growth factor and basic fibroblast growth factor: effects on an overlapping population of neocortical neurons in vitro. *Brain Res* 1990; 535: 255–263.
217. Morrison R, Sharma A, de Vellis J, Bradshaw R. Basic fibroblasts growth factor supports the survival of cerebral cortical neurons in primary cultures. *Proc Natl Acad Sci USA* 1986; 83: 7537–7541.
218. Schaudies RP, Christian EL, Savage CJ. Epidermal growth factor immunoreactive material in the rat brain. Localization and identification of multiple species. *J Biol Chem* 1989; 264: 10447–10450.
219. Rall LB, Scott J, Bell GI, et al. Mouse preproepidermal growth factor synthesis by the kidney and other tissues. *Nature* 1985; 313: 228–231.
220. Fallon JH, Seroogy KB, Loughlin SL, et al. Epidermal growth factor immunoreactive material in the central nervous system: location and development. *Science* 1984; 224: 1107–1109.
221. Nieto-Sampedro M, Gomez PF, Knauer DJ, Broderick JT. Epidermal growth factor receptor immunoreactivity in rat brain astrocytes. Response to injury. *Neurosci Lett* 1988a; 91: 276–282.
222. Adamson ED, Meek J. The ontogeny of epidermal growth factor receptors during mouse development. *Dev Biol* 1984; 103: 62–70.
223. Hadjiconstantiou M, Finkin JG, Dalia A, Neff NH. Epidermal growth factor enhances streatal dopaminergic parameters in the 1-methyl-4-phenyl-1,2,3,6-tetrahydropyridine-treated mouse. *J Neurochem* 1991; 57: 479–482.
224. Nieto-Sampedro M. Astrocyte mitogen inhibitor related to epidermal growth factor receptor. *Science* 1988b; 240: 1784–1786.
225. Giulian D, Lachman LB. Interleukin-1 stimu-

lates astroglial proliferation after brain injury. *Science* 1985; 228: 497–499.
226. Giulian D, Young DG, Woodward J, Brown DC, Lachman LB. Interleukin-1 is an astroglial growth factor in the developing brain. *J Neurosci* 1988; 8: 709–714.
227. Nieto-Sampedro M, Chandy KG. Interleukin-2-like activity in injured rat brain. *Neurochem Res* 1987b; 12: 723–727.
228. Farrar WL, Vinocour M, Hill JM. In situ hybridization histochemistry localization of interleukin-3 mRNA in mouse brain. *Blood* 1989; 73: 137–140.
229. Kamegai M, Niijima K, Kunishita T, et al. Interleukin 3 as a trophic factor for central cholinergic neurons in vitro and in vivo. *Neuron* 1990; 4: 429–436.
230. Hagg T, Varon S. Neurotropism of nerve growth factor for adult rat septal cholinergic axons in vivo. *Exp Neurol* (in press).
231. Stöckli KA, Lillian LE, Näher-Noé M, et al. Regional distribution, developmental changes, and cellular localization of CNTF-mRNA and protein in the rat brain. *J Cell Biol* 1991; 115: 447–459.

14
Pharmacology of Neuronal Regeneration

Alfredo Gorio, Anna Maria Di Giulio, and Paolo Mantegazza

Department of Medical Pharmacology, University of Milan, 20129 Milan, Italy

It is well established that neurons express dynamic properties such as synaptic and dendrite remodeling that are accelerated during development or as a consequence of injuries or degenerative disorders in the adult nervous system (1,2). These changes are strictly dependent on the typical neuronal morphology, and it is apparent that the convergence of the incoming signals upon the cell body and dendrites and the divergence of the outgoing signals via the axonal arborization regulate both cellular organization of the brain and neuronal reactive properties (Figs. 1,2). The morphological relationship between neuronal functions and plasticity is reinforced by several reports suggesting that maintenance of synaptic contacts, neuronal plasticity, and neurite outgrowth might be regulated also by neurotransmitters. It has been suggested that the environmental informations might be supplemented by synaptic regulations of membrane potential or of intracellular levels of second messengers such as calcium ions and cAMP (3). Neuronal regeneration is a morpho-functional process aiming at the reestablishment of the lost detailed neuronal organization by reconstructing the peripheral axon and its terminal arborization. The first description of the anatomical reconstruction of a damaged nerve was made in the XVIII century by Felice Fontana, personal medical doctor of the Grand Duke of Toscany (4) and famous scientist of his time. He described the peripheral nerve as constituted by long cylindrical discs containing a transparent gelatinous humour with moving particles (probably mitochondria). Twenty-nine days after axotomy caused by section of the rabbit hypoglossal nerve, he observed that the nerve was reconstituted and the lesion site was not obvious any more. Felice Fontana reached the conclusion that the hypoglossal nerve reproduced the injured parts. It is now well known that neuronal regeneration is different from that of other organs. The damaged or dead neurons cannot be substituted by others surviving the lesion by means of mitotic division, regeneration in the nervous system means reformation of the lost parts by re-elongation of the proximal portions with reformation of the degenerated processes. In addition to the regeneration of the injured neurons, there is another very important phenomenon of repair that takes place when an area is partially denervated. The surviving intact axons expand their territory of innervation by collateral sprouting and promote the recovery of functions of the denervated target (Colorplates 1-3).

The aim of any pharmacological or surgical manipulation for the treatment of neuronal injuries is to favor the achievement of the above-described reparatory events. It is generally accepted that the biology of neuronal regeneration is a complex phenomenon involving several other constituents of the nervous system in addition to the injured axons directly implicated in the de-

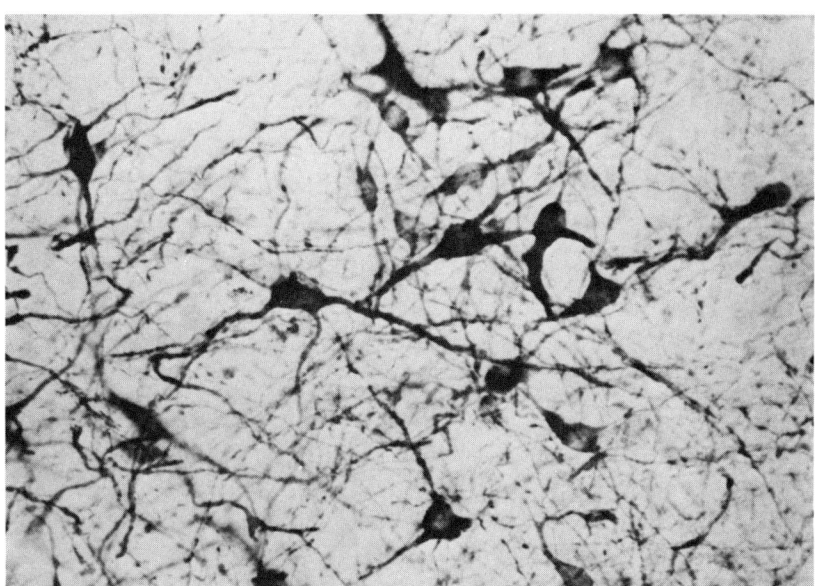

FIG. 1. Neurons, dendrites, and axons stained with antibodies to tyrosine hydroxylase in the pars reticulata of the substantia nigra.

generation and regeneration processes. Even for peripheral nerve injuries we must consider the retrograde changes implicating the lesioned neuron and others connected transsynaptically as in the case of the sensory system. Among nonneuronal structures a role is likely played by satellite and glial cells, the sheath cells of the peripheral nerves, and the microvasculature. The identification of those factors that act by limiting neuronal regeneration has been a primary target for the last two decades of research in this field. A major aim of this paper is to define some of these limiting factors as experimental tools for evaluating the efficacy of drugs that should be able to modify and overcome or circumvent them. A positive outcome would suggest the potential efficacy of the agent on neuronal regeneration. Ideally we have two goals: One is to enhance the intrinsic potential of a neuron to regenerate, and the other is to modify the environment (glial cells and substrates), improving its supporting capacity. The former is to identify a substance that would transform a neuron into a superpowerful machinery with regenerative properties significantly exceeding the normal rate of axonal regeneration. The latter aim would imply an alteration of the cellular and molecular composition of the neuronal and axonal environment increasing its supporting activity or by transforming a nonpermissive substrate into a permissive one. This problem might be particularly relevant for CNS neurons, since several recent reports have suggested that a modification of the environment may significantly improve axonal regeneration (1,2,5). In the past years several treatments were developed for degenerative diseases of the peripheral nervous system aiming at the improvement of nerve regeneration. The results are encouraging and some of them are reported in the second part of the paper.

RETROGRADE CHANGES FOLLOWING AXOTOMY

The survival of lesioned neurons is an obvious fundamental prerequisite for regen-

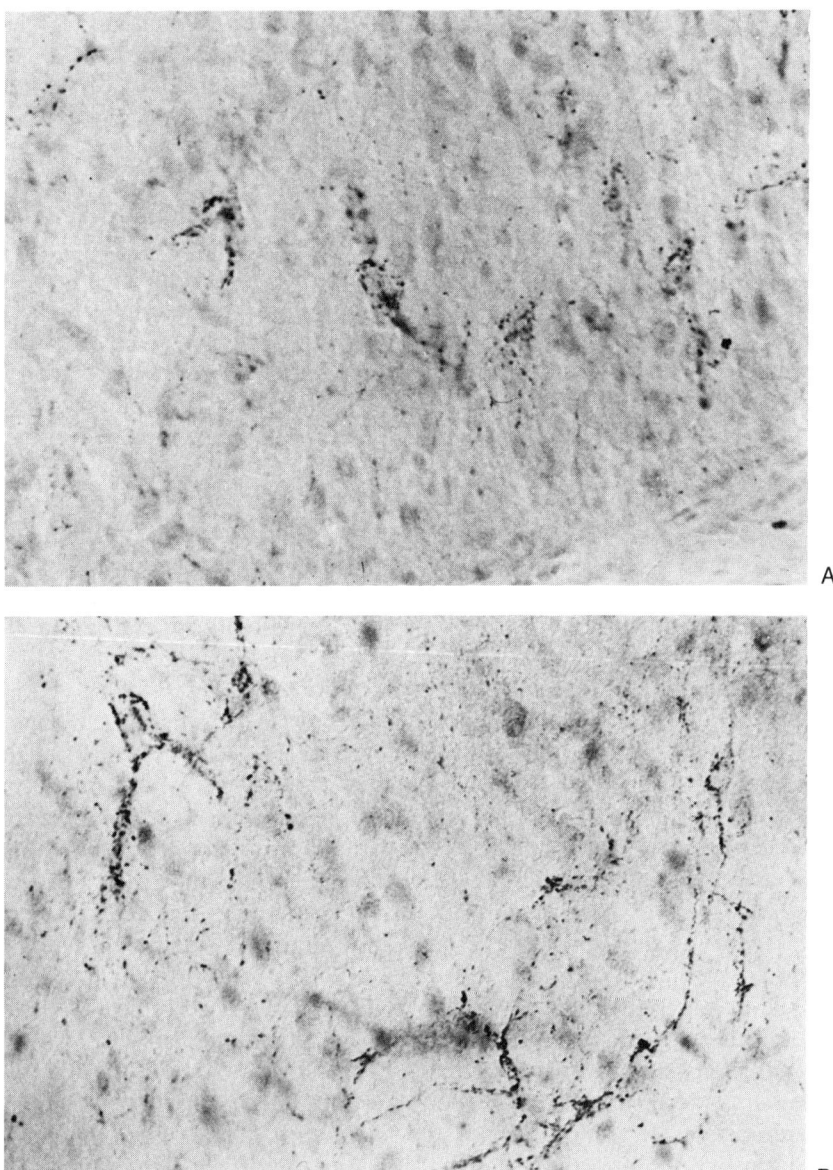

FIG. 2. Synaptic boutons stained with antibodies to tyrosine hydroxylase outline cell bodies and dendrites of neurons in the septum. **A:** In control animals such stains are contained at the level of the proximal portion of the dendrites. **B:** Following neonatal lesion with 6-OHDA, which depletes noradrenaline innervation, the number of tyrosine hydroxylase-positive boutons increases markedly, outlining also the upper portions of the dendrites.

eration. Many agents have shown activity by enhancing neuronal survival in vitro; however, the activity of these substances will become much more significant if the neuron survival test is further performed in vivo. The rescue of neurons otherwise destined for death or the reduction of retrograde degenerative events are equally important. The blockade of retrograde degeneration will prompt a more efficient regenerative process, while an effect on survival is desirable in the treatment of any neurological degenerative disorder. Such a goal was not even a hope 15–20 years ago; however, the discovery and the detailed description of site of synthesis and activity of several specific neurotrophic factors have changed the scene in a significant manner (6,7). Several research groups are directing their efforts in this direction in the hope of finding a cure for traumatic, vascular and, in general, degenerative diseases of the nervous system.

The time course and the extent of the retrograde changes following axotomy of peripheral nerves are well described in the literature. Sympathetic, sensory, and motor neurons are affected although with distinct differences. Perhaps the alterations occurring to the sensory system might be more useful to our purpose and will be discussed earlier. While crush is ineffective, sciatic nerve section causes degeneration in the dorsal root ganglion and intraspinally at the level of the dorsal horn. In the dorsal root ganglia there is a loss of about 30% of the axotomized sensory neurons, the cell death process taking place between 10 and 60 days after sciatic nerve section. Such a loss increases up to 75% if the nerve lesion is performed neonatally (8). There are also significant changes in the substantia gelatinosa ipsilaterally to the lesioned nerve. Between 10 and 15 days after sciatic nerve lesion there is a significant decrease of the order of 40–50% of substance P immunoreactivity as shown by immunocytochemistry and by radioimmunoassay (9). In addition to and concomitantly with substance P loss met-enkephalin boutons degenerate in the laminae I and II of the dorsal horn ipsilaterally to the lesion (9). The extent of the degeneration is similar for both peptidergic systems. Therefore peripheral nerve lesions cause direct degeneration of sensory neurons and of their central projections, and a transcellular intraspinal degenerative atrophy of axon terminals belonging to interneurons located in the substantia gelatinosa. These peptidergic denervations of the dorsal horn are gradually reverted by means of collateral sprouting of the surviving axons (8,9). In the dorsal horn the changes caused by the lesion can be visualized also using the fluoride-resistant acid phosphatase histological stain (Color Figure 4), which shows a significant loss of stain ipsilaterally to the lesion. The peptidergic alterations are preceded by a significant increase of 5-HT turnover in the lumbar cord; such an increase begins within 24 hours after axotomy and lasts over 7–10 days (11). 5-HT might play an important role in these changes. If rats are pretreated with para-chlorophenylalanine to deplete serotonin and then the sciatic nerve is lesioned there is no degeneration of met-enkephalin in the spinal cord while substance P loss occurs normally (11). The role of 5-HT in dorsal horn plasticity is further emphasized by its reduced turnover during the period of substance P and met-enkephalin restoration 60–90 days after sciatic nerve lesion (10). Another early signal triggered by axotomy is the ornithine decarboxylase (ODC) activity in dorsal root ganglia. Forty-eight hours after sciatic nerve resection there is a ten- to 20-fold increase in ODC activity in dorsal root ganglia ipsilaterally to the lesion (12).

In conclusion the above data suggest some parameters that can be utilized at various time after axotomy of sensory peripheral nerves for assessing potential efficacy on preventing retrograde degeneration by novel agents.

1. Short-term responses: effects upon ODC activity in DRG and 5-HT turnover in the lumbar cord 48 hours after axotomy
2. Intermediate-term responses: effects upon loss of substance P and met-enkephalin innervation of the substantia gelatinosa occurring 10–14 days after axotomy
3. Late-term responses: effects upon loss of neurons in the dorsal root ganglion 60–90 days after axotomy

Indeed a few substances have been tested in this experimental paradigm. NGF was applied for 3 weeks to the cut end of the proximal stump, while neuronal loss was evaluated 9 weeks after injury. It was found that the treatment reduced significantly the neuronal loss in the dorsal root ganglion (13). Recently it was shown that treatment with acetyl-l-carnitine prevents the changes in 5-HT turnover and peptidergic denervation of the substantia gelatinosa after chronic sciatic nerve axotomy (14). Also, gangliosides were tested, the result being that continuous treatment up to the day of sacrifice reduced the loss of spinal cord met-enkephalin with no effects on retrograde substance P sensory axon degeneration (10). These data suggest that NGF and acetyl-l-carnitine have neuroprotective activity on the injured neurons and intraspinally, while gangliosides might affect trans-synaptic degenerative processes with no protective effects upon the lesioned sensory neurons.

Similar tests on neuronal survival might be performed with sympathetic ganglia after axotomy or immunosympathectomy. With this experimental paradigm it was shown that polyamine treatment enhances survival of sympathetic neurons in vivo (15). The in vivo effects of neurotrophic factors were originally evaluated with this neuronal system looking at neuronal survival in the superior cervical and nodose ganglions (16–18). This in vivo test has differentiated BDNF and NGF from a variety of proteins and peptides that can promote neuronal survival in vitro but that were never tested or are lacking activity in these experimental conditions. In addition to the quantitative morphological evaluation of the cell number one can assay tyrosine hydroxylase activity and the enzyme mRNA levels that are reduced in the ganglion after axotomy (19).

Enhancement of motor neuron survival after axotomy in neonates also offers a good testing model. It is well known that developmentally regulated motor neuron death occurs during the embryological period and is completed before birth. On the other hand, axotomy of peripheral nerves causes a marked loss of motor neuron if performed in neonates, while in adults animals there are no alterations (20–22). It was recently reported that a 22 kD polypeptide extracted from the skeletal muscle was capable of preventing natural motor neuron death if supplied to the embryos during that critical period; such a substance is named choline acetyltransferase (ChAT) developmental factor (CDF) because it increases markedly ChAT activity when supplemented to motoneurons in culture (23). CDF does not prevent sensory and sympathetic neurons natural death (23).

In recent years, the role of neurotrophic substances in CNS injuries has been tested. It was found that after brain hypoxia the levels of NGF are elevated in several brain areas (24) and that NGF applied intraventricularly enhances survival of septal neurons after axotomy (for more extended informations on neurotrophic factors see Hagg et al., Chapter 13, and Gold and Spencer, Chapter 6, this volume). A similar rescuing effect on axotomized septal neurons was observed for basic fibroblast growth factor (bFGF) applied in situ (25,26). The local application of bFGF on the axons at the site of lesion also rescued from death retinal and sensory neurons (27). More recently it was shown that intra-

administration of bFGF prevents photoreceptor degeneration in rats with inherited retinal dystrophy; the survival effect of a single injection could last over 2 months (28).

NEURONAL REGENERATION: EXPERIMENTAL PARADIGMS AND TREATMENTS FOR ENHANCING REGENERATION IN THE NERVOUS SYSTEM

Regeneration in CNS

The same molecular and cellular mechanisms underlying reversal of degenerative events and rescue of dying neurons are likely linked to axonal regeneration. Therefore agents that might be capable of enhancing neuronal survival and of preventing retrograde degenerative events caused by trauma or by insults related to degenerative disorders hold the potential for being active on increasing the regenerative capacity of neurons. Indeed, as it will be shown later, several substances that have displayed activity by preventing neuronal retrograde degeneration are also capable of enhancing neuronal regeneration in a variety of experimental models.

Neuronal regeneration is believed to be restricted to peripheral nervous system; however many neurons in the brain and spinal cord are capable of significant axonal regeneration if the injured axons are exposed to a favorable environment such as the one provided by peripheral nerves (29). Such an observation was made originally by Santiago Ramón y Cajal early in the century: He reported that axons entered peripheral nerve stumps placed in the brain and spinal cord (30). With the application of neuroanatomical tracing techniques it was shown that the axons entering peripheral nerves grafts were originating from CNS neurons and not from axons innervating the blood vessels and meninges (31,32). These regenerating axons can elongate for several centimeters, a distance much longer than they normally attain, and are myelinated by the Schwann cells (31). By connecting a severed optic nerve with a peripheral nerve graft it has been possible to reconnect 10% of retinal ganglion cells with far and deep brain areas such as the superior culliculus (33). In addition to the regenerative effect, also the enhanced retinal ganglionic cell survival was likely due to the trophic action of the peripheral nerve graft (34). These data would suggest that the lesion itself may supply the initial stimulus capable of triggering the initial steps of axonal regeneration even in the case of central nervous system neurons, and that the peripheral nerve environment supplies both a proper substrate for outgrowth and some trophic factors required for neuronal survival.

Another experimental tool for improving axonal regeneration in CNS is the neuronal transplantation technique. At first it was shown that grafted neurons survive in the new environment and can restitute functions: The transplantation into the striatum of embryonic dopamine (DA) neurons reversed the behavioral abnormalities caused by the destruction of the DA nigrostriatal pathway. The grafted neurons form neurites reinnervating the denervated striatum of the host (35,36). The essential requirement for the donor is that the neurons transplanted must be fetal. The early transplantation experiments used solid pieces of selected brain areas that were placed in cavities surgically prepared in proximity of the target to be innervated (37–39). The subsequent development using dissociated neurons from younger fetuses (about 13–15 day old embryos for DA neurons) allowed the implantation in deeper structures and reduced the tissue damage caused by the cavitation method (40). In addition to the above advantages and the increased anatomical precision in placing the graft, the cell suspension technique gives behavioral changes at a much earlier time. The recovery is observed in a few weeks compared to months as in the case of the solid grafts. The behavioral recovery is correlated with

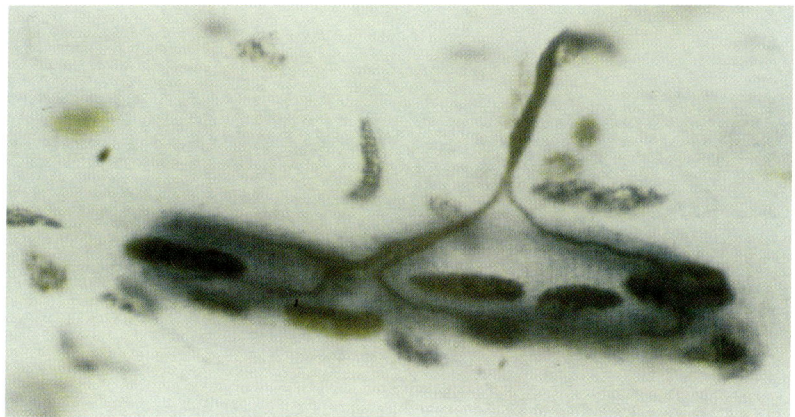

Colorplate 1. Axon terminals silver impregnated branching and making synapse on a muscle fiber. The end-plate is outlined by AChE stain. (From ref. 75, with permission of authors and editors.)

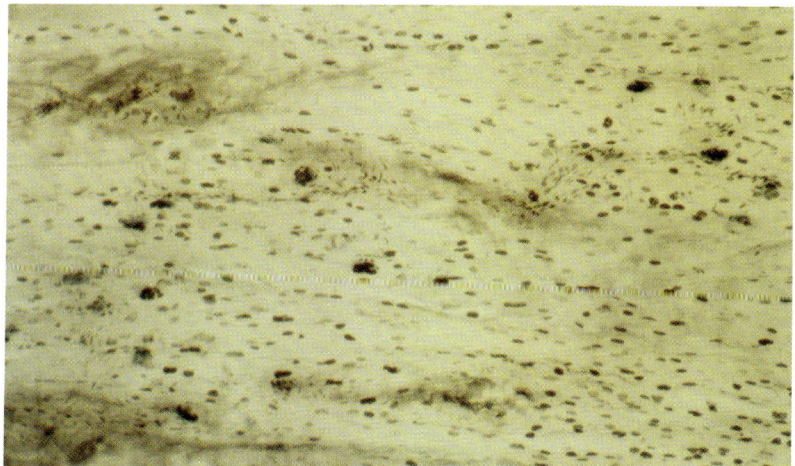

Colorplate 2. In a denervated muscle the blue spots indicate the former neuromuscular junctions, and the stream of small nuclei show the path of the degenerated nerve.

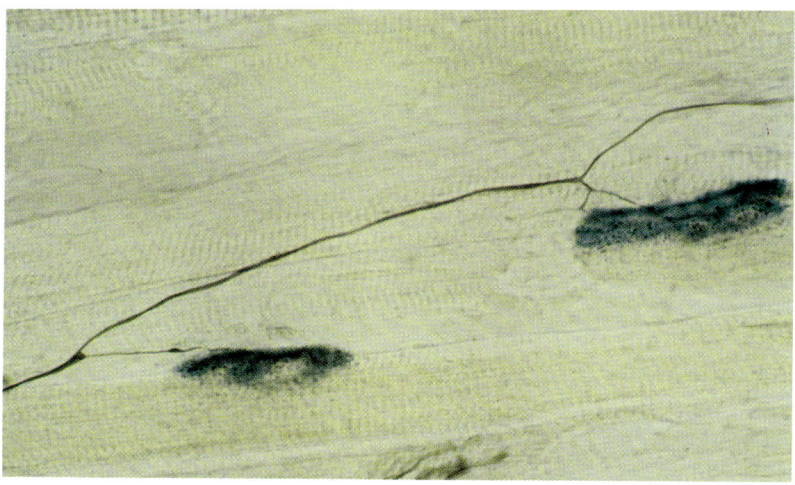

Colorplate 3. End-plates are reinnervated by thin collaterals originating from a regenerating axon. (From ref. 75, with permission of authors and editors.)

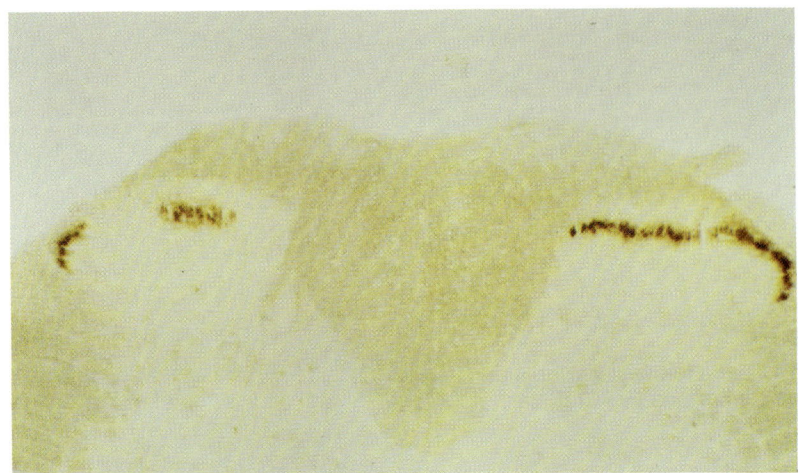

Colorplate 4. Loss of fluoride-resistant acid phosphatase (FRAP) stain in the substantia gelatinosa of the dorsal horn ipsilaterally to sciatic nerve resection.

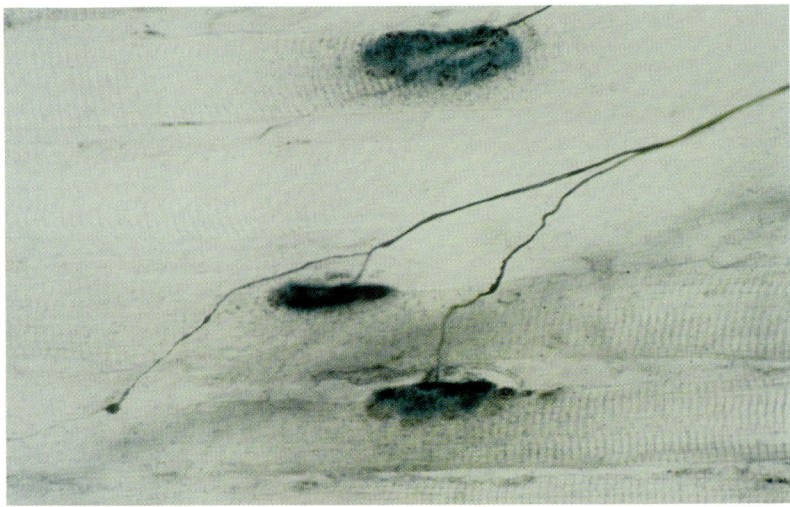

Colorplate 5. Regenerating axons evidenced by silver staining. The substained collateralization allows a faster reinnervation of the muscle. (From ref. 75, with permission of authors and editors.)

the fiber ingrowth and target reinnervation by the transplant; however, at a certain extent of reinnervation a peak for the behavioral recovery is reached and a further increased reinnervation does not correspond to an improved behavioral effect (39,41). The grafted neurons are electrically normal and their responses to drugs are also very similar to native ones (42,43). In the case of DA neurons, the resting release is on the order of 40–80% of control values (43,44) and the stimulation by amphetamine is similar to normal (44) even several months after transplantation. DA transplants are, however, less sensitive to apomorphine as if the autoreceptors might not be working normally (44). The fetal DA neurons grafted in primate brain reverse MPTP-induced parkinsonism (45). All together these results prepared the grounds for the clinical application of fetal dopaminergic grafts in Parkinson disease patients (46).

The studies above reported and, in general, the literature on transplantation indicate that implanted embryonic neurons can substitute quite well for the lost input to a denervated target brain area. As indicated above, in the case of reinnervation of the denervated host brain there are good indications suggesting that the behavioral recovery is likely due to neurite outgrowth into the denervated area. However, in the case of the grafts placed in the ventricles, the restorative effects are more likely due to the release of diffusible substances from the graft to the host brain. Often, however, the graft may serve as a bridge allowing regeneration of lesioned axons into the graft. In the case of the solid hippocampal transplants placed in the fimbria-fornix cavity, the graft serves as a bridge for septal fibers that either innervate or cross the graft reinnervating the hippocampus (47,48). The bridge phenomenon might be very important and crucial for spinal cord regeneration across the injury site that has been filled with the receptive graft (see M. Goldberger et al., Chapter 12, this volume). The embryonic tissue is therefore supplying substances that diffuse, reaching the target area and/or supplying extracellular substrates and a favorable environment essential for allowing axonal regrowth. The diffusable substances might be neurotrophic or neurotransmitters as clearly demonstrated for the DA and cholinergic transplants. It is possible that the tonic and likely nonphysiological and neuroanatomically inexact neurotransmitter release from the grafts exerts a regulatory effect that might compensate for the denervation, keeping dendrites and cell bodies of the denervated neurons in good health and function. Such a trophic action may reduce the degenerative atrophy of the denervated neurons. In conclusion, the reinnervation by the graft allows a normal functon for the reinnervated target area, in spite of the irregular anatomy of the reconstructed network that may completely lack the original and natural input.

One of the major problems for regeneration in CNS are the oligodendrocytes that are inhibitors of neurite growth in vitro and of axonal regeneration in vivo (49). Using frozen pieces of optic and sciatic nerve and neurons in culture, it was shown that several axons entered the sciatic nerve and no axons in the optic nerve (50). The inhibitory or nonpermissive effect of oligodendrocytes was further analyzed with dissociated neurons and CNS glial cells in culture (51,52). Looking at such dishes one can observe that neurites avoid contacts with the branched peripheral processes of the oligodendrocytes; in this way some areas are occupied by neurite networks and others by oligodendrocytes (52). However, if one looks at the dynamics of this process of separation, it may be seen that growing neurites upon contact with the oligodendrocytes processes either change direction and continue to grow or retract the filopodia of the growth cone and remain immobilized (53,54). The inhibitory effect was recovered with two proteins of molecular masses of 33–35 and 250 kDa purified on sodium dodecyl sulfate-polyacrylamide gel electrophoresis (SDS-PAGE); when incorporated into liposomes and added to dorsal root ganglion (DRG) neurons in cultures the neurite outgrowth was blocked in minutes (53). The two proteins were named NI-35 and NI-250. Monoclonal antibodies against these proteins were raised and added to the culture media with either myelin preparations or the liposomes with the inhibitory proteins incorporated. The antibodies prevented the inhibitory activity of both preparations (55). Such a preventive action by the antibodies is exerted also in vivo allowing axonal regeneration in the spinal cord to a certain extent. The hybridoma cells secreting the antibodies were placed unilaterally in contact with the lateral ventricle so that large amounts of antibodies were secreted in the CSF, and the corticospinal tract was bilaterally sectioned at the level of the upper thoracic region (56). At the site of lesion, sprouting was robust and several axons could go around the scar reaching a length of 5–10 mm in the animals bearing the hybridoma cells (56).

Taken together, the three types of experiments reviewed above suggest that in appropriate conditions CNS neurons can survive after lesion and may be capable of regenerating. In experimental animal models regeneration of peripheral nerves is normally very good; however, clinically the recovery from nerve lesions is frequently poor. Therefore there is also a need for developing treatments that can improve regeneration of injured peripheral nerves in humans. A few compounds of synthetic or natural origin were evaluated for their efficacy in this context. In the case of peripheral nerve lesions the rate of axonal regeneration and muscle reinnervation is fairly homogeneous among the animals used in the study and the progress can be evaluated step by step with precision using electrophysiological, morphological, and biochemical techniques. There are also simple and quite repeatable models of regeneration in CNS; some on the monoaminergic pathways will be described in the last portion of this chapter.

Nerve Regeneration

The acutely injured nerves display a premature and a much elevated return of newly synthetized proteins to the cell body; such an alteration is gradually normalized with nerve regeneration and muscle reinnervation (57,58). The normalization of transport does not occur if injured axons are not allowed to regrow (58). Such data would suggest that the retrograde transport might be a sort of feedback signaling on the progress of repair processes so that the cell body might regulate its metabolic and biosynthetic activity. A good example of such a feedback regulation is supplied by the changing fate of synaptic related material after axotomy of peripheral nerves. The changes are observable within 48 hrs after injury (59). Noradrenergic axons show reduced transport for noradrenaline (NA), dopamine-B-hydroxylase (DBH) and tyrosine hydroxylase (TH), and cholinergic neurons show a reduction for AChE and ChAT (60–66). The process of neuronal regeneration is supported by axonal transport (see Brady, Chapter 2, this volume), but some reactive processes such as collateral sprouting in the target areas may occur by direct utilization of the axoplasmic material (i.e., the cytoskeleton) present in the axon at the site of sprouting. This conclusion is suggested by the following experiment: If the axon of a DRG neuron in culture is amputated the distal portion disconnected from the cell body collapses forming a bid that after a short time re-elongates constituting a neurite with the shape and dimension similar to the original one before amputation (67). These data suggest that the distal portion of an axon has available all the biological machineries necessary for reorganizing its shape and is capable of reacting to a stimulus such as injury or denervation. It is also evident that we have two kinds of pharmacological targets for promoting regeneration: One is related to the intrinsic machineries regulating axonal shape, and the other is the environment or an improvement of the interaction between axons and environment (see Carbonetto and David, Chapter 5, and De Vellis, Chapter 4, this volume).

In order to define schematically the points of possible pharmacological intervention we must briefly summarize the major steps involved in axonal regeneration following axotomy.

Axonal reaction at the site of injury occurs usually within 72 hrs and is characterized by formations of new buds from the swollen proximal segment of the injured axons; the growth of the new sprouts was correlated with the extinction of the swelling (68). The parent axons can form one or more sprouts; however, the crossing of the site of lesion usually limits such a redundancy to a ratio of 1:2, in other words the regenerated nerve usually contains more axons than normal. Increasing the number of reactive sprouts at the site of lesion should increase the number of axons crossing the lesioned site and therefore enhance the chances of successful repair after nerve injury (Fig. 3).

Following the entry into the distal stump of the lesioned nerve, the newly formed axons begin the elongation process to reach the denervated muscle. Such an event has been extensively studied in the late 1970s and early 1980s showing that there is a direct correlation between slow axonal transport and rate of axonal regeneration (See Brady, Chapter 2, this volume). In particular it appeared a clear dependency of axonal elongation on the rate of cytoskeletal protein transport, a phenomenon verified across several species as rats, mice, fish, etc. (69–72). In the rat, axonal growth along the distal stump is a fast event and the latency between nerve injury and muscle reinnervation is of the order of 2–3 weeks; the elongation velocity is about 4 mm/day. Unfortunately the distance that has to be covered by human regenerating nerves is many fold longer than in rats and the rate of axonal regeneration is about 1 mm/day. Such a dual problem shows clearly that at best a reinnervation latency might be of the order of several months in humans, with deleterious consequences for the trophism of the denervated muscles and a successful reinnervation (73). Therefore a drug that would be able to increase the velocity of axonal elongation in humans even from 1 to 2 mm/day should be able to reduce muscle paralysis of several months with enormous advantages for the patient. This is a target of primary importance and of choice if anyone would aim at the therapy of peripheral neuropathies of the degenerative kind.

Elongation ceases after reinnervation of the muscle. The nerve terminals newly formed at the reinnervated neuromuscular junction are extremely small and immature functionally regarding transmitter release; in the rat the normalization of synaptic transmission occurs in 1 month while the morphological recovery of the neuromuscular junction may be as long as 90 days (74,75). If synaptic maturation is slow in rats. it would likely be even slower in humans. An eventual drug effect on synapse reformation should be tested on degenerative disorders of the nervous system.

The regenerating axons while reinnervating the muscle form several collateral branches aiming at the fastest possible reinnervation of the other denervated end-plate (Color Figure 5). Enhancing such a process would suggest an effect of the drug on axonal sprouting, which is highly desired in situations of partial denervation (75). Further validation should be performed with a specific partial denervation experimental model where the surviving and intact axons would form new collateral branches for reinnervating the denervated end-plates. One of the models that can be utilized for such an experiment is the partial denervation of the soleus muscle of the rat. Denervation may be caused by resection of a mixed nerve such as L5, which constitutes with L4 and L6 the sciatic nerve. Such a lesion eliminates all the motor axons belonging to the soleus nerve that are originating from L5 mixed nerve (76). The surviving axons innervating the soleus muscle within a few days start the reinnervation process by forming new collateral branches

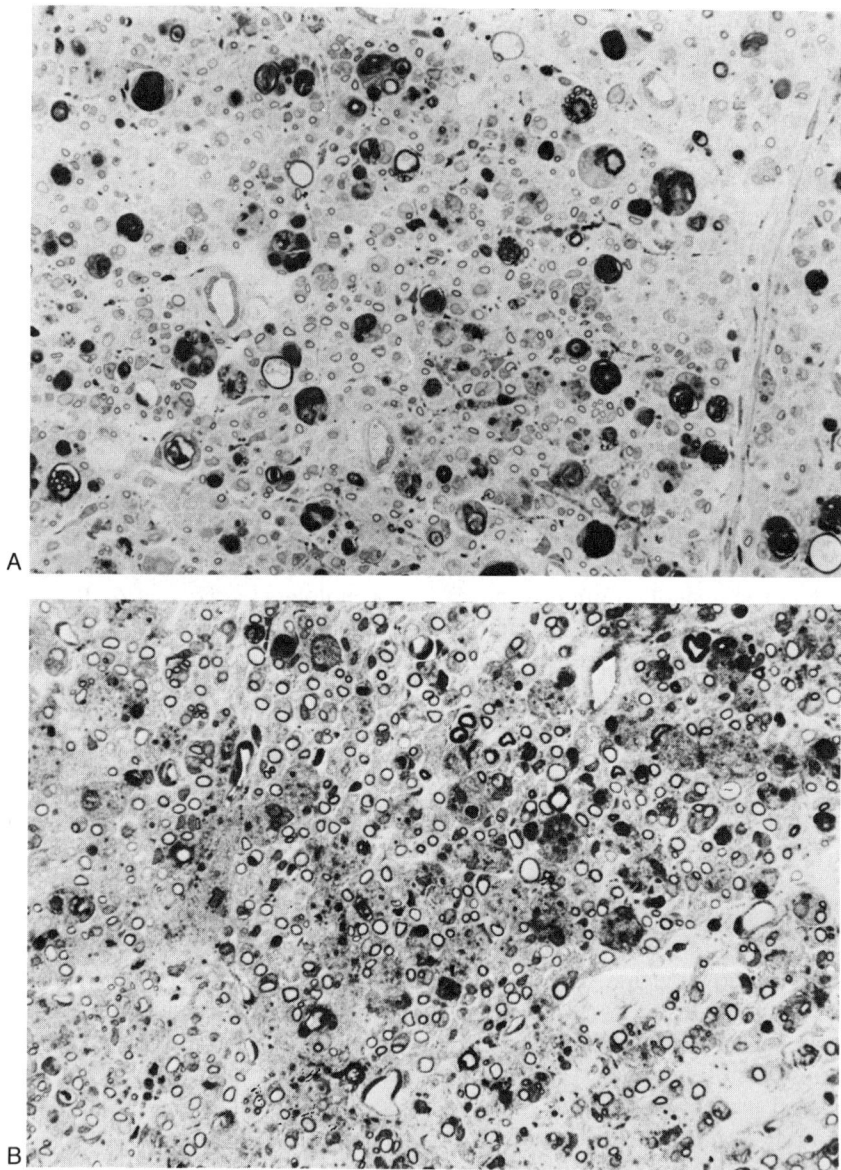

FIG. 3. Toluidine blue stain of semi-thin sections of sciatic nerve 5 mm distally from crush point. Nerve was fixed 15 days after lesioning. **A:** Note the relatively small number of regenerating axons in saline-treated rats. **B:** In Acetyl-l-carnitine-treated rats the number of new axons is far greater.

from the nodes of Ranvier (Fig. 4). The extent of the reinnervation can be assessed by indirect isometric tension stimulating the soleus nerve at gradually higher intensities so that each single soleus motor axon can be recruited (76). At 30 days after L5 resection the motor unit size expanded up to 4.5-fold as a maximum leaving part of the muscle denervated (76). The expansion of the motor unit size is an index of the extent of collateral sprouting and reinnervation by the surviving intact axons. In aged animals sprouting is repressed both in PNS (77) and CNS (78) experimental models. Some pharmacological treatments were capable of increasing sprouting and will be discussed later.

In summary the following four points are of interest for evaluating drugs active upon neuronal regeneration:

1. Reactivity at the site of lesion, sprout formation, and number of axons in the regenerating nerve. Morphological evaluation.
2. Rate of axonal elongation or velocity of regeneration. Evaluations can be performed with great accuracy with morphological techniques, with the pinch test for sensory axons and measuring the latency for recovery of muscle functions in the case of motor axons.
3. Synapse reformation and maturation. By means of electrophysiological and/or morphological techniques the event can be quantitatively assessed.
4. Sprouting. During nerve regeneration sprouting can be assessed by electrophysiological techniques, while the collateral sprouting should be evaluated after partial denervation of a muscle and by means of measuring isometric tension following gradual stimulation of the nerve.

Diabetic Peripheral Neuropathy

Diabetic peripheral neuropathy is a degenerative disorder that we have chosen to describe as an experimental model for assessing drug activity for two reasons. One is that the critical parameters to monitor are well described and characterized and the other is that most of the drugs undergoing basic and clinical research described in this report have also been tried in this pathological condition. Other kinds of peripheral neuropathies are described by Gold and Spencer (Chapter 6, this volume). Diabetic neuropathy is one of the most common correlates of diabetes mellitus. The onset is directly related to the length of diabetes; indeed the percentage of patients with neuropathy increases with the progression of the disease (79). The alterations most often involve the distal sensory nerves with significant functional impairment correlated with reduced nerve conduction velocity and axonal degeneration. In addition to the most common sensory loss, there are cases of painful neuropathies with paresthesia (spontaneous pins-and-needles sensations), dysesthesia (hypersensitivity to light touch), and deep and burning pain sensations (80). Also motor neuropathies are common particularly in patients over 50 years of age (80). The autonomic neuropathies are apparently very frequent; for instance most diabetic patients show gastrointestinal dysfunctions that might be correlated with the onset of enteric and autonomic nerve neuropathy (81–83). Changes in CNS functions have also been described, suggesting that the neuronal damage caused by diabetes may not be restricted to peripheral nerves (84,85). Diabetic neuropathy is a progressive axonal degenerative disease characterized by progressive axonal atrophy and reduced axonal transport (86–88). These changes are associated with reduced nerve conduction velocity and with minor alterations of myelin (89,90). These alterations have been found in all the available experimental models of diabetes either chemically induced with streptozotocin or alloxan or of genetic origin (79). The autonomic neuropathy of the gut is perhaps more complex, as some enteric neuronal

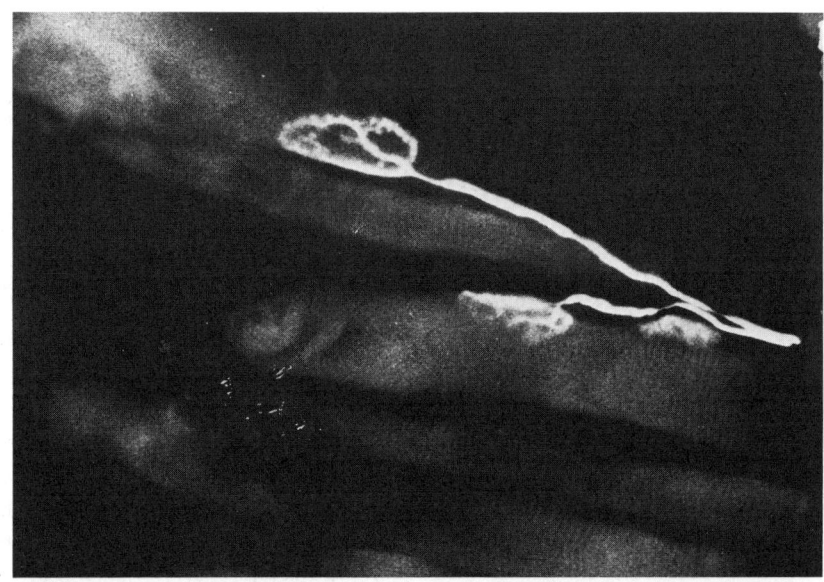
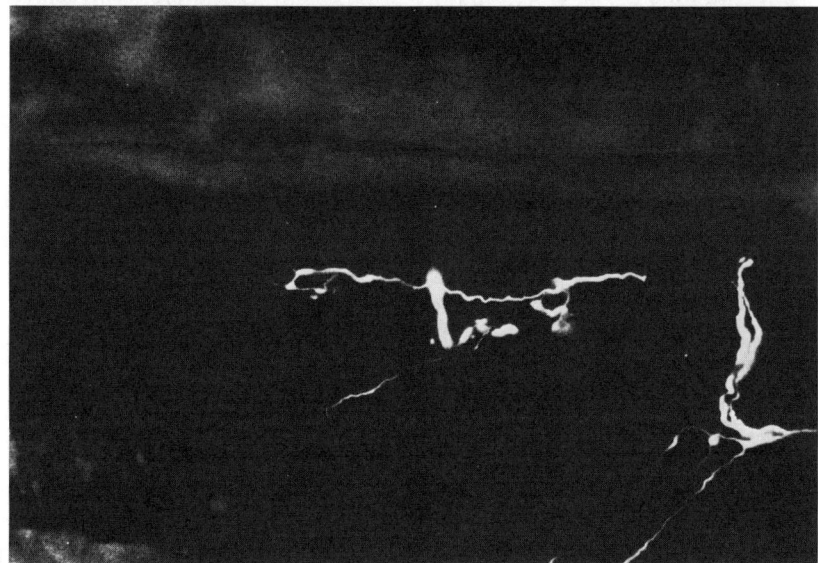

FIG. 4. Axons stained with antibodies to neurofilaments. **A:** Two axons and their terminals are shown; the thinning of the stain indicates nodes of Ranvier. **B:** After partial denervation of the soleus muscle, the new collateral branches appear thin and straight as at the node where the sprouts have just originated from. One can notice that old surviving axons maintained the normal structure as revealed by the anti-neurofilament antibodies.

systems undergo atrophy (met-enkephalin, substance P) while others undergo hypertrophy (VIP). This peptidergic rearrangement is accompanied by changes in the sympathetic innervation (83). Most recently we have described that in the retina and brain of diabetic animals there are functional changes in the transduction of synaptic signals mediated by G proteins (91,92). The dysfunction is apparently present in the systems utilizing Gi/Go proteins with consequent hyperfunction of the Gs-mediated systems (91,92). There might be several causes for these neurological abnormalities, although the microangiopathy is considered among the most important one (79,93). For assessing the potential efficacy of a new drug treatment, the use of experimental models of diabetic neuropathy is mandatory and according to the experience of these authors the following priority schedule of experiments is advised.

Axonal Transport Impairment

The reduced axonal transport can be considered a primary target for drug treatment, being the cause of axonal atrophy and likely of the subsequent degeneration. There are several relatively simple tests such as the rate of accumulation of AChE and ChAT at the point of ligature or section of the nerve, or the content and accumulation of peptides such as substance P and VIP (86,87,94). The accumulation occurs at both ends of nerve, giving information on anterograde and retrograde transport. The treatment should normalize such a loss. To avoid data variability it is our opinion that axonal transport and drug treatment should be evaluated 5–6 weeks after diabetes induction.

Axonal Atrophy

The quantitative evaluation of axonal atrophy is time consuming and has been positioned at a secondary place to axonal transport although both events might be interrelated and are most important correlates of diabetes. A simple distribution of axonal areas/frequency would indicate the development of diabetes and the effect of the treatment (95).

Nerve Conduction Velocity

As indicated above, diabetic neuropathy is characterized by reduced nerve conduction velocity that is on the average about 20% less than normal 8–9 weeks after diabetes induction. The assay can be performed in vivo or in vitro with dissected nerves (89,95). Drug treatment should prevent or limit the reduction in nerve conduction velocity.

Retrograde Degeneration of Sensory Neurones

Electrophysiological evaluations have shown that in chronic diabetic animals sensory conduction along the spinal cord decreases (84). Such a functional alteration is correlated by a retrograde degeneration of sensory nerves evidenced by the reduction of substance P content in the lumbar cord (85). The electrophysiological evaluation can be performed along the cord or by assessing the delay of the somatosensory potentials, and the retrograde degeneration in the cord can be quantitatively established by radioimmunoassay or immunocytochemistry with specific antibodies (85).

Autonomic Enteric Neuropathy

The typical alterations of gut innervation present in chronic diabetic neuropathy offer a good experimental model for further evaluating drugs in experimental peripheral diabetic neuropathy. The met-enkephalin and substance P loss is of the order of 50% throughout the gut, while VIP increases (about 50%) mainly in the small intestine and caecum. In our experience the alteration is very significant—perhaps the most difficult to be corrected by drug treatment. Peptidergic changes can be evaluated by radioimmunoassay with specific antibodies (83).

Diabetic Encephalopathy

As indicated above several changes in CNS sensory conduction can be found in diabetic animals. The alterations are reported for somatosensory, auditory, and visual evoked potentials (84,91). We have recently reported that such changes might be due to abnormal functions of G protein-mediated transduction systems with hypoactivity of the Gi/Go components and hyperactivity of the Gs (91,92). In the striatum the prevention of such a dysfunction might be monitored by stimulating D2 receptors, hypofunctional in diabetic rats, and D1 receptors, hyperfunctional in diabetic rats, and assaying cAMP production. The correction of such imbalance could be a primary biochemical target for diabetic encephalopathy. A further test would be the quantitative evaluation of ADP-ribosilation of G proteins mediated by the specific toxins (cholera for Gs, pertussis for Gi/Go). Indeed we have recently found that pertussis toxin mediated-ribosylation of Gi/Go proteins is reduced in the striatum of chronic diabetic rats (96).

TREATMENTS DEVELOPED FOR IMPROVING NERVE REPAIR AND REGENERATION

Gangliosides

Gangliosides are carbohydrate-rich complex lipids, that are found in cell membranes of a variety of cells, particularly neurons (97). They are constituted by a hydrophobic moiety, consisting of sphingosine and stearic acid, and a hydrophilic moiety, consisting of sialic acid and other carbohydrates. The lipid portion is inserted in the membranes, while the hydrophilic one protrudes toward the extracellular space (97). Treatment with mixed gangliosides (50 mg/kg) during muscle reinnervation after nerve crush stimulated sprouting in the muscle as suggested by the electrophysiological evaluation of increased polyneuronal innervation. No effects on nerve rate of regeneration and on the number of axons constituting the regenerating nerve were found (98,99). The effect of gangliosides on neuronal sprouting was also observed after partial denervation of the soleus muscle (76) and after poisoning with botulinum toxin or muscle paralysis (100). In diabetic neuropathy either induced by an injection of alloxan in rats or by genetic origin such as in the case of the mouse C57BL/Ks (db/db) the treatment with gangliosides ameliorated nerve conduction velocity and nerve ultrastructure, and in the case of alloxan-induced diabetes the treatment reversed the reduced transport rate of AChE (101,102). In spite of the positive results obtained in experimental models, several double blind clinical trials were performed in various kinds of degenerative and diabetic neuropathies. Overall the results were not clearly positive or quite inconsistent or very negative (103). The blind clinical studies published on medical and scientific journals are very few and except for the study by Bassi et al. based on alcoholic and diabetic neuropathies (104) there are no reported positive findings (105). The early open trial on diabetic neuropathy suggested positive effects on nerve conduction velocity (106); however other studies did not show any electrophysiological improvement (107) or showed byphasic effects with improvement during the treatment and worsening (compared to controls) during the wash-out period (108). No clinical or electrophysiological effects were observed in chronic peripheral neuropathies and spinocerebellar degeneration (103). The drug was also tested in amyotrophic lateral sclerosis with very minor effects (109,110). The results of ganglioside therapy in experimental peripheral neuropathies are consistent and suggestive of activity by the drug (see Gold and Spencer, Chapter 6, this volume, for further evaluations of ganglioside therapy), however the outcome of the clinical trials raised some concern for their inconsistency (111) or for the negative results (103). The clinical trials were performed with dosages ranging from 20 to 50 mg/patient and rarely as high as 100 mg. Perhaps the dosage should be adjusted to resemble more closely the experimental conditions, where the dosage most frequently used was 50 mg/kg. Recently some problems have arisen about the possibility that ganglioside treatment may cause antibody formation in susceptible patients with possible worsening of the clinical syndrome. Indeed several types of peripheral nerve disorders are associated with anti-GM1 antibodies (112–115). In the case of Guillain-Barré syndrome there is a correlation between the presence of anti-glycoconjugate antibodies and patient disability; on the other hand these antibodies bind to the sequence Gal(B1-3)GalNac that is shared by GM1, GD1b, and by several other glycolipids and glycoproteins (116). There might be a correlation between the presence of antibodies and infection with *Campylobacter jejuni* (116). On the other hand it is unclear if exogenous gangliosides applied in this pathological condition might promote further the antibody formation. Apparently parenteral administration of GM1 does not stimulate immunogenic processes in healthy patients (117).

Melanocortins

Among the various melanocortin peptides, ACTH and alpha-MSH at the dose of 10 µg/day have shown an interesting activity on experimental neuronal degeneration and regeneration. These peptides derive from a large polypeptide precursor, the proopiomelanocortin (POMC) that has been found in several brain areas (118). For these studies also a modified form of ACTH 4-10 (ORG 2766) was used. If ACTH is supplied during the first 8 days following peripheral nerve lesion there is an enhanced formation of sprout at the site of injury with no effect on the rate of axonal elongation (119). However the motor units formed after reinnervation are smaller in ACTH-treated rats as if more motor axons entered the muscle (120). Treatment with melanocortins also improves the recovery of nerve conduction velocity in regenerating nerves (121). The potential capacity of ORG 2766 of stimulating sprouting was also assessed after resection of L5 mixed nerve and partial denervation of the soleus muscle. The treatment enhanced sprouting by 50% (122). ORG 2766 is also effective in experimental toxic peripheral neuropathy induced by cis-platinum. If treatment was subsequent to intoxication there was an improvement of nerve conduction velocity (123); however, if treatment was concomitant with the intoxication no changes in conduction velocity were observed (121). Also beneficial effects on nerve conduction velocity were observed in diabetic neuropathy (124,125). ORG 2766 at the dose of 1 mg was used clinically in the prevention of cisplatin-induced neuropathy: The results are encouraging with a prominent prevention of neurologic symptoms without alteration of the chemiotherapic effects of cisplatinum (126). Unfortunately the number of patients treated with ORG 2766 is very small and further studies are required for better understanding the therapeutic value of this drug in peripheral neuropathies.

Acetyl-L-Carnitine

In the last 10 years several reports have shown that treatment with acetyl-l-carnitine (ALCAR) can reverse several biochemical and functional alterations in the aging brain (127). ALCAR is the acetyl ester of carnitine, which is an essential metabolite active in the transport of free fatty acids from the cytosol to the mitochondrial matrix (128). The studies on the biochemical effects of ALCAR treatment on the aging brain raised the hypothesis that a preferential site of action was the cholinergic system by raising both synthesis and release of ACh (129). In young rats the effect on the cholinergic system, induced by postnatal treatment with ALCAR, is accompanied by the increased expression of NGF receptor (130), which is also increased by ALCAR in adult and aged animals (131,132). The effects on trophic factors and on the cholinergic system might be correlated with the significant prevention of neuronal death (133,134) and with the improvement of cognitive deficits (135,136) in aged rats. Other clear effects of ALCAR are on the restoration of mitochondrial functions altered during aging (137,138); also the energy state of the brain is affected with a marked increase of phosphocreatine levels and a reduction of lactate (139). All together these data have prompted a series of clinical trials on Alzheimer disease: Over 600 patients were treated with ALC at a dose of 2 g/day and the results were overall positive (140).

More recently the effects of ALC treatment were assessed upon peripheral nerve degeneration and regeneration, muscle reinnervation, and diabetic neuropathy. The neuroprotective efforts of ALCAR treatment were assessed upon sensory and vagus nerve neurons following permanent axotomy. As indicated above chronic resection of rat sciatic nerve causes a significant degeneration of substance P sensory axons and of intraspinal met-enkephalin-containing nerve terminals, and ALCAR treatment prevents the degeneration of both neuronal systems (14). The neuroprotective action was also tested after permanent section of vagus nerve axons that cause shrinkage and degeneration of the respective cell bodies; in the treated animals no atrophy and no loss of neurons were observed (141). ALCAR treatment can stimulate peripheral nerve regeneration as the number of regenerating axons after sciatic nerve crush is markedly increased in treated animals. The enhanced nerve regeneration is correlated by an accelerated normalization of the morphology of regenerating nerves, as 60 days after crush no more degenerating bodies are present in treated rats while in control rats more than 20% of axonal profiles present in the regenerated nerve are degenerating (142). The same study showed that ALCAR stimulated intramuscular sprouting of the regenerating axons (142). The data reported above strongly indicate that ALCAR increases nerve reactivity at the site of injury, promotes normalization of the regenerating nerve by increasing both nerve regeneration and degeneration of the distal nerve stump, and stimulates intramuscular sprouting and muscle reinnervation. Also the regeneration of the catecholaminergic system is sensitive to treatment with ALC. Intravenous injection of 6-OHDA in neonate rats causes iris denervation, which is followed by slow reinnervation by the lesioned axons originating from the superior cervical ganglion. In ALCAR-treated rats the reinnervation process is increased by 50% (143).

Diabetic neuropathy was chemically induced with a single injection of alloxan or streptozotocine; subsequently nerve conduction velocity was evaluated 5 and 10 weeks after diabetes induction, while motor coordination (rotarod) was evaluated only at 10 weeks. ALCAR treatment normalized both parameters that are greatly reduced in diabetic animals (144). The autonomic neuropathy was estimated by assaying gastrointestinal peptides such as met-enkephalin (MET), substance P (SP), and vasoactive intestinal polypeptide (VIP). In 12 week old diabetic autonomic neuropathy there is a significant reduction of MET and SP, while VIP increases; ALCAR treatment normalizes these alterations in gut innervation (145). Such neuroprotective effect is also exerted on the sciatic nerve and on the lumbar spinal cord by preventing the loss of substance P occurring in diabetic animals

(145). It must be noted that the effects on nerve conduction velocity can also be observed in acute after a single injection of ALCAR (146). Neuronal aging is usually regarded as a brain problem; however, peripheral nerves are affected with reduction of nerve conduction velocity, axonal degeneration, and alterations of neuromuscular morphology. These changes are prevented by ALCAR (147). So far the clinical trials performed in a double blind randomized manner have involved the evaluation of ALCAR treatment effect on 60 patients affected by facial palsy, 50 by traumatic neuropathy and 200 by diabetic neuropathy. The outcome of the studies was positive. In the first two trials the drug-treated group of traumatic neuropathy patients showed faster recovery, while in diabetic neuropathy the treatment significantly reduced sensory loss, pain, and hyperpathia with a general improvement of clinical symptoms and autonomic functions (148–150).

Isaxonine and Other Agents

Isaxonine is a chemical compound (N-isopropyl-amino-2-pyrimidine orthophosphate) capable of promoting neuritogenesis and neuronal sprouting in vitro (151). When administered to rats after peripheral nerve lesion, the rate of nerve regeneration was reported to be increased by about 50%, from 1.6 mm/day to 2.3 mm/day (152,153); such an effect upon the rate of axonal elongation was confirmed later by other investigators (154). By means of intracellular electrophysiological measurements it was found that isaxonine stimulated polyneuronal innervation as a consequence of an enhanced axonal sprouting during muscle reinnervation (155). The effect of this substance was also apparent on the trophism of denervated muscle (156). Several clinical trials of vincristine on traumatic, leprosy, and diabetic neuropathies have been performed. In general the drug was considered to be active although the studies were clearly preliminary (157–162,154). Unfortunately the experiments ceased because isaxonine caused hepatitis in 28 per 100,000 patients and the drug was withdrawn from clinical use (154).

Agents such as pyronin and forskolin were also used in this experimental paradigm. The latter is an activator of adenylate cyclase, which was reported to be capable of enhancing nerve regeneration rate in frog preparations (163). Unfortunately these results could not be reproduced in rats after sciatic nerve lesion (Gorio A, unpublished data). The effects of pyronin on nerve regeneration were described in the mid-1950s by Hoffman; more recently it was shown that this substance can promote muscle reinnervation perhaps by accelerating degeneration of the distal stump (164,165). Degeneration and subsequent remyelination of regenerating axons in the distal stump might also be a novel and convenient site for studying pharmacological interventions for peripheral nerve diseases. A possible suggestion derives from the role played by apolipoprotein E (apo E) in nerve regeneration. It has been shown that apo E is expressed at higher levels by rat sciatic nerve during postnatal development and particularly during myelin formation (166,167). Similarly there is a marked endoneurial accumulation in the distal nerve stump following crush injury in adult animals (168–170). Such an increase is maintained as long as regeneration is prevented, otherwise it will decline within 8 weeks (169). The source of apo E in peripheral nerves are nonresident macrophages that likely penetrate the distal stump after axotomy (171,172). A possible role of apo E would be to prevent the loss of cholesterol from the degenerating myelin. The rescued cholesterol might then be taken up by Schwann cells and used for myelination or by growth cone; indeed the synthesis of cholesterol by sciatic nerve endoneurium is reduced during the entire period of remyelination of the regenerating axons (173).

Among the exogenous substances tested

in nerve regeneration, an important role was played by the thyroid hormones, which are able to stimulate protein synthesis in the developing nervous system but are no longer efficacious when the nervous system becomes mature. On the other hand nerve regeneration is retarded in adult animals affected by hypothyroidism (174) and is normally restored if a replacement therapy with T4 is applied (175). In experimental hyperthyroidism the rate of axonal regeneration and recovery from peripheral nerve injury is accelerated (176–180). Similarly in hyperthyroid animals the degenerative and regenerative events might be accelerated, as described above for ALCAR treatment (142). The mode of action of thyroid hormones in stimulating nerve regeneration is still not fully understood, although it is conceivable that these hormones might increase the rate of protein synthesis of lesioned neurons (181). It has been also reported that the effects of T4 treatment on axonal regeneration can be observed in spinal cord lesions (182). These data suggest that enhancing protein synthesis might be a good target to aim for in the improvement of nerve regeneration. Such an action might be interactive with endogenous trophic factors giving rise to greater effects as suggested by some in vitro experiments (183).

A variety of chemical agents such as vitamins, myo-inositol, phosphatidil-inositol, and to a much larger extent inhibitors of the enzyme aldose reductase have been used for the treatment of diabetic neuropathy; so far none of them has shown clear clinical efficacy (184). The field of aldose reductase inhibitors did receive an enormous impulse from pharmaceutical firms, but the promising early results were followed by increasing failures, partly owing to the adverse reactions caused by the drug treatment. Many of the biochemical and functional abnormalities present in the nerves of diabetic animals were corrected by this treatment; therefore, there is still hope for the development of an inhibitor of aldose reductase that might be clinically active in the treatment of diabetic neuropathy (184–186). On purely theoretical grounds one wonders if all the neurological alterations present in diabetes can be simply reconciled with the activity of the aldose reductase enzyme; on the other hand recent reports indicate that this line of drug development is still active and of interest (187–191). Several chemically different substances (gangliosides, ACTH and its derivatives, acetyl-l-carnitine, inositol derivatives, aldose reductase inhibitors, etc.) and even gamma linolenic acid (192) showed significant activity in improving or preventing the onset of the typical alterations of diabetic neuropathy. With all the limitations deriving from the animal models of diabetic neuropathy available, these data indicate that the points of pharmacological attack are perhaps multiple. Gangliosides and inositol derivatives likely are active at membrane and signal transduction level; acetyl-l-carnitine is active at enhancing energy production and at rescuing mithochondrial functions, and it displays neurotrophic activity; ACTH may act as a trophic factor. Therefore it is obvious that there is enormous room for drug development that goes beyond aldose reductase inhibitors: The secret aim appears to be the functional normalization of neurons and their environment, which might be achieved in different way.

Regeneration Chambers

The development of this device stems from the necessity of solving the basic problem of nerve regeneration across the gap formed after complete transection. Crossing the gap after a clean knife cut might be not a very difficult task for the regenerating sprouts of the rat sciatic nerve, but the task becomes extremely difficult and unlikely to succeed if such an accident occurs in a human patient. The problem is dual, stemming from the difference in size and from the much smaller nerve regeneration rate in man. The kind of injury may also worsen the situation if the two stumps are so separated that the re-entry into the distal stump by the regenerating sprouts is preceded by the formation of a scar interposed between the two stumps (1). Microsuture or use of fibrin glue is a common repair technique in microsurgery of peripheral nerves (1,193); however, joining the two stumps together may create problems if the distance between them is such that tension must be applied for a proper nerve coaptation. A possible over-stretching of the nerve may cause structural lesions to axons and vascular tissues above and or below the apposition point (1). For avoiding these problems and for reconnecting distal and proximal nerve segments separated by a large gap after lesion, autologous nerve grafts were developed. However, the development of chambers suitable for nerve regeneration would be a great help for solving the problem of crossing the distance between the two stumps. The use of the chamber is also very important as a tool for evaluating in vivo the cellular and molecular components of the peripheral nerve that are necessary for a successful repair process. Ideally one should be able to supply the chamber with all the materials necessary for promoting nerve regrowth and perhaps enhancing nerve regeneration rate. The chambers utilized are made up of various materials of biological origin (mesothelial cells, veins, nerve grafts, etc.), or synthetic (silicone, etc.) or semisynthetic materials such as chemically modified hyaluronic acid (194). The length of the gap between the two stumps is of the order of 10 mm and may differ according to the experimental conditions. Longer distances were achieved by filling the chamber with various saline solutions and additives (195–197). Extracellular matrix components are among the obvious additives that were tested; it was shown that laminin enhances nerve regrowth through the chamber (198), and likely other extracellular matrix constituents can as well (199). Also collagen film may act by forming a suitable surface for axonal regrowth: when applied into a biodegradable polyglycolic tube it was shown to be capable of promoting regeneration (200,201). Other substances of interest could be the glycosaminoglycans that are among the major constituents of the basal lamina and are transported at enhanced rate by regenerating axons (202). In addition it is well known that heparan sulfate binds to laminin and potentiates the neuritogenic effect of bFGF (203,204). The application of a trophic factor such as NGF into the chamber has promoting effects during the early stages of nerve regeneration; however, at 10 weeks after lesion there is no difference in axonal number and diameter, or in myelin thickness between saline and NGF treated groups (205). Similar early positive effects were observed by adding to the chamber a cocktail made of laminin and FGF, the enhanced regeneration was curtailed by an enormous fibrosis that had deleterious effects upon the regenerating axons (206). There are some necessary requirements for achieving growth in the chamber, the essential one being the presence of the distal stump or of a piece of nerve at the other end of the chamber (207–209). At first the chambers are filled with fluids, which gradually develop into a matrix of fibrin connecting the two stumps (210,211). Then cellular migration begins from both ends of the chamber, and gradually perineurial cells, fibroblasts, endothelial cells, and Schwann cells penetrate, forming the necessary environment for nerve entry. In a few weeks the axonal regeneration across the chambers takes place and muscle reinnervation occurs in 2–3 months (212).

Applied Electric Fields

Several reports have indicated that applied steady electric fields may affect neuritogenesis in vitro and neuronal regeneration in vivo. Explanted embryonic medullary tissue of the chick was grown in organ culture with an applied steady electric field of 100 mV/mm; it was found that neuritogenesis was accelerated toward the negative pole (213). The stimulated asymmetric neurite outgrowth induced by the electric field was also observed with chick DRG in culture (214); it is likely that such an effect is due to an improved orientation of growth but also to a probably higher number of neuroblasts forming neurites and to a higher number of neurites formed per cell (215,216). The effect was also reproduced on a single neurite if the electric field was applied via a pipette (217). The stimulatory effects of the electric fields were also observed in vivo; the rate and amount of nerve regeneration was enhanced in frog preparations (218), while neurite regeneration across the site of lesion was augmented in the cord of the lamprey (219). It has also been shown that applied electric fields can enhance collateral sprouting of sensory axons following partial denervation in mammalian preparations (220) and can facilitate regeneration after spinal cord hemisection in the guinea pig (221). The enhanced regeneration was correlated by an improved recovery of cutaneous sensory responses ipsilaterally, and below the lesion toe spreading also recovered (222,223). This research area would need further development for evaluating the clinical potential of this technique, although one can see quite promising data such as the increased capacity of regenerating exons to penetrate into or even to cross the injury tissue scar.

CNS CHEMICAL LESIONS: REGENERATION OF MONOAMINERGIC NEURONS AND THE INHIBITORY EFFECTS OF MORPHINE TREATMENT

Selective neurotoxins have become standard laboratory tools for experimental lesioning CNS and PNS monominergic pathways. Conventional lesion techniques are crude and nonselective at cellular and anatomical levels; consequently the lack of selectivity may cause other perturbations in addition to the changes caused by lesioning the chosen neuronal system. The discovery of 6-OH-DA selective for the catecholaminergic systems was the initial step in this direction (224,225), soon followed by the introduction of 5,6- and 5,7-dihydroxytryptamine (5,6-HT and 5,7-HT, respectively) as selective toxins for central serotoninergic neurons (226,227). The axon terminals are apparently the most susceptible to the neurotoxin action of all the neuronal components; such a cytological selectivity is likely due to the ratio cytoplasm size/number of monoamine uptake sites (228). The degenerative process is very rapid and within 2 days is mostly completed (228).

In the case of 6-OH-DA treatment there is a heterogeneous response between central and peripheral adrenergic systems, although the observed lesion is always dependent upon the route of toxin administration. When injected intravenously in mice at the dose of 20 mg/kg an efficient sympathetectomy can be achieved; regrowth of the axons is slow but within a few weeks the iris is reinnervated (229). The rate of recovery is likely dependent upon the extent of degeneration: The closer the cell body is to the lesion the longer is the lag time before reinnervation. Likely such a correlation may be achieved using different dosages of toxin, higher dosages means slower and poorer regeneration (230,231). However, at certain dosages the blood-brain barrier may be permeable to 6-OH-DA, so that with 100 mg/kg we might observe degeneration in the brain (232). While such an experimental condition may be optimal for PNS lesioning and regeneration, it is certainly not advisable for obtaining a repeatable CNS model of injury and regrowth. Intracisternal or intraventricular injections of 6-OH-DA cause significant catecholaminergic denervation throughout the brain; unfortunately the extent of such denervation may vary greatly from area to area, making such an experimental model not very suitable for our pur-

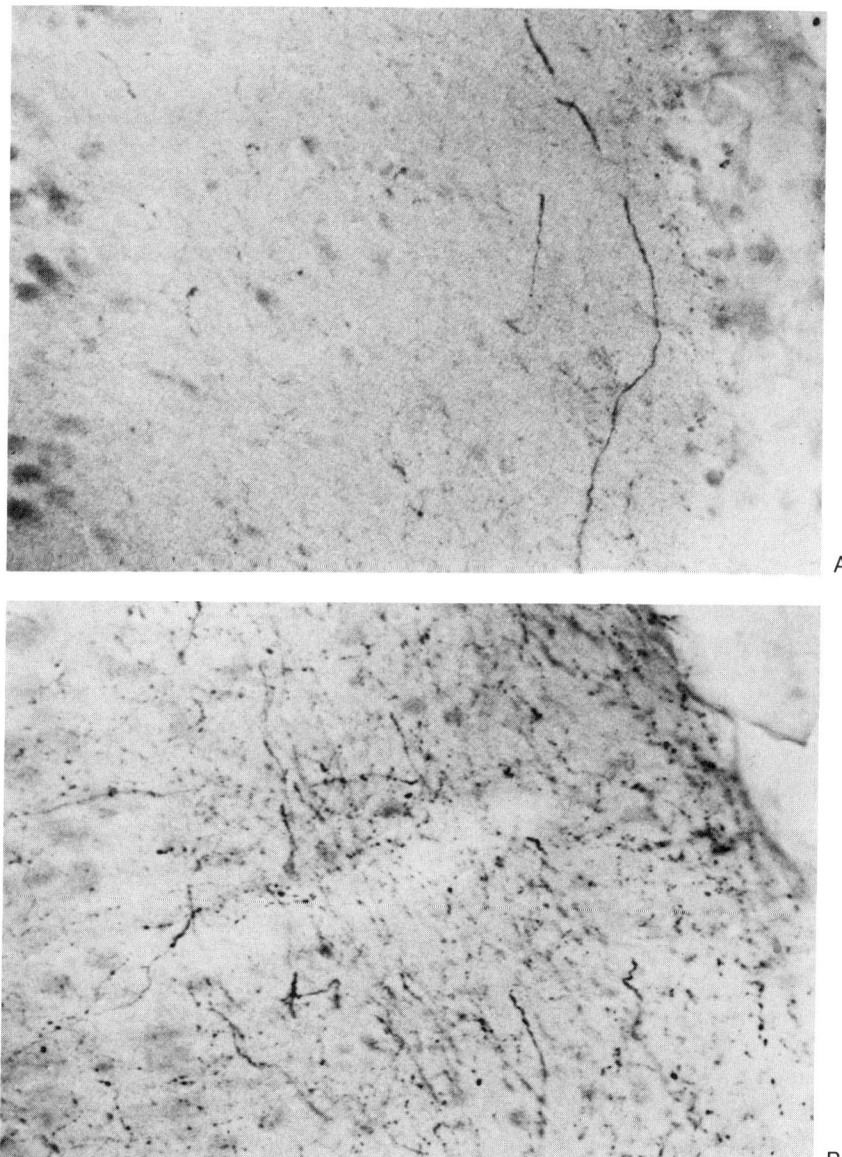

FIG. 5. Axons and terminals stained with antibodies to tyrosine hydroxylase in the frontal cortex. **A:** In control animals, long axons with rare branchings and few terminals are found. **B:** Following neonatal 6-OHDA and permanent noradrenergic denervation the tyrosine hydroxylase-positive axons and boutons are present at much higher density in the frontal cortex. **C:** In morphine-exposed rats the increase in density is very much contained.

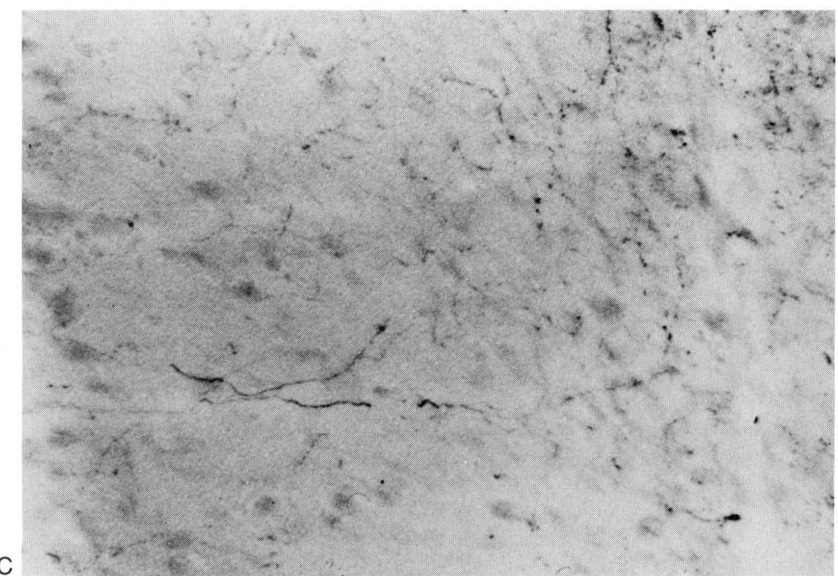

FIG. 5. Continued.

poses of evaluating drug activity. However, a more localized and repeatable lesion can be obtained using a minicannula inserted into cerebral cortex. The toxin is supplied by an osmotic minipump at the rate of 1 μl/hr and at the concentration of 2 mM. The infusion may last even 1 week, causing a profound noradrenergic denervation around the cannula and in the occipital cortex with normal innervation of the frontal (233). During the following weeks there is a gradual regrowth of NA axons in the cortex (233). In such a model we tested the efficacy of GM1 ganglioside treatment: No effect was observed if the drug was supplied during or after 6-OH-DA infusion. However if drug treatment began 3 days prior to lesioning there was a stimulation of NA regeneration in the cortex (233). Such an effect of GM1 might be due to prevention of retrograde degeneration, thereby allowing a more prompt regeneration. However the fact that GM1 administration was effective only when performed before neurotoxin infusion raises the question that the efficacy might derive from sequestration of the toxin by GM1. The lesion with 6-OH-DA in neonate rats offers another interesting model for assessing drug effects upon axonal regeneration in the brain. The neurotoxin is injected subcutaneously at the dose of 100 mg/kg in rats within 6 hrs from birth; such a treatment causes a permanent loss of noradrenergic innervation in the cortex that is followed by a hyperinnervation of the mesencephalon. In the frontal cortex the denervated targets are collaterally reinnervated by serotonergic, dopaminergic (229), and met-enkephalinergic axons, while substance P and GABAergic axons do not collaterally outgrow (author's unpublished results). The dopaminergic sprouting is also observed in the septum (Fig. 2). We have recently found that perinatal exposure to low dosages of morphine (1–5 mg/kg/day in drinking water) completely suppresses compensatory collateral sprouting in the frontal cortex after neonatal 6-OHDA (134), and in Fig. 5 the inhibitory action on dopaminergic axon outgrowth is shown.

The good regenerative capacity of the brain serotoninergic systems (135) and the selectivity of the lesions with 5,7-HT are very strong points for suggesting this experimental model as one of the favorites for testing drug efficacy upon CNS neuronal regeneration. Serotoninergic axons can regenerate and by collateral sprouting can reinnervate adjacent or contralateral territories previously denervated (236–239) and grow fibers out of fetal transplants into the spinal cord (240). In this case the neonatal lesion (229) also offers an excellent experimental method. Subcutaneous injection with 50 mg/kg of 5,7-HT within 6 hours from birth causes a rapid destruction of the most distal projections of 5-HT neurons, which leaves the spinal cord and cerebral cortex denervated. Gradually there is a regeneration of 5-HT axons that reinnervate sequentially the cervical cord, then the thoracic cord, and later, in about 8 weeks, also the lumbar spinal cord. In the cortex a similar regenerative process also takes place. The serotoninergic reinnervation of the distal territories is preceded by hyperinnervation of the pons-medulla by the short collaterals. This process, called "pruning effect," is already evident 1 week after lesioning, and recedes partially during regeneration of the distal axon terminals. Perinatal exposure to morphine as described above suppresses the pruning effect and strongly reduces regenerative capacity of serotoninergic axons (241–243).

CONCLUSIONS

In this report some basic issues related to neuronal regeneration and its pharmacology have been put forth, and the activity of many chemical agents has been described so that the hope of identifying a substance effective on neuronal regeneration or peripheral neuropathies may soon become a reality. The tissue culture methods offer the advantage of reducing the complexity of the approach and enable a direct visualization of the events and an easy manipulation of the environment and of the media. In recent years "in vitro" neuronal models have supplied the early information on a variety of substances such as ions, peptides, lipids, and unidentified proteins constituting conditioned media that promote neuronal survival and neurite outgrowth. It is conceivable that from tissue culture experiments we might extract information about new compounds that after more complex "in vivo" testing may be available for clinical testing in neuronal degenerative disorders. Nerve growth factor was shown recently to be active in experimental models of toxic sensory neuropathy (244,245), suggesting that treatment of peripheral neuropathies might be the first clinical goal for the first identified neurotrophic factor; however, it must be borne in mind that reaching the target will be difficult. Among the drugs described, melanocortins and gangliosides require further testing, perhaps at higher doses for the latter, while acetyl-L-carnitine appears promising by displaying a good correlation between preclinical and clinical performance.

REFERENCES

1. Gorio A, Millesi H, Mingrino S. *Posttraumatic peripheral nerve regeneration. Experimental basis and clinical implications.* New York: Raven Press; 1981.
2. Waxman SG, *Advances in neurology,* vol 47. New York: Raven Press; 1988.
3. Lipton SA, Kater SB. Neurotransmitter regulation of neuronal outgrowth, plasticity and survival. *TINS* 1989; 12: 265–270.
4. Fontana F. Treatise on the venom of the viper; . . . To which are annexed, observations on the primitive structure of the animal body. Different experiments on the reproduction of the nerves. Florence, 1787. Transl. from the French by J. Skinner. London: Murray.
5. David S, Bouchard C, Tsatas O, Giftochristos N. Macrophages can modify the nonpermissive nature of the adult mammalian central nervous system. *Neuron* 1990; 5:463–469.
6. Thoenen H. The changing scene of neurotrophic factors. *TINS* 1991; 14: 165–170.
7. Wetmore C, Ernfors P, Persson H, Olsson L. Localization of brain-derived neurotrophic factor mRNA to neurons in the brain by in situ hybridization. *Exp Neurol* 1990; 109: 141–152.
8. Himes BT, Tessler A. Death of some dorsal root ganglion neurons and plasticity of others following sciatic nerve section in adult and neonatal rats. *J Comp Neurol* 1989; 284: 215–230.
9. Di Giulio AM, Mantegazza P, Doná M, Gorio A. Peripheral nerve lesions cause simultaneous

9. alterations of substance P and enkephalin levels in the spinal cord. *Brain Res* 1985; 342: 405–408.
10. Di Giulio AM, Tenconi B, Mantegazza P, Gorio A. Reversibility and prevention of intraspinal peptidergic loss caused by sciatic nerve lesions. *J Neurosc Res* 1989; 22: 92–96.
11. Di Giulio AM, Tenconi B, Mannavola A, Mantegazza P, Schiavinato A, Gorio A. Spinal cord interneuron degenerative atrophy caused by peripheral nerve lesions is prevented by serotonin depletion. *J Neurosci Res* 1987; 18: 443–448.
12. Soiefer AI, Moretto A, Spencer PS, Sabri MI. Axotomy-induced ornithyne decarboxylase activity in the mouse dorsal root ganglion is inhibited by the vinca alkaloids. *Neurochem J* 1988; 13: 1169–1173.
13. Rich KM, Disch SP, Eichler ME. The influence of regeneration and nerve growth factor on the neuronal cell body reaction to injury. *J Neurocytol* 1989: 18: 569–576.
14. Tenconi B, Donadoni L, Germani E, Bertelli A, Mantegazza P, Di Giulio AM, Ramacci MT, Gorio A. Acetyl-l-carnitine prevents intraspinal degenerative atrophy caused by sciatic nerve lesions. *Int J Clin Pharmacol* 1992; (in press).
15. Gilad GM, Gilad VH. Early polyamine treatment enhances survival of sympathetic neurons after postnatal axonal injury or immunosympathectomy. *Brain Res* 1988; 466: 175–181.
16. Levi Montalcini R, Hamburger V. A diffusible agent of mouse sarcoma, producing hyperplasia of sympathetic ganglia and hyperneurotization of viscera in the chick embryo. *J Exp Zool* 1953; 123: 233–388.
17. Levi Montalcin R. The nerve growth factor 35 years later. *Science* 1987; 237: 1154–1162.
18. Hofer MM, Barde YA. Brain-derived neurotrophic factor prevents neuronal death in vivo. *Nature* 1988; 331: 261–262.
19. Koo EH, Hoffman PN, Price DL. Levels of neurotransmitter and cytoskeletal mRNA during nerve regeneration in sympathetic ganglia. *Brain Res* 1988; 449: 361–363.
20. Schmalbruch H. Motoneuron death after sciatic nerve section in newborn rats. *J Comp Neurol* 1984; 224: 252–258.
21. Kashihara Y, Kuno M, Miyata Y. Cell death of axotomized motoneurones in neonatal rats and its prevention by peripheral reinnervation. *J Physiol (Lond)* 1987; 350: 135–148.
22. Carlson J, Lais AC, Dyck PJ. Axonal atrophy from persistent peripheral axotomy in adult cat. *J Neuropathol Exp Neurol* 1979; 38: 579–585.
23. McManaman JL, Oppenheim RW, Prevette D, Marchetti D. Rescue of motoneurones from cell death by a purified skeletal muscle polypeptide: effects of the ChAT development factor, CDF. *Neuron* 1990; 4: 891–898.
24. Lorez H, Keller F, Ruess G, Otten U. Nerve growth factor increases in adult rat brain after hypoxic injury. *Neurosci Lett* 1989; 98: 339–344.
25. Otto D, Frotscher M, Unsicker K. Basic fibroblast growth factor and nerve growth factor administered in gel foam rescue medial septal neurons after fimbria fornix transection. *J Neurosci Res* 1989; 22: 83–91.
26. Anderson KJ, Dan D, Lee S, Cotman CW. Basic fibroblast growth factor prevents death of lesioned cholinergic neurons in vivo. *Nature* 1988; 332: 360–361.
27. Sievers J, Hausmann B, Unsicker K, Berry M. Fibroblast growth factors promote the survival of adult rat retinal ganglion cells after transection of the optic nerve. *Neurosci Lett* 1987; 76: 157–162.
28. Faktorovich EG, Steinberg RH, Yasumura D, Matthes MT, LaVail MM. Photoreceptor degeneration in inherited retinal dystrophy delayed by basic fibroblast growth factor. *Nature* 1990: 347: 83–86.
29. Bray BG, Vidal-Sanz M, Aguayo A. Regeneration of axons from the central nervous system of adult rats. In: Seil FJ, Herbert E, Carlson BM, eds. *Progress in brain research,* vol 71. Amsterdam: Elsevier; 1987: 373–379.
30. Ramón y Cajal S. Degeneration and regeneration of the nervous system (May RM translation). London: Oxford University Press; 1928.
31. Richardson PM, Issa VMK, Aguayo A. Regeneration of long spinal axons in the rat. *J Neurocytol* 1984; 11: 949:966.
32. Richardson PM, McGuinnes UM, Aguayo A. Axons from CNS neurons regenerate into PNS grafts. *Nature* 1980; 284: 264–265.
33. Vidal-Sanz M, Bray GM, Willegas-Perez MP, Thanos S, Aguayo A. Axonal regeneration and synapse formation in the superior culliculus by retinal ganglion cells in the adult rat. *J Neurosci* 197; 7: 2894–2902.
34. Villegaz-Perez MP, Vidal-Sanz M, Bray GM, Aguayo A. Influences of peripheral nerve grafts on the survival and regrowth of axotomized retinal ganglion cells in adult rats. *J Neurosci* 1988; 8: 265–280.
35. Bjorklund A, Stenevi U. Reconstruction of the nigrostriatal pathway by intracerebral nigral transplants. *Brain Res* 1979; 177: 555–560.
36. Perlow MJ, Freed WJ, Hoffer BJ, Seiger A, Olson L, Wyatt RJ. Brain grafts reduce motor abnormalities produced by destruction of nigrostriatal dopamine system. *Science* 1979; 204: 643–647.
37. Bjorklund A. Stenevi U, Svendgaard N-A. Growth of transplanted monoaminergic neurones into the adult hippocampus along the perforant path. *Nature* 1976; 262: 787–790.
38. Low WC, Lewis PR, Bunch ST, Dunnett SB, Thomas SR, Iversen SD, Bjorklund A, Stenevi U. Functional recovery following neural transplantation of embryonic septal nuclei in adult rats with septoippocampal lesions. *Nature* 1982; 300: 260–262.
39. Bjorklund A, Dunnet SB, Stenevi U, Lewis ME

and Iversen SD. Reinnervation of the denervated striatum by substantia nigra transplants: functional consequences as revealed by pharmacological and sensorimotor testing. *Brain Res* 1980; 199: 307–333.

40. Schmidt RH, Bjorklund A, Stenevi U. Intracerebral grafting of dissociated CNS tissue suspensions: a new approach for neuronal transplantation to deep brain sites. *Brain Res* 1981; 218: 347–356.

41. Brundin P, Isacson O, Gage FH, Prochiantz A, Bjorklund A. The rotating 6-hydroxydopamine lesioned mouse as a model for assessing functional effects of neuronal grafting. *Brain Res* 1986; 366: 346–349.

42. Wuerthele SM, Freed WJ, Olson L, Morihisa J, Spoor L, Wyatt RJ, Hoffer BJ. Effect of dopamine agonists and antagonists on the electrical activity of substantia nigra neurons transplanted into the lateral ventricle of the rat. *Exp Brain Res* 1981; 44: 1–10.

43. Strecker RE, Sharp T, Brundin P, Zetterstrom T, Ungerstedt U, Bjorklund A. Autoregulation of dopamine release and metabolism by intrastriatal nigral grafts as revealed by intracerebral dialysis. *Neuroscience* 1987; 22: 169–178.

44. Zettestrom T, Brundin P, Gage FH, Sharp T, Isacson O, Dunnett SB, Ungersted U, Bjorklund A. Spontaneous release of dopamine from intrastriatal nigra grafts as monitored by the intracerebral dialysis technique. *Brain Res* 1986; 362: 344–349.

45. Sladek JR, Redmond DE, Collier TJ, Haber SN, Elsworth JD, Deutsch AY, Roth RH. Transplantation of fetal dopamine neurons in primate brain reverses MPTP induced parkinsonism. In: Seil FJ, Herbert E, Carlson BM (eds). *Progress in Brain Research* vol 71. Amsterdam: Elsevier; 1987: 309–323.

46. Bjorklund A. Neural transplantation-an experimental tool with clinical possibilities. *TINS* 1991; 14: 319–322.

47. Kromer LF, Bjorklund A, Stenevi U. Innervation of hippocampal implants by regenerating axons of cholinergic septal neurons in the adult rat. *Brain Res* 1981; 210: 153–171.

48. Kromer LF, Bjorklund A, Stenevi U. Regeneration of the septo-hippocampal pathways in adults rats is promoted by utilizing embryonic hippocampal implants as bridges. *Brain Res* 1981; 210: 173–210.

49. Schwab ME. Myelin-associated inhibitors of neurite growth and regeneration in the CNS. *TINS* 1990; 13: 452–456.

50. Schwab ME, Thoenen H. Dissociated neurons regenerate into sciatic nerve but not optic nerve explants in culture irrespective of neurotrophic factors. *J Neurosci* 1985; 5: 2415–2423.

51. Savio T, Schwab ME. Rat CNS white matter, but not gray matter, is nonpermissive for neuronal cell adhesion and fiber outgrowth. *J Neurosci* 1989; 9: 1126–1133.

52. Schwab ME, Caroni P. Oligodendrocytes and CNS myelin are nonpermissive substrates for neurite growth and fibroblast spreading in vitro. *J Neurosci* 1988; 8: 2381–2393.

53. Bandtlow C, Zachleder T, Schwab ME. Oligodendrocytes arrest neurite growth by contact inhibition. *J Neurosci* 1990; 10: 3837–3848.

54. Fawcett JW, Rokos J, Bakst I. Oligodendrocytes repel axons and cause axonal growth cone collapse. *J Cell Sci* 1989; 92: 93–100.

55. Caroni P, Schwab ME. Antibody against myelin-associated inhibitor of neurite growth neutralizes non-permissive substrate properties of CNS white matter. *Neuron* 1988; 1: 85–96.

56. Schnell L, Schwab ME. Axonal regeneration in the rat spinal cord produced by an antibody against myelin-associated neurite growth inhibitors. *Nature* 1990; 343: 269–272.

57. Bisby MA, Bulger VT. Reversal of axonal transport at nerve crush. *J Neurochem* 1977; 29: 313–320.

58. Bulger VT, Bisby MA. Reversal of axonal transport in regenerating nerves. *J Neurochem* 1978; 31: 1411–1418.

59. Grafstein B. Role of slow axonal transport in nerve regeneration. *Acta Neuropathol [Suppl]* 1971; 5: 144–152.

60. Boyle FC, Gillespie JS. Accumulation and loss of noradrenaline central to a constriction of adrenergic nerves. *Eur J Pharmacol* 1970; 12: 77–84.

61. Cheah TB, Geffen LB. Effect of axonal injury on norepinephrine, tyrosine hydroxylase and monoamine oxidase levels in sympathetic ganglia. *J Neurobiol* 1973; 4: 443–452.

62. Kao CC, Wrathall JR, Kyoshima K. Axonal reaction to transection. In: Kao CC, Bunge RP, Rejer PJ, eds. *Spinal cord reconstruction*. New York: Raven Press; 1983: 41–58.

63. Reis DJ, Ross RA. Dynamic changes in brain dopamine-beta-hydroxilase activity during anterograde and retrograde reactions to injury of central noradrenergic axons. *Brain Res* 1973; 57: 307–326.

64. Reis DJ, Ross RA, Gilad G, Joh TH. Reaction of central catecholaminergic neurons to injury: model systems for studying the neurobiology of central regeneration and sprouting. In: Cotman CW, ed. *Neuronal plasticity*. New York: Raven Press; 1978: 197–226.

65. Di Giamberardino L, Couraud JY, Hassig R, Gorio A. Recovery of axonal transport of acetylcholinesterase in regenerating sciatic nerve precedes muscle reinnervation. In: Weiss DG, Gorio A, eds. *Axonal transport in physiology and pathology*. Berlin: Springer Verlag; 1982: 77–80.

66. Frizell M, Sjostrand J. Transport of proteins, glycoproteins and cholinergic enzymes in regenerating hypoglossal neurons. *J Neurochem* 1974; 22: 845–850.

67. Shaw G, Bray D. Movement and extension of isolated growth cones. *Exp Cell Res* 1977; 104: 55–62.

68. Friede RL, Bischausen R. The fine structure of

stumps of transected fibers in subserial sections. *J Neurol Sci* 1980; 44: 181–203.
69. Hoffman PN, Lasek RJ. Axonal transport of the cytoskeleton in regenerating motor neurons: constancy and change. *Brain Res* 1980; 202: 317–333.
70. Lasek RJ, Hoffman PN. The neuronal cytoskeleton, axonal transport and axonal growth. In: Goldman R, Pollard T, Rosenbaum J, eds. *Cell motility,* vol 3. *Cold Spring Harbor Conf* 1976; 1021–1049.
71. Lasek RJ, Garner JA, Brady ST. Axonal transport of the cytoplasmic matrix. *J Cell Biol* 1984; 99: 212–221.
72. Grafstein B, Forman D. Intracellular transport in neurons. *Physiol Rev* 1980; 60: 1167–1283.
73. Gorio A. Sprouting and regeneration of peripheral nerve. In: Zagoren JC, Fedoroff S, eds. *The node of ranvier.* New York: Academic Press; 1984: 353–388.
74. Carmignoto G, Finesso M, Siliprandi R, Gorio A. Muscle reinnervation—I. Restoration of transmitter release mechanisms. *Neuroscience* 1983; 8: 393–401.
75. Gorio A, Carmignoto G, Finesso M, Polato P, Nunzi MG. Muscle reinnervation—II. Sprouting, synapse formation and repression. *Neuroscience* 1983; 8: 402–416.
76. Gorio A, Marini P, Zanoni R. Muscle reinnervation—III. Motoneuron sprouting capacity, enhancement tby exogenous gangliosides. *Neuroscience* 1983; 8: 417–429.
77. Pestronk A, Drachman DB, Griffin JW. Effect of aging on nerve sprouting and regeneration. *Exp Neurol* 1980; 70: 65–82.
78. Cotman CW, Nieto-Sampedro M. Cell biology of synaptic plasticity. *Science* 1984; 225: 1287–1294.
79. Dyck PJ, Thomas PK, Asbury AK, Winegrad AI, Porte D, eds. *Diabetic neuropathy.* Philadelphia: Saunders; 1987.
80. Thomas PK, Brown M. Diabetic polyneuropathy. In: Dyck PJ, Thomas PK, Asbury AK, Winegrad AI, Porte D, eds. *Diabetic neuropathy.* Philadelphia: Saunders; 1987: 56–65.
81. Feldman M, Schiller LR. Disorders of gastrointestinal motility associated with diabetes mellitus. *Ann Int Med* 1983; 98: 380–384.
82. Belai A, Lincoln J, Milner P, Crowse R, Loesch H, Burnstock G. Enteric nerves in diabetic rats: increase in vasoactive intestinal peptide but not substance P. *Gastroenterology* 1985; 89: 967–976.
83. Di Giulio AM, Tenconi B, La Croix R, Mantegazza P, Abbracchio MP, Cattabeni F, Gorio A. Denervation and hyperinnervation in the nervous system of diabetic animals. I. The autonomic neuronal dystrophy of the gut. *J Neurosci Res* 1989; 24: 355–361.
84. Carsten RE, Whalen LR, Ishii DN. Impairment of spinal cord conduction velocity in diabetic rats. *Diabetes* 1989; 38: 730–736.
85. Di Giulio AM, Tenconi B, La Croix R, Mantegazza P, Abbracchio MP, Cattabeni F, Gorio A. Denervation and hyperinnervation in the nervous system of diabetic animals. II. Monoaminergic and peptidergic alterations in the diabetic encephalopathy. *J Neurosci Res* 1989; 24: 362–368.
86. Vitadello M, Couraud JY, Hassig R, Gorio A, Di Giamberardino L. Axonal transport of acetylcholinesterase in the mutant diabetic mouse. *Exp Neurol* 1983; 82: 143–147.
87. Vitadello M, Filliatreau G, Dupont JI, Hassig R, Gorio A, Di Giamberardino L. Altered axonal transport of cytoskeletal proteins in the mutant diabetic mouse. *J Neurochem* 1985; 45: 860–868.
88. Tomlison DR, Mayer JH. Defect of axonal transport in diabetes mellitus: a possible contribution to the etiology of diabetic neuropathy. *J Auton Pharmacol* 1984; 4: 59–72.
89. Eliasson SG. Nerve conduction changes in experimental diabetes. *J Clin Invest* 1964; 43: 2353–2358.
90. Schiavinato A, Morandin A, Gorio A. Quantitative analysis of myelin and axolemma particle distribution in C57BL/Ks diabetic mice and the effects of ganglioside treatment. *J Neurol Sci* 1985; 69: 301–317.
91. Abbracchio MP, Di Luca M, Di Giulio AM, Cattabeni F, Tenconi B, Gorio A. Denervation and hyperinnervation in the nervous system of diabetic animals. III. Functional alterations of G proteins in diabetic encephalopathy. *J Neurosci Res* 1989; 24: 517–523.
92. Abbracchio MP, Cattabeni F, Di Giulio AM, Paoletti AM, Finco C, Tenconi B, Gorio A. Early alterations of Gi/Go protein-dependent transductional processes in the retina of diabetic animals. *J Neurosci Res* 1991; 29: 196–200.
93. King RH, Llewelin JG, Thomas PK, Gilbey SG, Watkins PJ. Diabetic neuropathy: abnormalities of Schwann cell and perineurial basal laminae. Implications for diabetic vasculopathy. *Neuropathol Appl Neurobiol* 1989; 15: 339–355.
94. Noda K, Umeda F, Ono H, Hisatomi A, Chjiiwa Y, Nawata H, Ibayashi H. Decreased VIP content in peripheral nerve from streptozotocin-induced diabetic rats. *Diabetes* 1990; 39: 608–612.
95. Norido F, Canella R, Zanoni R, Gorio A. The development of diabetic neuropathy in the C57BL/Ks (db/db) mouse and its treatment with gangliosides. *Exp Neurol* 1984; 83: 221–233.
96. Finco C, Abbracchio MP, Malosio ML, Cattabeni F, Di Giulio AM, Paternieri B, Mantegazza P, Gorio A. Diabetes induced alterations of central nervous system G proteins: ADP-ribosylation, immunoreactivity and gene-expression studies in rat striatum. *J Chem Cell Neuropathol* 1992; (in press).
97. Ledeen R. Ganglioside structures and distribution: Are they located at the nerve ending? *J Supram Struct* 1978; 8: 1–17.
98. Gorio A, Carmignoto G, Facci L, Finesso M. Motor nerve sprouting induced by ganglioside

treatment. Possible implications for gangliosides on neuronal growth. *Brain Res* 1980; 197: 236–241.
99. Sparrow JR, Grafstein B. Sciatic nerve regeneration in ganglioside-treated rats. *Exp Neurol* 1982; 77: 230–235.
100. Robb G, Keynes RJ. Stimulation of nodal and terminal sprouting of mouse motor nerves by gangliosides. *Brain Res* 1983; 295: 368–371.
101. Norido F, Canella R, Zanoni R, Gorio A. The development of diabetic neuropathy in the C57 BL/Ks (db/db) mouse and its treatment with gangliosides. *Exp Neurol* 1984; 83: 221–232.
102. Marini P, Vitadello M, Bianchi R, Triban C, Gorio A. Impaired axonal transport of acetylcholinesterase in the sciatic nerve of alloxan-diabetic rats: effects of ganglioside treatment. *Diabetologia* 1986; 29: 254–258.
103. Bradley WG, Badger G, Tandan R, Fillyaw MJ, Young J, Fries TJ, Krusinski PB, Witarsa M, Boerman J, Blair BA. Double-blind controlled trials of Cronasadger sial in chronic neuromuscular diseases and ataxia. *Neurology* 1988; 38: 1732–1739.
104. Bassi S, Albizzati MG, Calloni F, Frattola L. Electromyographic study of diabetic and alcoholic polyneuropathic patients treated with gangliosides. *Muscle Nerve* 1982; 5: 531–536.
105. Horowitz SH. Therapeutic strategies in promoting peripheral nerve regeneration. *Muscle Nerve* 1989; 12: 314–322.
106. Pozza G, Saibene V, Comi G, Canal N. The effect of ganglioside administration in human diabetic peripheral neuropathy. In: Rapport MM, Gorio A, eds. *Gangliosides in neurological and neuromuscular function, development and repair.* New York: Raven Press; 1981: 253–257.
107. Hallet M, Flood T, Slater N, Dambrosia J. Trial of ganglioside therapy for dyabetic neuropathy. *Muscle Nerve* 1987; 10: 822–825.
108. Naarden A, Davidson J, Harris L, Moore J, De Felice S. Treatment of painful polyneuropathy with mixed gangliosides. In: Ledeen RW, Yu RK, Rapport MM, Suzuky K, eds. *Ganglioside structure, function, and biomedical potential.* New York: Plenum Press; 1984: 575–579.
109. Bradley WJ, Hedlund W, Cooper C, Desousa GJ, Gabbai A, Mora JS, Munsat TL, Scheife R. A double-blind controlled trial of bovine brain gangliosides in amyotrophic lateral sclerosis. *Neurology* 1984; 34: 1079–1082.
110. Harrington H, Hallett M, Tyler HR. Ganglioside therapy for amyotrophic lateral sclerosis: a double-blind controlled trial. *Neurology* 1984; 34: 1083–1085.
111. Suzuky K. Gangliosides and neuropathy. In: Rahmann H, ed. *Gangliosides and modulation of neuronal function.* Berlin: Springer-Verlag; 1987: 531–546.
112. Sadiq SA, Thomas FP, Kilidireas K, Protopsaltis S, Hays AP, Lee KW, Romas SN, Kumar N, van den Berg L, et al. The spectrum of neurologic diseases associated with anti-GM1 antibodies. *Neurology* 1990; 40: 1067–1072.
113. Quarles RH, Ilyas AA, Willison HJ. Antibodies to gangliosides and myelin proteins in Guillain-Barre syndrome. *Ann Neurol* [Suppl] 1990; 27: 48–52.
114. Latov N. Neuropathy and anti-GM1 antibodies. *Ann Neurol* 1990; 27 Suppl: 41–43.
115. Yu RK, Ariga T, Kohriyama T, Kusunoki S, Maeda Y, Miyatani N. Autoimmune mechanisms in peripheral neuropathies. *Ann Neurol* [Suppl] 1990; 27: 30–35.
116. Walsh FS, Cronin M, Koblar S, Doherty P, Winer J, Leon A, Hughes RAC. Association between glycoconjugate antibodies and Campylobacter infection in patients with Guillain-Barré syndrome. *J Neuroimmunol* 1991; 34: 43–51.
117. Gallo P, Piccinno MG, Tavolato B, Innocenti M, Callegaro L, Kirschner G, Bruno R, Chizzolini C, Fiori MG. Parenteral administration of GM1 does not affect cytokines and anti-ganglioside antibody pattern. *J Immunol* 1992; 36: 81–86.
118. Palkovits M. Distribution of neuropeptides in the central nervous system: a review of biochemical mapping studies. *Prog Neurobiol* 1984; 23: 151–189.
119. Verhaagen J, Edwards PM, Gispen WH. Pharmacological aspects of the influence of melanocortins on the formation of regenerative peripheral nerve sprouts. *Peptides* 1987; 8: 581–584.
120. Saint-Come C, Strand FL. ACTH/MSH4-10 improves motor unit reorganization during peripheral nerve regeneration in the rat. *Peptides* 1985; 6: 77–83.
121. Koning P de, Gispen WH. Org 2766 improves functional and electrophysiological aspects of regenerating schiatic nerve in the rat. *Peptides* 197; 8: 415–422.
122. Hoop RG van der, Brokkee J-H, Kopelle H, Samson M, Koning P de, Yispen WH. A new approach for the evaluation of recovery after peripheral nerve damage. *J Neurosci Meth* 1988; 26: 111–116.
123. Gerritsen van der Hoop R, Koning P de, Neijt JP, Jennekens FGI, Gispen WH. Efficacy of the neuropeptide ORG 2766 in the prevention and treatment of cisplatin-induced neurotoxicity in rats. *Eur J Cancer Clin Oncol* 1988; 24: 637–642.
124. Zee CEEM van der, Edwards PM, Koning P de, Gispen WH. Beneficial effects of melanocortins on axonal regeneration: possibility for treatment of diabetic-induced peripheral neuropathy. *Neurosci Lett* 1987, 22:254.
125. Zee CEEM van der, Buuse M van der, Gispen WH. Beneficial effect of an ACTH-(4-9) analog on peripheral neuropathy and blood pressure response to tyramine in streptozotocin diabetic rats. *Eur J Pharmacol* 1990; 177: 211–213.
126. Hoop RG van der, Vecht CJ, Burg ME van der, Elderson A, Boogerd W, Heimans JJ, Vries EP, Houwelingen JC van, et al. Prevention of cisplatin neurotoxicity with an ACTH (4-9) analogue in patients with ovarian cancer. *N Engl J Med* 1990; 322: 89–94.

127. Calvani M, Carta A. Clues to the mechanism of action of acetyl-l-carnitine in the central nervous system. *Dementia* 1991; 2: 1–6.
128. Fritz IB, Yue KTN. Effect of carnitine on acetyl-CoA oxidation by heart muscle mitochondria. *Am J Physiol* 1964; 206: 531.
129. Imperato A, Ramacci MT, Angelucci L. Acetyl-l-carnitine enhances acetylcholine release in the striatum and hippocampus of awake freely moving rats. *Neurosci Lett* 1989; 107: 251–255.
130. De Simone R, Ramacci MT, Aloe L. Effect of acetyl-l-carnitine on forebrain cholinergic neurons of developing rats. *Int J Dev Neurosci* 1991; 9: 39–46.
131. Angelucci L, Ramacci MT, Taglialatela G, Hulsebosch C, Morgan B, Werrbach-Perez K, Perez-Polo R. Nerve growth factor binding in aged rat central nervous system: effect of acetyl-l-carnitine. *J Neurosci Res* 1988; 20: 491–496.
132. Taglialatela G, Angelucci L, Ramacci MT, Foreman PJ, Perez-Polo JR. 125I-B-Nerve growth factor binding is reduced in rat brain after stress exposure. *J Neurosci Res* 1990; 25: 331–335.
133. Ramacci MT, De Rossi M, Lucreziotti MR, Mione MC, Amenta F. Effects of long-term treatment with acetyl-l-carnitine on structural changes of aging rat brain. *Drugs Exp Clin Res* 1988; 14: 112–115.
134. Napoleone P, Ferrante F, Ghirardi O, Ramacci MT, Amenta F. Age-dependent nerve cell loss in the brain of Sprague-Dawley rats: effects of long term acetyl-l-carnitine treatment. *Arch Gerontol Geriatr* 1990; 10: 173–185.
135. Barnes CA, Markowska AL, Ingram DK, Kameton H, Spangler EL, Lemken VJ, Olton DS. Acetyl-L-Carnitine 2: effect on learning and memory performance of aged rats in simple and complex mazes. *Neurobiol Aging* 1990; 11: 499–506.
136. Caprioli A, Ghirardi O, Ramacci MT, Angelucci L. Age-dependent deficit in radial maze performance in the rat: effect of chronic treatment with acetyl-l-carnitine. *Prog Neuropsychopharmacol Biol Psychiatry* 1990; 14: 359–369.
137. Curti D, Dagani F, Galmozzi MR, Marzatico F. Effect of aging and acetil-l-carnitine on energetic and cholinergic metabolism in rat brain regions. *Mech Aging Dev* 1989; 47: 39–45.
138. Gadaleta MN, Petruzzella V, Renis M, Fracasso F, Cantatore P. Reduced transcription of mitochondrial DNA in senescent rat: tissue dependence and effect of acetyl-l-carnitine. *Eur J Biochem* 1990; 187: 501–506.
139. Aureli T, Miccheli A, Ricciolini R, Di Cocco ME, Ramacci MT, Angelucci L, Ghirardi O, Conti F. Aging brain: effect of acetyl-l-carnitine treatment on rat brain energy and phospholipid metabolism. A study by 31P and 1H NMR spectroscopy. *Brain Res* 1990; 526: 108–112.
140. Carta A, Calvani M. Acetyl-l-carnitine: a drug able to slow the progress of Alzheimer's disease. In: Growdon JH, Corkin S, Ritter-Walker E, Wurtmann RJ, eds. *Proceedings of the sixth meeting of the International Study Group on the Pharmacology of Memory Disorders Associated with Aging.* 1991.
141. Fernandez A, Pallini R, Lauretti L, Marchese E, Gangitano C, Del Fa A, Olivieri-Sangiacomo C, Sbriccoli A, Rossi GF. Levocarnitina acetyl prevents cell death following chronic section of the vagus nerve in rats. *Int J Clin Pharmacol* 1992; (in press).
142. De Angelis C, Scarfó C, Falcinelli M, Reda E, Ramacci MT, Angelucci L. Levocarnitine acetyl stimulates peripheral nerve regeneration and neuromuscular junction remodeling following sciatic nerve injury. *Int J Clin Pharmacol Res* 1992; (in press).
143. De simone R, Aloe L, Ferraris L, Ramacci MT. Levocarnitine acetyl treatment promotes iris reinnervation following 6-OHDA induced noradrenergic denervation in rats. *Int J Clin Pharmacol* 1992; (in press).
144. Pacifici L, Bellucci A, Piovesan P, Maccari F, Gorio A, Ramacci MT. Levocanitine acetyl counteracts experimentally induced diabetic neuropathy. *Int J Clin Pharmacol Res* 1992; (in press).
145. Gorio A, Di Giulio AM, Tenconi B, Donadoni L, Germani E, Bertelli A, Mantegazza P, Maccari F, Ramacci MT. Acetyl-l-carnitine treatment prevents alterations in autonomic diabetic neuropathy. *Int J Clin Pharmacol* 1992; (in press).
146. Di Giulio AM, Gorio A, Bertelli A, Mantegazza P, Ferraris L, Ramacci MT. Acetyl-l-carnitine prevents substance P loss in the sciatic nerve and lumbar spinal cord of diabetic animals. *Int J Clin Pharmacol* 1992; (in press).
147. Scarfó C, Falcinelli M, Pacifici L, Bellucci A, Reda E, De Angelis C, Ramacci MT, Angelucci L. Levocarnitine acetyl prevents morphological and electrophysiological changes of peripheral nerve-muscle unit in the aged rat. *Int J Clin Pharmacol* 1992; (in press).
148. Mezzina C, De Grandis D, Calvani M, Marchionni A, Pomes A. Idiopathic facial paralysis: new therapeutic prospects with acetyl-l-carnitine. *Int J Clin Pharmacol* 1992; (in press).
149. Mezzina C, Frigato F, Virgili F, Pomes A, Donadoni W, Livolsi P, Onofrj M, Fulgente T, Verienti P, Marchionni A, Marchionni M, Calvani M. Acetyl-l-carnitine, a new treatment for diabetic neuropathy: a multicenter double blind trial. *Int J Clin Pharmacol* 1992; (in press).
150. Onofrj M, Colamartino P, Tomasello M, Alofaci C, De Sanctis E, Cudoni S, Espa E, Ventura F, Pennisi G, Bella R, Marchionni A, Colonna V, Calvani M. Acetyl-l-carnitine treatment of patients affected by peripheral neuropathies: a multicenter double blind trial. *Int J Clin Pharmacol* 1992; (in press).
151. Hantaz-Ambroise D, Koenig J. Etude in vitro de l'action de l'isaxonine sur la croissance des neurones de la moelle épinière de rat. *Nouv Press Med* 1982; 11: 1238–1242.

152. Hugelin A, Legrain Y, Bondoux-Jahan M. Nerve growth promoting action of isaxonine in rat. *Experientia* 1979; 35: 626–627.
153. Hugelin A, Tarrade T, Istin M, Coelho R. Acceleration de la vitesse de croissance de neurone par une nouvelle substance neurotrope: Le N-isopropyl-2-amino-pyrimidine. *C R Acad Sci Paris* 1977; 285: 1339–1341.
154. Le Quesne PM, Fowler CJ, Harding AE. A study of the effects of isaxonine on vincristine induced peripheral neuropathy in man and regeneration following peripheral nerve crush in the rat. *J Neurol Neurosurg Psychiatry* 1985; 48: 933–935.
155. Pecot-Dechavassine M, Mira JC. Effects of isaxonine on skeletal muscle reinnervation in the rat: an electrophysiological evaluation. *Muscle Nerve* 1985; 8: 105–114.
156. DeBleecker J, DeCoster W, DeReuck J, Blancquaert JP. Influence of isaxonine on the target phenomenon, muscle fiber size and neuromuscular junction in the tenotomized and denervated gastrocnemius muscle of the rat. *Acta Neuropathol* 1986; 69: 337–340.
157. Duhamel G, Parlier Y. Activité protectrice de l'isaxonine dans la neuropathie à la vincristine. *Nouv Press Med* 1982; 11: 1254–57.
158. Guiheneuc P, Ginet J, Grolleau J-Y, Rojouan J. Etude des effets de l'isaxonine sur les lesions de dégénérescence axonal rétrograde induites chez l'homme par la vincristine. *Nouv Press Med* 1982; 11: 1257–1261.
159. Cambier J, Dordain G. Essai controlé de l'isaxonine dans les neuropathies de cause traumatique ou ischemique (par compression). *Nouv Press Med* 1982; 11: 1272–1274.
160. Dehen H. Etude clinique et electrophysiologique de l'isaxonine dans les paralysies faciales periferiques. *Nouv Press Med* 1982; 11: 1262–1264.
161. Sebille A, Hugelin A. Muscle reinnervation enhanced by isaxonine in man. *Br J Clin Pharmacol* 1980; 9: 275–276.
162. Augustin P, Tathery M, Essai clinique de l'isaxonine dans les neuropathies diabetiques. *Nouv Press Med* 1982; 11: 1265–1268.
163. Kilmer SL, Carlsen RD. Forskolin activation of adenylate cyclase in vivo stimulates nerve regeneration. *Nature* 1984; 307: 455–457.
164. Hoffman H. Acceleration and retardation of the process of axon-sprouting in partially denervated muscle. *Aust J Exp Biol Med Sci* 1952; 30: 541–566.
165. Keynes RJ. The effects of pyronin on sprouting and regeneration of mouse motor nerves. *Brain Res* 1982; 254: 13–18.
166. Muller HW, Ignatius MJ, Hangen OH, Shooter EM. Expression of specific sheath cell proteins during peripheral nerve growth and regeneration in mammals. *J Cell Biol* 1986; 102: 293–402.
167. Muller WH, Shooter EM. Molecular approach to the role of macrophages and astrocytes in nerve growth and development. In: Althaus HH, Seifert W, eds. *Glial-neuronal communication in development and regeneration*. Berlin: Springer-Verlag: Nato ASI series H, vol 2: 630–640.
168. Skene JHP, Shooter EM. Denervated sheath cells secrete a new protein after nerve injury. *Proc Natl Acad Sci USA* 1983; 80: 4169–4173.
169. Muller HW, Gebicke-Harter PJ, Hangen OH, Shooter EM. A specific 37000-Dalton protein that accumulates in regenerating but not in nonregenerating mammalian nerves. *Science* 1985; 228: 499–501.
170. Snipes GJ, McGuire CB, Norden JJ, Freeman JA. Nerve injury stimulates the secretion of apolipoprotein E by nonneuronal cells. *Proc Natl Acad Sci USA* 1986; 83: 1130–1134.
171. Stoll G, Muller HW. Macrophages in the peripheral nervous system and astroglia in the central nervous system of rat commonly express apolipoprotein E during development but differ in their response to injury. *Neurosci Lett* 1986; 72: 233–238.
172. Muller HW, Minwegen P. Nonresident macrophages in peripheral nerve of rat: effect of silica on migration, myelin phagocytosis, and apolipoprotein E expression during wallerian degeneration. *J Neurosci Res* 1987; 18: 222–289.
173. Goodrum JF. Cholesterol synthesis is downregulated during regeneration of peripheral nerve. *J Neurochem* 1990; 54: 1709–1715.
174. Marmisco G, Minea J. Nouvelles recherches sur l'influence qu'exerce l'ablation du corps thiroide sur la degenerescence et la regenerescence des nerfs. *CR Soc Biol* 1910; 68: 188–190.
175. Isenscmid R. Ueder den einfluss von thymus und schilddrusse auf die nerven-regeneration. Versuche mit thymokreszin und thyroxin. *Schweiz Med Wochenschr* 1932; 62: 785–789.
176. McIsaac G, Kiernan JA. Accelerated recovery from peripheral nerve injury in experimental hyperthyroidism. *Exp Neurol* 1975; 48: 88–94.
177. McQuarrie IG. Nerve regeneration and thyroid hormone. *J Clin Neurol Sci* 1975; 26: 499–502.
178. Berenberg RA, Forman DS, Wood DK, De Silva A, Demaree J. Recovery of peripheral nerve function after axotomy: effect of triiodothyronine. *Exp Neurol* 1977; 57: 349–363.
179. Cockett SA, Kiernan JA. Acceleration of peripheral nervous regeneration in the rat by exogenous triiodothyronine. *Exp Neurol* 1973; 39: 389–394.
180. Kiernan JA, Heiniche EA. Estimation of lengths of regenerated axons in nerves. *Exp Neurol* 1977; 56: 431–434.
181. Cook RA, Kiernan JA. Effect of triiodothyronine on protein synthesis in regenerating peripheral neurons. *Exp Neurol* 1976; 52: 515–524.
182. Harvey JE, Srebnik HH. Locomotor activity and axonal regeneration following spinal cord compression in rats treated with l-thyroxin. *J Neuropathol Exp Neurol* 1967; 26: 661–668.
183. Hagashi M, Patel AJ. An interaction between thyroid hormone and nerve growth factor in the regulation of choline-acetyltransferase activity

183. ...in neuronal cultures, derived from the septal-diagonal band region of the embryonic rat brain. *Dev Brain Res* 1987; 36: 109–120.
184. Dyck PJD, Thomas PK, Asbury AK, Winegrad AI, Porte D, eds. *Diabetic neuropathy*. Philadelphia: Saunders; 1987.
185. Tomlison DR, Towsend J, Fretten P. Prevention of defective axonal transport in streptozotocin-diabetic rats by treatment with Statil (ICI 128436), an aldose reductose inhibitors. *Diabetes* 1985; 34: 970–972.
186. Canal N, Comi G. Aldose reductase inhibitors: pharmacological data and therapeutic perspectives. *TIPS* 1985; 6: 328–330.
187. Ao S, Shingu Y, Kikuchi C, Takano Y, Nomura K, Fujiwara T, Ohkubo Y, Notsu Y, Yamaguchi I. Characterization of a novel aldose reductase inhibitor, FRT74366, and its effects on diabetic cataract and neuropathy in the rat. *Metabolism* 1991; 40: 77–87.
188. Kato K, Nakayama K, Ohta M, Murakami N, Murakami K, Mizota M, Miwa I, Okuda J. Effect of novel aldose reductase inhibitors, M16209 and M16287, on streptozotocin-induced diabetic neuropathy in rats. *Eur J Pharmacol* 1991; 193: 185–191.
189. Greene DA, Lattimer SA, Carroll PB, Fernstrom JD, Finegold DN. A defect in sodium-dependent amino acid uptake in diabetic rabbit peripheral nerve. Correction by an aldose reductase inhibitor or Myo-inositol administration. *J Clin Invest* 1990; 85: 1657–1665.
190. Yagihashi, Kamijo M, Ido Y, Mirrlees DJ. Effect of long term aldose reductase inhibition on development of experimental diabetic neuropathy. Ultrastructural and morphometric studies of sural nerve in streptozotocin-induced diabetic rats. *Diabetes* 1990; 39: 690–696.
191. Jennings PE, Nightingale S, Le-Guen C, Lawson N, Williamson JR, Hoffman P, Barnett AH. Prolonged aldose reductase inhibition in chronic peripheral diabetic neuropathy: effects on microangiopathy. *Diabetic Med* 1990; 7: 63–68.
192. Jamal GA, Carmichael H. The effect of gamma-linolenic acid on human diabetic peripheral neuropathy: a double-blind placebo-controlled trial. *Diabetic Med* 1990; 7: 319–323.
193. Maragh H, Meyer BS, Davemport D, Gould JD, Terzis JK. Morphofunctional evaluation of fibrin glue versus microsuture nerve repair. *J Reconstr Microsurg* 1990; 6: 331–337.
194. Favaro G, Bortolami MC, Cereser S, Dona M, Pastorello A, Callegaro L, Fiori MG. Peripheral nerve regeneration through a novel bioresorbable nerve guide. *ASAIO Trans* 1990; 36: 291–294.
195. Lundborg G, Daklin LB, Danielson N, Gelberman RH, Longo FM, Powell HC, Varon S. Nerve regeneration in silicon chambers: influence of gap length and of distal stump components. *Exp Neurol* 1982; 76: 3361–3375.
196. Williams LR, Varon S. Modification of fibrin matrix formation in situ enhances nerve regeneration in silicone chambers. *J Comp Neurol* 1985; 231: 209–220.
197. Muller H, Williams LR, Varon S. Nerve regeneration chamber: evaluation of exogenous agents applied by multiple injections. *Brain Res* 1987; 413: 320–325.
198. Madison R, da Silva CT, Dikkes P, Chiu T-H, Sidman RL. Increased rate of peripheral nerve regeneration using bioresorbable nerve guides and a laminin-containing gel. *Exp Neurol* 1985; 88: 767–772.
199. Longo FM, Hayman EG, Davis GE, Ruoslahti E, Engvall E, Manthorpe M, Varon S. Neurite promoting factors and extracellular matrix components accumulating in vivo within nerve regeneration chambers. *Brain Res* 1984; 309: 105–117.
200. Rosen JM, Padilla JA, Nguyen KD, Padilla MA, Sabelman EE, Pham HN. Artificial nerve graft using collagen as an extracellular matrix for nerve repair compared with sutured autograft in a rat model. *Ann Plast Surg* 1990; 25: 375–387.
201. Takahashi M, Satou T, Hashimoto S. Experimental in vivo regeneration of peripheral nerve axons and perineurium guided by resorbable collagen film. *Acta Pathol Jpn* 1988; 38: 1489–1502.
202. Coughlin C, Elam JS. Enhanced axonal transport of glycosaminoglycans in regenerating goldfish optic nerve. *Brain Res* 1989; 493: 326–330.
203. Lander Ad, Fuji DK, Gospodarowicz D, Reichardt LF. Characterization of a factor that promotes neurite outgrowth: evidence linking activity to heparan sulfate proteoglycans. *J Cell Biol* 1982; 94: 574–585.
204. Walicke PA. Basic and acidic fibroblast growth factors have trophic effects on neurons from multiple CNS regions. *J Neurosci* 1988; 8: 2618–2627.
205. Hollowell JP, Villadiego A, Rich KM. Sciatic nerve regeneration across gaps within silicone chambers: long-term effects of NGF and consideration on axonal branching. *Exp Neurol* 1990; 110: 45–51.
206. Khouri RK, Chiu DT, Feinberg J, Tark KC, Harper A, Spielholz N. Effects of neurite-promoting factors on rat sciatic nerve regeneration. *Microsurgery* 1989; 10: 206–209.
207. Lundborg G, Daklin LB, Danielson N, Gelberman RG, Longo FM, Powell HC, Varon S. Nerve regeneration in silicon chambers: influence of gap length and of distal stump components. *Exp Neurol* 1982; 76: 361–375.
208. Lundborg G, Gelberman RG, Longo FM, Powell HC, Varon S. In vivo regeneration of cut nervesencased in silicone tubes: growth across a six millimeter gap. *J Neuropathol Exp Neurol* 1982; 41: 412–422.
209. Williams LR, Powell HC, Lundborg G, Varon S. Competence of nerve tissue as distal inert promoting nerve regeneration in a silicone chamber. *Brain Res* 1984; 293: 201–211.
210. Longo FM, Hayman EG, Davis GE, Ruoslahti E, Engvall E, Manthorpe M, Varon S. Neurite-promoting factors and extracellular matrix

components accumulating in vivo within nerve regeneration chambers. *Brain Res* 1984; 309: 105–117.
211. Williams LR, Longo FM, Powell HC, Lundborg G, Varon S. Spatial-temporal progress of peripheral nerve regeneration within a silicone chamber: parameters for a bioassay. *J Comp Neurol* 1983; 218: 460–470.
212. Varon S, Williams LR. Peripheral nerve regeneration in a silicone chamber: cellular and molecular aspects. *Peripheral Nerve Rep Reg* 1986; 1: 9–25.
213. Marsh G, Beams HW. In vitro control of growing chick nerve fibers by applied electric currents. *J Cell Comp Physiol* 1946; 27: 139–157.
214. Jaffe LF, Poo MM. Neurites grow faster towards the cathode than the anode in a steady field. *J Exp Zool* 1979; 209: 115–127.
215. Hinkle L, McCraig CD, Robinson KR. The direction of growth of differentiating neurons and myoblasts from frog embryos in an applied electric field. *J Physiol* 1981, 314: 121–135.
216. Patel NB, Poo MM. Orientation of neurite growth by extracellular electric fields. *J Neurosci* 1982; 2: 483–496.
217. Patel NB, Poo MM. Perturbation of the direction of neurite growth by pulsed and focal electric fields. *J Neurosci* 1984; 4: 2939–2947.
218. Borgens RB, Vanable JW Jr, Jaffe LF. Small artificial currents enhance *Xenopus* limb regeneration. *J Exp Zool* 1979; 200: 403–416.
219. Borgens RB, Roederer E, Cohen MJ. Enhanced spinal cord regeneration in lamprey by applied electric fields. *Science* 1981; 213: 611–617.
220. Pomeranz B, Mullen M, Markus H. Effect of applied electric fields on sprouting of intact saphenous nerve in adult rat. *Brain Res* 1984; 303: 331–336.
221. Borgens RB, Blight AR, Murphy DJ, Stewart L. Transected dorsal column axons within the guinea pig spinal cord regenerate in the presence of an applied electric field. *J Comp Neurol* 1986; 250: 168–180.
222. Borgens RB, Blight AR, McGinnis ME. Behavioral recovery induced by applied electric fields after spinal cord hemisection in guinea pig. *Science* 1987; 238: 366–369.
223. Borgens RB, Blight AR, McGinnis ME. Functional recovery after spinal cord hemisection in guinea pigs: the effects of applied electric fields. *J Comp Neurol* 1990; 296: 634–653.
224. Tranzer JP, Thoenen H. An electron-microscopic study of selective, acute degeneration of sympathetic nerve terminals after administration of 6-hydroxydopamine. *Experientia* 1968; 29: 314–315.
225. Bloom FE, Algeri S, Groppetti A, Revuelta A, Costa E. Lesions of central norepinephrine terminals with 6-OH-dopamine. *Science* 1969; 166: 1284–1286.
226. Baumgarten HG, Bjorklund A, Lachenmayer L, Nobin A, Stenevi U. Long-lasting selective depletion of brain serotonin by 5,6-dihydroxytryptamine. *Acta Physiol Scand [Suppl]* 1971; 373.
227. Baumgarten HG, Lachenmayer L. 5,7-dihydroxytryptamine: improvement in chemical lesioning of indolamine neurons in the brain. *Z Aellforsch* 1972; 135: 399–414.
228. Jonsson G, Sachs CH. Effects of 6-hydroxydopamine on the uptake and storage of noradrenaline in sympathetic adrenergic neurons. *Eur J Pharmacol* 1970; 9: 141–155.
229. Jonsson G, Gorio A, Hallman H, Janigro D, Kojima H, Luthman J, Zanoni R. Effects of GM1 ganglioside on developing and mature serotonin and noradrenaline neurons lesioned by selective neurotoxins. *J Neurosci Res* 1984; 12: 459–476.
230. Jonsson G, Sachs CH. Neurochemical properties of adrenergic nerves regenerated after 6-hydroxydopamine. *J Neurochem* 1972; 19: 2577–2585.
231. Jonsson G, Sachs CH. Histochemical and neurochemical studies on adrenergic nerves regenerated after chemical sympathectomy produced by 6 hydroxydopamine. In: Fujiwara, ed. *Fluorescence histochemistry of biogenic amines*. Tokyo: Igaku-Shoin; 1973: 67–81.
232. Sachs CH, Jonsson G. Changes in central noradrenaline neurons after systemic 6-hydroxydopamine administration. *J Neurochem* 1973; 21: 1517–1524.
233. Kojima H, Gorio A, Janigro D, Jonsson G. GM1 ganglioside has a regrowth enhancing effect on neurotoxin induced lesion of noradrenaline nerve terminals in rat cerebral cortex. *Neuroscience* 1984; 13: 1011–1022.
234. Gorio A, Tenconi B, Donadoni ML, Malosio ML, Finco C, Di Giulio AM, Mantegazza P. Reactive CNS compensatory events are inhibited by perinatal exposure to morphine. *J Pharmacol Toxicol* 1991; (in press).
235. Steinbusch HW, Van Lujitelaar MG, Dijkstra H, Nijssen A, Tonnaer JA. Aging and regenerative capacity of the rat serotoninergic system. A morphological, neurochemical and behavioral analysis after transplantation of fetal raphe cells. *Ann NY Acad Sci* 1990; 600: 384–402.
236. Frankfurt M, Azmitia E. Regeneration of serotoninergic fibers in the rat hypothalamus following unilateral 5,7-dihydroxytryptamine injection. *Brain Res* 1984; 298: 273–282.
237. Frankfurt M, Beaudet A. Reinnervation of dopamine neurons by regenerating serotonin axons in the rat medial zona incerta. A combined radioautographic and immunocytochemical ultrastructural study. *Exp Brain Res* 1988; 72: 473–480.
238. Frankfurt M, Beaudet A. Ultrastructural organization of regenerated serotonin axons in the dorsomedial hypothalamus of the adult rat. *J Neurocytol* 1987; 16: 799–809.
239. Luthman J, Bolioli B, Tsutsumi T, Verhofstad A, Jonsson G. Sprouting of striatal serotonin nerve terminals following selective lesions of

nigro-striatal dopamine neurons in neonatal rats. *Brain Res Bull* 1987; 19: 269–274.
240. Privat A, Mansour H, Pavy A, Geffard M, Sandillon F. Transplantation of dissociated foetal serotonin neurons into the transected spinal cord of adult rats. *Neurosci Lett* 1986; 66: 61–66.
241. Di Giulio AM, Restani P, Galli CL, Tenconi B, La Croix R, Gorio A. Modified ontogenesis of enkephalin and substance P containing neurons in rat after perinatal exposure to morphine. *Toxicology* 1988; 49: 197–201.
242. Gorio A, Malosio ML, Tenconi B, Donadoni ML, Mantegazza P, Di Giulio AM. Supression of reactive compensatory changes in the brain by morphine. *21st Annual Meeting of the Society of Neuroscience.* (abstract) New Orleans: 1991, p. 737.
243. Gorio A, Tenconi B, Zonta N, Mantegazza P, Di Giulio AM. Reactive sprouting (pruning effect) is altered in the brain of rats perinatally exposed to morphine. In: Timiras PS, et al. eds. *Plasticity and regeneration of the nervous system.* New York: Plenum Press; 1991: 61-67.
244. Apfel SC, Lipton RB, Arezzo JC, Kessler JA. Nerve growth factor prevents toxic neuropathy in mice. *Ann Neurol* 1991; 29: 87–90.
245. Apfel SC, Arezzo JC, Lipson LA, Kessler JA. Nerve growth factor prevents experimental cisplatin neuropathy. *Ann Neurol* 1992; 31: 76–80.

15

Future Directions on Neuroregeneration Research

Concluding Remarks

Alfredo Gorio, Anna Maria Di Giulio, and Paolo Mantegazza

Departments of Medical Pharmacology, Chemotherapy, and Toxicology, University of Milan, 20129 Milan, Italy

Neuroregeneration has been and will be again among the major topics of neuroscience research for two main reasons: One is social and is related to the marked increase in frequency of neurodegenerative disorders associated with the longer average life span, with the marked increase of traumatic injuries involving mainly young people, and with the dramatic increase in social costs; the other reason originates from the great advancement of research in the area, which is witnessed by the present volume. As is apparent, a further improved understanding of the mechanisms underlying neuroregeneration is necessary for the description of neuronal regeneration and for designing new approaches to treatment, which aims to improve neural repair in man affected by neurodegenerative disorders.

The role of cytoskeletal components in neurite sprouting and elongation is quite clear, with a critical involvement of actin and microfilaments in sprouting and microtubules in elongation. As S.T. Brady (Chapter 2, this volume) has well pointed out, the conditioning lesion paradigm triggers a change in neuronal protein synthesis associated with an increase of SCb rate of transport and with an increased amount of tubulin in the same cytoskeletal fraction. Such a change in axonal transport is correlated by a correspondent enhancement of nerve regeneration rate. Also the local disruption of myelination, as occurs in the trembler mouse, alters axonal cytoskeletal organization with changes in slow transport and in rate of regeneration. When transported neurofilaments enter a nerve graft originated from a trembler mouse, their transport velocity is slowed (see Brady, Chapter 2, this volume). These examples show that it is possible to up-regulate the expression and dynamics of cytoskeletal proteins such as microtubules and thereby affecting neuronal regeneration. The trembler mouse example has shown that a local alteration of axon-glia interaction alters locally the transport of cytoskeletal components. Future deeper research in this area would supply the needed knowledge on the basic transport mechanisms linking together dynamics and regeneration. Likely this would be a way to develop strategies of treatment for achieving faster neuronal regeneration, which is most desired in many cases of peripheral nerve disorders. Of the several agents reviewed in this volume (see Gorio et al.) none is capable of such effects. A novel approach to treatment that deserves further development comes from the experience from acetyl-1-carnitine, which is known to reverse several biochemical and behavioral parameters altered in aging brain by mechanisms affecting brain energy state and by preventing mitochondrial alterations (see Gorio et al., this volume). Perhaps a good target for improving nerve regeneration and for repairing nerve dysfunctions could be the mitochondria.

The role of neurotrophic factors in nerve regenerations and the advantages and problems raised by their use in the treatment of peripheral neuropathies are well discussed by Gold and Spencer (Chapter 6, this volume). In their article a broad literature derived from in vivo and in vitro data is reviewed; one can extrapolate that an early exogenous supplementation of these agents may prevent retrograde degeneration and neuronal death. On the other hand it is apparent from the data reported and from their comments that the systemic use of trophic factors may be difficult if the target is the enhancement of neuronal regeneration. For instance, nerve growth factor (NGF) acting locally on injured nerve might be useful while NGF reaching the cell bodies would give the false information of a normal trophic situation shutting down the biosynthesis of materials required for regeneration. Future research should make this point clear and suggest the way of overriding this problem. Hagg et al. (Chapter 13, this volume) have reviewed the entire field of neurotrophic factors, showing how several other trophic molecules have been identified in addition to neurotrophins. Their potential utility derives from a supposed reduced supply of trophic substances to the injured neuron. Therefore the same restrictions and requirements indicated for NGF apply also to them.

While axonal regeneration in the peripheral nervous system is possible and the goal of improving its efficiency might be forthcoming, in the central nervous system regeneration can be achieved only by the monoaminergic systems or by local synaptic rearrangements mediated by collateral sprouting in partially denervated areas. Future research for enhancing recovery from neural injuries stems from two basically different strategies: One aims to promote regeneration in the central nervous system, while the other one aims at developing treatments that may promote recovery without directly affecting regeneration. The former approach is based on devising means capable of stimulating regeneration by supplying the lesioned axons with an appropriate substrate for outgrowth. The attempts to identify cell surface molecules able to enhance or inhibit this process are well described by Carbonetto and David (Chapter 5, this volume). The extensive literature on n-CAM in nervous system development and the effects of sialo-glycolipids on neuronal regeneration are indicative of the potential role for cell surface agents in neural repair. There is a need for better understanding and for clear advancement in this area of research that has to be considered crucial to neuroregeneration in the central nervous system. A way of supplying a favorable substrate for regeneration has been elegantly described by Goldberger et al. (Chapter 12, this volume). In addition to describing the intrinsic anatomical and behavioral plasticity of neural networks in the spinal cord, they have shown the use of neural transplants for enhancing morphological and functional regeneration in the spinal cord after transection. In their chapter they have shown how the spinal cord can be the site of powerful processes of collateral sprouting and, in appropriate conditions, is even capable of sustaining axonal regeneration if the lesion gap is filled with a neural transplant. The nonregenerative approach to treatment of spinal injuries is documented by W. Young (Chapter 9, this volume). The starting point is that "complete" spinal cord lesions do not necessarily mean total loss of connections between spinal cord and higher centers. Most patients still have several axons surviving in the ventral portion of the cord; they are demyelinated and their excitability is altered. The author suggests that future research should aim at the prevention of excitability loss and/or to its restoration since it is known that remyelination can be obtained with Schwann cells and that some potassium channel blockers have shown early promising results. In addition, Schwann cells can supply a complex milieu that may enhance neuronal survival and regrowth; therefore Schwann cells may promote recovery of excitability and regeneration at the site of lesion. Another problem to solve in this issue is the source of Schwann cells, since the amounts of cells to be employed for filling the gap of a human spinal cord injury might be enormous.

As is well described by Cotman and colleagues (Chapter 11, this volume) brain neuronal plasticity is essential for normal functions such as learning and memory and plays a big role in the recovery after injury or disease. Such a process is present under several forms also in the brain of Alzheimer disease (AD) patients. In some instances compensatory neuroregenerative events are normal as in the case of cholinergic sprouting in the dentate gyrus of AD patients who have lost enthorinal cortex neurons; the same events are described in animals after enthorinal cortex lesion. On the other hand they also show that in the brain of AD patients regenerative outgrowth occurs around senile plaques and that several molecular markers of sprouting and synaptogenesis are present. The misdirected growth around the senile plaques is correlated by a local overexpression of basic fibroblast growth factor and of β-amyloid protein (see Cotman et al., this volume).

Therefore it appears that AD might be a miscellany of physiological compensatory plasticity processes and misdirected outgrowth stimuli as in the case of senile plaques. Future research must identify the mechanisms that lead to aberrant plasticity and to neuronal progressive degeneration.

The information assembled in this volume deals with the regulation of neuronal survival, regeneration, and plasticity, and special reference was placed on data related to the mammalian system, to in vivo experiments, and to treatments aimed at improving repair after nerve injuries. The available evidence was reviewed and, although we are aware that some issues are missing, we hope that the evidence gathered will foster new energy into the field. One point that was only lightly discussed is the possible role of neurotransmitters and of the signal transduction systems on neuronal survival and regeneration. The changes in content of second messengers and ions such as calcium might alter the cytoskeleton and thereby affect neurite outgrowth (see S.T. Brady, Chapter 2, this volume). It has been also reported by Gorio et al. (this volume) that functional alterations of G proteins occur in the retina of diabetic animals and that such changes are likely associated with the reduction of axonal transport rate in the optic nerve of diabetic rats. Accordingly there might be an intracellular mechanism that links G protein functions and neuron degeneration and plasticity. If such a hypothesis were true it would be possible to design new drugs aimed at G proteins for the prevention of degeneration and the treatment of neuropathies.

Subject Index

A

Acetyl-L-carnitine, in nerve repair, 303–305
Acetylcholine receptors. *See* Membranes.
Acetylcholinesterase
  in cholinergic neurons, 268, 270
  in diabetic peripheral neuropathy, 301
  marker of axon sprouting, 223, 226
  in nerve regeneration, 296
  in synaptogenesis, 159–160
Acrylamide, and axonal transport, 102–103
ACTH, in nerve repair, 303
Actin
  in growth cone motility, 267
  microfilaments, 14
  synthesis, in axon reaction, 104
Adenylyl-imidodiphosphate (AMP-PNP), and axonal transport, 18
Adhesive molecules. *See* Cell adhesion molecules.
Adrenal medulla, neurite-promoting factors, 266–267
Age factors
  brain, plasticity processes, 235–236
  peripheral neuropathy, axonal transport, 102–103
Agrin, in junctional membranes, 155–158
Aldose reductase, in nerve repair, 306
Alzheimer's disease
  β-amyloid, 229–230
  future directions, 323
  regenerative sprouting, 225
  senile plaques, 226
    bFGF, 227–228
    heparan sulfate, 228–229
4-Aminopyridine, and demyelination in spinal cord injury, 171
β-Amyloid
  in Alzheimer's disease, 229–230
  APP processing and formation, 232–234
  growth factor cascades, 230–232
Amyloid precursor protein (APP), 229–234
  organization and distribution, 232–234
Amyotrophic lateral sclerosis, axon reaction, 104
Anti-adhesive molecules, 88–91
Antibodies, monoclonal, basal lamina, 156
Antigens, major histocompatibility complex, in Schwann cell culture, 135–137
Apolipoprotein E, in nerve repair, 305
Astrocyte differentiation and function, 66–67
Astrotactin, 79
Atrophy
  axonal, in diabetic peripheral neuropathy, 301
  cellular, NGF effects, 272
Auditory system, transneuronal degeneration, 38–45
Autonomic nervous system, in diabetic peripheral neuropathy, 299, 301–302
Autoregeneration, historical background of neuroregeneration, 1
Axolemma, in brain trauma, 190–193
Axonal transport
  collateral sprouting, 242
  in diabetic peripheral neuropathy, 301
  molecular mechanisms, 14–20
    cytoskeletal structure movement, 16
    dyneins, 19
    kinesins, 18–19
    membrane bounded organelles, 16–17
    motors in nervous system, 17–18
    myosins, 19–20
    and physiological functions, 20
    structural hypothesis, 15–16
  in peripheral neuropathies, 102–103
  regulation and targeting, 20–22
Axonopathies, chemical-induced, trophic regulation, 108–110
Axons
  in brain trauma, 187–195
  caliber, in axon reaction, 104–105
  dynamics and regeneration, 7–36
    glial modulation, 22–28
    morphology, 8–14
      cytoskeletal structures, 10–14
      membrane components, 9–10
      protein synthesis, 8–9
      transport. *See* Axonal transport.
  fasciculation, cell adhesion molecules, 80
  regeneration
    in brain trauma, 202–206

Axons (*contd.*)
    cholinergic, and nerve growth factor, 271–275
  in spinal cord injury, 171
  transection (reaction), 104
    triggering of, 107–108
    trophic regulation, 105–106
Axotomy
  distal stump
    axon regeneration, 111–112
    and neural response to injury, 112–113
    Wallerian degeneration, 110–111
  retrograde changes, 290–294

B

Bands of Bungner, 110
Basal lamina of junctional membranes, 155–158
Blood-brain barrier
  astrocyte function, 67
  in brain trauma, 197–199
Blood flow, cerebral, in brain trauma, 197–199
Brain
  aging, plasticity processes, 235–236
  trauma, 185–216
    injury spectrum, 199–200
    lymphokines, 278
    parenchymal response, 185–199
      axonal damage, 187–195
      neuroexcitation/agonist receptor interaction, 186–187
      neuronal somatic changes, 195–196
    repair after CNS injury, 201–212
      axonal regeneration, 202–206
      brain reorganization, 202
      neuroplasticity, 206–212
      secondary insults, 200–201
      vascular changes, 196–199
Brain-derived neurotrophic factor (BDNF), 108, 115, 265, 276

C

Cadherins, 82
Calcitonin gene-related peptide (CGRP)
  in junctional membranes, 158–159
  marker for terminals, 244
  nerve growth factor control, 104
Calcium
  in brain trauma, 190
  and demyelination in spinal cord injury, 171
Calpains, and axonal transport, 21, 22
Carbon dioxide, in brain trauma, 197–199

Cell adhesion molecules, 78–82
  cadherins, 82
  and growth cone, 267
  immunoglobulins, 78–81
    F3/F11, TAG-1/axonin-1, contactin, 81
    L1, Ng-CAM, 80–81
    neural cell adhesion molecule, 78–80
    Nr-CAM, 81
    SC1/DM-GRASP, 81
Central nervous system (CNS)
  axon regeneration, 245–247
  chemical lesions, morphine effects, 308–311
  experimental regeneration, 294–296
  and PNS, axon comparison, 7–8
  regeneration. *See* Neurotrophic factors.
  sprouting pathways, 248–249
  supporting cells
    macroglia, 61–67
    microglia, 67–69
  transneuronal degeneration. *See* Degeneration, transneuronal; Brain trauma.
Chambers, regeneration, 306–307
Channels, acetylcholine receptors, 160–162
Choline acetyltransferase (ChAT)
  in diabetic peripheral neuropathy, 301
  in nerve regeneration, 296
  retrograde changes after axotomy, 293
Chromatolysis, 107–108
Ciliary-derived neurotrophic factor (CNTF), 115, 265, 276–277
Collagen
  in brain trauma, 203
  of extracellular matrix, 83–84
  of Schwann cells, 71
Collagenase, in Schwann cell tissue culture, 133
Complement, and demyelination in spinal cord injury, 171
Conduction, nerve, in diabetic peripheral neuropathy, 301
Cyclic AMP
  and antigenic expression by Schwann cells, 126–127
  in Schwann cell proliferation, 71
Cytoskeleton
  movement of structures, 16
  and neuronal growth, 10–14

D

Deafferentation, hindlimb, 252–253
Definitions, collateral sprouting, 241–243

Degeneration. *See also* Neurons, denervated.
  transneuronal, in CNS, 38–45
    cellular events, 40
    protein synthesis, 40–45
Demyelination in spinal cord injury, 171
Dendrites
  atrophy and remodeling. *See* Neurons, denervated.
  protein synthesis, 8–9
Denervation
  sensitivity, 146
  vs. paralysis
    long-term, 150–153
    short-term, 147–150
Dentate gyrus, in regenerative sprouting, 221–225
Diabetes mellitus
  axonal transport, 102–103
  peripheral neuropathy, 299–302
Dispase, in Schwann cell tissue culture, 133
Dopamine, in nerve repair, 294–295, 308–310
Dopamine-B-hydroxylase, in nerve regeneration, 296
Dorsal root ganglion
  axonal transport, 103
  sprouting, 243–245
    neonatal, 247–249
Dyneins
  cytoplasmic forms, 19
  as molecular motor, 17–18
Dysesthesia, in diabetic peripheral neuropathy, 299

E
Electric fields, in nerve repair, 307–308
Encephalopathy, diabetic, 302
End bulbs of Held, 38
Endothelium-derived relaxing factor, in brain trauma, 197
Entactin, of Schwann cells, 71
Entorhinal cortex, in regenerative sprouting, 221–225
Enzymes
  anterograde transport, 17
  in spinal cord injury, 169–170
Epidermal growth factor (EGF)
  and CNS regeneration, 265, 278
  Schwann cell mitogen, 127
Excitotoxicity, glutamate, neuronal dysfunction, 234–235
Extracellular matrix
  in neural regeneration, 82–88

  glycoproteins, 83–84
  proteoglycans, 84–85
  receptors, 85–88
    integrins, 85–87
    laminin, 87–88
    lectin-like, 88
    nonintegrin, 87
  neurite-promoting factors, 266–267
  in plasticity processes, 219

F
Fibroblast growth factor (FGF)
  acidic and basic, 277–278
  basic (bFGF)
    in animal models of sprouting and cell survival, 221–225
      after CNS injury, 223
    and heparan sulfate synergistic interaction, 219–221
    retrograde changes after axotomy, 293
    senile plaques in Alzheimer's disease, 227–228
  in oligodendrocyte differentiation, 65
  Schwann cell mitogen, 127
Fibronectin
  of extracellular matrix, 83–84, 89
  in plasticity processes, 219
  of Schwann cells, 71, 126
Fluoride-resistant acid phosphatase (FRAP), 244
Forskolin
  and antigenic expression by Schwann cells, 126, 129
  in nerve repair, 305

G
G proteins, in diabetic peripheral neuropathy, 301, 302
GABAergic fibers, in brain trauma, 207–209
Galactocerebroside, Schwann cell marker, 125, 126
Gamma aminobutyric acid, and spinal cord demyelination, 171, 172
Ganglion, dorsal root. *See* Dorsal root ganglion.
Gangliosides
  for axonal neuropathies, 113–114
  for nerve repair, 302–303
  in spinal cord injury, 169
GAP-43
  in Alzheimer's disease, 227
  in growth cone motility, 267

Genes, early response, and astrocyte function, 67
Glial cells, modulation of neuronal function, 22–28
Glial fibrillary acidic protein
  in macroglial development, 63, 66
  of neurofilaments, 14
Glial growth factor (GGF), Schwann cell mitogen, 126–129
Glial transcription factor, 128
Glucocorticoids
  in oligodendrocyte differentiation, 65, 128
  in spinal cord injury, 175
  in Wallerian degeneration, 111
Glucose metabolism
  in Alzheimer's disease, 234
  in brain trauma, 196
Glutamate
  excitotoxicity, neuronal dysfunction, 234–235
  NMDA interaction, in brain trauma, 186–187
Glutamine synthetase, astrocyte marker, 66
Glycoproteins
  acetylcholine receptor-inducer, 158
  of extracellular matrix, 83–84
  MHC genes, in Schwann cell tissue culture, 135–137
  Schwann cell markers, 125
Glycosaminoglycan. See also Heparan sulfate (HS).
  of extracellular matrix, 84–85
Grafts. See also Transplantation.
  and neurotrophic factors, 272–273
Granule cells, lesion-induced growth, 56–58
Growth cone
  integrin receptors, 86
  nerve growth factor, 267
  neural cell adhesion molecules, 79
  neuronal cytoskeleton, 14
Growth factors. See also Plasticity processes; specific factors.
  in oligodendrocyte differentiation, 63–65
  in Schwann cell proliferation, 71
  in sprouting mechanisms, 254
Guillain-Barré syndrome, 303

H
Hemorrhage, in brain trauma, 196–199
Heparan sulfate (HS)
  after CNS injury, 223–225
  and bFGF interaction, 219–221
  senile plaques in Alzheimer's disease, 228–229
2,5-Hexanedione, and axonal transport, 102
Hippocampus. See also Plasticity processes.
  remodeling during reinnervation, 50–58
  sprouting, NGF effects, 274
HIV particles, on microglia, 68
Horseradish peroxidase (HRP), dorsal root projections, 244
Hyaluronidase, in Schwann cell tissue culture, 133
5-Hydroxytryptamine (5-HT)
  brainstem pathways, 247
  in CNS chemical lesions, 308–311
  retrograde changes after axotomy, 292–293
Hypotension, in brain trauma, 200
Hypoxia, in brain trauma, 201

I
Immunoglobulins, cell adhesive. See Cell adhesion molecules.
Insulin, Schwann cell mitogen, 127
Insulin-like growth factor, in sprouting mechanisms, 254
Integrins of extracellular matrix, 85–87
Interleukin-1, in brain injury, 278
Ion channels, in neuronal membranes, 9–10
Isaxonine, 305–306

K
Kallman's syndrome, 83
Kinesins, 18–20
Kinetics, acetylcholine receptors, 160–162

L
Laminin, 79
  astrocyte marker, 66–67
  of extracellular matrix, 83–84, 89
  high affinity receptors, 87–88
  in plasticity processes, 219
  of Schwann cells, 71, 126
Lectin receptors, 88
Lipids, myelin, Schwann cell markers, 125
Lipopolysaccharide, and microglia, 68
Locomotion. See also Spinal cord.
  spinal pathways, 170–171
Lymphokines, in brain injury, 278

M
Macroglia
  astrocytes, 66–67
  development, 61–63
  oligodendrocytes, 63–66

SUBJECT INDEX

Macrophages
  and demyelination in spinal cord injury, 171
  in Wallerian degeneration, 111
Major histocompatibility complex (MHC), 135–137
Markers
  CNS cell types, 62
  Schwann cell differentiation, 70–71, 124–126
Melanocortins, 303
Membranes
  extrajunctional properties, 146–154
    denervation vs. paralysis
      long-term, 150–153
      short-term, 147–150
    nerve stump effects, nicotinic influences, 153–154
  junctional properties, 154–163
    acetylcholine receptor
      channel kinetics and metabolic stability, 160–163
      inducing activity, 158
    acetylcholinesterase, 159–160
    basal lamina, 155–158
    calcitonin gene-related peptide, 158–159
  neuronal components, 9–10
  organelle movement, 16–17
Merosin, of extracellular matrix, 84
Met-enkephalin, in nerve repair, 304
Methylprednisolone, in spinal cord injury, 169, 172
Microfilaments, and neuronal growth, 10–14
Microglia, 67–69
Microscopy, video-enhanced contrast, 17
Microtubule-associated protein (MAP)
  neurite-promoting factors, 267
  and neuronal growth, 12
Microtubules
  in dendritic atrophy, 47
  and neuronal growth, 10–14
Mitogens, Schwann cell, 126–127
MK-801, in brain trauma, 186–187
Monocytes, and microglia, 67–69
Monosialic gangliosides, in spinal cord injury, 169
Morphine, in CNS chemical lesions, 308–311
Mouse mutants, axonal transport, 23–28
Muscles, and nerve trophic interaction. *See* Nerves.
Myelin
  components in Schwann cells, 70
  nerve growth inhibition, 90–91
  in oligodendrocyte differentiation, 65
  protein gene transcription, 127–128
  protein synthesis, in Wallerian degeneration, 110
  sheath, Schwann cell markers, 125
Myelin-associated glycoprotein (MAG), 125, 128
Myelin basic protein, 125, 128
Myelination
  in axon regeneration, 113
  and axonal caliber, 23
Myo-inositol, in nerve repair, 306
Myosins
  as molecular motor, 17–18
  nonmuscle, 19–20

N

Nerve growth factor (NGF)
  in axon reaction, 106–107
    Schwann cell-derived, 107
  in axotomized distal stump, 110–111
  and cholinergic axonal regeneration, 271–275
  and noncholinergic CNS neurons, 275–276
  normal cholinergic CNS neurons, 267–268
  protective effects, 268–271
    nucleus basalis-cortex system, 271
    septohippocampal system, 268–271
  prototype of neurotrophic factors, 265
  in regenerative sprouting, 221
  future directions, 322
  historical background, 3
  and microglia, 68
  neonatal sprouting, 247–248
  receptors, 268–269
    in Schwann cell culture, 137–139
  retrograde transport, 17
  in Schwann cell proliferation, 71
  in sprouting mechanisms, 254
  in treatment of axonal neuropathies, 114
Nerves
  and muscle trophic interaction, 145–167
    extrajunctional membrane properties, 146–154
      denervation vs. paralysis
        long-term, 150–153
        short-term, 147–150
      nerve stump effects, 153–154
    junctional membrane properties, 154–163
      acetylcholine receptors, 158, 160–163
      acetylcholinesterase, 159–160
      basal lamina, 155–158

Nerves (*contd.*)
    calcitonin gene-related peptide, 158–159
Nestin, 62
Neurite outgrowth, growth factors and substrate molecules, 219–221
Neurofibromatosis, tissue culture studies, 139–140
Neurofilaments
    in axon reaction
        phosphorylated epitopes, 105
        triplet proteins, 104
    axonal transport, 102–103
    in brain trauma, 190–195
    in mouse mutants, 24–25
    and neuronal growth, 10–14
Neuroglia, 61
Neurons
    denervated, 37–60
        dendritic atrophy, 45–50
        remodeling during reinnervation, 50–58
            dendritic spines, 50–51
            deterioration and regrowth of dendrites, 51–56
            lesion-induced growth, 56–58
        transneuronal degeneration in CNS, 38–45
            cellular events, 40
            protein synthesis cessation, 40–45
    soma, and proximal axon, 103–108
        axon reaction, 104
            triggering of, 107–108
            trophic regulation, 105–106
        in brain trauma, 195–196
        nerve growth factor, 106–107
            Schwann cell-derived, 107
        phosphorylated neurofilament epitopes, 105
    somatofugal axonal atrophy, 101–105
Neuropathies, peripheral
    axonal transport, 102–103
    treatment, 113–115
Neuropeptides, anterograde transport, 17
Neuroplasticity. *See also* Plasticity processes.
    in brain trauma, 206–212
Neuroregeneration
    axonal dynamics, 7–36
        axonal transport, 14–20
            cytoskeletal structures, 16
            dyneins, 19
            kinesins, 18–19
            membrane bounded organelles, 16–17
            motors
                in nervous system, 17–18
                and physiological functions, 20
            myosins, 19–20
            regulation and targeting, 20–22
            structural hypothesis, 15–16
        glial modulation of neuronal function, 22–28
        neuronal morphology, 8–14
            cytoskeletal structures, 10–14
            dendritic and axonal protein synthesis, 8–9
            membrane components, 9–10
    historical background, 1–5
Neurotransmitters
    anterograde transport, 17
    and astrocyte function, 67
Neurotrophic factors, 265–287
    and CNS regeneration, 267–278
        cholinergic axonal regeneration, 271–275
        cholinergic CNS neurons, 267–268
        ciliary neuronotrophic factor, 276–277
        epidermal growth factor, 278
        fibroblast growth factor, 277–278
        lymphokines, 278
        nerve growth factor. *See* Nerve growth factor.
        NGF family members, 276
        noncholinergic CNS neurons, 275–276
    neurite-promoting effects, 266–267
    retrograde transport, 17
Neurotrophic inhibitory factor, 147
Neurotropin-3, 108, 115, 265, 276
Neurotropins, in treatment of axonal neuropathies, 115
Nexins, of Schwann cells, 71
Nissl bodies, in axon reaction, 104
N-methyl-D-aspartate (NMDA)
    and glutamate interaction in brain trauma, 186–187
    sprouting mechanisms, 254
Node of Ranvier
    astrocyte differentiation, 67
    and axonal transport, 25–27
    definition, 69
    sodium channels, 70–71
Noradrenaline, in nerve regeneration, 296
Nucleus basalis, cholinergic neurons, 271, 274
Nucleus laminaris, dendritic atrophy, 45–50
Nucleus magnocellularis, transneuronal degeneration, 38

O

Oligodendrocytes
    differentiation and function, 63–66
    inhibition of neurite outgrowth, 295

neurite outgrowth, 23
  remyelination of spinal axons, 171–172
Olive, medial superior, 45
Onuf's nucleus, 246–247
ORG 2766, 303
Organelles, membrane bounded, 16–17

P

P_0 glycoprotein, Schwann cell marker, 125–128
Pain
  in axonal neuropathies, 114
  in diabetic peripheral neuropathy, 299
Parenchyma, brain. *See* Brain trauma.
Paresthesia, in diabetic peripheral neuropathy, 299
Perikaryon, protein synthesis, 7, 8
Peripheral nervous system (PNS)
  axon regeneration, 245
  and CNS, axon comparison, 7–8
  neurotrophic function in neuropathies, 101–122
    axonal neuropathy treatment, 113–115
    axonal transport, 102–103
    chemical-induced axonopathies, 108–110
    distal stump, 110–112
      axon regeneration, 111–112
      and neuronal response to injury, 112–113
      Wallerian degeneration, 110–111
    myelination, 113
    neuronal soma and proximal axon, 103–108
      axon reaction, 104, 107–108
      nerve growth factor, 106–107
      phosphorylated neurofilament epitopes, 105
      Schwann cell-derived NGF, 107
      somatofugal axonal atrophy, 104–105
      trophic regulation of axon reaction, 105–106
  Schwann cell homografts, 172
  supporting cells
    cellular organization, 69
  Schwann cells
    differentiation, 69–71
    proliferation, 71–72
Peripherin, of neurofilaments, 14
Phencyclidine, in brain trauma, 186–187
Phosphatidyl inositol, in nerve repair, 306
Phosphorylation, and axonal transport, 21
Plaques, senile, 225–232
  β-amyloid peptides, 229–230

  bFGF, 227–228
  growth factor cascades, 230–232
  heparan sulfate, 228–229
Plasticity processes
  molecular cascades, 217–239
    AAP processing and formation of β-amyloid, 232–234
    aging brain, 235–236
    animal models of sprouting and cell survival, 221–225
      bFGF levels, 223
      HS levels, 223–225
    excitotoxicity, 234–235
    growth factors and substrate molecules, 219–221
      bFGF and HS synergistic interaction, 219–221
    senile plaques, 225–232
      β-amyloid peptide, 229–230
      bFGF, 227–228
      growth factor cascades, 230–232
      HS, 228–229
    sprouting in Alzheimer's disease, 225
  spinal cord, 243–247
    neonatal, 247–249
    sprouting
      of central pathways, 245–247
      of dorsal root axons, 243–245
Platelet-derived growth factor (PDGF)
  in oligodendrocyte differentiation, 63–65
  Schwann cell mitogen, 127
Polypeptide growth factor, 127
Polysialic acid, in neural cell adhesion molecule, 78–79
Potassium channels
  and axonal transport, 25
  in spinal cord injury, 171, 173
Pressure, intracranial, in brain trauma, 199
Proopiomelanocortin, in nerve repair, 303
Prostaglandins, and microglia, 68
Proteins
  myelin. *See also* Myelin.
  neurofilament triplet, 13–14
  synthesis
    dendritic and axonal, 8–9
    in perikaryon, 7, 8
    in transneuronal degeneration, 40–45
Proteoglycans
  of extracellular matrix, 83–85, 89
  of Schwann cells, 71
Proteolipid protein, Schwann cell marker, 125–128
Pyronin, 305

R

Receptors
  acetylcholine. *See* Membranes.
  in brain trauma, 186–187
  of extracellular matrix, 85–88
  low-affinity nerve growth factors (LNGFR), 268–269
  nerve growth factor, in Schwann cell culture, 124–125, 137–139
  in neuronal membranes, 9–10
  sprouting mechanisms, 253–254
Red nucleus, NGF effects, 275
Redundancy, of spinal pathways, 170–171, 175
Reflex function, spinal cord. *See* Spinal cord.
Regeneration. *See also* Plasticity processes; Spinal cord.
  adhesive molecules and extracellular matrix, 77–100
    anti-adhesive molecules, 88–91
      extracellular matrix, 89–90
      myelin-associated, 90–91
    cell adhesion molecules, 78–82
      cadherins, 82
      immunoglobulins, 78–81
    extracellular matrix, 82–88
      glycoproteins, 83–84
      proteoglycans, 84–85
      receptors, 85–88
  axonal, in brain trauma, 202–206
  chambers, 306–307
  future directions, 321–323
  in mouse mutants, 24
  neuronal, pharmacology of, 289–320
    CNS chemical lesions, morphine effects, 308–311
    experimental, 294–302
      CNS regeneration, 294–296
      diabetic peripheral neuropathy, 299–302
      nerve regeneration, 296–299
      retrograde changes after axotomy, 290–294
    treatment, 302–308
      acetyl-L-carnitine, 303–305
      electric fields, 307–308
      gangliosides, 302–303
      isaxonine and other agents, 305–306
      melanocortins, 303
      regeneration chambers, 306–307
  neurotrophic factors. *See* Neurotrophic factors.
Remodeling of denervated neuron, 50–58
  dendritic spines, 50–51
  deterioration and regrowth of dendrites, 51–56
Remyelination of spinal axons, 171–172
Retraction balls, in brain trauma, 187–190
Ribosomes, in transneuronal degeneration, 42–45

S

S-100 protein, astrocyte marker, 66
Satellite cells, 69
Schmidt-Lanterman clefts, 69
Schwann cells
  in axotomized distal stump, 110
  and CNS axon rejuvenation, 2
  definition, 69
  differentiation, 69–71
  nerve growth factor, 107
  proliferation, 71–72
  remyelination of spinal axons, 171–172
  tissue culture, 123–144
    antigenic expression, 126
    cell type specific markers, 124–126
    development and function, 124
    immortalized cell lines, 128–129
    major histocompatibility complex antigens, 135–137
    mitogens, 126–127
    neurofibromatosis, 139–140
    NGF receptor, 137–139
    techniques, 129–135
    transcription of myelin protein genes, 127–128
Scopolamine, in brain trauma, 186–187
Sensory neurons, in diabetic peripheral neuropathy, 301
Septohippocampal system, 268–274
Serotonin brainstem pathways, 247
Sidearms, neurofilaments, 13
Sodium channels. *See also* Membranes.
  and axonal transport, 25
  at node of Ranvier, 70–71
Spared root preparation, 243–245, 251–252
Spinal cord
  hemisection, 249–251
  nonregenerative injury, 169–184
    axonal dysfunction, 171
    functional recovery needs, 169–170
    mechanisms of recovery, 175
    recovery in humans, 172–173
    redundancy of spinal pathways, 170–171
    remyelination of spinal axons, 171–172
    time course of recovery, 173–175

sprouting and regeneration, 241–263
    plasticity, 241–254
        collateral sprouting, 241–249
        functional recovery, 249–253
        growth factors, 254
        sprouting mechanisms, 253–254
    transplants, 254–259
Spines, dendritic, in reinnervation, 50–51
Sprouting
    axonal reaction, 297
    future directions, 321–323
    intrahippocampal, NGF effects, 274
    isaxonine effects, 305
    regenerative
        in Alzheimer's disease, 225
        animal models, 221–225
    in spinal cord. *See* Spinal cord.
Stress proteins, 9
Structural Hypothesis of Axonal Transport, 15–16
Substance P
    in diabetic peripheral neuropathy, 301
    nerve growth factor control, 104
    in nerve repair, 304
    retrograde changes after axotomy, 292
    in sprouting, 253
    in treatment of axonal neuropathies, 114
    in visual system, 275
Sulfatide, Schwann cell markers, 125
Supporting cells, 61–75
    macroglia, 61–67
        development, 61–63
        differentiation and function
            of astrocytes, 66–67
            of oligodendrocytes, 63–66
    microglia, 67–69
    peripheral nervous system, 69–72
        nerves and ganglia, 69
        Schwann cells
            differentiation, 69–71
            proliferation, 71–72
Synaptogenesis. *See also* Membranes.
    in Alzheimer's disease hippocampus, 227
    historical background, 4
Synaptosomal-associated protein (SNAP-25), 227
Synpasin, and axonal transport, 21

T
Tau protein
    in Alzheimer's disease, 226–227
    and neuronal growth, 12, 21
Tenascin, 79, of extracellular matrix, 89–90
Tetrodotoxin. *See also* Membranes.
    transneuronal degeneration studies, 38–42
Thallium, and axonal transport, 102
Thrombospondin, 79, of extracellular matrix, 89–90
Thyroid hormone
    in nerve repair, 306
    in oligodendrocyte differentiation, 65
Tissue culture of Schwann cells. *See* Schwann cells.
Transferrin, in oligodendrocyte differentiation, 65
Transplantation
    neuronal technique, 294–295
    spinal cord, 254–259
Trophic functions, PNS. *See* Peripheral nervous system.
Tubulins
    in Alzheimer's disease, 226–227
    in axon reaction, 104
    isoforms, 11–12
Tumor necrosis factor, in spinal cord injury, 171
Tyrosine hydroxylase, in nerve regeneration, 296

V
Vasoconstriction, in brain trauma, 197–199
Vimentin
    in growth cone motility, 267
    of neurofilaments, 14
Vincullin, 267
Visual system, NGF effects, 275
Vitamin C, and myelination, 70
Vitamins
    in axonal transport, 102
    in nerve repair, 306
von Recklinghausen's disease, 139–140

W
Wallerian degeneration, 70
    in brain trauma, 187–190, 202–206
    distal stump, 110–111